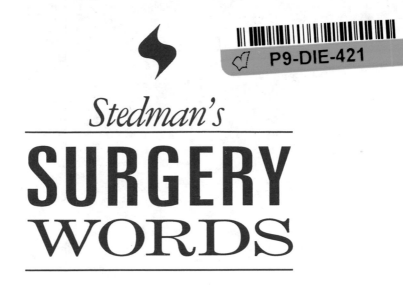

Stedman's

SURGERY
WORDS

Edited by
Sandy Kovacs, CMT

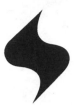

Stedman's

SURGERY

WORDS

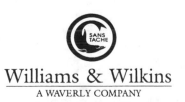

Williams & Wilkins
A WAVERLY COMPANY

BALTIMORE • PHILADELPHIA • LONDON • PARIS • BANGKOK
BUENOS AIRES • HONG KONG • MUNICH • SYDNEY • TOKYO • WROCLAW

Series Editor: Elizabeth B. Randolph
Managing Editor: Maureen Barlow Pugh
Editor: Sandy Kovacs, CMT
Production Coordinator: Marette Magargle-Smith
Printer & Binder: Vicks Lithograph & Printing
Copyright © 1998
Williams & Wilkins
351 West Camden Street
Baltimore, Maryland 21201-2436 USA

Printed in the United States of America

Library of Congress Cataloging-in-Publication Data
Stedman's surgery words / editor, Sandy Kovacs.
      p.   cm. — (Stedman's word book series)
   Companion v. to: Stedman's medical & surgical equipment words /
edited by Catherine S. Baxter. 2nd ed. c1996.
   ISBN 0-683-40190-4
   1. Surgery—Terminology. I. Kovacs, Sandy. II. Stedman's medical & surgical
equipment words. III. Series: Stedman's word books.
     [DNLM: 1. Surgery—terminology.   WO 15 S812 1997]
RD16.S74   1997
617'.001'4—dc21
DNLM/DLC
for Library of Congress
                                            97-20704
                                                  CIP

98 99
3 4 5 6 7 8 9 10

Contents

Acknowledgments

An important part of our editorial process is the involvement of medical transcriptionists — as advisors, reviewers and/or editors.

Special thanks are due Sandy Kovacs, CMT for editing and proofing the manuscript (and doing the necessary research involved with that large task). We also would like to extend our thanks to Helen Littrell who also edited the manuscript, and helped resolve many difficult content questions.

Thanks also to our *Stedman's Surgery Words* MT Editorial Advisory Board, consisting of Ellen Atwood; Darla Haberer, CMT; Anna Parr, CMT; and Christa Scott, CMT. These medical transcriptionists served as important contributors, editors, and advisors.

Barb Ferretti played an integral role in the process by reviewing the content files for format, updating the database and providing a final quality check.

As with all our *Stedman's* word references, we have benefitted from the suggestions and expertise of our many contacts in the medical transcriptionist community. Thanks to all our advisory board participants, reviewers and editors, AAMT meeting attendees, and others who have written in with requests and comments — keep talking, and we'll keep listening.

Publisher's Preface

Stedman's Surgery Words offers an authoritative assurance of quality and exactness to the wordsmiths of the health care professions — medical transcriptionists, medical editors and copy editors, health information management personnel, court reporters, and the many other users and producers of medical documentation.

For years we have received requests for a surgery word book, and for years we steered our customers to *Stedman's Medical & Surgical Equipment Words*, which contains a wealth of surgical equipment terms. Yet the requests continued, and we realized that medical language professionals needed to know more than just the equipment terms related to surgery, they needed to have a reference that covered other surgical terminology as well. They needed a handy, reliable reference for surgical anatomy and anesthesiology terms as well as procedure names, operations, methods, approaches, and types of incisions (to name just a few categories).

Although we considered including surgical vocabulary in our equipment book, it quickly became clear that the vast amount of terminology involved could not be contained in a handy word book-type reference. We then conceived of this "companion" book to the equipment word book: *Stedman's Surgery Words*. We hope that between *Stedman's Surgery Words* and *Stedman's Medical & Surgical Equipment Words, 2nd ed.*, users will find complete coverage of all types of terms related to surgery. Users will find listed thousands of diagnostic and therapeutic procedures, operations, new techniques and maneuvers, incisions, methods and approaches, and more from all the major specialties and subspecialties of medicine. Surgical anatomy and anesthesia terms are also included.

This compilation of over 85,000 entries, fully cross-indexed for quick access, was built from a base vocabulary of over 48,000 medical words, phrases, abbreviations and acronyms. The extensive A-Z list was developed from the database of *Stedman's Medical Dictionary* and supplemented by terminology found in current medical literature (please see list of References on page xiv).

We at Williams & Wilkins strive to provide you with the most up-to-date and accurate word references available. Your use of this word book will prompt new editions, which will be published as often as justified by updates and revisions. We welcome your suggestions for improvements, changes, corrections, and additions — whatever will make this *Stedman's* product more useful to you. Please use the postpaid card at the back of this book and send your recommendations care of "Stedmans" at Williams & Wilkins.

Explanatory Notes

Medical transcription is an art as well as a science. Both are needed to correctly interpret a physician's dictation, whose language is a product of education, training, and experience. This variety in medical language means that there are several acceptable ways to express certain terms, including jargon. *Stedman's Surgery Words* provides variant spellings and phrasings for many terms. This, in addition to complete cross-indexing, makes *Stedman's Surgery Words* a valuable resource for determining the validity of terms as they are encountered.

Alphabetical Organization

Alphabetization of entries is letter by letter as spelled, ignoring punctuation, spaces, prefixed numbers, Greek letters, or other characters. For example:

acid-fast staining methods
acid formaldehyde hematin
α-acid glycoprotein
acid hematin

In subentries, the abbreviated singular form or the spelled-out plural form of the noun main entry word is ignored in alphabetization.

Format and Style

All main entries are in **boldface** to speed up location of a sought-after entry, to enhance distinction between main entries and subentries, and to relieve the textual density of the pages.

Irregular plurals and variant spellings are shown on the same line as the singular or preferred form of the word. For example:

scolex pl. **scoleces**

curette, curet

Hyphenation

As a rule of style, multiple eponyms (e.g., Mears-Rubash approach) are hyphenated. Also, hyphens have been added between a manufacturer and one or more eponyms (e.g., Vital-Metzenbaum dissecting scissors). Please note that hyphenation is a question of style, not of accuracy, and thus is a matter of choice.

Possessives

Possessive forms have been dropped in this reference for the sake of consistency and to conform to the guidelines outlined by the American Association for Medical Transcription (AAMT) and other groups. Please note, however, that retaining the possessive is a question of style, not of accuracy, and thus is a matter of choice. To form the possessive of a word, simply add the apostrophe or apostrophe "s" to the end of the word.

Cross-indexing

The word list is in an index-like main entry-subentry format that contains two combined alphabetical listings:

(1) A *noun* main entry-subentry organization typical of the A-Z section of medical dictionaries like **Stedman's:**

approach
 abdominal a.
 acetabular extensile a.
 Alken a.
 anterior a.

dissection
 aortic d.
 arterial wall d.
 axillary d.
 balloon d.

(2) An *adjective* main entry-subentry organization, which lists words and phrases as you hear them. The main entries are the adjectives or modifiers in a multi-word term. The subentries are the nouns around which the terms are constructed and to which the adjectives or modifiers pertain:

congenital
 c. ectodermal defects
 c. erythropoietic porphyria
 c. ichthyosiform erythroderma
 c. syphilis

embolic
 e. abscess
 e. aneurysm
 e. pneumonia
 e. stroke

This format provides the user with more than one way to locate and identify a multi-word term. For example:

dissemination
    skin d.
disease
    Quincke d.
    Raynaud d.

skin
    s. dissemination
Quincke
    Q. disease
    Q. edema

It also allows the user to see together all terms that contain a particular descriptor as well as all types, kinds, or variations of a noun entity. For example:

balloon
    b. laser angioplasty
    b. occlusion
    Blue Max b.
    Brandt cytology b.
    Express b.

angioplasty
    balloon laser a.
    complex a.
    a. guiding catheter
    high-risk a.
    transluminal coronary a.

Wherever possible, abbreviations are separately defined and cross-referenced. For example:

PTCA
    percutaneous transluminal coronary angioplasty

percutaneous
    p. transluminal coronary angioplasty (PTCA)

angioplasty
    percutaneous transluminal coronary a. (PTCA)

References

In addition to the manufacturers' literature we gather at various medical meetings, scientific reports from hospitals, and our MT Editorial Advisory Board members' lists (from their daily transcription work), we used the following sources for new words for *Stedman's Surgery Words:*

Books

Klein SL. A glossary of anesthesia and related terminology, 2nd ed. New York: Springer-Verlag, 1993.

Lance LL. Quick look drug book. Baltimore: Williams & Wilkins, 1997.

Pyle V. Current medical terminology, 6th ed. Modesto: Health Professions Institute, 1996.

Sloane SB. The medical word book, 3ed. Philadelphia: WB Saunders Company, 1991.

Stedman's abbreviations, acronyms & symbols. Baltimore: Williams & Wilkins, 1992.

Stedman's cardiology & pulmonary words, 2 ed. Baltimore: Williams & Wilkins, 1997.

Stedman's dentistry words. Baltimore: Williams & Wilkins, 1993.

Stedman's dermatology & immunology Words. Baltimore: Williams & Wilkins, 1997.

Stedman's ENT words. Baltimore: Williams & Wilkins, 1993.

Stedman's GI & GU words, 2 ed. Baltimore: Williams & Wilkins, 1996.

Stedman's medical dictionary, 26th ed. Baltimore: Williams & Wilkins, 1995.

Stedman's medical & surgical equipment words, 2 ed. Baltimore: Williams & Wilkins, 1996.

Stedman's neurosurgery words. Baltimore: Williams & Wilkins, 1993.

Stedman's OB-GYN words, 2 ed. Baltimore: Williams & Wilkins, 1995.

Stedman's ophthalmology words. Baltimore: Williams & Wilkins, 1993.

Stedman's orthopaedic & rehab words, 2 ed. Baltimore: Williams & Wilkins, 1995.

Stedman's pathology & lab medicine words, 2 ed. Baltimore: Williams & Wilkins, 1997.

Stedman's psychiatry words. Baltimore: Williams & Wilkins, 1992.

Stedman's radiology & oncology words, 2 ed. Baltimore: Williams & Wilkins, 1995.

Szulec, Syllabus for the surgeon's secretary, 4th ed. Grosse Pointe: Medical Arts, 1990.

Tessier C. The surgical word book, 2ed. Philadelphia: WB Saunders Company, 1991.

Journals

Anesthesia & Analgesia. Baltimore: Williams & Wilkins, 1996–1997.

Anesthesiology. The Journal of the American Society of Anesthesiologists, Inc, 1996.

Journal of the American College of Surgeons. Chicago: The American College of Surgeons, 1995–1997.

Journal of the American Association for Medical Transcription. Modesto: American Association for Medical Transcription, 1995–1997.

The Latest Word. Philadelphia: WB Saunders Company, 1994–1996.

MT Monthly. Gladstone, MO: Computer Systems Management, 1994–1997.

Perspectives on the Medical Transcription Profession. Modesto: Health Professions Institute, 1993–1997.

Stedman's WordWatcher. Baltimore: Williams & Wilkins, 1995–1997.

A

A point
A ring
A ring of esophagus

AA

anterior apical
AA segment

AAA

abdominal aortic aneurysm
AAA bone graft

AACLR

arthroscopic anterior cruciate ligament
reconstruction

AANA

American Association of Nurse
Anesthetists

AB

anterior basal
AB segment

ab

a. externo filtering operation
a. externo incision
a. interno incision

ABA

American Board of Anesthesiology

Abbé

A. flap
A. operation
A. vaginal construction

Abbé-Estlander operation

Abbé-McIndoe

A.-M. procedure
A.-M. vaginal reconstruction

Abbé-McIndoe-Williams procedure

Abbé-Wharton-McIndoe procedure

Abbokinase

A. injection

Abbott

A. esophagogastroscopy
A. esophagogastrostomy
A. knee approach
A. method
A. tube

Abbott-Carpenter posterior approach

Abbott-Gill

A.-G. epiphyseal plate exposure
A.-G. osteotomy

Abbott-Lucas shoulder operation

Abbott-Miller tube

Abbott-Rawson

A.-R. double-lumen gastrointestinal
tube
A.-R. tube

Abbreviated Injury Scale

ABC

airway, breathing, and circulation

abdomen

acute surgical a.
boat-shaped a.
carinate a.
exquisitely tender a.
flat plate of a.
navicular a.
a. obstipum
pendulous a.
protuberant a.
scaphoid a.
soft a.
surgical a.

abdominal

a. adipose tissue
a. air collection
a. aorta
a. aortic aneurysm (AAA)
a. aortic plexus
a. approach
a. canal
a. cavity
a. colectomy
a. compartment syndrome
a. examination
a. external oblique muscle
a. fasciocutaneous flap
a. fat pad
a. fistula
a. guarding
a. gutter
a. hemorrhage
a. hysterectomy
a. hysteropexy
a. hysterotomy
a. incision
a. incision dehiscence
a. internal oblique muscle
a. irradiation
a. lipectomy
a. lymph node biopsy
a. muscle deficiency syndrome
a. myomectomy
a. nephrectomy
a. ostium of uterine tube
a. part of aorta
a. part of esophagus
a. part of thoracic duct
a. part of ureter
a. pressure
a. pressure technique
a. procedure
a. rectopexy

1

abdominal *(continued)*
    a. regions
    a. respiration
    a. ring
    a. sacropexy
    a. salpingo-oophorectomy
    a. salpingotomy
    a. section
    a. space
    a. stoma
    a. volume
    a. wall closure
    a. wall hernia
    a. wall lifting
    a. wall mass
    a. zone
abdominis
    diastasis recti a.
abdominocentesis
abdominocystic
abdominogenital
abdominohysterectomy
abdominohysterotomy
abdominoinguinal incision
abdominopelvic
    a. cavity
    a. irradiation
    a. mass
    a. splanchnic nerve
abdominoperineal
    a. excision
    a. resection (APR)
abdominoplasty
abdominosacral resection
abdominoscopy
abdominoscrotal
abdominothoracic
    a. arch
abdominovaginal
    a. hysterectomy
abdominovesical
abducens
    a. oculi
abducent
abduction
    a. deformity
    a. external rotation test
    a. osteotomy
    a. traction technique
abduction-external
    a.-e. rotation
    a.-e. rotation fracture
abductor
    a. digiti minimi muscle of foot
    a. digiti minimi muscle of hand
    a. digiti minimi opponensplasty
    a. digiti quinti opponensplasty
    a. hallucis muscle

    a. muscle of great toe
    a. muscle of little finger
    a. muscle of little toe
    a. osteotomy
    a. pollicis brevis muscle
    a. pollicis longus muscle
abductor-plasty
    flexor pollicis longus a.-p.
    Smith flexor pollicis longus a.-p.
abductory wedge osteotomy
Abell-Kendall method
Abell method
Aberdeen knot
Abernethy fascia
aberrancy
    acceleration-dependent a.
aberrant
    a. bile ducts
    a. degeneration of third nerve
    a. ductules
    a. ganglion
    a. obturator artery
    a. obturator vein
    a. regeneration
    a. regeneration of nerve
    a. tissue
aberration
    angle of a.
    chromatic lens a.
    color a.
    coma a.
    curvature a.
    dioptric a.
    distantial a.
    distortion a.
    intraventricular a.
    lateral a.
    lens a.
    longitudinal a.
    meridional a.
    monochromatic a.
    newtonian a.
    oblique a.
    optical a.
    regeneration a.
    sexual a.
    spherical lens a.
    ventricular a.
ability
    tumor-targeting a.
ABL
    ABL 330 analyzer
    ABL 30 blood gas analyzer
ablate
ablation
    accessory conduction a.
    adrenal a.
    androgen a.

A

atrioventricular junctional a.
carbon dioxide laser plaque a.
catheter a.
cold forceps a.
cold snare a.
continuous-wave laser a.
coronary rotational a.
cryogenic a.
cryosurgical a.
direct-current shock a.
electrical catheter a.
endometrial a.
ethanol a.
fast-pathway radiofrequency a.
His bundle a.
homogeneous a.
Kent bundle a.
laser uterosacral nerve a.
marrow a.
Nd:YAG laser a.
neoadjuvant total androgen a.
nerve rootlet a.
organ a.
ovarian a.
panretinal a.
parathyroid tumor a.
percutaneous ethanol a.
percutaneous radiofrequency
  catheter a.
percutaneous tumor a.
peripheral panretinal a.
pituitary a.
pulsed laser a.
radiofrequency catheter a. (RFCA)
rectoscopic endometrial a.
renal cyst a.
rollerball endometrial a.
rotational a.
slow-pathway a.
stereotactic surgical a.
surgical a.
a. therapy
thyroid nodule a.
tissue a.
toric a.
transcatheter a.
transurethral needle a.
tumor a.
valve a.
visual laser a.
ablative
a. cardiac surgery

a. laser angioplasty
a. laser therapy
a. procedure
a. surgery
a. technique
abnormal fetal urogenital tract
abnormality
caliceal a.
dislocation contour a.
diverticulation a.
electrical activation a.
extremity a.
limb reduction a.
migration a.'s
oral cavity a.
regional wall motion a. (RWMA)
reproductive tract a.
rostrocaudal extent signal a.
soft tissue a.
tissue texture a.
urinary tract a.
ventilation/perfusion a.
ventricular depolarization a.
ABO barrier
aborad
abortion
menstrual extraction a.
abortive infection
above-elbow amputation
above-knee
a.-k. amputation (AKA)
a.-k. amputation conversion
abrade
abraded wound
Abraham iridotomy
**Abraham-Pankovich tendo calcaneus
  repair**
abrasion
a. arthroplasty
bobby pin a.
a. chondroplasty
corneal a.
perioperative corneal a.
traumatic corneal a.
abrasive
a. point
abruption
abscess
acute a.
appendiceal a.
bicameral a.
buccal space a.

NOTES

3

abscess *(continued)*
    caseous a.
    chronic a.
    cold a.
    corneal a.
    crypt a.'s
    diffuse a.
    Douglas a.
    dry a.
    echinococcal liver a.
    enteroperitoneal a.
    extradural a.
    fecal a.
    a. formation
    gas a.
    gravitation a.
    hot a.
    hypostatic a.
    infraorbital space a.
    intra-abdominal a.
    intraperitoneal a.
    ischiorectal a.
    lacunar a.
    metastatic a.
    migrating a.
    miliary a.
    pancreatic a.
    paranephric a.
    parapharyngeal space a.
    pelvic a.
    perforating a.
    perianal fistula a.
    periappendiceal a.
    perineal a.
    perinephric a.
    perirectal a.
    peritoneal cavity a.
    periureteral a.
    periurethral a.
    phlegmonous a.
    point of a.
    premasseteric space a.
    prevertebral space a.
    pterygomandibular space a.
    residual a.
    retrocecal a.
    retroperitoneal-iliopsoas a.
    a. ring
    ring a.
    satellite a.
    soft tissue a.
    space of Retzius a.
    stercoral a.
    sterile a.
    stitch a.
    subdiaphragmatic a.
    subhepatic a.
    sublingual space a.
    submandibular space a.
    submasseteric space a.
    submental space a.
    subphrenic a.
    supralevator perirectal a.
    tuberculous a.
    wandering a.
abscission
    corneal a.
absconsio
absent respiration
Absidia infection
absolute
    a. construction
    a. curative resection
    a. noncurative resection
absorbable surgical suture
absorbent
    Baralyme CO_2 a.
    a. point
    soda lime CO_2 a.
    Sodasorb II CO_2 a.
    a. vessel
absorption
    external a.
    reservoir mucosal a.
    systemic a.
abut
abutment
    implant a.
    screw-type a.
    subperiosteal implant a.
acalculous cholecystitis
acantha
acanthion
acanthoid
acantholysis
accelerans
accelerated
    a. respiration
    a. transplant rejection
acceleration
    angular a.
    fetal growth a.
    fetal heart rate a.
    growth a.
    a. injury
    tibial a.
    a. time
acceleration/deceleration injury
acceleration-dependent aberrancy
accelerator
    a. fiber
    a. nerve
ACCEL stopcock
access
    a. cavity
    cavity a.

cutdown a.
exit a.
a. flap in osseous surgery
percutaneous a.
peritoneal a.
a. preparation
root canal a.
side-entry a.
accessorius
a. willisii
accessory
a. adrenal
a. cephalic vein
a. conduction ablation
a. duct stenting
a. flexor muscle of foot
a. hemiazygos vein
a. muscle activity
a. muscles of respiration
a. nerve
a. nerve lymph nodes
a. nerve trunk
a. obturator artery
a. palatine canal
a. pancreas
a. pancreatic duct
a. papillotomy
a. parotid gland
a. plantar ligaments
a. portion of spinal accessory
nerve
a. process
a. root canal
a. saphenous vein
a. spleen
a. suprarenal glands
a. thyroid gland
a. tubercle
a. vertebral vein
a. volar ligaments
accidental
a. hemorrhage
a. hypothermia
a. pulp exposure
accommodation
a. of crystalline lens
a. curve
a. disorder
a. of eye
a. of nerve
a. reflex
accordion graft

accretion line
AccuMark calibrated infant feeding tube
Accutracker blood pressure device
ACD resuscitator
Ace-Colles
A.-C. fracture frame
A.-C. frame technique
Ace-Fischer
A.-F. fracture frame
A.-F. ring frame
acellular pannus tissue
acentric relation
acestoma
acetabula (*pl. of* acetabulum)
acetabular
a. artery
a. augmentation graft
a. branch
a. cavity
a. cup arthroplasty
a. extensile approach
a. lip
a. protrusio deformity
a. rim fracture
acetabuloplasty
Albee a.
Pemberton a.
shelf a.
acetabulum, pl. acetabula
partial resection of the a.
acetohydroxamic acid irrigation
acetone chloroform
acetowhite lesion
acetylcholine (Ach)
a. receptor
acetylcysteine
10% a. 0.05% isoproterenol
hydrochloride solution
Ach
acetylcholine
achalasia balloon dilation
Achilles
A. bursa
A. tendon
A. tendon rupture
achondrogenesis
achondroplasia
homozygous a.
achondroplastic
achondroplasty

NOTES

5

acid
 ε-aminocaproic a.
 a. anhydride method
 a. aspiration
 5,5-diethylbarbituric a.
 epsilonaminocaproic a.
 a. etch bonding technique
 a. gland
 a. guanidine thiocyanate-phenol-
  chloroform method
 mefenamic a.
 methylhydroxymandelic a. (MOMA)
 phenylethylbarbituric a.
 trichloroacetic a.
acid-base
 a.-b. equilibrium
 a.-b. status
 a.-b. value
acid-citrate-dextrose solution
acid-etched restoration
acidification treatment
acinar tissue
acinic
 a. cell tumor of lung
 a. cell tumor of salivary gland
acinous gland
Ackerman-Proffitt classification of
 malocclusion
ACL
 anterior cruciate ligament
  ACL reconstruction
  ACL repair
acneform lesion
acne surgery
Acorn II nebulizer system
Acosta classification
acoupedic method
acoustic
 a. canal
 a. method
 a. nerve
 a. neuroma
 A. Neuroma Registry
 A. Pharyngometer two-microphone
  imaging system
 a. pressure
 a. quantification
 a. reflection measurement
 a. reflectometry
 a. stimulation study
 a. stimulation test
AC-PC line
acquired
 a. centric relation
 a. cornification disorder
 a. deformity
 a. eccentric jaw relation
acral

Acrel ganglion
acridine orange method
acrobrachycephaly
acrocephalia
acrocephalic
acrocephalopolysyndactyly
acrocephalosyndactyly type I-IV
acrocephalous
acrocephaly
acrodysplasia
acrofacial syndrome
acromial
 a. arterial network
 a. artery
 a. articular facies of clavicle
 a. articular surface of clavicle
 a. branch of suprascapular artery
 a. branch of thoracoacromial artery
 a. extremity of clavicle
 a. process
acromioclavicular
 a. articulation
 a. disk
 a. injury classification
 a. joint dislocation
 a. joint repair
 a. ligament
 a. space
acromiocoracoid
acromiohumeral
acromion
acromionectomy
 Armstrong a.
acromioplasty
 anterior a.
 McLaughlin a.
 McShane-Leinberry-Fenlin a.
 Neer a.
acromioscapular
acromiothoracic
 a. artery
acro-osteolysis
acro-osteolytica
 osteopetrosis a.-o.
acrylic graft
ACT
 activated clotting time
actinomycetoma
actinomycoma
actinomyoma
action
 anesthesia a.
 a. of anesthetic
 ball valve a.
 a. line
 nonstereospecific a.
 stereospecific a.

Activase injection
activated clotting time (ACT)
activating solution
activation
    baroreflex a.
    egg a.
    a. map-guided surgical resection
    a. moment
    very late a.
activation-sequence mapping
activator
    a. modification
    recombinant tissue-type
      plasminogen a. (rtPA)
active
    a. appliance therapy
    a. assistive motion therapy
    a. chronic inflammation
    a. core cooling
    a. reciprocation
    a. systemic bacterial infection
Activent-Sheehy tympanotomy tube
activity
    accessory muscle a.
    efferent nerve a.
    inspiratory intercostal a.
    a. pattern analysis
    sympathetic nerve a. (SNA)
actuation
    direct mechanical ventricular a.
actuator/adaptor
    endotracheal tube a.
acuminatum
    condyloma a.
acuology
acupuncture
    a. anesthesia
acus
acusection
Acuson echocardiographic equipment
acute
    a. abscess
    a. allergic extrinsic alveolitis
    a. allograft rejection
    a. calculous cholecystitis
    a. cellular rejection
    a. and chronic inflammation
    a. compression triad
    a. disconnection syndrome
    a. fracture
    a. gastric mucosal lesion
    a. graft-vs-host disease

    a. hemorrhagic inflammation
    a. hemorrhagic ulceration
    a. hepatic coma
    a. hepatic rupture
    a. inflammatory exudate
    a. inflammatory membrane
    a. intermittent porphyria
    a. lung rejection
    a. nonvariceal upper gastrointestinal
      hemorrhage
    a. normovolemic hemodilution
      (ANH)
    a. physiologic assessment and
      chronic health evaluation
    a. physiology and chronic health
      evaluation
    a. pyogenic membrane
    a. radiation pneumonitis
    a. recurrent rhabdomyolysis
    a. rejection of liver transplant
    a. respiratory distress syndrome
      (ARDS)
    a. subdural hematoma
    a. surgical abdomen
    a. traumatic lesion
    a. vascular rejection
ACUTENS transcutaneous nerve
  stimulator
Acutrol suture
acystia
adactylous
adactyly
adamantine membrane
adamantinoblastoma
adamantinocarcinoma
adamantinoma
adamantinum
    odontoma a.
Adamkiewicz
    artery of A.
Adams
    A. hip operation
    A. kidney stone filter
    A. procedure
Adam's apple
adaptation
    a. disease
    a. syndrome of Selye
adaptational approach
adapter
    circuit a.

NOTES

adapter *(continued)*
    Foregger-Racine a.
    pediatric Racine a.
adaptive
    a. correction
    a. relaxation
adaxial
Addison
    A. maneuver
    A. point
additional canal
additive interaction
additivity
adduction
    a. deformity
    a. osteotomy
    a. traction technique
adduction-internal rotation deformity
adductor
    a. canal
    a. hiatus
    a. longus muscle rupture
    a. tenotomy
    a. tenotomy and obturator
      neurectomy
adductovarus deformity
adenectomy
adenoacanthoma
adenoameloblastoma
adenocanthoma
adenocarcinoma
    alveolar a.
    ampullary a.
    anaplastic a.
    annular a.
    appendiceal a.
    bronchial a.
    bronchiolar a.
    bronchioloalveolar a.
    bronchogenic a.
    cervical a.
    colonic a.
    colorectal a.
    cystic a.
    duct cell a.
    duodenal a.
    endometrial a.
    esophageal a.
    gastric a.
    gastrointestinal tract a.
    infiltrating duct a.
    kidney a.
    medullary a.
    mesonephric a.
    metastatic a.
    ovarian clear cell a.
    pancreatic a.
    peritoneal a.

    prostatic a.
    renal a.
    sebaceous a.
    secretory a.
    serous a.
    signet-ring a.
    a. in situ
    stomach a.
    sweat gland a.
    undifferentiated a.
    vaginal a.
    vulvar adenoid cystic a.
Adenocard injection
adenochondroma
adenocystoma
adenodiastasis
adenoepithelioma
adenofibroma
adenofibromyoma
adenohypophysial
adenohypophysis
adenoidal pad
adenoidal-pharyngeal-conjunctival (A-P-C)
adenoidectomy
    lateral a.
    tonsillectomy and a.
adenoid tumor
adenoleiomyofibroma
adenolipoma
adenolymphocele
adenolymphoma
adenolysis
adenoma
    adnexal a.
    adrenal a.
    bile duct a.
    a. of breast
    bronchial a.
    colonic a.
    colorectal a.
    ductal a.
    duodenal a.
    fibroid a.
    hepatic a.
    kidney a.
    malignant a.
    papillary a. of large intestine
    parathyroid a.
    pituitary a.
    prostatic a.
    renal a.
    sessile a.
    sweat gland a.
    thyroid a.
    tracheal a.
adenoma-hyperplastic polyp ratio
adenoma-nonadenoma ratio

adenomatosis
    endocrine a.
adenomatous polyp
adenomectomy
adenomyoma
    a. of gallbladder
adenomyosarcoma
adenopathy
    retroperitoneal a.
adenosarcoma
adenose
adenosine triphosphate
adenosis
    sclerosing a.
adenotomy
adenotonsillectomy
adenoviral type 40/41 infection
adenovirus infection
adenylylation
adeps
    a. renis
adequate hydration
adherens
    leukoma a.
adherent leukoma
adhesed
adhesio
adhesiolysis
adhesion
    a. barrier
    cell-extracellular matrix a.
    fibrinous a.
    fibrous a.
    a. formation
    hard a.
    intra-abdominal a.
    intraperitoneal a.
    a. lysis
    lysis of a.'s
    peritoneal a.
    piano-wire a.
    primary a.
    secondary a.
adhesiotomy
adhesive
    a. arachnoiditis
    a. band
    a. bonding
    a. capsulitis
    a. disease
    a. foil
    a. ileus

    a. inflammation
    a. otitis media
    a. peritonitis
    a. resin-bonded bridge
    a. resin bonded cast restoration
    a. strapping
    a. syndrome
adipectomy
adipocele
adipodermal graft
adipolysis
adipose
    a. body
    a. capsule
    a. graft
    a. infiltration
    a. tissue
    a. tissue extract
aditus
    a. ad antrum
    a. ad saccum peritonei minorem
    a. glottidis inferior
    a. glottidis superior
    a. laryngis
    a. orbitae
    a. pelvis
adjunctive
    a. balloon angioplasty
    a. screw fixation
adjustable suture
adjuvant
    anesthesia a.
    a. chemoradiation therapy
    a. drug therapy
    a. irradiation
    a. nephrectomy
    a. whole-brain radiation therapy
Adkins
    A. spinal fusion
    A. technique spinal arthrodesis
Adler operation
Adlone injection
admaxillary gland
admedial
adminiculum
    a. lineae albae
administered
    spinally a.
administration
    drug a.
    epidural a.
    interpleural a.

NOTES

administration *(continued)*
    intraocular a.
    intraperitoneal drug a.
    intraspinal a.
    intrathecal a.
    intravenous a.
    oral a.
    oxygen a.
    parenteral a.
    route of a.
    sequential a.
    transdermal a.
    transnasal a.
    vasodilator a.
admixture
    a. lesion
    venous a.
adnexa (*pl. of* adnexum)
adnexal
    a. adenoma
    a. carcinoma
    a. infection
    a. mass
    a. metastasis
adnexectomy
adnexopexy
adnexum, pl. **adnexa**
    adnexa uteri
adrenal
    a. ablation
    accessory a.
    a. adenoma
    a. androgen
    a. body
    a. capsule
    a. carcinoma
    a. cortex
    a. cystic mass
    a. feminization syndrome
    a. gland
    a. gland biopsy
    a. hemorrhage
    Marchand a.'s
    a. medulla transplantation
    a. metastasis
adrenalectomy
    ipsilateral a.
    laparoscopic a.
    transperitoneal laparoscopic a.
adrenaline injection
α-adrenergic
    α-a. agent
    α-a. antagonist
    α-a. receptor
    α-a. receptor agonist
β-adrenergic
    β-a. agonist
    β-a. blockade

    β-a. blocking drug
    β-a. receptor
α₁-adrenergic
    α_1-a. agonist
    α_1-a. antagonist
α₂-adrenergic
    α_2-a. agonist
    α_2-a. receptor
    α_2-a. receptor antagonist
adrenergic blockade
β₂-adrenergic receptor
adrenic
adrenocortical
    a. extract
adrenoprival
α-adrenoreceptor
β-adrenoreceptor
α₂-adrenoreceptor agonist
Adrucil injection
Adson
    A. maneuver
    A. suction
    A. suction tube
    A. test
Adson-Coffey scalenotomy
Adsorbotear Ophthalmic solution
adsternal
adterminal
adult
    a. familial hyaline membrane
      disease
    a. respiratory distress syndrome
      (ARDS)
    a. scoliosis surgery
advanced
    A. Catheter Systems
    a. therapeutic endoscopy
    a. trauma life support (ATLS)
advancement
    a. flap graft
    Johnson pronator a.
    mandibular osteotomy a.
    a. procedure
    a. of rectal flap
Aebi-Etter-Coscia fixation dens fracture
Aeby
    A. muscle
    A. plane
aeration
    a. of lung
aerobic
    a. infection
    a. respiration
aerocele
aerocystoscopy
aerodigestive tract
aerodynamic size

aerosol
> DEY albuterol inhalation a.
> Fluro-Ethyl A.
> inhalation a.
> respirable a.
> a. therapy

aerosolized
> a. medication
> a. pollutant exposure
> a. prostacyclin

A-exotropia

AF
> aortofemoral
> AF tube

affection
> patellar a.

afferent
> a. glomerular arteriole
> a. loop syndrome
> a. projection

affrication

AFH
> anterior facial height

aftercooler

afterloading technique

afterload reduction

after-pain

after-root amputation restoration

agar diffusion method

age
> fertilization a.

Agee force-couple splint reduction

agenesis
> trachcal a.

agenetic fracture

agent
> α-adrenergic a.
> anesthetic induction a.
> antifibrinolytic a.
> cavity lining a.
> endogenous algogenic a.
> inhalation a.
> neuroleptic a.
> neuromuscular blocking a.
> Osteomark a.
> sympatholytic a.
> sympathomimetic a.
> β-sympathomimetic a.
> vasodilator a.
> ventilation a.
> volatile anesthetic a.

agent-specific filling device

agglutinant

agglutination technique

aggregate glands

aggressive lesion

Agliette supracondylar osteotomy

aglossia-adactylia syndrome

aglossostomia

agminate glands

agnathia

agnathous

Agnew
> A. canthoplasty
> A. operation

Agnew-Verhoeff incision

AgNOR staining

agonadal

agonal respiration

agonist
> α_2-a.
> β-adrenergic a.
> α_1-adrenergic a.
> α_2-adrenergic a.
> α-adrenergic receptor a.
> α_2-adrenoreceptor a.
> muscarinic a.
> opioid a.
> β-receptor a.

Agrikola operation

agrypnocoma

ahaustral

Ahern knot

AIO parenteral solution

air
> a. collection
> a. contrast barium enema
> a. cushion bed
> a. embolism
> a. entrainment
> a. entry
> a. exchange
> expiratory trapping of a.
> extrapleural a.
> a. filter
> a. injection
> a. insufflation
> intramyocardial a.
> intraperitoneal a.
> minimal a.
> oxygen in a.
> a. pressure driven apparatus
> a. sac
> a. space

NOTES

air *(continued)*
 a. space disease
 a. test
 a. tube
 a. vesicle
air/bone/tissue boundary
airborne infection
airbrasive technique
Aire-Cuf
 A.-C. endotracheal tube
 A.-C. tracheostomy tube
air-filled loop
air-fluid
 a.-f. exchange
 a.-f. line
air-gap technique
Air-Lon
 A.-L. laryngectomy tube
 A.-L. tracheal tube
airway
 anatomical a.
 a. compromise
 Concord/Portex a.
 a. elastance
 esophageal obturator a.
 a. gas monitoring
 a. heat and moisture exchanger
 laryngeal mask a. (LMA)
 Luomanen oral a.
 nasal a.
 a. occlusion technique
 oral pharyngeal a.
 pediatric a.
 pharyngeal a.
 a. pressure
 a. pressure release ventilation
 (APRV)
 a. protection
 a. reactivity
 a. responsiveness
 a. score
 a. shunting
 a. smooth muscle (ASM)
 a. suction
airway, breathing, and circulation
 (ABC)
Aitken epiphyseal fracture classification
AJCC TNM tumor classification
AKA
 above-knee amputation
AK-Dilate Ophthalmic solution
Akerlund deformity
Akin
 A. bunionectomy
 A. procedure
 A. proximal phalangeal osteotomy
AK-Nefrin Ophthalmic solution

Akwa Tears solution
ala, pl. alae
 a. major ossis sphenoidalis
 a. minor ossis sphenoidalis
 a. orbitalis
 a. ossis ilii
 sacral a.
 a. sacralis
 a. temporalis
Alanson amputation
alant starch
alar
 a. base reduction
 a. folds
 a. groove
 a. lamina of neural tube
 a. ligaments
 a. plate of neural tube
 a. reconstruction
 a. spine
 a. wedge excision
alarm
 ventilator a.
Albarran
 A. glands
 A. y Dominguez tubules
Albee
 A. acetabuloplasty
 A. bone graft
 A. spinal fusion
Albee-Delbert procedure
Albert
 A. suture
 A. suture technique
Albinus muscle
Albrecht bone
Albright-Chase arthroplasty
Albright synovectomy
albugineotomy
albumin-coated vascular graft
albuminized woven Dacron tube graft
Alcaine
Alcock canal
alcohol
 a. fixation
 a. injection
 polyvinyl a. (PVA)
 trichloroethyl a.
alcohol-fixed gastric biopsy
alcoholic coma
Alcon
 A. aspiration
 A. phacoemulsification
 A. suture
alcuronium chloride
aldehyde-tanned bovine carotid artery
 graft
Alden loop gastric bypass

Alder-Reilly anomaly
Aldrete score
Aldridge sling procedure
Aldridge-Studdefort urethral suspension
Alesen tube
Alexander
    A. incision
    A. operation
    A. technique
Alexander-Adams
    A.-A. hysteropexy
    A.-A. uterine suspension
Alexian Brothers overhead fracture frame
Alfenta injection
alfentanil
    a. hydrochloride
algesimeter
    coiled pressure a.
Al-Ghorab
    A.-G. modification
    A.-G. procedure
algology
algoscopy
alignment
    extramedullary a.
    a. of fracture fragment
    restoration of normal anatomic a.
alimentary
    a. apparatus
    a. canal
    a. tract
    a. tract duplication
alimentation
    central venous a.
    enteral a.
    forced a.
    intravenous a.
    peripheral intravenous a.
    rectal a.
    total parenteral a.
alinasal
A-line
aliquot
Alken approach
alkylation resistance
Alladin InfantFlow nasal continuous positive air pressure
Allain method
Allander air curtain

allantoic
    a. circulation
    a. sac
Allen
    A. correction
    A. maneuver
    A. operation
    A. reduction
    A. test
Allen-Ferguson Galveston pelvic fixation
allergen exposure
allergic
    a. inflammation
    a. manifestation
Allgöwer stitch
alligator skin
all-inside repair
Allis-Abramson breast biopsy
Allis maneuver
Allison
    A. gastroesophageal reflux repair
    A. hiatal hernia repair
Alliston procedure
Allman acromioclavicular injury classification
allobarbital
allocation
    dynamic storage a.
    fresh tissue a.
    static storage a.
    storage a.
    a. of treatment
allochezia
AlloDerm universal dermal tissue graft
allogeneic
    a. blood
    a. blood transfusion
    a. fetal graft
    a. transplantation
allogenic bone graft
allogenous bone graft
allograft
    a. corneal rejection
    cryopreserved heart valve a.
    femoral cortical ring a.
    organ a.
    osteoarticular a.
    osteochondral a.
    pancreaticoduodenal a.
    a. transplantation
allokeratoplasty
allongement

NOTES

allopathic keratoplasty
alloplast
alloplastic
    a. chin augmentation
    a. graft
alloplasty
allotransplantation
alloy restoration
Allport operation
allylbarbital
Alonso-Lej classification
alopecia
    pressure a.
    traction a.
alpha cell of hypophysis
alphadione
alpha-loop maneuver
alphaprodine
Alport syndrome
ALPSA lesion
already-threaded suture
Alsus-Knapp operation
Alsus operation
alteration
    dentin crystal a.
alterative inflammation
altercursive intubation
alternate-day therapy
alternation
alternative
    graft material a.
altitude simulation study
aluminum
    a. cranioplasty
    a. filter
    implant alloy a.
aluminum-bronze wire suture
alveodental suppuration
alveolar
    a. adenocarcinoma
    a. body
    a. canal
    a. carbon dioxide pressure
    a. cavity
    a. cleft graft
    a. dead space
    a. diffusion measurement
    a. ectasia
    a. end-capillary difference
    a. fistula
    a. foramina
    a. gas equation
    a. hemorrhage
    a. hyperventilation
    a. hypoventilation
    a. index
    a. oxygen partial pressure (PAO$_2$)
    a. partial pressure

    a. plateau
    a. plate fenestration
    a. point
    a. point-basion line
    a. point-meatus plane
    a. point-nasal point line
    a. point-nasion line
    a. process fracture
    a. rhabdomyosarcoma
    a. sac
    a. socket wall fracture
    a. ventilation
    a. ventilation per minute
    a. yoke
alveolar-arterial pressure difference
alveolar-capillary membrane
alveolarization
alveolectomy
    partial a.
alveolitis
    acute allergic extrinsic a.
    chronic extrinsic a.
    extrinsic allergic a.
alveolobasilar line
alveolocapillary
    a. membrane
    a. partial pressure gradient
alveolodental membrane
alveololabial groove
alveolomerotomy
alveolonasal line
alveoloplasty
    interradicular a.
    intraseptal a.
alveolotomy
alveolysis
alveoplasty
alveus
    a. urogenitalis
alvinolith
Alvis operation
AM
    anterior midpapillary
    AM segment
amalgam
    a. condensation
    a. restoration
Amato body
amaurosis
    intoxification a.
    pressure a.
Amberg lateral sinus line
ambiens
    cisterna a.
ambient
    a. cisterna
    a. oxygen concentration
    a. temperature

a. wing of the quadrigeminal cistern
AMBI fixation
ambifixation
ambiguous external genitalia
amblyopia
    deprivation a.
    eclipse a.
    ex a.
    exertional a.
Ambu
    A. infant resuscitator
    A. suction booster
ambulatory
    a. anesthesia
    a. gynecologic laparoscopy
    a. hemorrhoidectomy
    a. surgery
amebic infection
amelioration
ameloblastoma
Americaine
American
    A. Association of Nurse Anesthetists (AANA)
    A. Board of Anesthesiology (ABA)
    A. circle nephrostomy tube
    A. Heart Association classification
    A. laryngectomy technique
    A. Rheumatism Association index
    A. silk suture
    A. Society of Anesthesiologists classification
    A. tracheotomy tube
    A. Urological Association symptom index
A-methaPred injection
ametropia
    position a.
AMeX method
Amidate
    A. injection
amidation
Amikin injection
amino acid-based dialysate solution
ε-aminocaproic acid
Aminofusin L Forte amino acid solution
aminophylline
4-aminopyridine
amiodarone

Amis 2000 respiratory mass spectrometer
AMLR
    auditory middle-latency response
Ammon
    A. canthoplasty
    A. operation
amnesia
    patch a.
amnestic effect
amnioma
amnion
    a. ring
    a. rupture
amnioscopy
amniotic
    a. band amputation
    a. cavity
    a. infection syndrome
    a. membrane
    a. sac
amniotocele
amniotomy
amobarbital
A-mode echo-tracking device
amphibolic fistula
amphibolous fistula
amphoric respiration
amphotericin B lipid complex injection
Amplatz technique
amplitude
    a. of fusion
    a. modulation
amplitude-summation
    a.-s. interferential current
    a.-s. interferential current therapy
ampulla, pl. ampullae
    a. chyli
    a. of ductus deferens
    duodenal a.
    a. duodeni
    a. of gallbladder
    hepatopancreatic a.
    a. hepatopancreatica
    invagination of the a.
    a. of lacrimal canal
    rectal a.
    a. recti
    a. of rectum
    a. of the semicircular canals
    a. of the semicircular ducts
    Thoma a.

NOTES

ampulla *(continued)*
    a. tubae uterinae
    a. of uterine tube
    Vater a.
    a. of Vater
ampullary
    a. adenocarcinoma
    a. aneurysm
    a. crura of semicircular ducts
    a. granulation tissue
    a. sulcus
    a. tumor
ampulloma
amputation
    above-elbow a.
    above-knee a. (AKA)
    Alanson a.
    amniotic band a.
    Béclard a.
    below-elbow a.
    below-knee a. (BKA)
    Berger interscapular a.
    Bier a.
    bilateral a.
    birth a.
    bloodless a.
    border ray a.
    Boyd ankle a.
    Bunge a.
    Burgess below-knee a.
    Callander a.
    central ray a.
    cervical a.
    chop a.
    Chopart a.
    circular open a.
    closed flap a.
    congenital above-elbow a.
    congenital below-elbow a.
    consecutive a.
    corporectomy a.
    disarticular a.
    dry a.
    extremity a.
    fingertip a.
    fish-mouth a.
    forearm a.
    forequarter a.
    Gordon-Taylor hindquarter a.
    Gritti-Stokes a.
    guillotine a.
    hand a.
    hindfoot a.
    hindquarter a.
    immediate a.
    incomplete a.
    index ray a.
    interilioabdominal a.
    interinnominoabdominal a.
    intermediate a.
    interpelviabdominal a.
    interphalangeal a.
    intrapyretic a.
    intrauterine a.
    Jaboulay a.
    Kendrick method below-knee a.
    King-Steelquist hindquarter a.
    Lisfranc a.
    major a.
    middle finger a.
    midthigh a.
    minor a.
    multiple ray a.
    one-stage a.
    open a.
    pathologic a.
    penile a.
    Pirogoff a.
    primary a.
    pulp a.
    quadruple a.
    ray a.
    rectangular a.
    root a.
    secondary a.
    shoulder a.
    Sorondo-Ferré hindquarter a.
    spontaneous a.
    supracondylar a.
    Syme ankle disarticulation a.
    tarsal a.
    tarsometatarsal a.
    tendinomyoplastic a.
    tertiary a.
    through-knee a.
    transcarpal a.
    transiliac a.
    transmetatarsal a.
    transpelvic a.
    traumatic a.
    two-stage Syme a.
    Wagner modification of Syme a.
    Wagner two-stage Syme a.
    Wilms a.
amputee
Amreich vaginal extirpation
amrinone
Amsler
    A. corneal graft
    A. operation
Amspacher-Messenbaugh
    A.-M. closing wedge osteotomy
    A.-M. technique
Amstutz-Wilson osteotomy
Amussat
    A. incision

A. operation
A. valvula
Amvisc Plus solution
amygdaline
amygdalohippocampectomy
amygdalotomy
amylene
a. chloral
a. hydrate
amyl nitrite
amylocaine hydrochloride
amyloid
a. angiopathy
a. kidney
a. oral cavity disease
anaclitic therapy
anacrotic notch
anadidymus
anaerobic
a. ocular infection
a. respiration
anaeroplasty
anaesthesia (*var. of* anesthesia)
anaesthesiologist (*var. of* anesthesiologist)
anagenesis
Anagnostakis operation
anal
a. anastomosis
a. canal
a. cleft
a. column
a. condyloma
a. crypt
a. dilation
a. electrical stimulation
a. endoscopy
a. fascia
a. fistula
a. foreign body
a. HPZ
a. ileostomy with preservation of sphincter
a. orifice
a. pecten
a. pouch
a. region
a. sinuses
a. sphincter reconstruction
a. sphincter repair
a. sphincter squeeze pressure
a. squamous intraepithelial lesion
a. transitional zone (ATZ)

a. triangle
a. ulceration
a. verge
analgesia
a. algera
conduction a.
dermatomal level of a.
fentanyl-neostigmine a.
fixed-dose patient-controlled a. (FDPCA)
inhalation a.
interpleural a.
intrathecal opioid labor a.
level of a.
multimodal a.
opioid a.
parenteral a.
patient-controlled a. (PCA)
patient-controlled epidural a. (PCEA, PEA)
patient-controlled intranasal a. (PCINA)
perineal a.
a. permeation
postoperative a.
preemptive a.
preoperative a.
rescue a.
spinal a.
thoracic epidural a.
tracheal topical a.
analgesic
intranasal a.
intrathecal a.
intravenous a.
narcotic a.
nitrous oxide a.
NSAID a.
opioid a.
oral a.
pediatric a.
postoperative a.
spinal a.
transdermal a.
analgesimeter
analgetic
analgizer
Penthrane a.
analysis
activity pattern a.
blood-gas a.
body composition a.

NOTES

analysis *(continued)*
    body-fluid a.
    combined a.
    deformity a.
    displacement a.
    fixed-dose a.
    image a.
    isobologram a.
    isobolographic a.
    Kruskal-Wallis nonparametric a.
    neutron activation a.
    peak pressure a.
    power spectral a.
    pressure-volume a.
    p53 tumor suppressor gene a.
    restriction endonuclease a.
    saturation a.
    single strand conformation
      polymorphism a.
    slot-blot hybridization a.
    sound a.
    total space a.
    Tweed method of dentofacial a.
    Vindelov method flow cytometry a.
analytic
    a. method
    a. reconstruction
analyzer
    ABL 330 a.
    ABL 30 blood gas a.
    AVL Gas Check 939 blood gas a.
    Capnomac infrared a.
    Capnomac multiple gas a.
    Capnomac Ultima gas a.
    Corning 170 blood gas a.
    fast Fourier transformation
      spectrum a.
    Fourier transformation spectrum a.
    Gas Check blood a.
    halothane a.
    Ionalyzer a.
    iSTAT hand-held blood a.
    Myograph 2000 neuromuscular
      function a.
    Osteomeasure computer-assisted
      image a.
    oxygen a.
    pacing system a.
    Radiometer ABL 500 blood gas a.
    ULT-Svi calibrated end-tidal gas a.
    YSI 2300 STAT Plus glucose and
      lactose a.
anaphylactoid-type reaction
anaphylaxis
anaplastic
    a. adenocarcinoma
anaplasty
anapophysis

anastole
anastomose
anastomosed graft
anastomosis, pl. **anastomoses**
    anal a.
    aneurysm by a.
    antecolic a.
    aortic a.
    arterial a.
    arteriolovenular a.
    a. arteriovenosa
    arteriovenous a.
    Baffe a.
    Béclard a.
    beveled a.
    bidirectional superior
      cavopulmonary a.
    biliary-enteric a.
    biliodigestive a.
    Billroth I, II a.
    bladder neck-to-urethra a.
    Brackin ureterointestinal a.
    Braun a.
    carotid-basilar a.
    carotid-vertebral a.
    Carrel aortic patch a.
    cavopulmonary a.
    choledococaval a.
    circular a.
    Clado a.
    cobra-head a.
    Coffey ureterointestinal a.
    coloanal a.
    colocolonic a.
    coloendoanal a.
    colorectal a.
    conjoined a.
    Cooley intrapericardial a.
    Cooley modification of
      Waterston a.
    cornual a.
    Couvelaire ileourethral a.
    cross-facial nerve graft a.
    cruciate a.
    crunch-stick a.
    curved end-to-end a.
    Daines-Hodgson a.
    dismembered a.
    distal a.
    dog ear of a.
    elliptical a.
    endoanal a.
    end-to-end a.
    end-to-side a.
    end-weave a.
    esophagocolic a.
    extravesical a.
    fish-mouth a.

flexor tendon a.
Fontan atriopulmonary a.
Galen a.
gastrointestinal a.
Glenn a.
graft a.
grafting a.
hand-sewn a.
hand-sutured ileoanal a.
hepatojejunal a.
Hofmeister a.
Hofmeister-Pólya a.
Horsley a.
Hoyer anastomoses
H-shaped ileal pouch-anal a.
hypoglossal facial nerve a.
Hyrtl a.
ileal pouch-anal a.
ileal pouch-distal rectal a.
ileoanal a.
ilcorectal a.
ileotransverse colon a.
ileovesical a.
intercoronary a.
intermesenteric arterial a.
intestinal a.
intravesical a.
isoperistaltic a.
isthmointerstitial a.
jejunoileal a.
jejunojejunal a.
J-shaped ileal pouch-anal a.
Kocher a.
Kugel a.
leptomeningeal a.
Lich-Gregoire a.
lymphaticovenous a.
Martin-Gruber a.
mesocaval a.
microneurovascular a.
microsurgical tubocornual a.
microvascular surgical a.
mucosa-to-mucosa a.
Nakayama a.
nerve a.
nondismembered a.
onlay patch a.
pancreaticogastrointestinal a.
Parks ileoanal a.
percutaneous portocaval a.
Politano-Leadbetter a.
Pólya a.

portacaval a.
portal-systemic anastomoses
portoportal a.
portopulmonary venous a.
portosystemic a.
Potts a.
Potts-Smith a.
precapillary a.
primary end-to-end a.
rectosigmoid a.
Riche-Cannieu a.
right-angled end-to-side a.
Riolan a.
a. of Riolan
Roux-en-Y hepaticojejunal a.
Schmidel anastomoses
Schoemaker a.
side-to-side a.
spinal accessory nerve-facial
  nerve a.
splenorenal venous a.
S-shaped ileal pouch-anal a.
STA-MCA a.
stapled ileoanal a.
State end-to-end a.
stenotic esophagogastric a.
Sucquet a.
Sucquet-Hoyer a.
sutureless bowel a.
systemic to pulmonary artery a.
temporal-cerebral arterial a.
tension-free a.
termino-terminal a.
transanal mucosectomy with hand-
  sewn a.
transureteroureteral a.
two-layer a.
ureterocolonic a.
ureteroileal a.
ureterosigmoid a.
ureterotubal a.
ureteroureteral a.
urethrocecal a.
vascular a.
venous-to-venous a.
vesicourethral a.
Von Haberer-Finney a.
Waterston extrapericardial a.
wide elliptical a.
W-shaped ileal pouch-anal a.
anastomotic
a. failure

NOTES

anastomotic *(continued)*
    a. leakage
    a. stoma
    a. suture
    a. ulceration
    a. veins
anatomic
    a. barrier
    a. dead space
    a. equator
    a. fracture
    a. fracture reduction principle
    a. insertion
    a. integrity
    a. localization
    a. plane
    a. repair
Anatomica
    Basle Nomina A. (BNA)
anatomical
    a. airway
    a. dead space
    a. position
    a. radical retropubic prostatectomy
    a. snuffbox
    a. sphincter
anatomicosurgical
anatomique
    tabatière a.
anatomist
anatomy
    anomalous a.
    Billroth II a.
    cervicothoracic pedicle a.
    congenitally altered a.
    coronary vessel a.
    dental a.
    designed after natural a. (DANA)
    dorsalis pedis artery a.
    fetal intracranial a.
    gingival a.
    immune system a.
    intracranial a.
    knee a.
    Lowsley lobar a.
    native coronary a.
    neurovascular a.
    normal planar MR a.
    pathological a.
    pedicle a.
    peritoneal a.
    plantar compartmental a.
    surgical a.
    zonal a.
anatrophic
    a. nephrolithotomy
    a. nephroscopy
    a. nephrotomy

Ancap braided silk suture
anchor
    a. band
    a. molar
anchorage
    extramaxillary a.
    extraoral a.
anchoring
    a. point
    a. suture
anchovy procedure
ancipital
anconeal
anconeus muscle
Andersch
    A. ganglion
    A. nerve
Anderson
    A. ankle fusion
    A. flexible suction tube
    A. gastric tube
    A. modification of Berndt-Harty classification
    A. procedure
Anderson-D'Alonzo odontoid fracture classification
Anderson-Fowler
    A.-F. anterior calcaneal osteotomy for pes planus
    A.-F. calcaneal displacement osteotomy
    A.-F. procedure
Anderson-Hutchins
    A.-H. technique
    A.-H. unstable tibial shaft fracture
Anderson-Hynes pyeloplasty
Anderson-Keys method
Andrews
    A. iliotibial band reconstruction
    A. spinal frame
    A. technique
Andrews-Pynchon
    A.-P. suction tube
    A.-P. tube
Andrews-type nonorthodontic normal crown angulation
androblastoma
androgen
    a. ablation
    adrenal a.
    excess a.
androgenic
androgenization
android pelvis
Andy Gump deformity
anecdotal procedure
anechoic tissue

Anectine
    A. Chloride injection
    A. Flo-Pack
Anel
    A. method
    A. operation
anemia
anemometer
    hot-wire a.
    warm-wire a.
Anestacon
anesthesia, anaesthesia
    a. action
    acupuncture a.
    a. adjuvant
    ambulatory a.
    ankle block a.
    axillary block a.
    balanced a.
    barbiturate burst-suppression a.
    basal a.
    Bier block a.
    block a.
    bolus intravenous a.
    brachial a.
    bypass a.
    CABG a.
    cardiac a.
    cardiovascular a.
    a. cartridge
    caudal a.
    centroneuroaxis a.
    cervical a.
    circle absorption a.
    a. circuit
    a. circuit filter
    closed a.
    closed-circuit a.
    cocaine a.
    co-induction of a.
    combined epidural/general a.
    combined spinal/epidural a. (CSE)
    come-and-go a.
    compression a.
    computer-assisted a.
    conduction a.
    continuous epidural a.
    continuous lumbar peridural a.
    continuous spinal a.
    corneal a.
    crossed a.
    dental a.

    depth of a.
    diagnostic a.
    differential spinal a.
    digital block a.
    dissociated a.
    dissociative a.
    a. dolorosa
    duration of a.
    ear a.
    electric a.
    endotracheal a.
    enflurane a.
    epidural a. (EA)
    exam under a.
    extradural a.
    failed a.
    field block a.
    fractional epidural a.
    fractional spinal a.
    general a. (GA)
    general endotracheal a.
    geriatric a.
    girdle a.
    glove a.
    graded spinal a.
    gustatory a.
    gynecologic a.
    halothane a.
    halothane/narcotic/nitrous oxide a.
    high spinal a.
    high thoracic level epidural a.
    hyperbaric spinal a.
    hypobaric spinal a.
    hypotensive a.
    hypothermic a.
    hysterical a.
    induction of a.
    infiltration a.
    infraorbital a.
    inhalant a.
    inhalation a.
    inhalational a.
    insufflation a.
    intercostal a.
    interpleural a.
    intracavitary a.
    intraligamentary a.
    intramedullary a.
    intranasal a.
    intraoral a.
    intraorbital a.
    intraosseous a.

NOTES

anesthesia *(continued)*
 intraperitoneal a.
 intrapulpal a.
 intraspinal a.
 intrathecal a.
 intratracheal a.
 intravenous block a.
 intravenous regional a. (IVRA)
 isobaric spinal a.
 isoflurane a.
 isoflurane/narcotic/nitrous oxide a.
 isoflurane/nitrous oxide a.
 laryngeal a.
 ligamental a.
 local a.
 low-flow sevoflurane a.
 low spinal a.
 low thoracic level epidural a.
 lumbar epidural a.
 MAC a.
 MacIntosh blade a.
 Madajet XL local a.
 maintenance of a.
 management of a.
 maternal a.
 mechanisms of a.
 medial canthus single injection periocular a.
 methoxyflurane a.
 modified Van Lint a.
 muscular a.
 narcotic/nitrous oxide a.
 neonatal a.
 nerve block a.
 nerve compression a.
 neuroleptanalgesia a.
 neurosurgical a.
 newborn a.
 nitrous oxide/fentanyl a.
 nitrous oxide/isoflurane a.
 nitrous oxide/opioid/barbiturate a.
 nitrous oxide/opioid/midazolam/thiopental a.
 nonrebreathing a.
 N_2O/O_2/opioid a.
 nose a.
 O'Brien a.
 obstetric a.
 olfactory a.
 one-lung a.
 open drop a.
 ophthalmic a.
 ophthalmologic a.
 opioid a.
 opioid/nitrous oxide/oxygen a.
 orbital a.
 orthopedic a.
 outpatient a.
 painful a.
 paracervical block a.
 paravertebral a.
 parenteral a.
 patient-controlled epidural a.
 patient-controlled intravenous a.
 pediatric radiotherapy a.
 peribulbar a.
 peridural a.
 perineal a.
 perineural a.
 periodontal ligament a.
 peripheral nerve block a.
 pharyngeal a.
 Ponka technique for local a.
 post-cesarean a.
 postoperative a.
 preemptive a.
 pregnancy-induced a.
 preperitoneal a.
 presacral a.
 pressure a.
 pressure reversal of a.
 propofol/nitrous oxide a.
 pudendal a.
 rapid sequence induction of a.
 rebreathing a.
 a. record
 rectal a.
 refrigeration a.
 regional a. (RA)
 retrobulbar a.
 risk of a.
 risk management of a.
 sacral a.
 saddle block a.
 segmental epidural a.
 selective a.
 semiclosed a.
 semiopen a.
 a. simulator-recorder
 single-breath induction of a.
 spinal a. (SA)
 splanchnic a.
 stellate ganglion block a.
 stocking a.
 subarachnoid a.
 supraclavicular brachial block a.
 surgical a.
 tactile a.
 therapeutic a.
 thermal a.
 thermic a.
 thiopental/sufentanil/desflurane/nitrous oxide a.
 thoracic a.
 throat a.

to-and-fro a.
toe block a.
topical oropharyngeal a.
total intravenous a. (TIVA)
total spinal a.
transdermal a.
traumatic a.
unilateral a.
urologic a.
Van Lint a.
variable-dose patient-controlled a.
  (VDPCA)
visceral a.
volatile a.
anesthesiologist, anaesthesiologist
anesthesiology
American Board of A. (ABA)
critical care a.
a. critical care medicine
anesthesiometer
Semmes-Weinstein pressure a.
anesthetic
action of a.
a. blockade
cardiac a.
Cetacaine topical a.
a. circuit
a. cutoff
a. depth
a. emergence
EMLA a.
epidural a.
a. ether
eutectic mixture of local a.'s
  (EMLA)
flammable a.
fluorinated ether a.
gas a.
a. gas
a. gas exposure
general a.
halogenated volatile a.
halothane a.
a. hepatitis
a. hepatotoxicity
hyperbaric local a.
a. immediate recovery
a. index
a. induction agent
inhalation a.
inhalational a.
inhaled a.

injection of local a.
instillation of a.
intradermal a.
intramuscular a.
intraperitoneal a.
intrathecal a.
intravenous a.
a. leprosy
lidocaine topical a.
local a.
low-dose a.
methyl isopropyl ether a.
a. monitoring
multiple mechanism inhaled a.
multiple site inhaled a.
opioid a.
oral a.
pediatric a.
polymer a.
a. potency
preoperative a.
primary a.
a. record
rectal a.
regional a.
secondary a.
a. shock
Silverstein tetracaine base
  powder a.
single mechanism inhaled a.
single site inhaled a.
spinal a.
a. system
a. technique
a. tolerance
topical a.
trace a.
a. vapor
volatile a.
walking epidural a.
Xylocaine topical a.
anesthetic/hypnotic
anesthetist
certified registered nurse a.
  (CRNA)
nurse a.
Anesthetists
American Association of Nurse A.
  (AANA)
anesthetization
anesthetize
aneuploid cell line

NOTES

aneurysm
    abdominal aortic a. (AAA)
    ampullary a.
    a. by anastomosis
    aortic a.
    arteriosclerotic a.
    arteriovenous a.
    atherosclerotic a.
    axial a.
    basilar bifurcation a.
    basilar tip a.
    Bérard a.
    berry a.
    bifurcation a.
    clavicular fracture a.
    compound a.
    congenital cerebral a.
    consecutive a.
    cylindroid a.
    diffuse a.
    dissecting a.
    ectatic a.
    endogenous a.
    exogenous a.
    false a.
    fusiform a.
    hernial a.
    infraclinoid a.
    intracranial a.
    miliary a.
    mitral valve a.
    mycotic a.
    peripheral a.
    phantom a.
    Pott a.
    ruptured abdominal aortic a.
    saccular a.
    serpentine a.
    supraclinoid a.
    traction a.
    traumatic false a.
    true a.
    tubular a.
    varicose a.
aneurysmal
    a. dilatation
    a. dilation
    a. hematoma
    a. hemorrhage
    a. rupture
    a. sac
    a. varix
aneurysmectomy
    Matas a.
aneurysmoplasty
aneurysmorrhaphy
aneurysmotomy
Angelucci operation

angel-wing deformity
angiectasia
angiectatic
angiectopia
angiitis
    necrotizing a.
angina
angina-guided therapy
angioblastoma
angiocentric
    a. immunoproliferative lesion
    a. lymphoproliferative lesion
angiodysplastic lesion
angioendothelioma
angiofibrolipoma
angiofibroma
angiogenesis
angiogram
    multigated a. (MUGA)
angiographically occult intracranial vascular malformation (AOIVM)
angiographic road-mapping technique
angioinvasive lesion
angiokeratoma
angioleiomyoma
angiolipofibroma
angiolipoma
angiolith
angiolithic
angiolysis
angioma
    arterial a.
    bleeding a.
    capillary a.
    cerebral a.
    cherry a.
    conjunctival a.
    gastric a.
    orbital a.
    pulmonary a.
    spider a.
    spinal a.
    strawberry a.
    superficial a.
    venous a.
angiomatosis
    skeletal-extraskeletal a.
angiomatous neoplastic tissue
angiomyofibroma
angiomyolipoma
angiomyoma
    a. of oviduct
angiomyoneuroma
angiomyxoma
angioneurectomy
angioneuromyoma
angioneurotomy

angio-osteohypertrophy
   a.-o. syndrome
angiopathy
   amyloid a.
   radiation a.
angioplany
angioplasty
   ablative laser a.
   adjunctive balloon a.
   aortoiliac a.
   balloon catheter a.
   balloon coarctation a.
   balloon coronary a.
   balloon dilation a.
   balloon laser a.
   bootstrap two-vessel a.
   brachiocephalic vessel a.
   complementary balloon a.
   coronary artery a.
   coronary balloon a.
   culprit lesion a.
   excimer laser coronary a.
   facilitated a.
   high-risk a.
   Ho:YAG laser a.
   infrapopliteal transluminal a.
   Kinsey rotation atherectomy extrusion a.
   kissing balloon a.
   laser-assisted balloon a.
   low-speed rotational a.
   Osypka rotational a.
   patch-graft a.
   percutaneous balloon a.
   percutaneous low-stress a.
   percutaneous transluminal coronary a. (PTCA)
   percutaneous transluminal renal a.
   peripheral balloon a.
   peripheral laser a.
   renal a.
   rescue a.
   salvage balloon a.
   subclavian vein patch a.
   Tactilaze a.
   thermal/perfusion balloon a.
   thulium:YAG laser a.
   tibioperoneal trunk a.
   tibioperoneal vessel a.
   transluminal coronary a.
   vein patch a.
   vibrational a.

angioplasty-related vessel occlusion
angioproliferative lesion
angioreticuloma
angiorrhaphy
angiorrhexis
angiosarcoma
angioscopy
   fluorescein fundus a.
   percutaneous transluminal a.
angioscotoma
angiostomy
angiotelectasis
angiotomy
angle
   a. of aberration
   a. of anomaly
   anomaly a.
   anorectal a.
   anterior angulation a.
   axial line a.
   biorbital a.
   a. bisection technique
   Böhler calcaneal a.
   Broca basilar a.
   Broca facial a.
   bucco-occlusal line a.
   calcaneal inclination a.
   calcaneal-second metatarsal angle inclination a.
   cavity line a.
   A. classification of malocclusion
   costal a.
   Daubenton a.
   declination a.
   deformity a.
   a. of direction
   distobuccal line a.
   distobucco-occlusal point a.
   distolabial line a.
   distolabioincisal point a.
   distolingual line a.
   distolinguoincisal point a.
   distolinguo-occlusal point a.
   disto-occlusal point a.
   duodenojejunal a.
   elevation a.
   epigastric a.
   facial a.
   a. of femoral torsion
   filtration a.
   Frankfort mandibular incisor a.
   Frankfort mandibular plane a.

NOTES

angle *(continued)*
   frontal a. of parietal bone
   a. of greatest extension
   hypsiloid a.
   incisal mandibular plane a.
   inferior a. of scapula
   infrasternal a.
   iridocorneal a.
   Jacquart facial a.
   a. of jaw
   labioincisal line a.
   lateral deviation a.
   lateral a. of eye
   lateral a. of scapula
   lateral a. of uterus
   line a.
   linguoincisal line a.
   linguo-occlusal line a.
   Louis a.
   Ludwig a.
   lumbosacral a.
   magnetization precession a.
   a. of mandible
   mastoid a. of parietal bone
   medial a. of eye
   mesiobuccal line a.
   mesiobucco-occlusal point a.
   mesiolabial line a.
   mesiolabioincisal point a.
   mesiolingual line a.
   mesiolinguoincisal point a.
   mesiolinguo-occlusal point line a.
   mesio-occlusal line a.
   metafacial a.
   a. of mouth
   nail-to-nail bed a.
   occipital a. of parietal bone
   occlusal plane a.
   ophryospinal a.
   a. of orientation
   parietal a.
   pelvivertebral a.
   Pirogoff a.
   point a.
   a. port pump
   pubic a.
   Quatrefages a.
   a. of reflection
   Serres a.
   space of iridocorneal a.
   sphenoid a.
   sphenoidal a. of parietal bone
   sternal a.
   sternoclavicular a.
   subpubic a.
   substernal a.
   superior a. of scapula
   talocalcaneal a.

   a. of thoracic inclination
   tip a.
   Topinard facial a.
   tracheal bifurcation a.
   venous a.
   y-a.
angled
   a. blade plate fixation
   a. pleural tube
   a. suction tube
angle-tip
angular
   a. acceleration
   a. artery
   a. deformity
   a. incision
   a. line
   a. notch
   a. osteotomy
   a. position
   a. spine
angularis body
angulated
   a. buccal tube
   a. fracture
angulation
   Andrews-type nonorthodontic normal crown a.
   anterior a.
   apex dorsal a.
   a. at the fracture site
   bracket slot a.
   built-in a.
   caudal a.
   coronal a.
   a. deformity
   a. fracture
   horizontal a.
   kyphotic a.
   limb length a.
   lower incisor a.
   a. motion
   a. osteotomy
   palmar a.
   plantar a.
   radius of a.
   RAO a.
   screw a.
   upper incisor a.
   valgus a.
   vertical a.
   volar a.
angulus, pl. anguli
   a. costae
   a. frontalis ossis parietalis
   a. inferior scapulae
   a. infrasternalis
   a. iridis

a. iridocornealis
a. lateralis scapulae
a. mandibulae
a. mastoideus ossis parietalis
a. occipitalis ossis parietalis
a. oculi lateralis
a. oculi medialis
a. oculi nasalis
a. oculi temporalis
a. oris
a. sphenoidalis ossis parietalis
a. sterni
a. subpubicus
a. superior scapulae

ANH
acute normovolemic hemodilution
anhepatic stage of liver transplantation
anhydration
anhydrous facial foundation
ani
levator a.
anileridine
animal graft
anisocoria
postoperative a.
anisotropic
a. rotation
a. tissue
ankle
a. block
a. block anesthesia
a. fusion
a. mortise diastasis
a. mortise fracture
Nélaton dislocation of a.
pronation-eversion-external rotation
injury of a.
a. region
ankle-brachial
a.-b. blood pressure ratio
a.-b. pressure measurement
ankyloglossia superior syndrome
ankylosis
extra-articular a.
extracapsular a.
Ann
A. Arbor classification
A. Arbor classification of Hodgkin
disease staging
ANNE
A. anesthesia inducer
A. anesthesia infuser

annexectomy
annexopexy
annular
a. adenocarcinoma
a. cartilage
a. constricting lesion
a. corneal graft
a. corneal graft operation
a. sphincter
annuloplasty
Carpentier a.
DeVega tricuspid valve a.
Gerbode a.
prosthetic ring a.
tricuspid valve a.
Wooler-type a.
annulorrhaphy
annulotomy
annulus
a. abdominalis
a. femoralis
a. fibrosus disci intervertebralis
a. fibrosus of intervertebral disk
a. of fibrous sheath
Haller a.
a. hemorrhoidalis
a. inguinalis profundus
a. inguinalis superficialis
a. iridis
a. iridis major
a. iridis minor
mitral valve a.
tricuspid valve a.
a. umbilicalis
a. urethralis
ano
fistula in a.
anociassociation
anococcygeal
a. body
a. ligament
anocutaneous
a. line
a. stimulation
anoderm
anodyne
anogenital
a. raphe
anomalous
a. anatomy
a. fixation

NOTES

27

anomalous *(continued)*
    a. innominate artery compression syndrome
    a. insertion
    a. rectification
anomaly
    Alder-Reilly a.
    a. angle
    angle of a.
    anorectal a.
    atrioventricular connection a.
    atrioventricular junction a.
    Axenfeld a.
    branchial a.
    cardiac a.
    cervical a.
    Chiari a.
    coloboma a.'s
    congenital conotruncal a.
    conjoined nerve-root a.
    conotruncal a.
    coronary artery a.
    craniofacial a.
    Cruveilhier-Baumgarten a.
    dental a.
    dentofacial a.
    double-inlet ventricle a.
    Duane a.
    duplication a.
    dysgnathic a.
    Ebstein cardiac a.
    eugnathic a.
    facet a.
    fetal cardiac a.
    fetal chest a.
    fetal gastrointestinal a.
    fetal vascular a.
    fixation a.
    Freund a.
    genetic a.
    genitourinary a.
    gestant a.
    hand a.
    heart a.
    intracranial dural vascular a.
    jugular bulb a.
    kidney a.
    Kimerle a.
    Klippel-Feil a.
    lacrimal angle duct a.
    laryngeal a.
    limb reduction a.
    maxillofacial a.
    megadolichovertebrobasilar a.
    Michel a.
    Moebius a.
    Mondini a.
    morning glory optic disk a.
    müllerian duct a.
    nevoid a.
    numerary renal a.
    occipitoatlantoaxial a.
    oculocephalic vascular a.
    oral a.
    orthopaedic a.
    osseous a.
    Peters a.
    Poland a.
    presacral a.
    pulmonary valve a.
    pulmonary venous connection a.
    pulmonary venous return a.
    renal a.'s
    reticulate pigmented a.
    root a.
    segmentation a.
    Shone a.
    Sprengel a.
    structural a.
    Taussig-Bing a.
    tracheobronchial a.
    Uhl a.
    umbilical cord a.
    Undritz a.
    urinary tract a.
    urogenital a.
    uterine a.
    VACTERL a.
    vaginal a.
    vascular a.
    vena cava a.
    ventricular inflow a.
    viscerobronchial cardiovascular a.
    vitelline duct a.
    a. of Zahn
anopia
anoplasty
    cutback a.
    House advancement a.
    House flap a.
    Martin a.
    a. treatment
    Y-V a.
anopsia
anorchia
anorchism
anorectal
    a. angle
    a. anomaly
    a. carcinoma
    a. fistula
    a. flexure
    a. foreign body
    a. junction
    a. lymph nodes
    a. malformation

a. myectomy
a. ring
a. space
a. surgery
anorectoplasty
Laird-McMahon a.
anorectum
anoscopy
anosigmoidoscopy
anospinal
anotia
anovesical
anovulation
persistent a.
anoxemia
anoxia
anoxic a.
diffusion a.
histotoxic a.
stagnant a.
anoxic
a. anoxia
ANP
autonomic nerve preservation
ansa, pl. **ansae**
a. cervicalis
Haller a.
a. hypoglossi
ansae nervorum spinalium
a. sacralis
a. subclavia
Vieussens a.
anserine
a. bursa
Anson-McVay hernia repair
ansotomy
antagonist
α-adrenergic a.
α₁-adrenergic a.
α₂-adrenergic receptor a.
antimuscarinic a.
β-receptor a.
antagonistic muscles
antagonize
antalgesia
antalgic
ant ax line (*var. of* anterior axillary line)
antebrachial
a. fascia
a. fascial graft
a. flexor retinaculum

antecolic
a. anastomosis
a. long-loop isoperistaltic gastrojejunostomy
antecubital
a. approach
a. arteriovenous fistula
a. space
antegrade
a. approach
a. catheterization
a. continence enema procedure
a. double balloon/double wire technique
a. method
a. puncture
antegrade/retrograde cardioplegia technique
antenatal dislocation
antenna procedure
antepartum hemorrhage
anteposition
anteprostate
anterior
a. acromioplasty
a. acromioplasty approach
a. angulation
a. angulation angle
a. antebrachial region
a. apical (AA)
a. articular surface of dens
a. aspiration
a. atlanto-occipital membrane
a. auricular groove
a. auricular muscle
a. auricular nerve
a. auricular vein
a. axillary approach
a. axillary fold
a. axillary line, ant ax line
a. basal (AB)
a. basal branch
a. basal segment
a. belly of digastric muscle
a. border of lung
a. border of pancreas
a. border of radius
a. border of testis
a. border of tibia
a. border of ulna
a. brachial region
a. calcaneal osteotomy

NOTES

anterior *(continued)*
a. capsulolabral reconstruction
a. capsulotomy
a. cardiac veins
a. cecal artery
a. cerebral artery
a. cerebral vein
a. cervical diskectomy and fusion
a. cervical intertransversarii muscles
a. cervical intertransverse muscles
a. cervical spine surgery
a. cervical surgery vocal cord damage
a. cervicothoracic junction surgery
a. chamber tube
a. choroidal artery
a. ciliary artery
a. circumflex humeral artery
a. clear space
a. column
a. column fracture
a. column osteosynthesis
a. commissure-posterior commissure line
a. communicating artery
a. complete dislocation
a. condylar canal
a. condyloid canal of occipital bone
a. condyloid foramen
a. cord compression
a. corneal curvature
a. corpectomy
a. correction
a. corticospinal tract
a. costotransverse ligament
a. cranial base
a. cranial fossa
a. cruciate ligament (ACL)
a. crus of stapes
a. cutaneous branches of intercostal nerves
a. cutaneous branch of iliohypogastric nerve
a. cutaneous nerve of abdomen
a. deep cervical lymph nodes
a. descending artery
a. diskectomy
a. epineurotomy
a. ethmoidal nerve
a. ethmoidectomy
a. extensile approach
a. extradural clinoidectomy
a. extremity
a. extremity of caudate nucleus
a. facial height (AFH)
a. facial vein
a. focal point

a. fontanel
a. fontanel pressure monitoring
a. ground bundle
a. group of axillary lymph nodes
a. helical rim free flap
a. hip dislocation
a. humeral circumflex artery
a. humeral line
a. hyaloid membrane
a. inferior cerebellar artery
a. inferior iliac spine
a. inferior segment
a. inferior segmental artery of kidney
a. innominate osteotomy
a. innominate rotation
a. intercostal arteries
a. intercostal veins
a. internal fixation
a. internal stabilization
a. intraoccipital joint
a. intraoccipital synchondrosis
a. jugular lymph nodes
a. jugular vein
a. junction line
a. knee region
a. labial arteries
a. labial commissure
a. labial nerve
a. labrum periosteum shoulder arthroscopic lesion
a. layer of rectus abdominis sheath
a. limb of stapes
a. limiting ring
a. lingual gland
a. lip of uterine os
a. lobe of hypophysis
a. lower cervical spine surgery
a. lumbar vertebral interbody fusion
a. median line
a. mediastinal arteries
a. mediastinal lymph nodes
a. mediastinal mass
a. mediastinum
a. meningeal artery
a. metallic fixation
a. midpapillary (AM)
a. nephrectomy
a. oblique projection
a. parietal artery
a. part of anterior commissure of brain
a. part of diaphragmatic surface of liver
a. part of fornix of vagina
a. partial laryngectomy
a. pelvic exenteration

A

a. pituitary extract
a. plate fixation
a. Pólya procedure
a. and posterior (A&P)
a. and posterior repair
a. primary division
a. pronator teres
a. puncture
a. pyramidal tract
a. quadriceps musculocutaneous flap
  technique
a. quadrilateral triplane frame
a. rectopexy
a. rectus muscle of head
a. region of arm
a. region of forearm
a. region of leg
a. region of neck
a. region of thigh
a. resection
a. retroperitoneal decompression
a. retroperitoneal flank approach
a. rhizotomy
a. root
a. sacrococcygeal ligament
a. sacroiliac ligaments
a. sacrosciatic ligament
a. sandwich patch technique
a. scalene muscle
a. sclerotomy
a. screw fixation
a. scrotal nerve
a. scrotal veins
a. semicircular canals
a. seromyotomy
a. serratus muscle
a. short-segment stabilization
a. shoulder dislocation
a. sliding tibial graft
a. spinal artery
a. spinal artery syndrome
a. spinal fixation
a. spinal fusion
a. spinocerebellar tract
a. spinothalamic tract
a. stabilization procedure
a. sternoclavicular ligament
a. sternomastoid approach
a. superficial cervical lymph nodes
a. superior alveolar arteries
a. superior iliac spine
a. superior segment

a. superior segmental artery of
  kidney
a. supraclavicular nerve
a. surface of cornea
a. surface of eyelids
a. surface of kidney
a. surface of maxilla
a. surface of pancreas
a. surface of prostate
a. surface of suprarenal gland
a. surface of ulna
a. surgical exposure
a. synechia formation
a. talofibular ligament rupture
a. temporal artery
a. temporal lobectomy
a. tibial artery
a. tibial bursa
a. tibial lymph node
a. tibial muscle
a. tibial recurrent artery
a. transabdominal approach
a. translation
a. transthoracic approach
a. triangle of neck
a. tubercle of atlas
a. tubercle of cervical vertebrae
a. urethra
a. vertebral vein
a. vertical canal
a. vitrectomy
a. wall of stomach
a. wall of vagina

anterior-inferior dislocation
anterior-posterior
  a.-p. compression
  a.-p. fusion with SSI
  a.-p. repair
anterograde transseptal technique
anterolateral
  a. approach
  a. compression fracture
  a. cordotomy
  a. dislocation
  a. fontanel
  a. thalamostriate arteries
  a. thoracotomy incision
  a. tractotomy
anterolisthesis
anteromedial
  a. bundle

NOTES

anteromedial *(continued)*
    a. retropharyngeal approach
    a. thalamostriate arteries
anteromesial temporal lobectomy
antero-oblique position
anteroposterior (A&P)
    a. compression
    a. correction
    a. nail
    a. projection
    a. translation
anterosuperior
    a. external ilium movement
    a. iliac spine graft
antevesical hernia
anthelix *(var. of* antihelix)
Anthony suction tube
anthrone method
anthropoid pelvis
anthropometric evaluation
antianalgesia
antiantibody formation
antiarrhythmic therapy
antibasement membrane
antibiotic
    a. bead pouch
    a. and saline solution
antibody
    fluorescent a. (FA)
antibody linkage method
anticalculous
anticholinergic medication
anticipatory coarticulation
anticoagulant
anticoagulation
    prophylactic a.
antidote
antidromic stimulation
antiembolic position
antiemetic
    rescue a.
    a. therapy
antifibrinolytic
    a. agent
    a. drug
antifog tube
antifungal esophageal infection
antifungal-resistant opportunistic infection
antigen
    human leukocyte a. (HLA)
antigen-extracted allogeneic bone
antigenic modulation
antiglaucoma surgery
antiglomerular
    a. basement membrane
    a. basement membrane antibody disease

antigravity muscles
antihelix, anthelix
antihemorrhagic
antihormonal therapy
anti-incontinence procedure
anti-inflammatory medication
antimesenteric
    a. enterotomy
    a. fat pad
antimicrobial filter
antimuscarinic antagonist
antimycotic
antinephritic
antiniad
antinial
antinion
antinociception
    intrathecal a.
antinociceptive
antipyogenic
antipyrine and benzocaine
antireflux
    a. flap-valve mechanism
    a. operation
    a. procedure
    a. surgery
    a. therapy
    a. ureteral implantation technique
antirefluxing colonic conduit
Anti-Sept bactericidal scrub solution
anti-shock military trousers
antisialagogue
antitension line
antithrombin
    a. III (ATIII)
antithrombotic therapy
antitragicus muscle
antitubular basement membrane
antra (*pl. of* antrum)
antral
    a. biopsy
    a. irrigation
    a. membrane
    a. sphincter
    a. web
antrectomy
    Roux-en-Y biliary bypass with a.
antroduodenectomy
antropyloric canal
antroscopy
antrostomy
    inferior meatal a.
    inferior meatus a.
    intraoral a.
    middle meatal a.
    nasal a.
antrotomy
antrum, pl. **antra**

antra ethmoidalia
a. of Highmore
mastoid a.
a. mastoideum
maxillary a.
pyloric a.
a. pyloricum
Antyllus method
anum
per a.
anuria
anuric
anus
artificial a.
ectopic a.
melanocarcinoma of a.
vaginal ectopic a.
a. vesicalis
vesicalis a.
Anustim electronic neuromuscular stimulator
AO
AO classification
AO compression
AO dynamic compression plate construct
AO external fixation
AO procedure
AO rigid fixation
AO spinal internal fixation
AO technique
AOD
aortic occlusive disease
AOIVM
angiographically occult intracranial vascular malformation
aorta, pl. **aortae**
abdominal a.
a. abdominalis
bifurcation of a.
coarctation of a.
dissection of a.
postductal coarctation of a.
pseudocoarctation of a.
recoarctation of a.
thoracic a.
a. thoracica
aortectomy
aortic
a. anastomosis
a. aneurysm
a. bifurcation

a. blood pressure
a. body
a. body tumor
a. cuff
a. dicrotic notch pressure
a. dissection
a. foramen
a. hiatus
a. intramural hematoma
a. knob
a. laceration
a. nipple
a. node metastasis
a. occlusive disease (AOD)
a. patch
a. pressure gradient
a. pullback pressure
a. regurgitation murmur
a. ring
a. root reconstruction
a. root velocity waveform
a. rupture
a. sac
a. sump tube
a. transection
a. tube graft
a. valve area
a. valve atresia
a. valve disease
a. valve gradient
a. valve insufficiency
a. valve leaflet
a. valve lesion
a. valve repair
a. valve replacement
a. valve resistance
a. valve restenosis
a. valve velocity profile
a. valvotomy
a. valvuloplasty
aortica
glomera a.
aorticorenal
a. ganglia
a. graft
aortic-pulmonic window
aortocaval fistula
aortocoronary
a. bypass graft
a. snake graft
aortoduodenal fistula

NOTES

aortoenteric
    a. fistula
    a. graft
aortoesophageal fistula
aortofemoral (AF)
    a. bypass
    a. bypass graft
aortogastric fistula
aortograft duodenal fistula
aortohepatic arterial graft
aortoiliac
    a. angioplasty
    a. bypass
    a. bypass graft
    a. occlusive disease
aorto-ostial lesion
aortoplasty
aortopulmonary
    a. fenestration
    a. window
aortorenal
    a. bypass
    a. reimplantation
aortorrhaphy
aortosigmoid fistula
aortotomy
AP
    area postrema
A&P
    anterior and posterior
    anteroposterior
    A&P projection
    A&P repair
APAAP technique
APACHE-II point
apatite calculus
A-P-C
    adenoidal-pharyngeal-conjunctival
apellous
Apert syndrome
apertura
    a. pelvis inferior
    a. pelvis minoris
    a. pelvis superior
    a. sinus frontalis
    a. sinus sphenoidalis
    a. thoracis inferior
    a. thoracis superior
aperture
    inferior pelvic a.
    inferior thoracic a.
    laryngeal a.
    a. of orbit
    superior pelvic a.
    superior thoracic a.
apex, pl. **apices**
    corneal a.
    a. dorsal angulation

    a. of external ring
    a. fracture
    a. of orbit
    a. ossis sacri
    a. partis petrosae ossis temporalis
    a. of petrous part of temporal
       bone
    a. prostatae
    a. of prostate
    a. of sacrum
    a. of urinary bladder
    a. vesicae
Apgar score
aphakia
    extracapsular a.
aphakic correction
aphthous-type lesion
aphthous ulceration
apical
    anterior a. (AA)
    a. fenestration
    a. gland
    a. group of axillary lymph nodes
    a. infection
    inferior a. (IA)
    lateral a. (LA)
    a. left ventricular puncture
    a. ligament of dens
    a. lordotic projection
    a. polar nephrectomy
    a. puncture
    a. ramification
    a. segment
    septal a. (SA)
    a. space
    a. transverse (AP-T)
apically repositioned flap in
    mucogingival surgery
apiceotomy
apices (*pl. of* apex)
apicoectomy
apicolysis
    extrapleural a.
    Semb a.
apicoposterior segment
apicostomy
apicotomy
Apley
    A. compression test
    A. maneuver
apnea
    induced a.
    obstructive a.
    posthyperventilation a.
    postoperative a.
apneic
    a. oxygenation
    a. threshold

A

apneustic
    a. breathing
    a. respiration
apocrine gland
aponeurectomy
aponeurorrhaphy
aponeurosis
    Denonvilliers a.
    epicranial a.
    a. epicranialis
    a. of external oblique
    external oblique a.
    Petit a.
    temporal a.
    thoracolumbar a.
aponeurotic
aponeurotomy
apophysary point
apophyseal fracture
apophysial point
apophysis, pl. apophyses
    iliac a.
    medial epicondylar a.
    ring a.
    slipped vertebral a.
    temporal a.
    vertebral ring a.
apophysitis
    calcaneal a.
apoplectic coma
apostaxis
apotreptic therapy
apparatus
    air pressure driven a.
    alimentary a.
    digestive a.
    a. digestorius
    eye-movement measuring a.
      (EMMA)
    genitourinary a.
    hyoid a.
    a. hyoideus
    Jackson-Rees a.
    lacrimal a.
    a. lacrimalis
    a. ligamentosus weitbrechti
    urinary a.
    urogenital a.
    a. urogenitalis
appendage
    epiploic a.
    a. of eye

    testicular a.
    vermiform a.
    vesicular a.
appendectomy, appendicectomy
    auricular a.
    colonoscopic a.
    emergency a.
    emergent a.
    incidental a.
    interval a.
    inversion a.
appendiceal
    a. abscess
    a. adenocarcinoma
    a. cancer
    a. fecalith
    a. mass
    a. opening
    a. orifice
    a. perforation
appendices (*pl. of* appendix)
appendicitis
appendicocele
appendicocystostomy
    continent cutaneous a.
    dismembered reimplanted a.
    nonplicated a.
    orthotopic a.
    plicated a.
    reversed reimplanted a.
appendicoenterostomy
appendicolithiasis
appendicolysis
appendicostomy
appendicovesicostomy
    Mitrofanoff a.
appendicular
    a. artery
    a. lymph nodes
    a. muscle
    a. skeleton
    a. vein
appendix, pl. appendices
    a. ceci
    a. epididymidis
    a. of epididymidis
    epiploic a.
    a. epiploica
    a. fibrosa hepatis
    fibrous a. of liver
    a. mucocele
    a. testis

NOTES

appendix *(continued)*
    a. of the testis
    a. vesiculosa
apperceptive mass
applanation
    a. pressure
    tension by a.
    a. tonometry
apple
    Adam's a.
apple-core lesion
appliance modification
application
    arch bar a.
    cast a.
    clip a.
    cold a.
    force a.
    frame a.
    Harrington rod instrumentation
      force a.
    heat a.
    ice a.
    interpleural a.
    Isola spinal implant system a.
    Kumar a.
    laparoscopic clip a.
    paraspinal rod a.
    pilot a.
    topical iodine a.
    traction a.
    transverse fixator a.
Appolito suture
apponensplasty
    ring sublimis a.
appose
apposition
    a. of skull suture
    stent a.
approach
    Abbott-Carpenter posterior a.
    Abbott knee a.
    abdominal a.
    acetabular extensile a.
    adaptational a.
    Alken a.
    antecubital a.
    antegrade a.
    anterior acromioplasty a.
    anterior axillary a.
    anterior extensile a.
    anterior retroperitoneal flank a.
    anterior sternomastoid a.
    anterior transabdominal a.
    anterior transthoracic a.
    anterolateral a.
    anteromedial retropharyngeal a.
    axillary a.

Bailey-Badgley anterior cervical a.
Banks-Laufman a.
basal subfrontal a.
Bennett posterior shoulder a.
Berger-Bookwalter posterior a.
Berke a.
bilateral ilioinguinal a.
bilateral sacroiliac a.
Bosworth a.
Boyd a.
Boyd-Sisk a.
brachial artery a.
Brackett-Osgood posterior a.
Brodsky-Tullos-Gartsman a.
Broomhead medial a.
Brown knee a.
Brown lateral a.
Bruner a.
Bruser knee a.
Bruser lateral a.
Bryan-Morrey elbow a.
Bryan-Morrey extensive posterior a.
buccopharyngeal a.
buttonhole a.
Caldwell-Luc a.
Callahan a.
Campbell posterior shoulder a.
Campbell posterolateral a.
Carnesale acetabular extensile a.
Carnesale hip a.
case-by-case a.
Cave hip a.
Cave knee a.
central a.
cerebellopontine angle a.
cervical a.
choledochofiberoscopic a.
Cloward cervical disk a.
cochleovestibular a.
Codman saber-cut shoulder a.
Colonna-Ralston ankle a.
Colonna-Ralston medial a.
combined anterior and posterior a.
combined low cervical and
    transthoracic a.
combined presigmoid-
    transtransversarium intradural a.
combined transsylvian and middle
    fossa a.
consortial a.
Coonse-Adams knee a.
Cubbins shoulder a.
curved a.
deltoid-splitting shoulder a.
deltopectoral a.
Dickinson a.
distal interphalangeal joint a.
dorsal finger a.

dorsal midline a.
dorsalward a.
dorsolateral a.
dorsomedial a.
dorsoplantar a.
dorsoradial a.
dorsorostral a.
dorsoulnar a.
Duran a.
DuVries a.
extended iliofemoral a.
extended subfrontal a.
extensile a.
extrabursal a.
extralaryngeal a.
extraperitoneal a.
extrapharyngeal a.
extreme lateral transcondylar a.
Fahey a.
far lateral inferior suboccipital a.
fascial sling a.
femoral artery a.
Fernandez extensile anterior a.
flank a.
foraminal a.
fornix a.
Fowler-Philip a.
frontotemporal a.
gasless laparoscopic a.
Gatellier-Chastang ankle a.
Gatellier-Chastang posterolateral a.
genetic a.
Gibson a.
Gordon a.
Guleke-Stookey a.
Hardinge lateral a.
Harmon cervical a.
Harmon modified posterolateral a.
Harmon shoulder a.
Harris anterolateral a.
Harris lateral a.
Hay lateral a.
Henderson posterolateral a.
Henderson posteromedial a.
Henry anterior strap a.
Henry anterolateral a.
Henry extensile a.
Henry posterior interosseous
  nerve a.
Henry radial a.
Hoffmann a.
Hoppenfeld-Deboer a.

Howorth a.
idiographic a.
Iliff a.
iliofemoral a.
ilioinguinal acetabular a.
inferior extradural a.
inferior-lateral endonasal
  transsphenoidal a.
inferior transvermian a.
infralabyrinthine a.
infratemporal fossa a.
infratentorial supracerebellar a.
inguinal a.
interfascial a.
interforniceal a.
interhemispheric a.
interscalene a.
intradural a.
intratentorial supracerebellar a.
keyhole a.
Kikuchi-MacNap-Moreau a.
Kocher curved L a.
Kocher-Gibson posterolateral a.
Kocher-Langenbeck a.
Kocher lateral J a.
Koenig-Schaefer medial a.
Kraske parasacral a.
labioglossomandibular a.
labiomandibular a.
lateral deltoid splitting a.
lateral extracavitary a.
lateral Gatellier-Chastung a.
lateral intradural a.
lateral J a.
lateral Kocher a.
lateral Ollier a.
lateral parapatellar a.
Lazepen-Gamidov anteromedial a.
Leslie-Ryan anterior axillary a.
Letournel-Judet a.
limbal a.
lingual a.
long deltopectoral a.
Lortat-Jacob a.
low cervical a.
Ludloff medial a.
lumbar a.
Mayo a.
McAfee a.
McConnell extensile a.
McConnell median and ulnar
  nerve a.

NOTES

approach *(continued)*
McFarland-Osborne lateral a.
McLaughlin a.
McWhorter posterior shoulder a.
Mears-Rubash a.
medial extradural a.
medial parapatellar a.
medial parapatellar capsular a.
middle fossa a.
midlateral a.
midline medial a.
midline spinal a.
Minkoff-Jaffe-Menendez posterior a.
Mize-Bucholz-Grogen a.
Molesworth-Campbell elbow a.
Moore posterior a.
neurosurgical a.
Ollier arthrodesis a.
Ollier lateral a.
operative a.
orbitozygomatic temporopolar a.
oropharyngeal a.
Osborne posterior a.
otomicrosurgical transtemporal a.
palmar a.
paramedian a.
pararectus a.
paraspinal a.
pars plana a.
patella turndown a.
PEACH a.
percutaneous transhepatic a.
peroral a.
Perry extensile anterior a.
petrosal a.
Pfannenstiel transverse a.
plantar a.
Pogrund lateral a.
posterior costotransversectomy a.
posterior inverted U a.
posterior lumbar a.
posterior midline a.
posterior occipitocervical a.
posterior transolecranon a.
posterolateral a.
posteromedial a.
preperitoneal a.
presigmoid-transtransversarium intradural a.
proprioceptive neuromuscular facilitation a.
proximal interphalangeal joint a.
pterional a.
pulp a.
Putti posterior a.
Redman a.
regressive-reconstructive a.
Reinert acetabular extensile a.

retrograde endoscopic a.
retrograde femoral a.
retrolabyrinthine presigmoid a.
retroperitoneal a.
retropharyngeal a.
retrosigmoid a.
rhinoseptal a.
Risdon a.
Roberts a.
Roos a.
Rowe posterior shoulder a.
saber-cut a.
sacral-foraminal a.
screw-plate a.
sensorimotor stimulation a.
Smith-Petersen a.
Smith-Petersen-Cave-Van Gorder anterolateral a.
Smith-Robinson cervical disk a.
Somerville anterior a.
Southwick-Robinson anterior cervical a.
Spetzler anterior transoral a.
split-heel a.
split-patellar a.
stabilization a.
sternum-splitting a.
subchoroidal a.
subclavicular a.
subfrontal a.
subfrontal-transbasal a.
sublabial midline rhinoseptal a.
suboccipital-subtemporal a.
suboccipital-transmeatal a.
subtemporal-intradural a.
superior-intradural a.
supine-oblique a.
supracerebellar a.
supraclavicular a.
supraduodenal a.
supraorbital-pterional a.
supratentorial a.
surgical a.
Swedish a.
sylvian a.
Taylor a.
therapeutic a.
Thompson anterolateral a.
Thompson anteromedial a.
Thompson posterior radial a.
thoracic a.
thoracoabdominal extrapleural a.
thoracoabdominal intrapleural a.
thoracolumbar retroperitoneal a.
thoracotomy a.
thumb metacarpophalangeal joint a.
transacromial a.
transantral ethmoidal a.

transaxillary a.
transbrachioradialis a.
transcallosal transventricular a.
transcanine a.
transcavernous transpetrous apex a.
transcerebellar hemispheric a.
transcervical a.
transclavicular a.
transcochlear a.
transcortical transventricular a.
transcranial frontal-temporal-
  orbital a.
transcranial-supraorbital a.
transcubital a.
transduodenal a.
transfibular a.
transfrontal a.
transgluteal a.
transhiatal a.
translabyrinthine and suboccipital a.
transmandibular-glossopharyngeal a.
transmastoid a.
transmeatal a.
transmural a.
transolecranon a.
transoral a.
transpalatal a.
transpapillary a.
transpedicular a.
transperitoneal a.
transradial a.
transrectal a.
transseptal a.
transsinus a.
transsphenoidal a.
transsternal a.
transsylvian a.
transtentorial a.
transthoracic a.
transtorcular a.
transtrochanteric a.
transvaginal a.
transvenous a.
transverse a.
transxiphoid a.
trap-door a.
triradiate acetabular extensile a.
triradiate transtrochanteric a.
unilateral sacroiliac a.
vaginal wall a.
volar finger a.
volar midline a.

volar radial a.
volar ulnar a.
volarward a.
Wadsworth elbow a.
Wadsworth posterolateral a.
Wagoner posterior a.
Watson-Jones anterior a.
Watson-Jones lateral a.
Wiltberger anterior cervical a.
Wiltse-Spencer paraspinal a.
Yee posterior shoulder a.
zig-zag a.
Z-plasty a.

approximate
  a. entropy
  a. lethal concentration
approximation
  Friedewald a.
  successive a.
  a. suture
  tissue a.
  vocal fold a.
  wound a.
APR
  abdominoperineal resection
  APR cement fixation
Apresoline injection
aprobarbital
aproctia
apron
  a. flap
  a. skin incision
aprotinin
APRV
  airway pressure release ventilation
AP-T
  apical transverse
  AP-T image
apudoma
AquaMEPHYTON injection
aquapuncture
AquaSite Ophthalmic solution
aquatic stabilization program
aqueduct
  Cotunnius a.
  a. veil
  a. of vestibule
aqueductal intubation
aqueductus
  a. cotunnii
  a. vestibuli

NOTES

aqueous
    a. extract
    a. solution
    a. vein
arachnoid
    arachnoid a.
    a. of brain
    a. granulation
    a. hemorrhage
    a. mater cranialis
    a. mater encephali
    a.'s mater spinalis
    a. membrane
    a. retrocerebellar pouch
    a. space
    a. of spinal cord
arachnoidea
arachnoiditis
    adhesive a.
Araki-Sako technique
araldehyde-tanned bovine carotid artery graft
Arantius
    A. body
    canal of A.
    A. ligament
arborization
    a. block
    pattern a.
    pulmonary a.
arc
    bregmatolambdoid a.
    flexion-extension a.
    longitudinal a. of skull
    nasobregmatic a.
    naso-occipital a.
    Riolan a.
arcade
    intestinal arterial a.'s
    pancreaticoduodenal arterial a.'s
    Riolan a.'s
arch
    abdominothoracic a.
    arterial a.'s of colon
    arterial a.'s of ileum
    arterial a.'s of jejunum
    arterial a. of lower eyelid
    arterial a. of upper eyelid
    axillary a.
    a. bar application
    cortical a.'s of kidney
    crural a.
    deep crural a.
    expansion of the a.
    extramedullary alignment a.
    femoral a.
    a. fracture
    hemal a.'s

    iliopectineal a.
    jugular venous a.
    Langer a.
    lateral lumbocostal a.
    medial lumbocostal a.
    neural a.
    posterior a. of atlas
    pubic a.
    Simon expansion a.
    superciliary a.
    supraorbital a.
    tendinous a.
    tendinous a. of levator ani muscle
    tendinous a. of pelvic fascia
    a. of thoracic duct
    Treitz a.
    vertebral a.
    wire a.
    zygomatic a.
archenteronoma
architecture
    tissue a.
arch-loop-whorl
"arch and slouch" position
arciform veins of kidney
ArCom compression-molded polyethylene
arctation
arcuate
    a. arteries of kidney
    a. eminence
    a. line of ilium
    a. line of rectus sheath
    a. nerve fiber bundle
    a. pubic ligament
    a. transverse keratotomy
    a. veins of kidney
    a. zone
arcuation
arcus
    corneal a.
    a. ductus thoracici
    a. inguinalis
    a. lumbocostalis lateralis
    a. lumbocostalis medialis
    a. pubis
    a. superciliaris
    a. tendineus
    a. tendineus fasciae pelvis
    a. tendineus musculi levatoris ani
    a. tendineus of obturator fascia
    a. unguium
    a. vertebrae
    a. zygomaticus
ARDS
    acute respiratory distress syndrome
    adult respiratory distress syndrome
Arduan

area
> aortic valve a.
> articulation a.
> bare a. of liver
> bare a. of stomach
> body surface a. (BSA)
> cribriform a. of the renal papilla
> a. cribrosa papillae renalis
> denture foundation a.
> end-diastolic cross-sectional a. (EDA)
> end-systolic cross-sectional a.
> a. of facial nerve
> fusion a.
> gastric a.
> a. gastrica
> a. of interest magnification
> left ventricular end-diastolic a. (LVEDa)
> left ventricular end-systolic a. (LVESa)
> mitral valve a.
> a. nervi facialis
> a. nuda hepatis
> Panum fusion a.
> pericolostomy a.
> a. postrema (AP)
> pressure a.
> pressure-sensitive a.
> proliferation a.
> pulmonary valve a.
> skip a.'s
> Stroud pectinated a.
> tissue-bearing a.
> tricuspid valve a.
> valve orifice a.
> visual association a.

area-length method
areflexia
> detrusor a.

areola, pl. **areolae**
> a. papillaris

areolar
> a. complex
> a. connective tissue
> a. glands

Arfonad injection
argon
> a. beam coagulation
> a. laser endophotocoagulation
> a. laser iridectomy
> a. laser photocoagulation
> a. laser therapy
> a. laser trabeculopexy
> a. laser trabeculoplasty

Argyle
> A. chest tube
> A. endotracheal tube
> A. feeding tube
> A. Sentinel Seal chest tube

Argyle-Dennis tube
Argyle-Salem sump tube
Argyll-Robertson
> A.-R. operation
> A.-R. suture technique

argyrophilic
> a. nucleolar organizer region
> a. nucleolar organizer region staining

arhinia
Aries-Pitanguy
> A.-P. breast reduction
> A.-P. mammaplasty
> A.-P. operation

Arion operation
aristotelian method
ARKIVE automated anesthesia record-keeper
Arlt
> A. epicanthus repair
> A. eyelid repair
> A. line
> A. operation

Arlt-Jaesche
> A.-J. excision
> A.-J. operation

arm
> brawny a.
> dissected tissue a.
> endosteal implant a.
> a. flap
> a. position

Armaly-Drance technique
Arm-a-Med endotracheal tube
armamentarium
> endodontic a.

Armistead
> A. technique
> A. ulnar lengthening operation

armored endotracheal tube
Armstrong
> A. acromionectomy
> A. grommet ventilation tube
> A. V-Vent tube

NOTES

Arneth classification
Arnold
  A. body
  A. bundle
  canal of A.
  A. canal
  A. ganglion
  A. tract
Arnold-Chiari
  A.-C. deformity
  A.-C. malformation
  A.-C. syndrome
Aronson-Prager technique
around-the-clock oral maintenance bronchodilator therapy
arrangement
  lesion a.
array
  64-lead epidural electrode a.
  64-lead subdural electrode a.
  PRx Endotak-Sub-Q a.
arrector, pl. arrectores
  a. pili muscle
  arrectores pilorum
  a. pilus
arrest
  circulatory a.
  deep hypothermic circulatory a.
  hypothermic circulatory a.
  hypothermic hypokalemic cardioplegic a. (HHCA)
  profoundly hypothermic circulatory a. (PHCA)
  traumatic cardiac a.
  vagal a.
arrhenoblastoma
Arrhigi
  point of A.
arrhythmia
  exercise-induced a.
arrhythmogenic
Arrow
  A. EID
  A. emergency infusion device
  A. percutaneous sheath introducer with integral side port
  A. tube
Arrowhead operation
arrow-point
Arroyo
  A. cataract extraction
  A. dacryostomy
  A. encircling suture
  A. keratoplasty
  A. operation
  A. tenotomy
Arruga
  A. cataract extraction

  A. dacryostomy
  A. keratoplasty
  A. operation
  A. tenotomy
Arruga-Berens operation
arteria, pl. arteriae
  a. angularis
  a. appendicularis
  a. basilaris
  a. bulbi penis
  a. bulbi urethrae
  a. bulbi vaginae
  a. bulbi vestibuli
  a. calcarina
  a. caudae pancreatis
  a. cecalis anterior
  a. cecalis posterior
  a. celiaca
  a. centralis brevis
  a. centralis longa
  a. cerebelli inferior anterior
  a. cerebelli inferior posterior
  a. cerebelli superior
  a. cerebri anterior
  a. cerebri media
  a. cerebri posterior
  a. cervicalis ascendens
  a. cervicalis profunda
  a. cervicalis superficialis
  a. cervicovaginalis
  a. circumflexa femoris lateralis
  a. circumflexa femoris medialis
  a. circumflexa scapulae
  a. colica dextra
  a. colica media
  a. colica sinistra
  a. comes nervi phrenici
  a. comitans nervi ischiadici
  a. comitans nervi mediani
  a. communicans anterior
  a. communicans posterior
  a. cystica
  a. deferentialis
  a. dorsalis clitoridis
  a. dorsalis pedis
  a. dorsalis penis
  a. dorsalis scapulae
  a. ductus deferentis
  a. epigastrica inferior
  a. epigastrica superficialis
  a. epigastrica superior
  a. facialis
  a. femoralis
  a. fibularis
  a. frontalis
  a. frontobasalis lateralis
  a. frontobasalis medialis
  a. gastrica dextra

arteriae gastricae breves
a. gastrica sinistra
a. gastroduodenalis
a. gastroepiploica dextra
a. gastroepiploica sinistra
a. gastro-omentalis dextra
a. gastro-omentalis sinistra
a. genus descendens
a. genus inferior lateralis
a. genus inferior medialis
a. genus media
a. genus superior lateralis
a. genus superior medialis
a. glutea inferior
a. glutea superior
a. gyri angularis
arteriae helicinae penis
a. hepatica communis
a. hepatica propria
a. hypogastrica
a. hypophysialis inferior
a. hypophysialis superior
arteriae ileales
a. ileocolica
a. iliaca communis
a. iliaca externa
a. iliaca interna
a. iliolumbalis
arteriae insulares
arteriae intercostales posteriores I
  et II
arteriae intercostales posteriores III-
  XI
a. intercostalis suprema
arteriae interlobares renis
arteriae interlobulares
a. interlobulares (hepatis)
a. interlobulares (renis)
a. intermesenterica
a. interossea anterior
a. interossea communis
a. interossea posterior
a. interossea recurrens
a. interossea volaris
arteriae intestinales
a. ischiadica
arteriae jejunales
arteriae labiales anteriores
a. labialis inferior
a. labialis superior
a. lienalis
a. ligamenti teretis uteri

a. lobi caudati
arteriae lumbales imae
a. lumbalis
a. mammaria interna
a. masseterica
arteriae mediastinales anteriores
a. mentalis
a. mesenterica inferior
a. mesenterica superior
a. metacarpea dorsalis
a. metacarpea palmaris
a. metatarsae
a. metatarsea dorsalis
a. metatarsea plantaris
a. musculophrenica
a. nervorum
a. obturatoria
a. obturatoria accessoria
a. occipitalis
a. occipitalis lateralis
a. occipitalis medialis
a. ovarica
arteriae palpebrales
a. pancreatica dorsalis
a. pancreatica inferior
a. pancreatica magna
a. pancreaticoduodenalis inferior
a. pancreaticoduodenalis superior
a. paracentralis
arteriae parietales
a. parietales anterior
a. parietales posterior
a. parieto-occipitalis
a. pericallosa
a. pericardiacophrenica
a. perinealis
a. peronea
a. pharyngea ascendens
a. phrenica inferior
a. phrenica superior
a. plantaris lateralis
a. plantaris medialis
arteriae pontis
a. poplitea
a. precunealis
a. princeps pollicis
a. profunda brachii
a. profunda clitoridis
a. profunda femoris
a. profunda linguae
a. profunda penis
arteriae pudendae externae

NOTES

43

arteria *(continued)*
- a. pudenda interna
- a. pulmonalis
- a. radialis
- a. radialis indicis
- a. radicularis magna
- a. rectalis inferior
- a. rectalis media
- a. rectalis superior
- a. recurrens radialis
- a. recurrens tibialis anterior
- a. recurrens tibialis posterior
- a. recurrens ulnaris
- a. renalis
- arteriae renis
- a. retroduodenalis
- a. sacralis lateralis
- a. sacralis mediana
- a. scapularis descendens
- a. scapularis dorsalis
- a. segmenti anterioris inferioris renis
- a. segmenti anterioris superioris renis
- a. segmenti inferioris renis
- a. segmenti posterioris renis
- a. segmenti superioris renis
- arteriae sigmoideae
- a. spermatica interna
- a. sphenopalatina
- a. spinalis anterior
- a. spinalis posterior
- a. splenica
- a. stylomastoidea
- a. subclavia
- a. subcostalis
- a. sublingualis
- a. submentalis
- a. subscapularis
- a. sulci centralis
- a. sulci postcentralis
- a. sulci precentralis
- a. supraduodenalis
- a. supraorbitalis
- arteriae suprarenales superiores
- a. suprarenalis inferior
- a. suprarenalis media
- a. suprascapularis
- a. suralis
- a. tarsea lateralis
- a. tarsea medialis
- a. temporalis anterior
- a. temporalis intermedia
- a. temporalis media
- a. temporalis posterior
- a. temporalis profunda
- a. temporalis superficialis
- a. testicularis

- arteriae thalamostriatae anterolaterales
- arteriae thalamostriatae anteromediales
- a. thoracica interna
- a. thoracica lateralis
- a. thoracica superior
- a. thoracoacromialis
- a. thoracodorsalis
- arteriae thymicae
- a. thyroidea ima
- a. thyroidea inferior
- a. thyroidea superior
- a. tibialis anterior
- a. tibialis posterior
- a. transversa cervicis
- a. transversa colli
- a. transversa faciei
- a. ulnaris
- a. umbilicalis
- a. urethralis
- a. uterina
- a. vaginalis
- a. vertebralis
- a. vesicalis inferior
- a. vesicalis superior
- a. volaris indicis radialis
- a. zygomatico-orbitalis

arterial
- a. anastomosis
- a. angioma
- a. arches of colon
- a. arches of ileum
- a. arches of jejunum
- a. arch of lower eyelid
- a. arch of upper eyelid
- a. blood collection
- a. blood gas
- a. blood pressure
- a. bypass graft
- a. cannulation anesthetic technique
- a. carbon dioxide
- a. carbon dioxide pressure
- a. circulation
- a. decortication
- a. dicrotic notch pressure
- a. dissection
- a. entry site
- a. flap
- a. grooves
- a. hemorrhage
- a. line, art line
- a. line filter
- a. line pressure bag
- a. mean line
- a. oxygen desaturation
- a. oxygen partial pressure (PaO_2)
- a. oxygen saturation (SaO_2)

a. oxyhemoglobin saturation (SpO_2)
a. partial pressure
a. partial pressure of CO_2
a. ring
a. segments of kidney
a. silk suture
a. switch operation
a. switch procedure
a. transfusion
umbilical a. (UA)
a. vein
a. wall dissection
a. wedge

arterial-arterial fistula
arterial-enteric fistula
arterialization
arterialized flap
arterial-portal fistula
arterial-selective intravenous vasodilator
arteriectomy
arteriobiliary fistula
arteriocapillary
arteriococcygeal gland
arteriodilator
arteriola, pl. arteriolae
a. glomerularis afferens
a. glomerularis efferens
a. temporalis retinae inferior
a. temporalis retinae superior
arteriolar attenuation
arteriole
afferent glomerular a.
capillary a.
copper-wire a.
efferent glomerular a.
silver-wire a.
arteriolith
arteriolosclerotic kidney
arteriolovenular anastomosis
arterionephrosclerosis
arterioplasty
arterioportal fistula
arterioportobiliary fistula
arteriorrhaphy
arteriorrhexis
arteriosclerotic
a. aneurysm
a. kidney
arteriosinusoidal penile fistula
arteriostenosis
arteriosus
patent ductus a. (PDA)

arteriotomy
brachial a.
end-to-side a.
arteriovenous
a. anastomosis
a. aneurysm
a. dialysis
a. fistula (AVF)
a. hemofiltration
a. malformation
artery
aberrant obturator a.
accessory obturator a.
acetabular a.
acromial a.
acromiothoracic a.
a. of Adamkiewicz
angular a.
a. of angular gyrus
anterior cecal a.
anterior cerebral a.
anterior choroidal a.
anterior ciliary a.
anterior circumflex humeral a.
anterior communicating a.
anterior descending a.
anterior humeral circumflex a.
anterior inferior cerebellar a.
anterior inferior segmental a. of kidney
a. of anterior inferior segment of kidney
anterior intercostal a.'s
anterior labial a.'s
anterior mediastinal a.'s
anterior meningeal a.
anterior parietal a.
anterior spinal a.
anterior superior alveolar a.'s
anterior superior segmental a. of kidney
a. of anterior superior segment of kidney
anterior temporal a.
anterior tibial a.
anterior tibial recurrent a.
anterolateral thalamostriate a.'s
anteromedial thalamostriate a.'s
appendicular a.
arcuate a.'s of kidney
ascending cervical a.
ascending pharyngeal a.

NOTES

artery *(continued)*

axillary a.
azygos a. of vagina
basilar a.
brachial a.
bronchial a.'s
buccinator a.
a. of bulb of penis
a. of bulb of vestibule
calcaneal a.'s
calcarine a.
a. of calf
callosomarginal a.
caroticotympanic a.'s
carpal a.
caudal pancreatic a.
a. of caudate lobe
cecal a.'s
celiac a.
central sulcal a.
a. of central sulcus
cerebellar a.'s
cerebral a.'s
a. of cerebral hemorrhage
cervicovaginal a.
chief a. of thumb
circumflex femoral a.'s
circumflex humeral a.'s
circumflex iliac a.'s
circumflex scapular a.
coarctation of pulmonary a.
colic a.'s
collateral digital a.
common hepatic a.
common iliac a.
common interosseous a.
common palmar digital a.
common peroneal a.
common plantar digital a.
communicating a.
companion a. to sciatic nerve
copper-wire a.
costocervical a.
cricothyroid a.
cystic a.
deep brachial a.
deep cervical a.
deep a. of clitoris
deep epigastric a.
deep a. of penis
deep temporal a.
deep a. of thigh
deep a. of tongue
deferential a.
descending genicular a.
descending a. of knee
descending palatine a.
descending scapular a.

digital collateral a.
D-loop transposition of the great a.'s
dolichoectatic a.
dorsal a. of clitoris
dorsal digital a.
dorsal interosseous a.
dorsalis pedis a.
dorsal pancreatic a.
dorsal a. of penis
dorsal scapular a.
dorsal thoracic a.
a. of ductus deferens
a. ectasia
ectatic carotid a.
endometrial spiral a.
esophageal a.'s
external carotid a. (ECA)
external iliac a.
external mammary a.
external maxillary a.
external pudendal a.'s
external spermatic a.
extradural vertebral a.
facial a.
femoral a.
frontal a.
gastric a.'s
gastroduodenal a.
gastroepiploic a. (GEA)
gastro-omental a.'s
genicular a.'s
great anastomotic a.
greater palatine a.
great pancreatic a.
great radicular a.
great superior pancreatic a.
helicine a.'s of the penis
hepatic a.'s
a. of Heubner
highest intercostal a.
highest thoracic a.
humeral a.
hypogastric a.
ileal a.'s
ileocolic a.
iliac a.'s
iliofemoral flap a.
iliolumbar a.
inferior epigastric a. (IEA)
inferior gluteal a.
inferior hemorrhoidal a.
inferior hypophysial a.
inferior internal parietal a.
inferior labial a.
inferior laryngeal a.
inferior lateral genicular a.
inferior medial genicular a.

inferior mesenteric a.
inferior pancreatic a.
inferior pancreaticoduodenal a.
inferior phrenic a.
inferior rectal a.
inferior segmental a. of kidney
a. of inferior segment of kidney
inferior suprarenal a.
inferior thyroid a.
inferior ulnar collateral a.
inferior vesical a.
infraorbital a.
infrascapular a.
insular a.'s
intercostal a.'s
interlobar a.'s of kidney
interlobular a.'s
interlobular a.'s of kidney
interlobular a.'s of liver
intermediate temporal a.
internal iliac a.
internal mammary a.
internal pudendal a.
internal spermatic a.
internal thoracic a. (ITA)
intestinal a.'s
jejunal a.'s
a.'s of kidney
lateral circumflex femoral a.
lateral circumflex a. of thigh
lateral femoral circumflex a.
lateral frontobasal a.
lateral inferior genicular a.
lateral occipital a.
lateral plantar a.
lateral sacral a.
lateral striate a.'s
lateral superior genicular a.
lateral tarsal a.
lateral thoracic a.
left colic a.
left coronary a.
left gastric a.
left gastroepiploic a.
left gastro-omental a.
left hepatic a.
lenticulostriate a.'s
lesser palatine a.
lienal a.
lingual a.
long thoracic a.
lowest lumbar a.'s

lowest thyroid a.
lumbar a.
marginal a. of colon
masseteric a.
medial circumflex femoral a.
medial circumflex a. of thigh
medial femoral circumflex a.
medial frontobasal a.
medial inferior genicular a.
medial occipital a.
medial plantar a.
medial superior genicular a.
median sacral a.
mediastinal a.'s
medium-sized a.
medullary spinal a.'s
mental a.
metatarsal a.
middle cerebral a.
middle colic a.
middle collateral a.
middle genicular a.
middle hemorrhoidal a.
middle meningeal a.
middle rectal a.
middle sacral a.
middle suprarenal a.
middle temporal a.
muscular a.
musculophrenic a.
mylohyoid a.
myometrial arcuate a.'s
myometrial radial a.'s
Neubauer a.
nutrient a.
nutrient a. of femur
nutrient a. of fibula
nutrient a.'s of humerus
nutrient a. of the tibia
obturator a.
occipital a.
orbitofrontal a.
ovarian a.
palmar interosseous a.
a. of the pancreatic tail
parietal a.'s
parietooccipital a.
a.'s of penis
perforating a.'s of internal
  mammary
pericallosal a.
pericardiacophrenic a.

NOTES

artery *(continued)*
perineal a.
peroneal a.
pontine a.'s
popliteal a.
postcentral sulcal a.
a. of postcentral sulcus
posterior alveolar a.
posterior cecal a.
posterior cerebral a.
posterior choroidal a.
posterior circumflex humeral a.
posterior communicating a.
posterior humeral circumflex a.
posterior inferior cerebellar a.
posterior intercostal a.'s 1–2
posterior intercostal a.'s 3-11
posterior interosseous a.
posterior labial a.'s
posterior mediastinal a.'s
posterior meningeal a.
posterior pancreaticoduodenal a.
posterior parietal a.
posterior segmental a. of kidney
a. of posterior segment of kidney
posterior spinal a.
posterior superior alveolar a.
posterior temporal a.
posterior tibial a.
posterior tibial recurrent a.
posterolateral central a.'s
posteromedial central a.'s
precentral a.
precentral sulcal a.
a. of precentral sulcus
precuneal a.
pre-Rolandic a.
princeps cervicis a.
princeps pollicis a.
principal a. of thumb
profunda brachii a.
profunda femoris a.
proper hepatic a.
proper palmar digital a.
proper plantar digital a.
pubic a.'s
a. of pulp
pyloric a.
radial collateral a.
radial index a.
radialis indicis a.
radial recurrent a.
radicular a.'s
recurrent interosseous a.
recurrent radial a.
recurrent ulnar a.
renal a.
retroduodenal a.

retrograde vascularization of
superior mesenteric a.
right colic a.
right gastric a.
right gastroepiploic a.
right gastro-omental a.
right hepatic a.
Rolandic a.
a. of round ligament of uterus
a. to sciatic nerve
scrotal a.'s
segmental a.'s of kidney
sheathed a.
short central a.
short gastric a.'s
sigmoid a.'s
spinal a.'s
splenic a. (SA)
sternal a.'s
sternomastoid a.
stylomastoid a.
subclavian a.
subcostal a.
submental a.
subscapular a.
sulcal a.
superficial brachial a.
superficial cervical a.
superficial circumflex iliac a.
superficial epigastric a.
superficial external pudendal a.
superficial palmar a.
superficial temporal a.
superficial temporal artery to
middle cerebral a. (STA-MCA)
superficial volar a.
superior cerebellar a.
superior epigastric a.
superior gluteal a.
superior hemorrhoidal a.
superior hypophysial a.
superior intercostal a.
superior internal parietal a.
superior labial a.
superior lateral genicular a.
superior medial genicular a.
superior mesenteric a. (SMA)
superior pancreaticoduodenal a.
superior phrenic a.
superior rectal a.
superior segmental a. of kidney
a. of superior segment of kidney
superior suprarenal a.'s
superior thoracic a.
superior thyroid a.
superior ulnar collateral a.
superior vesical a.
supraduodenal a.

A

supraorbital a.
suprascapular a.
supreme intercostal a.
sural a.
testicular a.
thoracoacromial a.
thoracodorsal a.
thymic a.'s
thyroid ima a.
transverse cervical a.
transverse facial a.
transverse a. of neck
transverse pancreatic a.
transverse scapular a.
ulnar a.
umbilical a.
urethral a.
uterine a.
vaginal a.
vertebral a.
volar interosseous a.
Wilkie a.
zygomatico-orbital a.

arthritis, pl. **arthritides**
arthrocele
arthrodesis

Adkins technique spinal a.
Batchelor-Brown extra-articular
  subtalar a.
beak modification with triple a.
Brockman-Nissen wrist a.
Charnley compression a.
compression a.
excisional a.
extension injury posterior
  atlantoaxial a.
extra-articular a.
resection a.
tarsometatarsal truncated-wedge a.
tibiocalcaneal a.
tibiotalocalcaneal a.
truncated tarsometatarsal wedge a.
truncated-wedge a.

arthrodial

a. articulation
a. cartilage
a. joint

**arthrographic capsular distension and
rupture technique**
arthrology

arthropathy

osteopulmonary a.
rotator cuff a.

arthrophyte
arthroplasty

abrasion a.
acetabular cup a.
Albright-Chase a.
Ashworth hand a.
Ashworth implant a.
Aufranc cup a.
Austin-Moore a.
autogenous interpositional
  shoulder a.
Bechtol a.
bipolar hip a.
Bryan a.
Campbell interpositional a.
Campbell resection a.
capitellocondylar total elbow a.
capsular interposition a.
carpometacarpal a.
Carroll a.
Castle-Schneider resection
  interposition a.
cemented total hip a.
cementless total hip a.
Charnley total hip a.
Clayton forefoot a.
Colonna trochanteric a.
condylar implant a.
constrained ankle a.
constrained shoulder a.
convex condylar implant a.
Coonrad-Morrey total elbow a.
Coonrad total elbow a.
Cracchiolo forefoot a.
Crawford-Adams cup a.
Cubbins a.
cuff tear a.
cup a.
Dewar-Barrington a.
distraction a.
duToit-Roux a.
Eaton implant a.
Eaton volar plate a.
Eden-Hybbinette a.
elbow a.
Ewald capitellocondylar total
  elbow a.
Ewald-Walker kinematic knee a.
excision a.

NOTES

arthroplasty *(continued)*
  fascial a.
  finger joint a.
  forefoot a.
  Girdlestone resection a.
  Gristina-Webb total shoulder a.
  Gunston a.
  Harrington total hip a.
  Head hip a.
  Helal flap a.
  hemiresection interposition a.
  hip a.
  Hungerford-Krackow-Kenna knee a.
  ICLH double cup a.
  implant a.
  Inglis triaxial total elbow a.
  Insall-Burstein-Freeman knee a.
  interpositional elbow a.
  interpositional shoulder a.
  intracapsular temporomandibular
    joint a.
  Jones resection a.
  Kates a.
  Keller resection a.
  knee a.
  Kocher-McFarland hip a.
  Kutes a.
  Larmon forefoot a.
  Mann-DuVries a.
  Matchett-Brown hip a.
  Mayo modified total elbow a.
  Mayo resection a.
  Memford-Gurd a.
  metacarpophalangeal joint a.
  Meuli a.
  Millender a.
  Miller-Galante knee a.
  modified mold and surface
    replacement a.
  mold acetabular a.
  monospherical total shoulder a.
  Morrey-Bryan total elbow a.
  Mould a.
  Mueller hip a.
  Mumford-Gurd a.
  NEB hip a.
  Neer unconstrained shoulder a.
  Niebauer trapeziometacarpal a.
  noncemented total hip a.
  Post total shoulder a.
  Press-Fit condylar knee a.
  prosthetic a.
  Putti-Platt a.
  resection a.
  revision hip a.
  rotator cuff tear a.
  Schlein elbow a.
  semiconstrained total elbow a.
  shoulder a.
  Silastic lunate a.
  silicone implant a.
  silicone rubber a.
  silicone wrist a.
  Smith-Petersen cup a.
  Speed a.
  Stanmore shoulder a.
  Steffee thumb a.
  Suave-Kapanje a.
  surface replacement hip a.
  Swanson Convex condylar a.
  Swanson radial head implant a.
  Swanson silicone wrist a.
  tendon interposition a.
  total ankle a.
  total articular replacement a.
  total articular resurfacing a.
  total elbow a.
  total hip a.
  total knee a.
  total patellofemoral joint a.
  total shoulder a.
  total wrist a.
  triaxial total elbow a.
  Tupper a.
  ulnar hemiresection interposition a.
  unconstrained shoulder a.
  unicompartmental knee a.
  Vaino MP a.
  Vitallium cup a.
  volar plate a.
  Volz a.
  Wilson-McKeever a.
arthroscopic
  a. abrasion chondroplasty
  a. anterior cruciate ligament
    reconstruction (AACLR)
  a. augmentation
  a. entry portal
  a. examination
  a. laser surgery
  a. meniscectomy
  a. microdiskectomy
  a. synovectomy
arthroscopy
  diagnostic and operative a.
  Gilquist a.
  laser a.
  lateral hip a.
  midcarpal a.
  needle a.
  operative a.
  radiocarpal a.
  Ringer a.
  total knee a. (TKR)
arthrosia
  exanthesis a.

arthrotomy
> diagnostic arthroscopy, operative arthroscopy, and possible operative a.
> Magnuson-Stack shoulder a.
> operative a.
> parapatellar a.

articular
> a. branches
> a. capsule
> a. cartilage
> a. cartilage lesion
> a. cavity
> a. crescent
> a. crests
> a. disk of temporomandibular joint
> a. eminence of temporal bone
> a. facet
> a. fossa of temporal bone
> a. fragment
> a. mass separation fracture
> a. muscle of elbow
> a. muscle of knee
> a. pillar fracture
> a. process
> a. surface of acromion
> a. surface of head of rib
> a. surface of tubercle of rib
> a. tubercle of temporal bone
> a. vascular circle
> a. vascular network
> a. vascular network of elbow
> a. vascular network of knee

articularis
> a. cubiti muscle
> a. genu muscle

articulate
articulated
articulating stylet
articulatio, pl. articulationes
> a. acromioclavicularis
> a. atlantoaxialis lateralis
> a. atlantoaxialis mediana
> a. atlanto-occipitalis
> a. bicondylaris
> a. capitis costae
> articulationes carpometacarpeae
> a. cartilaginis
> articulationes cinguli membri inferioris
> articulationes cinguli membri superioris
> a. complexa
> a. composita
> a. condylaris
> a. costochondralis
> a. costotransversaria
> articulationes costovertebrales
> a. cotylica
> a. coxae
> a. cricothyroidea
> a. cubiti
> a. dentoalveolaris
> a. ellipsoidea
> a. fibrosa
> a. genus
> a. humeri
> a. humeroradialis
> a. humeroulnaris
> a. incudomallearis
> articulationes intercarpeae
> articulationes interchondrales
> articulationes intermetacarpeae
> articulationes intermetatarseae
> articulationes interphalangeae manus
> articulationes interphalangeae pedis
> articulationes intertarseae
> a. lumbosacralis
> a. mandibularis
> articulationes manus
> a. mediocarpea
> articulationes membri inferioris liberi
> articulationes membri superioris liberi
> articulationes metacarpophalangeae
> articulationes metatarsophalangeae
> a. ossis pisiformis
> a. ovoidalis
> articulationes pedis
> a. plana
> a. radiocarpea
> a. sacrococcygea
> a. sacroiliaca
> a. sellaris
> a. simplex
> a. spheroidea
> a. sternoclavicularis
> articulationes sternocostales
> a. synovialis
> a. temporomandibularis
> articulationes zygapophyseales

articulation
> acromioclavicular a.

NOTES

articulation *(continued)*
    a. area
    arthrodial a.
    articulator a.
    atlantoaxial a.
    atlanto-occipital a.
    balanced a.
    bicondylar a.
    calcaneocuboid a.
    carpometacarpal a.
    Chopart a.
    condylar a.
    coracoclavicular a.
    coxofemoral a.
    cricothyroid a.
    a. curve
    dental a.
    deviant a.
    a. disorder
    external ligament of mandibular a.
    external ligament of
      temporomandibular a.
    glenohumeral a.
    humeral a.
    humeroradial a.
    humeroulnar a.
    incudomalleolar a.
    a. index
    infantile a.
    intercarpal a.
    interchondral a.'s
    intermetacarpal a.
    interphalangeal a.
    lateral ligament of
      temporomandibular a.
    Lisfranc a.
    mandibular a.
    metacarpophalangeal a.
    metatarsocuneiform a.
    metatarsophalangeal a.'s
    patellofemoral a.
    peg-and-socket a.
    a. of pisiform bone
    place of a.
    point of a.
    proximal radioulnar a.
    radiocapitellar a.
    radiocarpal a.
    radioulnar a.
    sacroiliac a.
    scapuloclavicular a.
    secondary a.
    spheroid a.
    sternocostal a.'s
    subtalar a.
    superior tibial a.
    talocalcaneal a.
    talocalcaneonavicular a.

    tarsometatarsal a.
    temporomandibular joint a.
    a. test
    tibiofemoral a.
    tibiofibular a.
    triquetropisiform a.
    trochoid a.
    Vermont spinal fixator a.
articulator articulation
articulatory procedure
Articulose-50 injection
artifact
    pacemaker a.
artificial
    a. anus
    a. classification cavity
    a. erection test
    a. fat pad
    a. fistulation
    a. intravaginal insemination
    a. kidney
    a. method
    a. nose
    a. respiration
    a. sphincter
    a. ventilation
    a. vertebral body
artifistulation
art line *(var. of* arterial line)
Arvidsson dimension-length method
arycorniculate synchondrosis
aryepiglottic
    a. fold
    a. muscle
arytenoid
    a. glands
arytenoidal articular surface of cricoid
arytenoidectomy
arytenoideus
arytenoidopexy
Asahi pressure controller
A.S.A.-induced gastric ulceration
ASA physical status
A-scan
    cross-vector A.-s.
ascending
    a. anterior branch
    a. aortic pressure
    a. branch
    a. branch of the inferior
      mesenteric artery
    a. cervical artery
    a. colon
    a. lumbar vein
    a. part of duodenum
    a. pharyngeal artery
    a. pharyngeal plexus

a. posterior branch
a. technique
Ascher
A. glass-rod phenomenon
A. syndrome
Aschoff body
ascites
a. adiposus
chyliform a.
chylous a.
a. drainage tube
exudative a.
fatty a.
gelatinous a.
hemorrhagic a.
milky a.
mucinous a.
mucoid a.
pseudochylous a.
tumor a.
ascitic
ascitogenous
Aselli pancreas
asepsis
aseptic
a. surgery
a. technique
asepticism
Asepto suction tube
Ashby differential agglutination method
Ashford retracted nipple operation
Ashhurst-Bromer classification of ankle fractures
ash leaf patch
Ashworth
A. hand arthroplasty
A. implant arthroplasty
ASIF screw fixation technique
Ask-Upmark kidney
ASM
airway smooth muscle
Asnis technique
aspect
buccal a.
dorsal a.
inferomedial a.
laminar cortex posterior a.
medial a.
paraspinous a.
plantar a.
posterolateral a.

spinous a.
volar a.
aspergilloma
a. formation
aspergillosis infection
Aspergillus **infection**
aspermatogenic
aspermia
asphyxia
asphyxial
asphyxiant
asphyxiate
asphyxiating
a. thoracic dysplasia
asphyxiation
intrapartum a.
aspirate
endotracheal a.
transtracheal a.
aspirated foreign body
aspiration
acid a.
Alcon a.
anterior a.
a. biopsy cytology
bone marrow a.
breast cyst a.
cataract a.
corporeal a.
a. of cortex
CT-guided fine-needle a.
cyst a.
endoscopic transesophageal fine-needle a.
epididymal sperm a.
fine-needle a. (FNA)
fluid a.
foreign body a.
a. of foreign body
a. of gastric contents
gastric fluid a.
guided fine-needle a.
irrigation and a.
joint a.
lateral a.
a. of lens
level of a.
meconium a.
medial a.
menstrual a.
microscopic epididymal sperm a.
microsurgical epididymal sperm a.

NOTES

aspiration *(continued)*
  mineral oil a.
  mucosal needle a.
  myringotomy with a.
  needle a.
  a. needle biopsy
  negative a.
  percutaneous balloon a.
  percutaneous CT-guided a.
  percutaneous epididymal sperm a.
  percutaneous fine-needle a.
  peritoneal a.
  pleural fluid a.
  a. pneumonia
  a. pneumonitis
  a. portal
  a. prophylaxis
  pulmonary a.
  real-time endoscopic ultrasound-
    guided fine-needle a.
  recurrent a.
  seminal vesicle a.
  silent a.
  sonography-guided a.
  sperm a.
  stereotactic a.
  suction a.
  suprapubic needle a.
  tracheal a.
  transbronchial needle a.
  transthoracic needle a.
  transtracheal a.
  ultrasonic a.
  ultrasound-guided fine-needle a.
  uterine a.
  vacuum a.
  vitreous a.
Aspisafe nasogastric tube
assay
  a. normalization
  a. technique
assessment
  awake neurological a.
  echocardiographic a.
  endoscopic color Doppler a.
  extrapyramidal function a.
  jugular bulb catheter placement a.
  nutritional a.
  weight estimation and a.
Assézat triangle
assimilation
  a. pelvis
  a. sacrum
assist-control mode ventilation
assisted
  a. circulation
  a. medical procreation
  a. reproductive technique

  a. respiration
  a. ventilation
associated myofascial trigger point
association
  auditory-vocal a.
  CHARGE a.
  a. cortex
  a. fiber
  law of a.
  a. mechanism
  megacystis-megaureter a.
  noncausal a.
  a. time
  a. tract
  VATER a.
asterion
asternal
asteroid body
asthma
  exercise-induced a.
  extrinsic a.
asthmoid respiration
astigmatic keratotomy
astigmatism
  corneal a.
  a. correction
Astler-Coller
  A.-C. A, B1, B2, C1, C2
    classification
  A.-C. modification of Dukes
    classification
astragalar
astragalocalcanean
astragaloscaphoid
astragalotibial
Astramorph PF injection
Astrand 30-beat stopwatch method
astriction
astringent
astroblastoma
astrocyte
  fibrillary a.
astrocytoma
Astwood-Coller staging system for
  carcinoma
asymmetric
  a. surgery
  a. unit membrane
asymmetry
asymptomatic
  a. infection
  a. mass
asynclitic
  a. position
  a. position of fetus
ataractic
Atasoy
  A. triangular advancement flap

A. volar V-Y flap
A. V-Y technique
Atasoy-type flap for nail injury repair
atavistic epiphysis
ataxia
respiratory a.
atelectasis
atherectomy
Auth a.
coronary angioplasty versus
  excisional a.
coronary rotational a.
directional coronary a.
high-speed rotational a.
a. index
Kinsey a.
percutaneous coronary rotational a.
rotational coronary a.
Simpson a.
transluminal extraction a.
atheroma
a. embolism
atheromatous plaque
atherosclerosis
atherosclerotic
a. aneurysm
a. lesion
ATIII
antithrombin III
Atkin epiphyseal fracture
Atkins-Cannard
A.-C. tracheal tube
A.-C. tracheotomy tube
Atkinson
A. lid block
A. silicone rubber tube
A. technique
atlantad
atlantal
a. fracture
atlantic part of vertebral artery
atlantoaxial
a. articulation
a. dislocation
a. fracture-dislocation
a. fusion
a. joint
a. lesion
a. rotatory fixation
a. stabilization
atlantoepistrophic

atlanto-occipital
a.-o. articulation
a.-o. extension
a.-o. fusion
a.-o. joint
a.-o. joint dislocation
a.-o. membrane
a.-o. stabilization
atlanto-odontoid
atlas
a. fracture
Jefferson fracture of a.
atlas-axis combination fracture
atloaxoid
atloid
atlo-occipital
ATLS
advanced trauma life support
**ATL Ultramark 7 echocardiographic
  device**
atmospheres of pressure
atomic mass
atonic bladder
atopic line
ATP hydrolysis
atrabiliary capsule
atracurium
a. besylate
Atraloc suture
atraumatic
a. braided silk suture
a. chromic suture
atresia
aortic valve a.
extrahepatic biliary a.
suprapubic cystotomy tract
  urethral a.
atretocystia
atretogastria
atrial
a. activation mapping
a. baffle operation
a. balloon septostomy
a. defibrillation threshold
a. dissociation
a. ectopic tachycardia
a. extrastimulus method
a. fibrillation
a. fibrillation-flutter
a. filling pressure
a. natriuretic peptide
a. ring

NOTES

atrial *(continued)*
    a. septal resection
    a. septectomy
    a. septostomy
    a. stasis index
atrial-well technique
atriocommissuropexy
atriodextrofascicular tract
atriofascicular tract
atrio-Hisian bypass tract
atrionodal bypass tract
atriotomy
    pursestring a.
atrioventricular
    a. bundle
    a. canal
    a. canal defect
    a. conduction tissue
    a. connection anomaly
    a. dissociation
    a. junctional ablation
    a. junction anomaly
    a. malformation
    a. nodal function
    a. node
    a. ring
    a. sulcus
    a. valve insufficiency
atrium
    a. glottidis
atrophic
    a. excavation
    a. fenestration
    a. fracture
    a. inflammation
    a. kidney
atrophy
    brown a.
    endometrial a.
    exhaustion a.
    multiple system a.
    peroneal muscle a.
    pressure a.
    scapular peroneal a.
    traction a.
Atrostim phrenic nerve stimulator
Atrovent Inhalation solution
attached
    a. cranial section
    a. craniotomy
    a. gingiva extension
attenuating tissue
attenuation
    arteriolar a.
    beam a.
    broadband a.
    a. correction
    digital beam a.

    heterogeneous a.
    interaural a.
    a. level
    signal a.
    a. of tendon
    ultrasonic a.
attollens
Attwood staining method
atypical
    a. dislocation
    a. mycobacterial infection
    a. regeneration
ATZ
    anal transitional zone
audioanalgesia
audiological evaluation
auditory
    a. canal
    a. closure
    a. method
    a. middle-latency response (AMLR)
    a. tract
    a. tube
auditory-vocal association
Auerbach
    A. ganglia
    A. plexus
Aufranc cup arthroplasty
augmentation
    alloplastic chin a.
    arthroscopic a.
    bladder a.
    breast a.
    chin a.
    connective tissue a.
    a. cystoplasty
    extra-articular a.
    gastroileac a.
    a. genioplasty
    gingival a.
    a. graft
    hamstring ligament a.
    ileocecocystoplasty bladder a.
    iliotibial band graft a.
    Leach-Schepsis-Paul a.
    Mainz pouch a.
    a. mammaplasty
    oxytocin a.
    Pitocin a.
    a. plaque
    reverse a.
    slotted acetabular a.
    submucosal urethral a.
    synthetic a.
    a. therapy
    thiol a.
    ureteral bladder a.
augmentor nerve

Augustine boat nail
aural fistula
aurem
retrahens a.
Aureomycin suture
auricular
a. appendectomy
a. branch of occipital artery
a. canaliculus
a. cartilage
a. cartilage graft
a. fibrillation
a. fissure
a. ganglion
a. index
a. ligaments
a. notch
a. point
a. surface of ilium
a. surface of sacrum
a. triangle
a. tubercle
a. veins
auriculocranial
auriculo-infraorbital plane
auriculotemporal
a. nerve
auriculoventricular groove
auscultation
Austin
A. bunionectomy
A. osteotomy
Austin-Flint respiration
Austin-Moore
A.-M. arthroplasty
A.-M. head
Autenrieth and Funk method
Auth atherectomy
autoamputation
autoaugmentation
bladder a.
autocastration
autocatheterization
autoclaved graft
autoclave sterilization
autocystoplasty
autocytolysis
autodermic
a. graft
autodilation
Frank nonsurgical perineal a.
autodrainage

autogeneic graft
autogenous
a. bone graft
a. cable graft interposition VII-VII neuroanastomosis
a. dermis fat graft
a. fibular graft
a. interpositional shoulder arthroplasty
a. keratoplasty
a. tooth transplantation
a. tunica vaginalis graft
a. vein
a. vein bypass graft
autograft
cultured epithelial a.
Russell fibular head a.
autografting
autoimmune
a. connective tissue disorder
a. demyelination
autoimmunization
surgical a.
autoinflation
autoinfusion
autokeratoplasty
autolesion
autologous
a. blood
a. blood donation
a. blood stem cell transplantation
a. fat graft
a. iliac crest bone graft
a. pericardial patch
a. rib bone graft
a. vein graft
autolytic débridement
automated
a. analysis instrument
a. anesthesia record
a. boundary protection
a. endoscopic system for optimal positioning
a. large-core breast biopsy
a. percutaneous diskectomy
automatic ectopic tachycardia
autonephrectomy
silent a.
autonomic
a. blockade
a. ganglion block
a. modulation

NOTES

autonomic *(continued)*
    a. nerve
    a. nerve block
    a. nerve preservation (ANP)
    a. neurogenic bladder
    a. plexuses
autonomous
auto-ophthalmoscopy
auto-PEEP
autoplast
autoplastic
    a. graft
autoplasty
autopod
autopodium
autopsy
autoreinfection
autorrhaphy
autosuture technique
autotransfusion
    massive a.
autotransplant
autotransplantation
    colostomy pyloric a.
    posttraumatic a.
    pyloric a.
    renal a.
    a. of splenic fragment
autotrophic fixation
autovaccination
Auvray incision
auxiliary
    a. canal
    a. implant rest
AV
    AV Gore-Tex fistula
    AV Gore-Tex graft
    AV malformation
A-V
    A-V bundle
    A-V dissociation
    A-V nodal modification
avascular
    a. fragment
    a. necrosis of the femoral head
avascularization
average
    a. flow rate
    a. mean pressure
AVF
    arteriovenous fistula
avidin-biotin-peroxidase complex method
Avila technique
Avitene
    Syringe A.
AVL Gas Check 939 blood gas
    analyzer
avoidance maneuver

avulse
avulsed
    a. fragment
    a. wound
avulsion
    a. stress fracture
    a. technique
awake
    a. craniotomy
    a. neurological assessment
awaken
    failure to a.
awakening
    planned a.
awareness
    body a.
Axenfeld
    A. anomaly
    A. suture technique
Axer
    A. lateral opening wedge
        osteotomy
    A. varus derotational osteotomy
Axer-Clark procedure
axes (*pl. of* axis)
axial
    a. aneurysm
    a. calcaneal projection
    a. compression
    a. compression injury
    a. compression principle
    a. compression test
    a. fixation
    a. hiatal hernia
    a. illumination
    a. inclination
    a. line angle
    a. loading fracture
    a. muscle
    a. pattern scalp flap
    a. plane
    a. point
    a. rotation
    a. rotation joint
    a. section
    a. sesamoid projection
    a. skeleton
    a. spin-echo image
    a. surface cavity
axil
axile
axilla, pl. axillae
    a. temperature
axillary
    a. approach
    a. arch
    a. artery
    a. block

A

a. block anesthesia
a. block anesthetic technique
a. dissection
a. fascia
a. flap
a. fold
a. fossa
a. hematoma
a. line
a. lymph nodes
a. nerve
a. node metastasis
a. perivascular technique
a. plexus
a. region
a. sheath
a. skin lesion
a. space
a. sweat glands
a. thoracotomy
a. triangle
a. vein
axillobifemoral bypass graft
axiobuccolingual plane
axiolabiolingual plane
Axiom double sump tube
axiomesiodistal plane
axis, pl. **axes**
basibregmatic a.
basicranial a.
basifacial a.
a. bulbi externus
celiac a.
cephalocaudal a.
conjugate a.
craniofacial a.
facial a.
a. fixation

flexion-extension a.
a. fracture
hypothalamic-hypophyseal-ovarian-
 endometrial a.
long a.
long a. of body
pelvic a.
a. pelvis
a. of rotation
thoracic a.
thyroid a.
axis-atlas combination fracture
axofugal
axonal
a. demyelination
a. regeneration
Axostim nerve stimulator
axotomy
Aylett operation
Ayoub-Shklar method
Ayre
A. spatula-Zelsmyr cytobrush
 technique
A. T-piece
A. tube
azaperone
azeotrope
halothane-ether a.
azeotropic solution
azure lunula of nail
azygoesophageal
a. line
a. recess
azygos
a. artery of vagina
a. fissure
a. vein
azygous

NOTES

B

B cell line
B point
B ring
B ring of esophagus
Babcock
B. operation
B. tube
Bachmann
B. bundle
internodal tract of B.
Baci-IM injection
bacitracin
b. irrigation
b. solution
bacitracin, neomycin, polymyxin B, and lidocaine
backbone
backfire fracture
backflow
pyelovenous b.
background illumination
back-knee deformity
back projection
back-up position
backward
b. coarticulation
b. position
Bacon-Babcock operation
bacteremia
bacterial
b. agar method
b. complication
b. contamination
b. endotoxin
b. filter
b. infection
b. mucosal infiltration
bactericidal concentration
bacteriolysis
bacteriopexy
bacteriospermia
bacteriostasis
bacteriostatic barrier
bacteriuria
Bactocill injection
Badal operation
Badenoch urethroplasty
Baden procedure
Badgley
B. combination procedure
B. iliac wing resection
B. resection of iliac wing
B. technique
Bado classification

BA-EDTA solution
Baehr-Lohlein lesion
Baerveldt glaucoma implant tube
Baffe anastomosis
baffle fenestration
bag
arterial line pressure b.
breathing b.
Cardiff resuscitation b.
GEM nonlatex medical b.
Hope resuscitation b.
Infu-Surg pressure infuser b.
Lifesaver disposable resuscitator b.
manual resuscitation b.
rebreathing b.
replacement collection b.
reservoir b.
bag-and-mask ventilation
BagEasy disposable manual resuscitator
bagged mask ventilation
bag-of-bones technique
bag-valve-mask (B-V-M)
bag-valve-mask-assisted ventilation
bag-valve resuscitator
Bailey-Badgley
B.-B. anterior cervical approach
B.-B. cervical spine fusion
B.-B. technique
Bailey-Dubow
B.-D. nail
B.-D. osteotomy
B.-D. technique
bailout valvuloplasty
Bailyn classification
Bain circle
Bair Hugger
B. H. fluid-warming device
B. H. forced-air warmer
B. H. patient heating unit
Bakamjian flap
Baker
B. jejunostomy tube
B. patellar advancement operation
B. pyridine extraction
B. self-sumping tube
B. Sudan black method
B. technique
B. translocation operation
Baker-Hill osteotomy
baking soda
Balacescu closing wedge osteotomy
Balacescu-Golden technique
Balamuth buffer solution
balance
heat b.

balance *(continued)*
    B. lavage solution
    thermal b.
balanced
    b. anesthesia
    b. anesthetic technique
    b. articulation
    b. electrolyte solution
    b. saline solution
    b. salt solution
balanic
balanitis
balanocele
balanoplasty
balanoposthitis
balanus
Balbiani
    B. body
    B. ring
Baldwin butterfly ventilation tube
Baldy operation
Baldy-Webster
    B.-W. procedure
    B.-W. uterine suspension
Balfour gastroenterostomy
Balkan
    B. fracture frame
    B. nephrectomy
ball
    B. operation
    b. valve action
    b. wedge
ball-and-socket
    b.-a.-s. epiphysis
    b.-a.-s. joint
    b.-a.-s. trochanteric osteotomy
Ballard examination
Ball-Hoffman operation
balloon
    b. aortic valvotomy
    b. aortic valvuloplasty
    b. atrial septostomy
    b. bronchoplasty
    b. catheter angioplasty
    b. catheter technique
    b. cell formation
    b. coarctation angioplasty
    b. coronary angioplasty
    b. counterpulsation
    b. dilatation
    b. dilation
    b. dilation angioplasty
    b. dilation of the papilla
    b. dilation valvuloplasty
    b. dissection
    b. epiphysis
    b. expulsion test
    b. inflation

    b. laser angioplasty
    b. mitral commissurotomy
    b. mitral valvotomy
    b. mitral valvuloplasty
    b. occlusive intravascular lysis enhanced recanalization
    b. photodynamic therapy
    b. pulmonary valvotomy
    b. pulmonary valvuloplasty
    b. rupture
    b. septectomy
    b. septostomy
    b. tricuspid valvotomy
    b. tube tamponade
    b. tuboplasty
    B. Valvuloplasty Registry
    b. valvulotomy
balloon-catheter and basket-retrieval technique
balloon-expandable
balloon-occluded retrograde transvenous obliteration
ball-valve obstruction
banana fracture
band
    adhesive b.
    anchor b.
    ciliary body b.
    Clado b.
    b.'s of colon
    fracture b.
    Fränkel head b.
    iliotibial b.
    Ladd b.
    Lane b.
    b. ligation
    longitudinal b.'s of cruciform ligament
    Lyon ring-constrictive b.
    Maissiat b.
    Meckel b.
    moderator b.
    pecten b.
    peritoneal b.
    Simonart b.'s
    traction b.
    ventricular b. of larynx
    zonular b.
Band-Aid operation
Bandi
    B. procedure
    B. technique
Bandl ring
Banff classification
Bangerter
    B. method of pleoptics
    B. pterygium operation

bank
- shoulder dislocation bone b.
- staple capsulorraphy bone b.
- tissue b.
- Traumatic Coma Data B.

Bankart
- B. fracture
- B. operation
- B. procedure
- B. reconstruction
- B. shoulder dislocation
- B. shoulder lesion
- B. shoulder repair

Bankart-Putti-Platt operation

banking
- cryopreserved tissue b.

Banks bone graft

Banks-Laufman
- B.-L. approach
- B.-L. incision
- B.-L. technique

bar
- b. of bladder
- b. bolt fixation
- median b. of Mercier
- Mercier b.
- b. resection
- b. section

Baralyme CO$_2$ absorbent

barber
- b. chair position
- b. pole stripe transfer

barbital

barbiturate
- b. burst-suppression anesthesia
- b. coma

barbiturate-related hyperalgesia

barbotage

Barbour technique

Barcat technique

Bard
- B. Ambulatory PCA device
- B. Extra Ilco B pouch
- B. gastrostomy feeding tube
- B. Infus OR syringe-type infusion pump
- B. Integrale pouch
- B. Neurostim peripheral nerve stimulator
- B. PCA pump
- B. PEG tube
- B. PTFE graft

Bardelli lid ptosis operation

Bardenheurer ligation

Bardic tube

bare
- b. area of liver
- b. area of stomach
- b. scleral technique

bariatric
- b. operation
- b. surgery

barium
- b. enema
- b. examination
- b. hydroxide

Barkan
- B. double cyclodialysis operation
- B. goniotomy operation
- B. membrane
- B. technique

Barkan-Cordes linear cataract operation

Barlow maneuver

Barnard operation

Barnes suction tube

Barnett-Bourne acetic alcohol-silver nitrate method

Barnhart repair

barometric pressure

Baron ear tube

Baron-Frazier suction tube

baroreceptor
- b. nerve
- b. test

baroreflex
- b. activation
- b. response

barostat method

barotrauma

Barr
- B. body
- B. nail
- B. open reduction and internal fixation
- B. tendon transfer operation
- B. tibial fracture fixation

barrage cryopexy

Barraquer
- B. enzymatic zonulolysis operation
- B. keratomileusis operation
- B. method
- B. silk suture
- B. zonulolysis

barrel-hooping compression

NOTES

barrel-shaped lesion
Barrett esophagus
Barrie-Jones canaliculodacryorhinostomy
    operation
barrier
    ABO b.
    adhesion b.
    anatomic b.
    bacteriostatic b.
    blood-air b.
    blood-brain b. (BBB)
    blood-cerebral b.
    blood-cerebrospinal fluid b.
    blood-liquor b.
    blood-ocular b.
    blood-optic nerve b.
    blood-retina b.
    blood-retinal b.
    blood-thymus b.
    blood-urine b.
    cerebrospinal fluid-brain b.
    elastic b.
    endothelial b.
    epithelial b.
    gastric mucosal b.
    integumentary b.
    b. layer
    b. method
    motion b.
    mucosal b.
    ocular b.
    pathologic b.
    physical b.
    physiologic b.
    placental b.
    posterior capsular zonular b.
    b. protection
    side-bending b.
    sterile field b.
    b. technique
    b. zone
Barrio operation
Barrnett-Seligman
    B.-S. dihydroxydinaphthyl disulfide
      method
    B.-S. indoxyl esterase method
Barron ligation
Barroso-Moguel and Costero silver
    method
Barsky
    B. cleft closure
    B. macrodactyly reduction
    B. procedure
    B. technique
Barth hernia
Bartholin
    B. cystectomy

    B. duct
    B. gland
Bartlett
    B. nail fold
    B. nail fold excision
    B. procedure
Barton-Smith fracture
Barton suction
basad
basal
    b. anal canal pressure
    b. anal sphincter pressure
    b. anesthesia
    anterior b. (AB)
    b. body temperature
    b. body thermometer
    b. cell carcinoma of eyelid
    b. cell membrane
    b. cistern
    b. ganglia hematoma
    b. ganglionic lesion
    inferior b. (IB)
    b. iridectomy
    b. lamina of ciliary body
    b. lamina of neural tube
    b. lamina of semicircular duct
    lateral b. (LB)
    b. layer of ciliary body
    b. line
    b. neck fracture
    b. part of occipital bone
    b. plate of neural tube
    septal b. (SB)
    b. skull fracture
    b. sphincter
    b. subfrontal approach
    b. tentorial branch of internal
      carotid artery
    b. veins
basalis
    cisterna b.
    norma b.
base
    anterior cranial b.
    b. of bladder
    cavity preparation b.
    cement b.
    cranial b.
    extension b.
    external b. of skull
    fixation b.
    b. of flap
    b. of hyoid bone
    internal b. of skull
    b. line
    b. of lung
    b. medication
    b. of phalanx

B

b. plane
b. projection
b. of prostate
b. of renal pyramid
b. of sacrum
saddle connector b.
b. of skull
b. of stapes
tissue-supported b.
tissue-tissue-supported b.
b. of tongue
b. wedge osteotomy
baseball
b. finger fracture
b. stitch
b. suture technique
baseline capacity evaluation
basement
b. membrane
b. membrane zone
base-of-the-neck osteotomy
base-ring tilt
bas-fond
basialis
basialveolar
basibregmatic axis
basicranial
b. axis
basic technique
basifacial
b. axis
basihyal
basihyoid
basilar
b. artery
b. bifurcation
b. bifurcation aneurysm
b. bone
b. cartilage
b. femoral neck fracture
b. fibrocartilage
b. index
b. invagination
b. lamina
b. membrane
b. osteotomy
b. part of the occipital bone
b. plexus
b. process of occipital bone
b. skull fracture
b. tip aneurysm
b. vertebra

basilateral
basilic
b. vein
b. vein graft
basinasal
b. line
basioccipital
b. bone
basiocciput
basioglossus
basion
basipetal
basipharyngeal canal
basis
b. cranii
b. cranii externa
b. cranii interna
b. mandibulae
b. modioli
b. ossis sacri
b. patellae
b. phalangis
physicochemical b. of gallstone
formation
b. prostatae
b. pyramidis renis
basisphenoid
b. bone
basitemporal
basivertebral
b. vein
basket fragmentation technique
basketing technique
basket-weave vacuolization
Basle Nomina Anatomica (BNA)
basolateral membrane
Bass
B. method
B. technique
Basset radical vulvectomy
Bassett electrical stimulation device
Bassini
B. inguinal hernia repair
B. inguinal herniorrhaphy
B. method
B. operation
B. procedure
B. technique
bastard suture
Basterra operation
Bastiaanse-Chiricuta procedure

NOTES

Batchelor-Brown extra-articular subtalar arthrodesis
Batch least-squares method
Batch-Spittler-McFaddin
  B.-S.-M. knee disarticulation
  B.-S.-M. technique
bat ear surgery
Bateman
  B. hemiarthroplasty
  B. modification of Mayer transfer operation
batrachian position
Batson plexus
batten graft
Battle
  B. incision
  B. operation
battledore incision
Baudelocque operation
Bauer-Jackson classification
Bauer-Tondra-Trusler
  B.-T.-T. operation
  B.-T.-T. technique
Bauhin
  B. gland
  valve of B.
Baume classification
Baumgard-Schwartz tennis elbow technique
Baumgartner method
Baxter
  B. PCA pump
  B. VAMP
  B. VAMP Jr.
  B. VAMP Sr.
  B. volumetric infusion pump
Baxter-D'Astous procedure
Baxter-PCA-on-demand system
Baylor
  B. cardiovascular sump tube
  B. intracardiac sump tube
Bayne-Klug centralization
bayonet
  b. canal
  b. dislocation
  b. fracture position
  b. position of fracture
bayonet-curved canal
BBB
  blood-brain barrier
B-B graft
BB to MM examination
beach chair position
bead
  b. bed
  b. chain study
  b. pouch
  b. technique filling

beak
  b. fracture
  b. modification with triple arthrodesis
  b. nail
beaking of head of talus
Beall-Feldman-Cooley sump tube
Beall-Webel-Bailey technique
beam attenuation
Beard-Cutler operation
Beard operation
Beardsley empyema tube
Beatson ovariotomy
beat-to-beat variation of fetal heart rate
Beau line
Beaver direct smear method
Bechterew
  line of B.
Bechtol arthroplasty
Beck
  B. cardiopericardiopexy
  B. gastrostomy
  B. I, II operation
  B. method
  B. triad
Beckenbaugh
  B. correction
  B. technique
Becker technique
Béclard
  B. amputation
  B. anastomosis
  B. hernia
  B. suture technique
  B. triangle
Becton
  B. open reduction
  B. technique
bed
  air cushion b.
  bead b.
  bone graft b.
  b. of breast
  fracture b.
  graft b.
  mud b.
  nail b.
  parotid b.
  Roto-Rest b.
  b. of stomach
  TheraPulse b.
  tumor b.
bedroom fracture
bedside spirometer
Beer operation
Begg light wire differential force technique

Behçet
    B. skin puncture test
    B. syndrome
bell
    b. clapper deformity
    B. muscle
    B. respiratory nerve
    B. suture
Bell-Buettner hysterectomy
Bell-Dally cervical dislocation
Bellemore-Barrett closing wedge osteotomy
Bellemore-Barrett-Middleton-Scougall-Whiteway technique
Bellocq tube
Bell-Tawse open reduction technique
Bell-Tawse procedure
Bellucci suction tube
belly
    anterior b. of digastric muscle
    b. bath therapy
    b. button
    b. button to medial malleolus examination
    b.'s of digastric muscle
    frontal b. of occipitofrontalis muscle
    inferior b. of omohyoid b.
    occipital b. of occipitofrontalis muscle
    b.'s of omohyoid muscle
    posterior b. of digastric muscle
Bel-O-Pak suction tube
below-elbow amputation
below-knee amputation (BKA)
Belsey
    B. esophagoplasty
    B. fundoplication method
    B. fundoplication procedure
    B. fundoplication technique
    B. Mark II, IV fundoplication
    B. Mark IV antireflux operation
    B. Mark IV 240-degree fundoplication
    B. Mark IV repair
    B. partial fundoplication
    B. two-thirds wrap fundoplication
Belt-Fuqua hypospadias repair
Belt technique
Belzer UW liver preservation solution
Bena-D injection
Benadryl injection

Benahist injection
Bence Jones body
bench
    b. examination
    b. surgery
    b. surgical technique
Benchekroun
    B. pouch
    B. stoma
Benedict
    B. orbit operation
    B. solution
Benedict-Talbot body surface area method
Benelli mastopexy
Bengston method
benign
    b. bone lesion
    b. duodenocolic fistula
    b. fasciculation
    b. giant cell synovioma
    b. lymphoepithelial lesion
    b. lymphoproliferative lesion
    b. mass
    b. mesothelioma of genital tract
    b. papillomavirus infection
    b. pneumatic colonoscopy complication
    b. prostatic hypertrophy
    b. vascular lesion
Bennett
    B. classification
    B. comminuted fracture
    B. dislocation
    B. fracture-dislocation
    B. lesion
    B. nail biopsy
    B. posterior shoulder approach
    B. sulfhydryl method
Bennhold Congo red method
Benoject injection
Bensley aniline-acid fuchsin-methyl green method
Bentall
    B. inclusion technique
    B. procedure
Bentley
    B. Duraflo II extracorporeal perfusion circuit
    B. Oxi-Sat Meter SM-0100
    B. oxygenator
bent nail

B

NOTES

bent-nail syndrome
benzethonium
benzocaine
> antipyrine and b.
> b., butyl aminobenzoate, tetracaine, and benzalkonium chloride
> b., gelatin, pectin, and sodium carboxymethylcellulose
> Orabase with b.

benzodiazepine conscious sedation
benzodiazepine-induced hypoventilation
benzo sky blue method
benzpyrinium bromide
benzquinamide
benzstigminum bromidum
benzyl
> b. alcohol

Bérard aneurysm
Berci-Shore choledochoscopy
Berens
> B. graft
> B. pterygium transplant operation
> B. sclerectomy operation

Berens-Smith
> B.-S. cul-de-sac restoration
> B.-S. operation

Berg chelate removal method
Berger
> B. disease
> B. interscapular amputation
> B. operation
> B. space

Berger-Bookwalter posterior approach
Bergey classification
Bergmann incision
Bergmann-Israel incision
Berke
> B. approach
> B. operation

Berke-Krönlein orbitotomy
Berkeley Bioengineering infusion terminal port
Berke-Motais operation
Berman-Gartland
> B.-G. metatarsal osteotomy
> B.-G. procedure

Bernard
> B. canal
> B. duct
> B. puncture

Berndt-Harty classification
berry
> b. aneurysm
> B. ligaments

Bertel position
Bertin columns
Bertrandi suture technique

besylate
> atracurium b.
> cisatracurium b.

beta
> b. cell of hypophysis
> b. hemolytic streptococci infection

beta-blocker medication
Beta-Cap II catheter closure
Betadine
> B. Helafoam solution
> B. scrub solution

Betagan
Bethesda
> B. Pap smear classification
> B. System for cervicovaginal sample

Bethke
> B. iridectomy
> B. operation

Bettman empyema tube
Bevan
> B. abdominal incision
> B. orchiopexy

bevel
beveled anastomosis
Beverly-Douglas lip-tongue adhesion technique
Bevin-Aurglass technique
BeWo choriocarcinoma cell line
bezoar
> medication b.

Bezold-Jarisch reflex
B_0-**gradient method**
B.H. Moore procedure
biarticular
biasterionic
biaxial joint
bicameral abscess
bicanalicular sphincter
BICAP coagulation
biceps
> b. interval lesion
> long head of b.
> short head of b.

bicepsplasty
Bichat
> B. canal
> B. fat pad
> B. fossa
> B. membrane

Bicillin
> B. C-R 900/300 injection
> B. L-A injection

bicipital
> b. groove
> b. rib
> b. ridges

bicipitoradial bursa

bicitrate
   sodium b.
Bickel-Moe procedure
Bickel ring
Bick procedure
bicondylar
   b. articulation
   b. graft
   b. joint
   b. T-shaped fracture
   b. Y-shaped fracture
bicoronal scalp flap
bicortical screw fixation
bicycle spoke fracture
bidirectional
   b. ligation
   b. superior cavopulmonary
   anastomosis
Biebl loop
Bielschowsky
   B. maneuver
   B. method
   B. operation
   B. three-step head-tilt test
Bielschowsky-Parks head-tilt, three-step test
Bier
   B. amputation
   B. block
   B. block anesthesia
   B. method
Biesiadecki fossa
bifemoral graft
bifid
   b. graft
   b. penis
   b. rib
   b. thumb deformity
bifocal fixation
bifoveal fixation
bifrontal craniotomy
bifurcated
   b. vascular graft
   b. vein graft for vascular reconstruction
bifurcatio
   b. tracheae
bifurcation
   b. aneurysm
   b. of aorta
   aortic b.
   basilar b.

   carotid artery b.
   b. of common bile duct
   coronary b.
   b. involvement
   b. lesion
   b. lymph nodes
   b. osteotomy
   b. of pulmonary trunk
   b. of root
   b. of trachea
Bigelow
   B. litholapaxy
   B. maneuver
   B. septum
bikini skin incision
bilaminar membrane
bilateral
   b. amputation
   b. bundle branch block
   b. frame
   b. ilioinguinal approach
   b. inguinal hernia repair
   b. inguinal hernia repair method
   b. inguinal hernia repair procedure
   b. inguinal hernia repair technique
   b. interfacetal dislocation
   b. intrafacetal dislocation
   b. lithotomy
   b. lymphadenectomy
   b. myocutaneous graft
   b. neck dissection
   b. nephroureterectomy
   b. sacroiliac approach
   b. salpingo-oophorectomy
   b. subcostal incision
   b. subcutaneous mastectomy
   b. temporary tarsorrhaphy
   b. transabdominal incision
   b. ureterostomy takedown
   b. vagotomy
   b. ventral rhizotomy
   b. V-Y Kutler flap
bile
   b. acid-EDTA solution
   b. duct
   b. duct adenoma
   b. duct cannulation
   b. duct carcinoma
   b. duct dilatation
   b. duct ligation
   b. duct manipulation
   b. duct pressure

NOTES

bile *(continued)*
    b. encrustation
    b. fluid examination
    b. papilla
    b. pigment demonstration in tissue
bile-plug syndrome
bi-level positive airway pressure
   (BiPAP)
Bilhaut-Cloquet procedure
biliary
    b. calculus
    b. canaliculus
    b. cannulation
    b. carcinoma
    b. dilation
    b. duct
    b. ductules
    b. endoprosthesis insertion
    b. endoscopy
    b. fistula
    b. lithiasis
    b. lithotripsy
    b. saturation index
    b. sphincterotomy
    b. stent patency
    b. tract
    b. tract cancer
    b. tract disease
    b. tract obstruction
    b. tract pressure
    b. tract stone
    b. tract torsion
    b. tract tumor
biliary-bronchial fistula
biliary-cutaneous fistula
biliary-duodenal
    b.-d. fistula
    b.-d. pressure gradient
biliary-enteric
    b.-e. anastomosis
    b.-e. anastomosis operation
    b.-e. fistula
biliodigestive anastomosis
bilious vomit
Billings method
Bill maneuver
billowing mitral valve syndrome
Billroth
    B. I gastroduodenostomy
    B. II anatomy
    B. II gastrojejunostomy
    B. I, II anastomosis
    B. I, II gastrectomy
    B. I, II gastroenterostomy
    B. I, II operation
    B. I, II procedure
    B. I, II reconstruction
    B. I, II technique
    B. I method
    B. I partial gastrectomy
    B. tube
bilobate
bilobectomy
bilobed
    b. polypoid lesion
    b. skin flap
    b. transposition flap
bilobular
bilocular
    b. femoral hernia
    b. joint
    b. stomach
bimalleolar ankle fracture
bimanual
    b. pelvic examination
bimastoid line
bimodal method
binaural
    b. fusion
    b. integration
bind
Binet system of classification
Bing-Siebenmann malformation
Bing-Taussig heart procedure
binocular
    b. eye patch
    b. fixation
    b. fusion
    b. indirect ophthalmoscopy
    b. microscopy
Binova Medical Technologies customized
   tracheostomy tube
Biobrane/HF experimental skin
   substitute
biochemical
    b. metastasis
    b. modulation
biocompatibility
    implant b.
Biocoral graft
biofragmentable anastomotic ring
Biofreeze with Ilex topical analgesic
   ointment
Biogenex antigen retrieval method
Biograft graft
Bioject injector system
Biolite ventilation tube
biologic fixation
biomagnetic therapy
biomechanical preparation
Bio-Medicus centrifugal pump
Bionit vascular graft
Bion Tears solution
BioPolyMeric
    B. femoropopliteal bypass graft
    B. vascular graft

B

bioprogressive technique
biopsy
    abdominal lymph node b.
    adrenal gland b.
    alcohol-fixed gastric b.
    Allis-Abramson breast b.
    antral b.
    aspiration needle b.
    automated large-core breast b.
    Bennett nail b.
    bite b.
    blind percutaneous liver b.
    bone marrow aspiration and b.
    brain b.
    breast b.
    bronchial brush b.
    bronchoscopic needle b.
    brush b.
    catheter-guided b.
    cervical cone b.
    channel and core b.
    chorionic villus b.
    CLO b.
    coin b.
    cold cup b.
    colonoscopic b.
    colorectal b.
    cone b.
    core needle b.
    corporal b.
    Crosby-Kugler capsule for b.
    CT-guided liver b.
    CT-guided needle-aspiration b.
    cytobrush b.
    cytologic b.
    diathermic loop b.
    digitally-guided b.
    direct vision liver b.
    Dunn b.
    elliptical b.
    embryo b.
    endometrial b.
    endomyocardial b.
    endoscopic small bowel b.
    endoscopic sphenoidal b.
    ERCP-guided b.
    esophageal b.
    excisional b.
    fetal liver b.
    fetal skin b.
    fine-needle aspiration b.
    FNA b.

    forage core b.
    Fosnaugh nail b.
    four-point b.
    b. of gastric mucosa
    guided transcutaneous b.
    guillotine needle b.
    hilar b.
    hot b.
    ileal b.
    image-guided stereotactic brain b.
    incisional b.
    intestinal b.
    intramedullary tumor b.
    jumbo b.
    Kevorkian punch b.
    Keyes punch b.
    kidney b.
    laparoscopic b.
    large-core needle b.
    large-particle b.
    lift-and-cut b.
    liver b.
    lumbar spine b.
    lung b.
    lymph node b.
    mediastinal lymph node b.
    Menghini technique for
      percutaneous liver b.
    minimally invasive b.
    mirror-image breast b.
    mucosal b.
    multiple core b.
    muscle b.
    nasopharyngeal b.
    native renal b.
    needle b.
    open lung b.
    open surgical b.
    out-of-phase endometrial b.
    outpatient b.
    pancreatic b.
    paracollicular b.
    parathyroid b.
    pelvic aspiration b.
    percutaneous fine-needle
      aspiration b.
    percutaneous fine-needle
      pancreatic b.
    percutaneous liver b.
    percutaneous native renal b.
    percutaneous needle b.
    percutaneous pancreas b.

NOTES

biopsy *(continued)*
pericardial b.
peritoneal b.
peroral intestinal b.
PET-guided b.
pinch b.
Pipelle b.
pleural b.
pouch b.
punch b.
random bladder b.
rectal b.
renal b.
saucerized b.
scalene fat pad b.
scalene lymph node b.
scan-directed b.
Scher nail b.
shave b.
skeletal b.
skin b.
skinny-needle b.
small bowel b.
snap-frozen b.
snare excision b.
snare loop b.
sonoguided b.
spinal infection b.
sponge b.
stereotactic breast b.
stereotactic core b.
stereotactic percutaneous needle b.
strip b.
suction b.
supraclavicular lymph node b.
surgical excision b.
synovial b.
systematic sextant b.
tangential b.
temporal artery b.
testicular b.
thin-needle b.
thoracic spine b.
thyroid needle b.
total b.
transbronchial lung b.
transcutaneous b.
transgastric fine-needle-aspiration b.
transitional zone b.
transjugular hepatic b.
transjugular liver b.
transpapillary b.
transrectal ultrasound-guided-
   sextant b.
transthoracic needle aspiration b.
transthoracic percutaneous fine-
   needle aspiration b.
transvenous liver b.

trephine needle b.
trophectoderm b.
ultrasound-guided automated large-
   core breast b.
ultrasound-guided core breast b.
vaginal cone b.
Valls-Ottolenghim-Schajowicz
   needle b.
ventricular endomyocardial b.
vertical lip b.
video-assisted excisional b.
Vim-Silverman technique for
   liver b.
vulvar b.
Watson capsule b.
wedge hepatic b.
Zaias nail b.
biopsy-proven metastasis
biorbital
   b. angle
Biosystems feeding tube
Biot
   B. breathing
   B. respiration
biotransformation
BiPAP
   bi-level positive airway pressure
   BiPAP nasal continuous positive
      airway pressure
biparietal
   b. diameter
bipedicle dorsal flap
bipennate
   b. muscle
biperforate
biphase pin fixation
biplane
   b. fluoroscopy
   b. scan
   b. trochanteric osteotomy
bipolar
   b. cauterization
   B. Circumactive Probe coagulation
   b. coagulation
   b. electrocoagulation
   b. hip arthroplasty
biramous
Bircher-Weber technique
Birch-Hirschfeld entropion operation
bird-beak deformity
bird's nest
   b.-n. lesion
   b.-n. vena cava filter
birth
   b. amputation
   b. canal
   b. canal laceration
   b. fracture

birthmark
bisacromial
bisaxillary
Bischof myelotomy
bisecting
    b. angle cone position
    b. angle technique
bisecting-the-angle technique
bisection
bisector line
bisegmentectomy
bisensory method
bisexual
Bishop classification
bisiliac
bismuth
    b. aluminate
    b. ammonium citrate
    b. benign bile duct stricture
      classification
    b. carbonate
    b. chloride oxide
    b. injection
    b. line
    b. oxide
    b. oxycarbonate
    b. oxychloride
    b. oxynitrate
    b. salicylate
    b. sodium tartrate
    b. subcarbonate
    b. subnitrate
    b. subsalicylate
    b. trichloride
bismuthyl
    b. carbonate
    b. chloride
bisubcostal incision
bisulfite
    sodium b.
bite
    b. biopsy
    16-b. nylon suture
    b. plane
    b. plane therapy
bitemporal
bitewing technique
biting pressure
bitrochanteric
biventer
    b. cervicis
biventral

Bivona
    B. Fome-Cuff tube
    B. sleep apnea tracheostomy tube
    B. TTS tracheostomy tube
bizygomatic
Björk method of Fontan procedure
Björk-Shiley graft
BKA
    below-knee amputation
black
    b. braided nylon suture
    b. braided silk suture
    B. classification
    b. epidermoidoma
    b. line
    b. patch syndrome
    b. periodic acid method
    B. peroneal tendon sheath injection
    B. repair
    b. silk sling suture
    B. technique
    b. twisted suture
Black-Broström staple technique
Blackburn technique
bladder
    atonic b.
    b. augmentation
    b. autoaugmentation
    autonomic neurogenic b.
    b. calculi
    b. carcinoma
    b. catheterization
    b. chimney procedure
    b. diverticulectomy
    exstrophy of b.
    b. fistula
    b. flap
    b. flap hematoma
    b. hemorrhage
    b. hernia
    hyperreflexic b.
    hypertonic b.
    ileal b.
    b. laceration
    b. neck elevation test
    b. neck preserving technique
    b. neck suspension
    b. neck-to-urethra anastomosis
    neurogenic b.
    neuropathic b.
    b. outlet reconstruction
    b. perforation

NOTES

bladder *(continued)*
    poorly compliant b.
    b. pressure
    pseudoneurogenic b.
    reflex neurogenic b.
    b. replacement urinary pouch
    b. stone
    b. temperature
    trabeculated b.
    transurethral resection of b.
    uninhibited neurogenic b.
    unstable b.
    urinary b.
    valve b.
blade
    b. atrial septostomy
    b. bone
    MacIntosh laryngoscope b.
    b. plate fixation
    shoulder b.
Blair
    B. epicanthus repair
    B. fusion
    B. incision
    B. modification of Gellhorn pessary
    B. operation
    B. technique
Blair-Brown
    B.-B. procedure
    B.-B. skin graft
Blair-Byars hypospadias technique
Blakemore
    B. esophageal tube
    B. nasogastric tube
Blakemore-Sengstaken tube
Blake pouch
Blalock-Hanlon
    B.-H. atrial septectomy
    B.-H. operation
    B.-H. procedure
Blalock-Taussig
    B.-T. operation
    B.-T. procedure
    B.-T. shunt ligation
blanchable red lesion
blanched cutaneous elevation
Bland-Altman method
Blandin gland
blanket
    CareDrape b.
    b. suture
    b. suture technique
Blaschko line
Blasius
    B. duct
    B. lid flap operation

Blaskovics
    B. canthoplasty operation
    B. dacryostomy operation
    B. flap
    B. inversion of tarsus operation
    B. lid operation
    B. tarsectomy
blastic
    b. lesion
    b. metastasis
blast injury
blastocele
blastocytoma
blastolysis
blastoma
    pulmonary b.
blastotomy
Blatt
    B. operation
    B. procedure
Blatt-Ashworth procedure
bleb
    endothelial b.
    b. resection
Bleck
    B. method
    B. recession technique
bleed
    postgastrectomy b.
    postpolypectomy b.
bleeder in tumor mass
bleeding
    b. angioma
    esophageal variceal b.
    esophagogastric variceal b.
    excessive b.
    gastric variceal b.
    implantation b.
    b. lesion
    placentation b.
    b. point
    b. site ligation
    b. site localization
    b. tumor
    variceal b.
Blenderm patch technique
blenorrhagic inflammation
blepharal
blepharectomy
blepharochalasis repair
blepharon
blepharoplasty
    Davis-Geck b.
    reoperative b.
blepharoptosis repair
blepharorrhaphy
    Elschnig b.
blepharosphincterectomy

blepharostat ring
blepharotomy
blind
    b. fistula
    b. foramen of frontal bone
    b. foramen of the tongue
    b. gut
    b. lithotripsy
    b. loop syndrome
    b. nasal intubation
    b. nasal intubation anesthetic
      technique
    b. nasotracheal intubation
    b. nasotracheal intubation anesthetic
      technique
    b. osteotomy
    b. percutaneous liver biopsy
    b. pouch syndrome
    b. upper esophageal pouch
blind-spot projection technique
blister
    fracture b.
    pressure b.
    subcorneal b.
bloc
    en b.
Bloch-Paul-Mikulicz operation
block
    b. anesthesia
    ankle b.
    arborization b.
    Atkinson lid b.
    autonomic ganglion b.
    autonomic nerve b.
    axillary b.
    Bier b.
    bilateral bundle branch b.
    brachial plexus b.
    Brightbill corneal cutting b.
    bundle-branch b.
    caudal b.
    celiac plexus b.
    central b.
    ciliovitrectomy b.
    complete left bundle-branch b.
    complete right bundle-branch b.
    depolarization b.
    depolarizing b.
    differential nerve b.
    differential spinal b.
    direct obturator nerve b.
    epidural b.

exit b.
extradural b.
femoral nerve b.
field b.
Hara infiltration b.
His bundle heart b.
iliohypogastric nerve b.
ilioinguinal/iliohypogastric nerve b.
  (IINB)
ilioinguinal nerve b.
3-in-1 b.
incomplete right bundle-branch b.
indirect obturator nerve b.
infiltration b.
b. injection
intercostal nerve b.
interscalene brachial plexus b.
intrapleural b.
lateral antebrachial cutaneous
  nerve b.
left bundle-branch b.
lower extremity nerve b.
lumbar plexus b.
lumbar sympathetic b.
motor point b.
nerve b.
neurolytic celiac plexus b.
neuromuscular b.
New Orleans corneal cutting b.
nondepolarizing b.
obturator nerve b.
b. osteotomy
paracervical b.
paravertebral lumbar sympathetic b.
penile b.
peripheral nerve b.
phase I, II b.
phrenic nerve b.
preganglionic sympathetic b.
regional b.
retrobulbar nerve b.
right bundle branch b.
sciatic nerve b.
sensory b.
sinoatrial exit b.
sinus exit b.
skull b.
Smith modification of Van Lint
  lid b.
Southern Eye Bank corneal
  cutting b.
spinal b.

NOTES

block *(continued)*
    Steinberg infiltration b.
    stellate ganglion b.
    subarachnoid b.
    subclavian perivascular b.
    subdural b.
    supraclavicular b.
    sympathetic b.
    sympathetic nerve b.
    Tanne corneal cutting b.
    therapeutic nerve b.
    tibial augmentation b.
    tracheal b.
    two-point nerve b.
    upper extremity nerve b.
    uterosacral b.
    wrist b.
    yoke b.
Block-Ace solution
blockade
    β-adrenergic b.
    adrenergic b.
    anesthetic b.
    autonomic b.
    cholinergic b.
    epidural neural b.
    flickering b.
    ganglionic b.
    gasserian ganglion b.
    interscalene b.
    lytic b.
    myoneural b.
    neuromuscular b. (NMB)
    onset of b.
    preganglionic cardiac sympathetic b.
    pulmonary sympathetic b.
    sensory b.
    sympathetic b.
blockage
    ganglion b.
    shunt b.
blocker
    calcium entry b.
    dihydropyridine calcium channel b.
    ganglion b.
    use-dependent sodium channel b.
blocking
    b. procedure
    tissue b.
    vecuronium neuromuscular b.
Blom-Singer tracheoesophageal fistula
blood
    b. alcohol concentration
    allogeneic b.
    autologous b.
    b. calculus
    b. coagulation
    b. coagulation disorder

    b. donation
    intraoperatively donated autologous b.
    mediastinal shed b. (MSB)
    MV b.
    occult b.
    b. oxygenation level-dependent
    b. oxygenation level-dependent contrast
    oxygen concentration in pulmonary capillary b.
    oxygen saturation of the hemoglobin of arterial b.
    b. patch
    b. patch injection
    preoperatively donated autologous b.
    b. pressure
    b. pressure cuff
    b. pressure monitoring
    b. stream infection
    b. substitute
    b. tumor
    UA b.
    UV b.
    b. vessel formation
    b. vessel tumor
blood-air barrier
blood-borne infection
blood-brain
    b.-b. barrier (BBB)
    b.-b. equilibration time
blood-cerebral barrier
blood-cerebrospinal fluid barrier
blood-gas
    b.-g. analysis
    b.-g. exchange
Bloodgood syndrome
bloodless
    b. amputation
    b. decerebration
    b. operation
    b. phlebotomy
bloodletting
    general b.
    local b.
blood-liquor barrier
blood-ocular barrier
blood-optic nerve barrier
blood-retina barrier
blood-retinal barrier
blood-thymus barrier
blood-tinged CSF
blood-urine barrier
bloody peritoneal fluid
Bloomberg SuperNumb anesthetic ring
Bloom-Raney
    B.-R. modification

B.-R. modification of Smith-
Robinson technique
blot hemorrhage
Blount
B. displacement osteotomy
B. technique for osteoclasis
B. tracing technique
blow-hole ileostomy
blow-in fracture
blow-out
b.-o. fracture
b.-o. fracture of orbit
blue
b. cotton suture
b. line
B. Line cuffed endotracheal tube
methylene b.
b. ring pessary
b. twisted cotton suture
blue-black monofilament suture
blue-gray lesion
Blumenbach clivus
Blumensaat line
Blumenthal lesion
Blumer shelf
Blundell-Jones technique
blunderbuss apical canal
blunt
b. eversion carotid endarterectomy
b. and sharp dissection
b. suction tube
b. trauma
blur point
blush
tumor b.
BMI
body mass index
BNA
Basle Nomina Anatomica
BNP
brain natriuretic peptide
Boari
B. bladder flap
B. bladder flap procedure
B. ureteral flap repair
Boari-Ockerblad flap
Boas point
boat nail
boat-shaped abdomen
Bobath method
bobbin myringotomy tube
bobby pin abrasion

Bochdalek
B. gap
B. hernia
Bock
B. ganglion
B. nerve
Boden-Gibb tumor staging
Bodian method
body
adipose b.
adrenal b.
alveolar b.
Amato b.
anal foreign b.
angularis b.
anococcygeal b.
anorectal foreign b.
aortic b.
Arantius b.
Arnold b.
artificial vertebral b.
Aschoff b.
aspirated foreign b.
aspiration of foreign b.
asteroid b.
b. awareness
Balbiani b.
Barr b.
basal layer of ciliary b.
Bence Jones b.
Bracht-Wachter b.
brassy b.
cancer b.
carotid b.
cartilaginous loose b.
b. cast syndrome
caudate b.
cavernous b. of clitoris
cavernous b. of penis
b. cavity
b. cell mass
central fibrous b.
chromaffin b.
chromatinic b.
ciliary b.
b. of clavicle
b. of clitoris
coccidian b.
coccygeal b.
colloid b.
colonic foreign b.
b. composition analysis

B

NOTES

body *(continued)*
  compressed b.
  compressible cavernous b.'s
  corneal foreign b.
  Creola b.
  crescent b.
  cystoid b.
  cytoid b.
  dense b.
  duodenal foreign b.
  Dutcher b.
  Ehrlich inner b.
  electromagnetic removal of
    foreign b.
  Elschnig b.
  b. of epididymis
  esophageal foreign b.
  esophageal Lewy b.
  external geniculate b.
  F b.
  b. fat
  fat b. of cheek
  fat b. of ischiorectal fossa
  fibrous loose b.
  b. fluid
  foreign b.
  b. of fornix
  b. of gallbladder
  Gamna-Gandy b.
  gastric foreign b.
  gelatin compression b.
  geniculate b.
  glomus b.
  Goldmann-Larson foreign b.
  Gordon b.
  Gordon elementary b.
  b. habitus
  Hamazaki-Wesenberg b.
  Harting b.
  Hassall b.
  Heinz b.
  Heinz-Ehrlich b.
  b. hematocrit-venous hematocrit
    ratio
  hematoxylin b.
  Henle b.
  Hensen b.
  Highmore b.
  Hirano b.
  hyaline b.
  hyaloid b.
  b. of hyoid bone
  b. of ilium
  b. image
  infrapatellar fat b.
  ingested foreign b.
  intra-articular loose b.
  intraluminal foreign b.

intraocular foreign b.
intraorbital foreign b.
intrauterine foreign b.
intravascular foreign b.
b. of ischium
Jaworski b.
juxtaglomerular b.
juxtarestiform b.
Kelvin b.
Lallemand b.'s
Lallemand-Trousseau b.
Landolt b.
lateral geniculate b.
lenticular fossa of vitreous b.
Lieutaud b.
loose b.
loose intra-articular b.
lower GI tract foreign b.
Luys b.
lyssa b.'s
malpighian b.
mamillary b.
b. of mammary gland
Maragiliano b.
b. mass index (BMI)
Maxwell b.
May-Hegglin b.
medial geniculate b.
melon seed b.
metallic foreign b.
mineral oil foreign b.
Mott b.
Müller duct b.
multilamellar b.
Neill-Mooser b.
newtonian b.
nigroid b.
nucleus of the mamillary b.
nucleus of medial geniculate b.
olivary b.
osteocartilaginous loose b.
osteochondral loose b.
owl eye inclusion b.
pampiniform b.
b. of pancreas
paranephric b.
paraterminal b.
pectinate b.
peduncle of mamillary b.
pedunculated loose b.
pedunculus of pineal b.
b. of penis
perineal b.
b. of phalanx
pigmented layer of ciliary b.
pineal b.
pituitary b.
b. position

Prowazek-Greeff b.
psammoma b.
pubic b.
b. of pubis
pyknotic b.
radiopaque foreign b.
rectal foreign b.
refractile b.
Reilly b.
removal of foreign b.
residual b.
restiform b.
retained foreign b.
b. of rib
rice b.
b. righting reflex
rigid b.
Rosenmüller b.
Ross b.
round b.
Rucker b.
sand b.
Sandström b.'s
Savage perineal b.
b. scanning
Schaumann b.
b. schema
Schiller-Duvall b.
sclerotomy removal of foreign b.
Seidelin b.
selenoid b.
b. side integration
b. of sphenoid bone
spongy b. of penis
S-shaped b.
b. stalk
b. of sternum
b. of stomach
striate b.
suprarenal b.
b. surface area (BSA)
b. surface burned
b. surface Laplacian mapping
b. of sweat gland
Symington anococcygeal b.
b. of talus
b. temperature
b. of thigh bone
thoracic vertebral b.
thyroid b.
b. of tibia
b. of tongue

tracheobronchial foreign b.
trapezoid b.
b. of ulna
upper GI tract foreign b.
b. of urinary bladder
b. of uterus
vagal b.
vaginal foreign b.
ventral nucleus of trapezoid b.
vermiform b.
b. of vertebra
vertebral b.
vitreous foreign b.
b. weight
Wesenberg-Hamazaki b.
Winkler b.
wolffian b.
X b.
Y b.
yellow b.
body-exhaust suit
body-fluid
   b.-f. analysis
   b.-f. exchange
Boerema
   B. anterior gastropexy
   B. hernia repair
Boerhaave
   B. glands
   B. syndrome
Bogros space
Böhler
   B. calcaneal angle
   B. reducing fracture frame
Böhler-Braun fracture frame
Bohlman
   B. anterior cervical vertebrectomy
   B. cervical fusion technique
   B. triple-wire technique
Böhm operation
Bohr
   B. effect
   B. equation
   B. isopleth method
Boitzy open reduction
bolster
   b. suture
   b. suture technique
bolt fixation
Bolton-nasion line
Bolton point

NOTES

bolus
    b. injection
    b. intravenous anesthesia
    b. intravenous anesthetic technique
Bonaccolto-Flieringa
    B.-F. scleral ring
    B.-F. scleral ring operation
    B.-F. vitreous operation
Bonaccolto scleral ring
bonded cast restoration
bonding
    adhesive b.
bone
    Albrecht b.
    antigen-extracted allogeneic b.
    b. autogenous graft
    basilar b.
    basioccipital b.
    basisphenoid b.
    blade b.
    b. block procedure
    breast b.
    Breschet b.'s
    bundle b.
    calcaneal b.
    calf b.
    capitate b.
    central b.
    cheek b.
    b. chip
    collar b.
    compact b.
    cortical b.
    coxal b.
    cranial b.'s
    cuboid b.
    cuneiform b.
    b. cyst excision
    b. cyst fracture probability
    b. destruction
    b.'s of digits
    b. dissection
    dorsal talonavicular b.
    ear b.'s
    ectopic b.
    enchondroma of b.
    endochondral b.
    eosinophilic granuloma of b.
    epactal b.'s
    epipteric b.
    episternal b.
    ethmoid b.
    exoccipital b.
    b. exposure
    facial b.'s
    first cuneiform b.
    flank b.
    b. flap

Flower b.
b. formation
b. fragment
frontal b.
giant cell tumor of b.
Goethe b.
b. graft bed
b. graft collapse
b. graft decompression
b. graft extrusion
b. graft incorporation
b. graft placement
b. graft repair
greater multangular b.
hamate b.
heel b.
hip b.
hollow b.
hooked b.
horizontal plate of palatine b.
hyoid b.
iliac b.
incarial b.
innominate b.
intermediate cuneiform b.
interparietal b.
irregular b.
ischial b.
jaw b.
jugal b.
Krause b.
lateral cuneiform b.
lentiform b.
b. lesion
lesser multangular b.
lingual b.
long b.
b.'s of lower limb
lunate b.
lyophilization of b.
malignant giant cell tumor of b.
b. marrow aspiration
b. marrow aspiration and biopsy
b. marrow examination
b. marrow graft
b. marrow infiltration
b. marrow lesion
b. marrow pressure
b. marrow puncture
b. marrow transplantation
b. mass
b. matrix
maxillary surface of perpendicular plate of palatine b.
medial cuneiform b.
mesethmoid b.
b. metastasis
metatarsal b.

B

middle cuneiform b.
multangular b.
navicular b.
occipital b.
orbital plane of frontal b.
orbital plate of ethmoid b.
orbital plate of frontal b.
osteonal lamellar b.
osteoporotic b.
parietal b.
b. peg graft
periotic b.
petrosal b.
pipe b.
Pirie b.
pisiform b.
pneumatic b.
postsphenoid b.
preinterparietal b.
presphenoid b.
pubic b.
pyramidal b.
b. resection
Riolan b.'s
sacred b.
scaphoid b.
second cuneiform b.
semilunar b.
sesamoid b.
shank b.
shin b.
short b.
sieve b.
b.'s of skull
sphenoid b.
sphenoidal turbinated b.'s
superior surface of horizontal plate
  of palatine b.
suprainterparietal b.
suprasternal b.
sutural b.'s
tail b.
b. technique
temporal b.
thigh b.
three-cornered b.
tongue b.
triangular b.
triquetral b.
b. tumor
tympanic b.
tympanohyal b.

unciform b.
upper jaw b.
Vesalius b.
b.'s of visceral cranium
b. wax suture
b. wedge
wedge b.
wormian b.'s
yoke b.
zygomatic b.
bone-cement interface
bone-implant interface
bone-ingrowth fixation
bone/ligament dissection
bone-patellar tendon-bone preparation
bone-screw interface strength
bone-tendon-bone graft
bone-to-bone graft
Bonferroni correction
Bonfiglio
  B. bone graft
  B. modification
  B. modification of Phemister
    technique
Bonfiglio-Bardenstein technique
Bongort urinary diversion pouch
Bonnaire method
Bonner position
Bonnet
  B. capsule
  B. enucleation operation
Bonney
  B. abdominal hysterectomy
  B. test
Bonola technique
bony
  b. bridge resection
  b. canal
  b. deformity
  b. demineralization
  b. dissection
  b. element destruction
  b. excrescence
  b. exposure
  b. fragment
  b. labyrinth
  b. landmark
  b. lesion
  b. mass
  b. metastasis
  b. necrosis and destruction
  b. procedure

NOTES

bony *(continued)*
    b. projection
    b. semicircular canals
Bonzel operation
boomerang-shaped lesion
booster
    Ambu suction b.
boost technique
bootstrap
    b. dilation
    b. two-vessel angioplasty
    b. two-vessel technique
boot-top fracture
Boplant graft
Bora
    B. centralization
    B. operation
    B. technique
Borchgrevink method
border
    anterior b. of lung
    anterior b. of pancreas
    anterior b. of radius
    anterior b. of testis
    anterior b. of tibia
    anterior b. of ulna
    free b. of ovary
    frontal b.
    frontal b. of parietal bone
    frontal b. of sphenoid bone
    inferior b. of liver
    inferior b. of lung
    inferior b. of pancreas
    interosseous b.
    interosseous b. of fibula
    interosseous b. of radius
    interosseous b. of tibia
    interosseous b. of ulna
    lambdoid b. of occipital bone
    lateral b. of forearm
    lateral b. of humerus
    lateral b. of kidney
    lateral b. of scapula
    mastoid b. of occipital bone
    medial b. of forearm
    medial b. of humerus
    medial b. of kidney
    medial b. of scapula
    medial b. of suprarenal gland
    medial b. of tibia
    mesovarian b. of ovary
    nasal b. of frontal bone
    occipital b.
    occipital b. of parietal bone
    occipital b. of temporal bone
    parietal b.
    parietal b. of frontal bone
    parietal b. of sphenoid bone

    parietal b. of temporal bone
    posterior b. of petrous part of
      temporal bone
    posterior b. of radius
    posterior b. of testis
    posterior b. of ulna
    radial b. of forearm
    b. ray amputation
    right b. of heart
    sagittal b. of parietal bone
    sphenoidal b. of temporal bone
    squamous b.
    squamous b. of parietal bone
    squamous b. of sphenoid bone
    superior b. of pancreas
    superior b. of petrous part of
      temporal bone
    superior b. of scapula
    superior b. of spleen
    superior b. of suprarenal gland
    b. tissue
    b. tissue of Jacoby
    b. tissue movement
    b. of uterus
    vermilion b.
    vertebral b. of scapula
    zygomatic b. of greater wing of
      sphenoid bone
Bores twist fixation ring
Borggreve
    B. limb rotation
    B. method
Borggreve-Hall technique
Borg treadmill exertion scale
boric acid solution
boron neutron-capture therapy
Borrmann gastric cancer classification
Borthen iridostasis operation
Bose
    B. nail fold excision
    B. procedure
Bosniak classification
Bossalino blepharoplasty operation
bosselation
Boston Advance conditioning solution
Bosworth
    B. approach
    B. bone peg insertion
    B. femoroischial transplantation
    B. fracture
    B. spinal fusion
    B. tendo calcaneus repair
both-bone fracture
both-column fracture
Böttcher
    B. canal
    B. space

bottle
    Mariotte b.
    b. operation
botulinum A toxin
Bouchut
    B. laryngeal tube
    B. respiration
bougienage technique
Bouin fixative solution
bounce point
boundary
    air/bone/tissue b.
Bourdon
    B. tube
    B. tube pressure gauge
boutonnière
    b. deformity
    b. hand dislocation
    b. incision
Bovero muscle
Bovie
    B. cauterization
    B. coagulation
bovine
    b. dialyzable leukocyte extract
    b. graft
    b. lavage extract surfactant
    b. pericardial heart valve xenograft
bowel
    b. bypass
    b. bypass syndrome
    b. dilation
    loop of b.
    b. loop
    b. movement
    Noble surgical plication of b.
    b. perforation
    b. preparation
    b. refashioning procedure
    b. resection
    b. stoma
    b. wall hematoma
Bowen
    B. cavity primer
    B. patch
    B. suction
Bower PEG tube
Bowers technique
bowing
    b. deformity
    b. fracture
    b. of mitral valve leaflet

bowleg deformity
Bowles technique
bowl fistula
Bowman
    B. gland
    B. membrane
    B. operation
    B. space
    B. tube
bow-tie
    b.-t. knot
    b.-t. stitch
boxer fracture
Box technique
Boyce
    longitudinal nephrotomy of B.
    B. modification of Sengstaken-Blakemore tube
    B. position
Boyce-Vest procedure
Boyd
    B. ankle amputation
    B. approach
    B. classification
    B. dual onlay bone graft
    B. hip disarticulation
    B. operation
    B. point
Boyd-Anderson
    B.-A. biceps tendon repair
    B.-A. technique
Boyd-Bosworth procedure
Boyden
    B. chamber technique
    B. sphincter
Boyd-Griffin trochanteric fracture classification
Boyd-Ingram-Bourkhard treatment
Boyd-McLeod
    B.-M. procedure
    B.-M. tennis elbow technique
Boyd-Sisk
    B.-S. approach
    B.-S. posterior capsulorrhaphy
    B.-S. procedure
Boyer bursa
Boyes brachioradialis transfer technique
Boytchev procedure
Bozeman
    B. operation
    B. position

NOTES

Bozeman *(continued)*
    B. suture
    B. suture technique
BP
    bronchopleural
    bronchopulmonary
    BP fistula
BPCF
    bronchopleurocutaneous fistula
BPD
    bronchopulmonary dysplasia
Braasch bulb technique
brachia (*pl. of* brachium)
brachial
    b. anesthesia
    b. arteriotomy
    b. artery
    b. artery approach
    b. fascia
    b. gland
    b. lymph nodes
    b. muscle
    b. plexus
    b. plexus block
    b. plexus block anesthetic
       technique
    b. plexus infiltration
    b. plexus repair
    b. plexus traction injury
brachialis muscle
brachioaxillary bridge graft fistula
brachiocephalic
    b. trunk
    b. veins
    b. vessel angioplasty
brachioradialis
    b. flap
    b. muscle
brachioradial muscle
brachiosubclavian bridge graft fistula
brachium, pl. **brachia**
Bracht maneuver
Bracht-Wachter
    B.-W. body
    B.-W. lesion
brachybasocamptodactyly
brachybasophalangia
brachycheilia
brachydactyly
brachyfacial
brachygnathia
brachymorphic
brachypellic pelvis
brachyprosopic
brachyrhinia
brachyrhynchus
brachystaphyline
brachysyndactyly

brachytherapy
    endobronchial b.
    interstitial b.
bracing
    external b.
    fracture b.
bracket
    b. modification
    b. slot angulation
Brackett-Osgood posterior approach
Brackett-Osgood-Putti-Abbott technique
Brackett osteotomy
Brackin
    B. incision
    B. technique
    B. ureterointestinal anastomosis
Bradford
    B. fracture frame
    B. fusion
Bradley method of prepared childbirth
Brady-Jewett technique
Bragg peak proton-beam therapy
Brahms procedure
braided
    b. Ethibond suture
    b. Mersilene suture
    b. Nurolon suture
    b. nylon suture
    b. polyamide suture
    b. silk suture
    b. Vicryl suture
    b. wire suture
braid-like lesion
Brailey operation
brain
    b. biopsy
    compression of b.
    b. concussion
    b. congestion
    b. contusion
    b. edema
    b. herniation
    b. infection
    b. laceration
    b. lesion
    b. mass
    b. metastasis
    b. natriuretic peptide (BNP)
    b. puncture
    respirator b.
    b. revascularization
    b. stem evoked response
    b. stimulation
    b. temperature
    b. transplantation
    b. tumor
    b. tumor headache
brain-dead patient

brainstem
    b. compression
    b. hemorrhage
Brain Tumor Registry
braking radiation
Bralon suture
branch
    acetabular b.
    acromial b. of suprascapular artery
    acromial b. of thoracoacromial
      artery
    anterior basal b.
    anterior cutaneous b. of
      iliohypogastric nerve
    anterior cutaneous b.'s of
      intercostal nerves
    articular b.'s
    ascending b.
    ascending anterior b.
    ascending b. of the inferior
      mesenteric artery
    ascending posterior b.
    auricular b. of occipital artery
    basal tentorial b. of internal
      carotid artery
    buccal b.'s of facial nerve
    calcarine b. of medial occipital
      artery
    capsular b.'s of renal artery
    carotid sinus b.
    caudate b.'s
    celiac b.'s of vagus nerve
    cervical b. of facial nerve
    clavicular b. of thoracoacromial
      artery
    communicating b.'s of spinal
      nerves
    communicating b.'s of sympathetic
      trunk
    deep b. of the lateral plantar
      nerve
    deep b. of the medial femoral
      circumflex artery
    deep b. of the medial plantar
      artery
    deep palmar b. of ulnar artery
    deep plantar b. of dorsalis pedis
      artery
    deep b. of the radial nerve
    deep b. of the transverse cervical
      artery
    deep b. of the ulnar nerve

    deltoid b.
    descending anterior b.
    descending b. of occipital artery
    descending posterior b.
    digastric b. of facial nerve
    dorsal lingual b.'s of lingual artery
    dorsal b. of the lumbar artery
    dorsal b. of the posterior
      intercostal arteries 3–11
    dorsal b. of the posterior
      intercostal veins 4–11
    dorsal b. of the subcostal artery
    dorsal b. of the superior intercostal
      artery
    dorsal b. of the ulnar nerve
    epiploic b.'s
    esophageal b.'s of the inferior
      thyroid artery
    esophageal b.'s of the left gastric
      artery
    esophageal b.'s of the thoracic
      aorta
    esophageal b.'s of the vagus nerve
    external b. of accessory nerve
    external b. of superior laryngeal
      nerve
    faucial b.'s of lingual nerve
    femoral b. of genitofemoral nerve
    frontal b. of superficial temporal
      artery
    ganglionic b. of internal carotid
      artery
    ganglionic b.'s of lingual nerve
    ganglionic b.'s of maxillary nerve
    gastric b.'s of anterior vagal trunk
    gastric b.'s of posterior vagal b.
    genital b. of genitofemoral nerve
    genital b. of iliohypogastric nerve
    glandular b.'s
    glandular b.'s of facial artery
    glandular b.'s of inferior thyroid
      artery
    glandular b.'s of submandibular
      ganglion
    hepatic b.'s of vagus nerve
    iliac b. of iliolumbar artery
    inferior cervical cardiac b.'s of
      vagus nerve
    inferior labial b.'s of mental nerve
    inferior b. of pubic bone
    inferior b. of superior gluteal
      artery

B

NOTES

branch *(continued)*

inferior b.'s of transverse cervical nerve

infrahyoid b. of superior thyroid artery

infrapatellar b. of saphenous nerve

inguinal b.'s of external pudendal arteries

internal b. of accessory nerve

internal b. of superior laryngeal nerve

joint b.'s

lateral basal b.

lateral calcaneal b.'s of sural nerve

lateral costal b. of internal thoracic artery

lateral cutaneous b.

lateral cutaneous b.'s of intercostal nerves

lateral mammary b.'s

lateral nasal b.'s of anterior ethmoidal nerve

lateral orbitofrontal b.

b. lesion

lingual b.'s

lingual b. of facial nerve

lingular b.

lumbar b. of iliolumbar artery

mammary b.'s

marginal mandibular b. of facial nerve

marginal tentorial b. of internal carotid artery

mastoid b. of occipital artery

mastoid b.'s of posterior auricular artery

medial calcaneal b.'s of tibial nerve

medial cutaneous b.

medial mammary b.'s

medial nasal b.'s of anterior ethmoidal nerve

mediastinal b.'s

mediastinal b.'s of thoracic aorta

meningeal b. of internal carotid artery

meningeal b. of mandibular nerve

meningeal b. of occipital artery

meningeal b. of ophthalmic nerve

meningeal b. of spinal nerves

meningeal b. of vagus nerve

mental b.'s of mental nerve

middle lobe b.

middle meningeal b. of maxillary nerve

occipital b.

omental b.'s

orbital b. of middle meningeal artery

orbital b.'s of pterygopalatine ganglion

ovarian b. of uterine artery

b. pad

palmar b. of median nerve

palmar b. of ulnar nerve

palpebral b.'s of infratrochlear nerve

pancreatic b.'s

parietal b.

parietal b. of medial occipital artery

parietal b. of middle meningeal artery

parietal b. of superficial temporal artery

parotid b.'s

pectoral b.'s of thoracoacromial artery

perforating b.'s of internal thoracic artery

pericardial b. of phrenic nerve

pericardial b.'s of thoracic aorta

petrosal b. of middle meningeal artery

pharyngeal b.'s

pharyngeal b. of descending palatine artery

pharyngeal b. of glossopharyngeal nerve

pharyngeal b. of inferior thyroid artery

pharyngeal b. of pterygopalatine ganglion

pharyngeal b. of vagus nerve

phrenicoabdominal b.'s of phrenic nerve

posterior basal b.

posterior b. of great auricular nerve

posterior b. of lateral cerebral sulcus

posterior b. of obturator artery

posterior b. of obturator nerve

posterior b. of recurrent ulnar artery

posterior b. of renal artery

posterior b. of right branch of portal vein

posterior b. of right hepatic duct

posterior b. of spinal nerves

posterior b. of superior thyroid artery

pterygoid b.'s of maxillary artery

pubic b. of inferior epigastric artery

pubic b. of obturator artery
recurrent meningeal b. of spinal
nerves
renal b. of lesser splanchnic b.
renal b.'s of vagus nerve
right b. of portal vein
right b. of proper hepatic artery
saphenous b. of descending
genicular artery
sectorial b.
b.'s of segmental bronchi
sinoatrial nodal b. of right
coronary artery
b. to sinoatrial node
splenic b.'s of splenic artery
sternal b.'s of internal thoracic
artery
stylohyoid b. of facial nerve
subscapular b.'s of axillary artery
superficial b. of the lateral plantar
nerve
superficial b. of the medial plantar
artery
superficial palmar b. of radial
artery
superficial b. of the radial nerve
superficial b. of the superior
gluteal artery
superficial b. of the ulnar nerve
superior cervical cardiac b.'s of
vagus nerve
superior labial b.'s of infraorbital
nerve
superior laryngeal nerve external b.
superior b. of the pubic bone
superior b. of the superior gluteal
artery
superior b. of the transverse
cervical nerve
suprahyoid b. of lingual artery
sympathetic b. to submandibular
ganglion
temporal b.'s of facial nerve
thoracic cardiac b.'s of vagus
nerve
thymic b.'s of internal thoracic
artery
tonsillar b. of the facial artery
tonsillar b.'s of glossopharyngeal
nerve
tracheal b.'s
b. to trigeminal ganglion

tubal b. of the uterine artery
ulnar communicating b. of
superficial radial nerve
ulnar b. of medial antebrachial
cutaneous nerve
ureteral b.'s
ureteric b.'s
ureteric b.'s of the ovarian artery
ureteric b.'s of the renal artery
ureteric b.'s of the testicular artery
zygomatic b.'s of facial nerve
zygomaticofacial b. of zygomatic
nerve
zygomaticotemporal b. of zygomatic
nerve
branched
b. calculus
b. vascular graft
branchial
b. anomaly
b. fistula
branching
b. canal
b. tubule formation
branchiomeric muscles
Brandt-Andrews maneuver
Brand tendon transfer technique
Brandy
B. scalp stretcher I, front closure
B. scalp stretcher II, rear closure
Brannon-Wickström technique
Brantigan procedure
Brantigan-Voshell procedure
Brasdor method
brassy body
Braun
B. anastomosis
B. procedure
B. shoulder tenotomy
Braune
B. canal
B. muscle
Braun-Jaboulay gastroenterostomy
Braun-Wangensteen graft
Brawley nasal suction tube
brawny
b. arm
b. induration
break point
breast
adenoma of b.
b. augmentation

NOTES

87

breast *(continued)*
- b. biopsy
- b. biopsy tissue
- b. bone
- B. Cancer Detection Demonstration Project
- b. carcinoma
- compression of b.
- b. cyst aspiration
- fibroadenoma of b.
- b. lesion
- male b.
- b. metastasis
- b. mucocele
- b. preservation
- b. reconstruction
- b. stimulation contraction test
- supernumerary b.

breast-conserving
- b.-c. method
- b.-c. procedure
- b.-c. surgery
- b.-c. technique

breath
- b. excretion test
- b. stacking

breathing
- apneustic b.
- b. bag
- Biot b.
- b. circuit
- continuous positive pressure b. (CPPB)
- intermittent positive pressure b. (IPPB)
- b. method
- negative inspiratory b.
- pattern of b.
- positive-negative pressure b. (PNPB)
- sign mechanism for ventilator b.
- spontaneous b.
- work of b. (WOB)

Brecher
- B. new methylene blue technique

Brecher-Cronkite
- B.-C. method
- B.-C. technique

breech
- b. extraction
- b. head

bregma

bregma-mentum projection

bregmatic
- b. fontanel

bregmatolambdoid arc

Brenner gastrojejunostomy technique

brephoplastic graft

Breschet
- B. bones
- B. canal
- B. hiatus

Brescia-Cimino
- B.-C. AV fistula
- B.-C. graft

Breslow thickness

Brethine injection

Bretschneider histidine tryptophan solution

Bretschneider-HTK cardioplegic solution

Brett bone graft

Brett-Campbell tibial osteotomy

Breuer-Hering inflation reflex

Brevibloc
- B. injection

brevis
- extensor carpi radialis b. (ECRB)
- extensor digitorum b.
- extensor pollicis b.
- extensor tensor pollicis b.

Brevital Sodium

Bricanyl injection

Bricker
- B. operation
- B. pouch
- B. procedure
- B. ureteroileostomy

Brickner position

bridge
- adhesive resin-bonded b.
- catheter-deflecting b.
- ceramometal implant b.
- colostomy b.
- conjugation b.
- extension b.
- Gaskell b.
- b. graft
- loop ostomy b.
- membrane b.
- B. operation
- b. pedicle flap
- b. pedicle flap operation
- b. plate fixation
- retention suture b.
- b. suture
- suture b.

bridgeless mask

bridge-like
- b.-l. lesion
- b.-l. septum

bridging syndesmophyte

bridle
- B. procedure
- b. suture

Briggs strabismus operation

Brightbill corneal cutting block

Bright disease
brightness modulation
brim
  pelvic b.
brine flotation method
Brinell hardness indenter point
Brisbane method
brisement therapy
Bristow-Helfet procedure
Bristow-May procedure
Bristow operation
brittle
  b. nail
  b. nail syndrome
broad
  b. fascia
  b. ligament hernia
broadband attenuation
Broadbent registration point
Broadbent-Woolf four-limb Z-plasty
broadest muscle of back
Broca
  B. basilar angle
  B. facial angle
  B. pouch
  B. visual plane
Brock
  B. infundibulectomy
  B. operation
  B. procedure
Brockenbrough
  B. technique
  B. transseptal commissurotomy
Brockhurst technique
Brockman
  B. incision
  B. procedure
Brockman-Nissen wrist arthrodesis
Brödel bloodless line
Broders classification
Brodie bursa
Brodie-Trendelenburg tourniquet test
Brodsky-Tullos-Gartsman approach
Broesike fossa
Bromage scale
bromide
  benzpyrinium b.
  decamethonium b.
  hexafluorenium b.
  pancuronium b.
  pipecuronium b.

  rocuronium b.
  vecuronium b.
bromidum
  benzstigminum b.
bromination
Bromley foreign body operation
bromocriptine dopaminergic medication
Brompton solution
Brom repair
bronchi (pl. of bronchus)
bronchia
bronchial
  b. adenocarcinoma
  b. adenoma
  b. arteries
  b. brush biopsy
  b. brushing
  b. carcinoma
  b. fracture
  b. glands
  b. inflammation
  b. inhalation challenge test
  b. mucous membrane
  b. respiration
  b. sleeve resection
  b. tract
  b. tubes
  b. veins
bronchial-associated lymphoid tissue
bronchiogenic
bronchiolar adenocarcinoma
bronchiole
  respiratory b.'s
  terminal b.
bronchioli (pl. of bronchiolus)
bronchioloalveolar adenocarcinoma
bronchiolopulmonary
bronchiolus, pl. bronchioli
  bronchioli respiratorii
  b. terminalis
bronchitis
bronchium
bronchoalveolar
bronchobiliary fistula
Broncho-Cath
  B.-C. double-lumen endotracheal
    tube
  B.-C. endobronchial tube
bronchocavernous respiration
bronchoconstriction
bronchodilatation
bronchodilation

NOTES

bronchoesophageal
   b. fistula
   b. muscle
bronchoesophagoscopy
bronchogenic
   b. adenocarcinoma
bronchomediastinal trunk
bronchoplasty
   balloon b.
bronchopleural (BP)
   b. fistula
   b. leak squeak
bronchopleurocutaneous fistula (BPCF)
bronchopneumonia
   sequestration b.
bronchoprovocation test
bronchopulmonary (BP)
   b. dysplasia (BPD)
   b. fistula
   b. foregut malformation
   b. lymph nodes
   b. segment
bronchorrhaphy
bronchoscope
   single-channel fiberoptic b.
bronchoscope-guided intubation
bronchoscopic needle biopsy
bronchoscopy
   b. anesthetic technique
   b. disposable suction tube
   fiberoptic b.
   flexible fiberoptic b.
   rigid b.
   ultrasound-guided b.
bronchospasm
   exercise-induced b.
bronchospirography
bronchospirometer
bronchospirometry
bronchostomy
bronchotomy
bronchotracheal
bronchovesicular
   b. respiration
bronchus, pl. bronchi
   ectatic b.
   eparterial b.
   hyparterial bronchi
   intermediate b.
   b. intermedius
   left main b.
   lobar bronchi
   bronchi lobares
   b. principalis dexter
   b. principalis sinister
   right main b.
   segmental b.

   b. segmentalis
   stem b.
Bronkephrine injection
Bronkhorst High Tec controller
Bronson foreign body removal
   operation
bronze wire suture
Brooke ileostomy
Brooker frame
Brooker-Wills nail
Brooks
   B. technique
   B. type fusion
Brooks-Jenkins atlantoaxial fusion
   technique
Brooks-Seddon transfer technique
Broomhead medial approach
Brophy operation
Broström
   B. injection technique
   B. procedure
brow
   b. fixation
   b. position
brow-anterior position
brow-down position
browlift
brown
   b. adipose tissue
   b. atrophy
   B. dietary method for colon
     preparation
   b. fat tumor
   b. induration of lung
   B. knee approach
   B. knee joint reconstruction
   B. lateral approach
   B. technique
   b. tumor of hyperparathyroidism
   B. and Wickham pressure profile
     method
Brown-Beard technique
brown-black lesion
Brown-Brenn technique
Brown-Dodge method
Browning vein
Brown-McHardy pneumatic mercury
   bougie dilation
Brown-Roberts-Wells
   B.-R.-W. base ring
   B.-R.-W. head frame
Brown-Sharp gauge suture
Brown-Wickham technique
brow-posterior position
brow-up position
Bruce bundle
Bruch membrane
Bruecke tube

Bruger
    cul-de-sac of B.
Bruhat
    B. laser fimbrioplasty
    B. technique
Bruhn method
bruit
Bruner approach
Brunner glands
Brunn nests
Brunschwig operation
Bruser
    B. knee approach
    B. lateral approach
    B. skin incision
    B. technique
brush
    b. biopsy
    b. technique filling
brush-border
    b.-b. membrane
    b.-b. membrane vesicle
brushing
    bronchial b.
brusque dilatation of esophagus
Bryan
    B. arthroplasty
    B. procedure
Bryan-Morrey
    B.-M. elbow approach
    B.-M. extensive posterior approach
    B.-M. technique
BSA
    body surface area
B-scan frame
B&S gauge suture
BTF-37 arterial blood filter
bubble
    b. jar
    b. oxygenation
    b. oxygenator
bubbly bone lesion
bucca
buccal
    b. aspect
    b. branches of facial nerve
    b. cavity
    b. fat pad
    b. lymph node
    b. mucosal flap
    b. mucosal patch graft
    b. nerve

b. ostectomy
b. restoration
b. smear for sex chromatin
    evaluation
b. space
b. space abscess
b. space infection
b. surface
b. transmucosal delivery
b. tube
buccinator
    b. artery
    b. crest
    b. muscle
    b. nerve
    b. node
    b. plication
    b. space
buccolingual
    b. plane
    b. relation
bucconeural duct
bucco-occlusal line angle
buccopharyngeal
    b. approach
    b. fascia
    b. space
Buck
    B. extension frame
    B. fascia
    B. method
bucket-handle
    b.-h. fracture
    b.-h. incision
    b.-h. tear
Buck-Gramcko
    B.-G. pollicization
    B.-G. technique
buckle fracture
bucrylate
Bucy-Frazier suction tube
Bucy suction tube
Budde halo ring
Budin-Chandler method
Budinger blcpharoplasty operation
buffered saline solution
buffer solution
Bugg-Boyd technique
Buie
    B. position
    B. rectal suction tube
built-in angulation

NOTES

Buist method
bulb
    b. of corpus spongiosum
    b. deformity
    duodenal b.
    irrigation b.
    jugular b.
    b. of jugular vein
    jugular venous b.
    b. of penis
    Rouget b.
    self-inflating b.
    b. suction
    b. suture
    b. tip retrograde study
    b. of urethra
    b. of vestibule
bulbar
    b. cephalic pain tractotomy
    b. tractotomy
bulbi
    endothelium camerae anterioris b.
bulbocavernosus
    b. fat flap
    b. fat pad
    b. muscle
bulboid
bulbourethral
    b. gland
bulbous internal auditory canal
bulboventricular tube
bulbus
    b. penis
    b. urethrae
    b. venae jugularis
    b. vestibuli vaginae
bulk
    b. graft
    b. pack technique
    tumor b.
bulkhead method
bulldog head
bullectomy
    transaxillary apical b.
bullous
    b. edema
    b. edema vesicae
    b. granulomatous inflammation
    b. skin lesion
bull's-eye macular lesion
bullular canal
bumper fracture
bunching maneuver
Buncke technique
bundle
    anterior ground b.
    anteromedial b.
    arcuate nerve fiber b.

Arnold b.
atrioventricular b.
A-V b.
Bachmann b.
b. bone
b. branch reentry
Bruce b.
cingulum b.
coherent b.
commissural b.
b. of Drualt
Drualt b.
fiber b.
b. fiber
fiberoptic b.
Gierke respiratory b.
Held b.
Helweg b.
b. of His
His b.
Hoche b.
IG b.
image guide b.
inferior arcuate b.
intermediate b.
b. of Itis
James b.
Keith b.
Kent b.
Kent-His b.
Killian b.
Krause respiratory b.
lateral ground b.
LG b.
light guide b.
Lissauer b.
Loewenthal b.
maculopapillary b.
maculopapular b.
Mahaim b.
main b.
master IG b.
medial forebrain b.
medial longitudinal b.
medial neurovascular b.
Meynert retroflex b.
microfilament b.
Monakow b.
neovascular b.
nerve fiber b.
neurovascular b.
olfactory b.
olivocochlear b.
papillomacular nerve fiber b.
paracentral nerve fiber b.
Pick b.
posterior longitudinal b.
posterolateral b.

precommissural b.
predorsal b.
principal fiber b.
Rathke b.'s
Schütz b.
sensory nerve fiber b.
solitary b.
b. of Stanley Kent
superior arcuate b.
superior gluteal neurovascular b.
Thorel b.
Türck b.
vascular b.
Vicq d'Azyr b.
bundle-branch
  b.-b. block
  b.-b. reentrant tachycardia
Bunge amputation
bunion
  b. deformity
  b. formation
bunionectomy
  Akin b.
  Austin b.
  chevron b.
  DuVries-Mann modified b.
  Hauser b.
  Joplin b.
  Keller b.
  Kreuscher b.
  Lapidus b.
  Ludloff b.
  Mayo-Heuter b.
  McBride b.
  Peabody-Mitchell b.
  Reverdin b.
  Reverdin-Laird b.
  Reverdin-McBride b.
  Silver b.
  tailor b.
  tricorrectional b.
  Wilson b.
bunk-bed fracture
Bunnell
  B. atraumatic technique
  B. crisscross suture
  B. figure-eight suture
  B. modification of Steindler
    flexorplasty
  B. opponensplasty
  B. solution
  B. stitch

B. tendon repair
B. tendon transfer technique
Bunnell-Williams procedure
bupivacaine
  b. hydrochloride
  hyperbaric b.
  meperidine with b.
buprenorphine
  b. hydrochloride
  b. narcotic analgesic therapy
Burch
  B. bladder suspension
  B. bladder suspension method
  B. bladder suspension procedure
  B. bladder suspension technique
  B. colpourethropexy
  B. eye evisceration operation
  B. modification
Burdach tract
burden
  tumor b.
**Burger technique for scapulothoracic
  disarticulation**
Burgess
  B. below-knee amputation
  B. method
  B. technique
buried
  b. flap
  b. lock suture
  b. mass far-and-near suture
    technique
  b. penis
Burkhalter
  B. modification of Stiles-Bunnell
    technique
  B. transfer technique
**Burkhalter-Reyes method of phalangeal
  fracture**
burn
  b. boutonnière deformity
  corneal alkali b.
  first degree b.
  full-thickness b.
  irrigation b.
  partial-thickness b.
  plaster cast application b.
  radiation b.
  second degree b.
  superficial b.
  third degree b.

NOTES

burned
> body surface b.

Burnet-Talmadge-Lederberg theory of antibody formation

Burnett syndrome

burning
> b. dysesthesia
> b. pain

burn-out procedure

Burns
> space of B.
> B. space

Burns-Haney incision

Burow
> B. flap operation
> B. quantitative method
> B. solution
> B. triangle
> B. vein

Burr corneal ring

Burron Discofix stopcock

Burrows technique

bursa, pl. **bursae**
> Achilles b.
> b. achillis
> b. of acromion
> b. anserina
> anserine b.
> anterior tibial b.
> bicipitoradial b.
> b. bicipitoradialis
> Boyer b.
> Brodie b.
> Calori b.
> coracobrachial b.
> deep infrapatellar b.
> Fleischmann b.
> b. of gastrocnemius
> gluteofemoral b.
> gluteus medius bursae
> gluteus minimus b.
> b. of great toe
> b. of hyoid
> iliac b.
> b. iliopectinea
> iliopectineal b.
> inferior b. of biceps femoris
> infrahyoid b.
> b. infrahyoidea
> b. infrapatellaris profunda
> infraspinatus b.
> intermuscular gluteal b.
> b. intermuscularis musculorum gluteorum
> b. intratendinea olecrani
> b. ischiadica musculi glutei maximi
> b. ischiadica musculi obturatoris interni

ischial b.
laryngeal b.
lateral malleolar subcutaneous b.
lateral malleolus b.
b. of latissimus dorsi
medial malleolar subcutaneous b.
b. of Monro
b. mucosa
b. musculi bicipitis femoris superior
b. musculi coracobrachialis
b. musculi extensoris carpi radialis brevis
b. musculi piriformis
b. musculi semimembranosi
b. musculi tensoris veli palatini
b. of obturator internus
b. of olecranon
omental b.
b. omentalis
ovarian b.
b. ovarica
b. of the piriformis muscle
b. of popliteus
prepatellar b.
b. quadrati femoris
radial b.
retrocalcaneal b.
retrohyoid b.
b. retrohyoidea
sartorius bursae
b. of semimembranosus muscle
subacromial b.
b. subacromialis
subcoracoid b.
b. subcutanea acromialis
b. subcutanea calcanea
b. subcutanea infrapatellaris
b. subcutanea malleoli lateralis
b. subcutanea malleoli medialis
b. subcutanea olecrani
b. subcutanea prepatellaris
b. subcutanea prominentiae laryngeae
b. subcutanea trochanterica
b. subcutanea tuberositatis tibiae
subcutaneous acromial b.
subcutaneous calcaneal b.
subcutaneous infrapatellar b.
subcutaneous b. of the laryngeal prominence
subcutaneous b. of lateral malleolus
subcutaneous b. of medial malleolus
subcutaneous olecranon b.
subcutaneous b. of tibial tuberosity
subdeltoid b.
b. subdeltoidea

b. subfascialis prepatellaris
subfascial prepatellar b.
subhyoid b.
sublingual b.
b. sublingualis
subscapular b.
b. subtendineae musculi gastrocnemii
bursae subtendineae musculi sartorii
b. subtendinea iliaca
b. subtendinea musculi bicipitis femoris inferior
b. subtendinea musculi infraspinati
b. subtendinea musculi latissimus dorsi
b. subtendinea musculi obturatoris interni
b. subtendinea musculi subscapularis
b. subtendinea musculi teretis majoris
b. subtendinea musculi tibialis anterioris
b. subtendinea musculi trapezii
b. subtendinea musculi tricipitus brachii
b. subtendinea prepatellaris
subtendinous b. of gastrocnemius muscle
subtendinous iliac b.
subtendinous prepatellar b.
subtendinous b. of the tibialis anterior muscle
superior b. of biceps femoris
suprapatellar b.
b. suprapatellaris
synovial b.
b. synovialis
b. tendinis calcanei
b. of tendo calcaneus
b. of tensor veli palatini muscle
b. of teres major
tibial intertendinous b.
b. of trapezius
triceps b.
trochanteric b.
bursae trochantericae musculi glutei medii
b. trochanterica musculi glutei maximi
b. trochanterica musculi glutei minimi
trochlear synovial b.
ulnar b.
bursa-equivalent tissue
bursal
b. projection
b. sac
b. tissue
bursectomy
burst fracture
bursting dislocation
burst-type laceration
Burton line
Burwell-Scott modification of Watson-Jones incision
butabarbital
butacaine
b. sulfate
butalbital
butamben
butane
butanol-extractable
b.-e. iodine
Butchart staging classification
butethal
butethamine hydrochloride
Butler
B. fifth toe operation
B. procedure to correct overlapping toes
B. tonsillar suction tube
butorphanol tartrate
butter
b. of bismuth
butterfly
b. flap
b. fracture
b. fracture fragment
b. patch
buttocks
b. pad
button
belly b.
b. one-step gastrostomy
b. suture
b. technique
buttonhole
b. approach
b. deformity
b. fracture
b. incision
b. iridectomy
buttressing in internal fixation

NOTES

butyl
    b. aminobenzoate
butyrophenone
Buxton bolus suture technique
Buyes air-vent suction tube
Buzard-Thornton fixation ring
Buzzard maneuver
Buzzi operation
B-V-M
    bag-valve-mask
B-W graft
Byers flap
bypass
    Alden loop gastric b.
    b. anesthesia
    aortofemoral b.
    aortoiliac b.
    aortorenal b.
    bowel b.
    cardiac b. (CBP)
    cardiopulmonary b.
    extra-anatomic b.
    extracorporeal venous b.
    extracranial-intracranial b.
    femoral-tibial-peroneal b.

    femoropopliteal b.
    gastric b.
    b. graft
    b. graft catheterization
    jejunoileal b. (JIB)
    loop gastric b.
    b. method
    nonanatomic renal b.
    b. operation
    partial ileal b.
    b. procedure
    Roux-en-Y gastric b.
    saphenous vein b.
    in situ b.
    b. surgery
    b. technique
    b. tract
    venovenous b. (VVB)
    venovenous extracorporeal b.
Byrd-Drew method
Byron
    B. Smith ectropion operation
    B. Smith lazy-T correction
Bywaters lesion
Byzantine arch palate

C

C graft
C sliding osteotomy
C2-C3 cervical disk excision
CABG ˋ
coronary artery bypass graft
coronary artery bypass grafting
CABG anesthesia
redo CABG
cable
c. graft
c. wire suture
Cabot-Nesbit orchiopexy
Cabot ring
Cabral coronary reconstruction
cachexia exophthalmica
CACT
celite-activated clotting time
cadaver
c. graft
c. renal preservation
CADD PCA device
CAF
coronary artery fistula
caffeine
c. and halothane contracture test
(CHCT)
cage
thoracic c.
Cairns
C. maneuver
C. operation
C. trabeculectomy
Cajal
C. formol ammonium bromide
solution
C. gold-sublimate method
C. uranium silver method
Calandriello procedure
Calandruccio fixation
calcaneal
c. apophysitis
c. arterial network
c. arteries
c. avulsion fracture
c. bone
c. displaced fracture
c. fracture reduction
c. inclination angle
c. L osteotomy
c. process of cuboid bone
c. region
c. spur syndrome
c. sulcus
c. tendon

c. tenodesis
c. tuber
c. tubercle
calcaneal-second metatarsal angle
inclination angle
calcanean tendon
calcaneoastragaloid
calcaneocavovarus deformity
calcaneocavus deformity
calcaneocuboid articulation
calcaneonavicular
c. bar resection
calcaneoscaphoid
calcaneotibial
c. fusion
calcaneovalgus deformity
calcaneovarus deformity
calcaneum
calcaneus
calcar
c. femorale
c. pedis
calcareous
c. degeneration of cornea
c. infiltration
c. metastasis
calcarine
c. artery
c. branch of medial occipital
artery
calces (*pl. of* calx)
Calciferol injection
calcification
c. line
c. lines of Retzius
c. zone
calcified
c. granulomatous inflammation
c. lesion
c. liver metastasis
c. renal mass
calcifying metastasis
calciotraumatic line
calcipexy
Calcitite bone graft
calcium
c. alginate
c. entry blocker
c. entry blocking drug
c. hydroxide
calculous formation
calculus, pl. calculi
apatite c.
biliary c.
bladder calculi

calculus *(continued)*
    blood c.
    branched c.
    caliceal diverticular c.
    cat's eye c.
    cerebral c.
    combination c.
    coral c.
    cystine c.
    dendritic c.
    encysted c.
    fibrin c.
    gastric c.
    hard c.
    hemic c.
    infection c.
    intestinal c.
    matrix c.
    c. migration
    mulberry c.
    nephritic c.
    oxalate c.
    pancreatic c.
    pleural c.
    pocketed c.
    preputial c.
    primary renal c.
    prostatic c.
    renal c.
    secondary renal c.
    staghorn c.
    struvite c.
    urethral c.
    urinary c.
    vesical c.
    weddellite c.
    whewellite c.
Caldwell-Coleman flatfoot technique
Caldwell-Luc
    C.-L. approach
    C.-L. incision
    C.-L. operation
    C.-L. window procedure
Caldwell-Moloy
    C.-M. classification
    C.-M. method
Caldwell projection
calf
    c. bone
    c. lung surfactant extract
    c. pump
Calhoun-Hagler lens extraction
  operation
calibrated electrical stimulation
calibration
    c. of the cardia
    c. curve

    oscillometric c.
    c. overshoot
caliceal
    c. abnormality
    c. diverticular calculus
    c. diverticulum
    c. extension
    c. fornix
    c. infundibulum
    c. nephrostolithotomy
calicectasis
calicectomy
calices (*pl. of* calix)
caliciform
calicine
calicoplasty
calicotomy
caliectasis
caliectomy
caligation
calioplasty
caliorrhaphy
caliotomy
calix, pl. **calices**
    major calices
    minor calices
    c. puncture
    calices renales majores
    calices renales minores
Callahan
    C. approach
    C. extension of cervical injury
    C. fusion technique
    C. operation
    C. root canal filling method
Callander amputation
Callender cell type classification
callosal disconnection syndrome
callosomarginal artery
callosotomy
    corpus c.
callus
    c. formation
    fracture c.
    irritation c.
Calori bursa
caloric
    c. expenditure
    c. irrigation
calorimetry
Calot triangle
Caluso
    C. PEG gastrostomy tube
    C. PEG tube
calvaria, pl. **calvariae**
calvarial
calvarium
calx, pl. **calces**

calyceal
    c. fistula
calycectomy
calyces (*pl. of* calyx)
calyciform
calycine
calycle
calycoplasty
calycotomy
calyoplasty
calyorrhaphy
calyotomy
calyx, pl. calyces
Cambridge classification
cameral fistula
Cameron femoral component removal
Camey
    C. enterocystoplasty
    C. enterocystoplasty urinary
    diversion
    C. I, II operation
    C. ileocystoplasty
    C. procedure
    C. urinary pouch
Camino
    C. catheter technique
    C. intracranial pressure monitoring
    device
Camitz technique
Campbell
    C. interpositional arthroplasty
    C. onlay bone graft
    C. osteotomy
    C. posterior shoulder approach
    C. posterolateral approach
    C. resection arthroplasty
    C. screw fixation
    C. technique
    C. triceps reflection
Campbell-Akbarnia procedure
Campbell-Goldthwait procedure
Camper
    C. chiasm
    C. fascia
    C. ligament
    C. line
    C. plane
Camp-Gianturco method
camphorated phenol
Campodonico
    C. canal
    C. operation

campotomy
camptomelic syndrome
camsylate
    trimetaphan c.
    trimethaphan c.
Canadian Cardiovascular Society
   classification
canal
    abdominal c.
    accessory palatine c.
    accessory root c.
    acoustic c.
    additional c.
    adductor c.
    Alcock c.
    alimentary c.
    alveolar c.
    ampulla of lacrimal c.
    anal c.
    anterior condylar c.
    anterior condyloid c. of occipital
    bone
    anterior semicircular c.'s
    anterior vertical c.
    antropyloric c.
    c. of Arantius
    Arnold c.
    c. of Arnold
    atrioventricular c.
    auditory c.
    auxiliary c.
    basipharyngeal c.
    bayonet c.
    bayonet-curved c.
    Bernard c.
    Bichat c.
    birth c.
    blunderbuss apical c.
    bony c.
    bony semicircular c.'s
    Böttcher c.
    branching c.
    Braune c.
    Breschet c.
    bulbous internal auditory c.
    bullular c.
    Campodonico c.
    carotid c.
    cartilage c.
    caudal c.
    central c. of spinal cord
    cervical c.

C

NOTES

canal (*continued*)
cervicoaxillary c.
ciliary c.
Cloquet c.
collateral pulp c.
common c.
condylar c.
cortical bone primary c.
Cotunnius c.
C-shaped c.
c. curvature
curved c.
c. of Cuvier
c. débridement
defalcated root c.
deferent c.
dehiscent mandibular c.
dental c.
dentinal c.
dilacerated c.
diploic c.'s
Dorello c.
Dupuytren c.
ear c.
endocervical c.
epidermoanal c.
ethmoid c.
external auditory c.
facial c.
fallopian c.
femoral c.
Ferrein c.
filling c.
Fontana c.
furcation c.
galactophorous c.'s
Gartner c.
gastric c.
gubernacular c.
Guyon c.
Hannover c.
haversian c.
Hensen c.
c. of Hering
Hirschfeld c.
His c.
horizontal c.
Hovius c.
Hoyer c.'s
c. of Huguier
Huguier c.
humeral c.
Hunter c.
hyaloid c.
hypoglossal c.
identifying c.
incisal c.
incisive c.

infraorbital c.
inguinal c.
c. innominate osteotomy
inoperable c.
interdental c.
interfacial c.
internal auditory c.
intramedullary c.
c. irrigation
Kovalevsky c.
lacrimal c.
Lambert c.
large c.
lateral c.
Lauth c.
locating c.
longitudinal c.'s of modiolus
Löwenberg c.
lumbar c.
lumbosacral c.
lymphatic c.
mandibular c.
maxillary c.
medullary c.
mental c.
mesiobuccal c.
musculotubal c.
nasal c.
nasolacrimal c.
neural c.
neurenteric c.
Nuck c.
nutrient c.
c. obturation
obturator c.
optic c.
orbital c.
overfilled c.
palatine c.
palatomaxillary c.
palatovaginal c.
pancreatobiliary c.
partial atrioventricular c.
parturient c.
pelvic c.
perivascular c.
persistent common
  atrioventricular c.
Petit c.
pharyngeal c.
plane of pelvic c.
pleuroperitoneal c.
posterior vertical c.
pterygoid c.
pterygopalatine c.
pudendal c.
pulmoaortic c.
pulp c.

pyloric c.
radicular c.
c. resonance response
Rivinus c.'s
root c.
ruffed c.
sacral c.
Santorini c.
Schlemm c.
c. of Schlemm
scleral c.
scleroticochoroidal c.
semicircular c.
sickle-shaped c.
Sondermann c.
sphenopalatine c.
spinal c.
c. of Stilling
straight c.
subsartorial c.
Sucquet c.
Sucquet-Hoyer c.
supplementary c.
supraciliary c.
supraoptic c.
supraorbital c.
talar c.
tarsal c.
temporal c.
Tourtual c.
tympanic c.
type I–IV c.
uniting c.
urogenital c.
uterovaginal c.
Van Hoorne c.
Velpeau c.
ventricular c.
Verneuil c.
vertebral c.
c. of Vesalius
vesicourethral c.
vestibular c.
vidian c.
Volkmann c.
vomerine c.
vomerobasilar c.
vomerorostral c.
vomerovaginal c.
Walther c.'s
Wirsung c.
zipped c.

Zuckerkandl perforating c.
zygomaticofacial c.
zygomaticotemporal c.
Canale
　　C. osteotomy
　　C. technique
canales (*pl. of* canalis)
canalicular
　　c. ducts
　　c. laceration
　　c. sphincter
canaliculi (*pl. of* canaliculus)
canaliculodacryocystostomy
canaliculodacryorhinostomy
canaliculorhinostomy
canaliculus, pl. **canaliculi**
　　auricular c.
　　biliary c.
　　c. innominatus
　　c. rod and suture
canalis, pl. **canales**
　　c. analis
　　c. carpi
　　c. centralis medullae spinalis
　　c. cervicis uteri
　　c. condylaris
　　canales diploici
　　c. femoralis
　　c. gastrici
　　c. gastricus
　　c. infraorbitalis
　　c. inguinalis
　　c. musculotubarius
　　c. nervi facialis
　　c. nervi petrosi superficialis
　　minoris
　　c. nutricius
　　c. obturatorius
　　c. pterygoideus
　　c. pudendalis
　　c. pyloricus
　　c. sacralis
　　c. umbilicalis
　　c. vertebralis
　　c. vomerorostralis
　　c. vomerovaginalis
canalith repositioning procedure
canalization
canaloplasty
canal-wall-up technique
cancellectomy
cancellization

C

NOTES

cancellous
- c. chip bone graft
- c. and cortical bone graft
- c. insert graft
- c. tissue

Cancell therapy

cancer
- appendiceal c.
- biliary tract c.
- c. body
- early gastric c.
- endobronchial c.
- endometrial c.
- extrahepatic bile duct c.
- fulguration in bladder c.
- hard palate c.
- head and neck c.
- International Union Against C. (UICC)
- islet cell c.
- c. juice
- nasal cavity c.
- c. pain
- peritoneal c.
- postgastrectomy c.
- soft palate c.
- C. Surveillance Program
- suture line c.
- Union Internationale Contre le C. (UICC)
- urologic system c.

canceration

cancerization
- field c.

candela lithotripsy

Candida **infection**

candidal infection

canine fossa

canister
- carbon dioxide absorption c.

Cannon point

cannulated nail

cannulation
- bile duct c.
- biliary c.
- c. of the biliary tree
- duct c.
- endoscopic retrograde c.
- endoscopic transpapillary c.
- ERCP c.
- ex vivo c.
- intravenous c.
- percutaneous arterial c.
- peripheral venous c.
- postsphincterotomy ERCP c.
- retrograde c.
- selective ductal c.
- transpapillary c.

- unilateral pedicle c.
- vascular c.

cannulization

canonical
- c. correlation
- c. univariate parameter

canthal

canthectomy

canthi (*pl. of* canthus)

cantholysis

canthomeatal line

canthopexy

canthoplasty
- Agnew c.
- Ammon c.
- Imre lateral c.

canthorrhaphy
- Elschnig c.

canthotomy
- external c.
- lateral c.

canthus, pl. canthi
- external c.
- internal c.
- lateral c.
- medial c.

cantilevered bone graft

Cantlie line

Cantor
- C. intestinal tube
- C. tube

Cantwell-Ransley
- C.-R. epispadias repair
- C.-R. urethroplasty

cap
- corneal c.
- duodenal c.
- metanephric c.
- phrygian c.
- syringe c.

capacity
- exercise c.
- forced expiratory c.
- functional residual c. (FRC)
- maximum breathing c. (MBC)

Capello technique

Capener
- C. lateral rhachotomy
- C. nail

Cape Town technique

capillaroscopy
- nail fold c.

capillary
- c. angioma
- c. arteriole
- c. dilation
- c. drainage
- c. endothelium

c. fracture
c. hemangioma of eyelid
c. hyperfiltration
c. malformation
c. vein
c. wedge pressure
capillus, pl. **capilli**
Capiox-E bypass system oxygenator
Capiox hollow flow oxygenator
capita (*pl. of* caput)
capital
c. femoral epiphysis
c. fragment
c. operation
capitate
c. bone
c. fracture
capitation
capitellar fracture
capitellocondylar total elbow arthroplasty
capitellum
Hahn-Steinthal fracture of c.
Kocher-Lorenz fracture of c.
capitonnage suture
capitopedal
capitular
c. epiphysis
c. joint
capitulum, pl. **capitula**
c. humeri
c. of humerus
c. radiale humeri fracture
capnograph
Nellcor N-2500 c.
capnography
spectral edge frequency c.
Capnomac
C. infrared analyzer
C. multiple gas analyzer
C. Ultima gas analyzer
C. Ultima sidestream spirometer
capnometer
Cardiocap c.
capnometry
volumetric c.
capping technique
CAPRI
Cardiopulmonary Research Institute
CAPRI program
Caprolactam suture
capsula, pl. **capsulae**

c. adiposa renis
c. articularis
c. articularis cricothyroidea
c. extrema
c. fibrosa glandulae thyroideae
c. fibrosa renis
c. lienis
capsular
c. branches of renal artery
c. exfoliation syndrome
c. fixation
c. flap pyeloplasty
c. imbrication
c. incision
c. interposition arthroplasty
c. ligament
c. shift procedure
c. space
c. support tissue
capsule
adipose c.
adrenal c.
articular c.
atrabiliary c.
Bonnet c.
cricothyroid articular c.
Crosby c.
Crosby-Kugler biopsy c.
exfoliation of lens c.
external c.
extreme c.
fatty renal c.
fibrous articular c.
fibrous c. of kidney
fibrous c. of liver
fibrous c. of parotid gland
fibrous c. of spleen
fibrous c. of thyroid gland
c. flap technique
c. forceps technique
Gerota c.
Glisson c.
glomerular c.
hepatic c.
joint c.
Müller c.
pseudoexfoliation of lens c.
suprarenal c.
tumor c.
capsulectomy

NOTES

capsulitis
  adhesive c.
  glenohumeral adhesive c.
capsuloplasty
  Zancolli c.
capsulorrhaphy
  Boyd-Sisk posterior c.
  duToit-Roux staple c.
  medial c.
  pants-over-vest c.
  posterior c.
  Rockwood posterior c.
  Roux-duToit staple c.
  staple c.
  Tibone posterior c.
capsulotomy
  anterior c.
  Castroviejo c.
  Curtis PIP joint c.
  Darling c.
  dorsal transverse c.
  dorsolateral and medial c.
  posterior c.
  renal c.
  triangular c.
  T-shaped c.
  Vannas c.
  Verhoeff-Chandler c.
capture
  c. cross section
  pacemaker c.
Capuron points
caput, pl. capita
  c. breve
  c. breve musculi bicipitis brachii
  c. breve musculi bicipitis femoris
  c. costae
  c. epididymidis
  c. epididymis
  c. femoris
  c. gallinaginis
  c. humerale
  c. humeri
  c. infraorbitale quadrati labii
    superioris
  c. laterale
  c. laterale musculi gastrocnemii
  c. laterale musculi tricipitis brachii
  c. longum
  c. longum musculi bicipitis brachii
  c. longum musculi bicipitis femoris
  c. longum musculi tricipitis brachii
  c. mallei
  c. mediale
  c. mediale musculi gastrocnemii
  c. mediale musculi tricipitis brachii
  c. obliquum
  c. ossis femoris

  c. pancreatis
  c. phalangis
  c. radiale
  c. radii
Carabelli endobronchial tube
carbamate
carbaril
carbetapentane citrate
carbidopa dopaminergic medication
Carbocaine
  C. injection
carbolfuchsin-methylene blue staining
  method
carbol-fuchsin solution
carbon
  c. dioxide (CO_2)
  c. dioxide absorption canister
  c. dioxide concentration
  c. dioxide dissociation curve
  c. dioxide elimination ($VECO_2$)
  c. dioxide fixation
  c. dioxide laser plaque ablation
  c. dioxide pressure
  c. dioxide response
  c. fiber graft
  c. gelatin mass
  c. monoxide (CO)
  c. tetrachloride-induced liver
    regeneration
carbonization
Carbo-Seal cardiovascular composite
  graft
carboxymethylcellulose
  benzocaine, gelatin, pectin, and
    sodium c.
carbuncle
  kidney c.
Carcassone perineal ligament
carcinogenesis
  foreign body c.
carcinoid
  nonappendiceal c.
  c. valve disease
carcinoma
  adnexal c.
  adrenal c.
  anorectal c.
  bile duct c.
  biliary c.
  bladder c.
  breast c.
  bronchial c.
  cecal c.
  cervical c.
  c. of cervix
  clear cell c. of kidney
  colon c.
  colonic c.

colorectal c.
duct c.
ductal c.
Dukes classification of c.
Edmondson grading system for
  hepatocellular c.
c. en cuirasse
endometrial c.
esophageal c.
ethmoid sinus c.
c. of eyelid
fallopian tube c.
false cord c.
follicular c.'s
gallbladder c.
gastric c.
gastrointestinal c.
genital c.
giant cell c. of thyroid gland
glandular c.
glottic c.
gynecological c.
hilar c.
large bowel c.
laryngeal c.
lung c.
maxillary sinus c.
meibomian gland c.
meningeal c.
metastatic c.
metastatic prostatic c.
metastatic renal cell c.
napkin-ring c.
nasopharyngeal c.
oat cell c.
orofacial c.
oropharyngeal c.
ovarian c.
pancreatic c.
parathyroid c.
parotid c.
penile c.
periampullary c.
pharyngeal wall c.
c. of prostate
prostatic c.
radiation-induced c.
rectal c.
renal c.
renal cell c.
renal pelvis c.
salivary duct c.

salivary gland c.
scar c.
sigmoid colon c.
signet-ring c.
sinonasal c.
c. in situ (CIS)
splenic flexure c.
stage B, C c.
terminal duct c.
testicular c.
thymic c.
thyroid c.
c. of uncertain primary site
urachal c.
ureteral c.
urethral c.
urothelial c.
uterine papillary serous c.
vaginal c.
vulvar c.
vulvovaginal c.
wolffian duct c.
carcinomatosis
  peritoneal c.
carcinosarcoma
Carden bronchoscopy tube
Cardene I.V.
cardia
  calibration of the c.
  gastric c.
cardiac
  c. anesthesia
  c. anesthetic
  c. anomaly
  c. bypass (CBP)
  c. catheterization
  c. compression
  c. decompression
  c. defibrillation
  c. dilatation
  c. dilation
  c. examination
  c. fibrillation
  c. fibrous skeleton
  c. glands of esophagus
  c. herniation
  c. impression of liver
  c. impression of lung
  c. irradiation
  c. lymphatic ring
  c. mass
  c. metastasis

C

NOTES

cardiac *(continued)*
    c. muscle wrap
    c. output (CO)
    c. part of stomach
    c. patch
    c. perforation
    c. plexus
    c. position
    c. resuscitation
    c. rupture
    c. segment
    c. surgery
    c. symphysis
    c. tumor
    c. tumor plop
    c. valvular malformation
    c. veins
cardiectomy
Cardiff resuscitation bag
cardinal
    c. ligament
    c. point
    c. position
    c. suture
Cardiocap capnometer
Cardio-Cool myocardial protection
  pouch
cardioesophageal
    c. relaxation
Cardioflon suture
cardiohepatic
cardiomyopathy
cardiomyoplasty
    dynamic c.
cardiomyotomy
    Heller c.
cardio-omentopexy
cardiopericardiopexy
    Beck c.
cardiopexy
    ligamentum teres c.
cardiophrenic angle mass
cardioplasty
cardioplegia
cardioplegic solution
cardiopressor reflex
cardioprotective effect
cardiopulmonary
    c. bypass
    c. complication
    c. manifestation
    c. resuscitation (CPR)
Cardiopulmonary Research Institute
  (CAPRI)
cardiorespiratory complication
cardiorrhaphy
cardiothoracic surgery
cardiotomy

cardiotoxic
    c. effect
    c. myolysis
cardiovalvotomy
cardiovalvulotomy
cardiovascular
    c. adverse effect
    c. anesthesia
    c. complication
    c. imaging technique
    c. malformation
    c. pressure
    c. Prolenc suture
    c. silk suture
    c. stability
cardiovasculorenal
cardioversion
cardiovert
care
    monitored anesthesia c. (MAC)
    c. and protection proceedings
CareDrape blanket
Carey Ranvier technique
caricarb
caries
    c. classification
carina
    c. tracheae
    c. urethralis vaginae
    urethral c. of vagina
    c. vaginae
carinal lymph nodes
carinate abdomen
carious
    c. pulp exposure
    c. restoration margin
Carlens
    C. double-lumen endotracheal tube
    C. endotracheal induction
Carlo Traverso maneuver
Carl Zeiss myringotomy tube
Carmeda BioActive surface
  extracorporeal circuit
C-arm fluoroscopy
Carmody-Batson operation
Carnesale
    C. acetabular extensile approach
    C. hip approach
    C. technique
Carnesale-Stewart-Barnes classification of
  hip dislocation
caro
    c. quadrata sylvii
Caroli-Sarles classification
Caroli syndrome
caroticoclinoid ligament
caroticotympanic arteries

carotid
>   c. ablative procedure
>   c. arterial blood flow
>   c. artery bifurcation
>   c. artery compression
>   c. artery dissection
>   c. body
>   c. body tumor
>   c. canal
>   c. circulation
>   c. ejection time
>   c. endarterectomy
>   external c.
>   c. foramen
>   c. ganglion
>   c. groove
>   c. preservation
>   c. preservation technique
>   c. sheath
>   c. sinus branch
>   c. space
>   c. sulcus
>   c. triangle
>   c. tubercle
>   c. wall of middle ear

carotid-basilar anastomosis
carotid-cavernous sinus fistula
carotid-dural fistula
carotid-vertebral
>   c.-v. anastomosis
>   c.-v. vein bypass graft

carpal
>   c. artery
>   c. bone stress fracture
>   c. compression test
>   c. synovectomy

carpectomy
>   distal-row c.
>   Omer-Capen c.
>   proximal-row c.

Carpentier
>   C. annuloplasty
>   C. ring
>   C. tricuspid valvuloplasty

carpet lesion
carpi (*pl. of* carpus)
carpocarpal
carpometacarpal
>   c. arthroplasty
>   c. articulation
>   c. fracture-dislocation

>   c. joint dislocation
>   c. joint fracture

carpopedal
Carpue method
carpus, pl. **carpi**
Carrel
>   C. aortic patch
>   C. aortic patch anastomosis
>   C. treatment
>   C. tube

Carrell
>   C. fibular substitution technique
>   C. resection

Carroll arthroplasty
Carstan reverse wedge osteotomy
Cartam-Treander reverse wedge osteotomy
Carter operation
cartilage
>   annular c.
>   arthrodial c.
>   articular c.
>   auricular c.
>   basilar c.
>   c. canal
>   connecting c.
>   costal c.
>   cuneiform c.
>   diarthrodial c.
>   ensiform c.
>   falciform c.
>   c. graft
>   hypsiloid c.
>   c. inflammation
>   interosseous c.
>   intervertebral c.
>   intra-articular c.
>   intrathyroid c.
>   investing c.
>   Jacobson c.
>   c.'s of larynx
>   Luschka c.
>   c. matrix
>   meatal c.
>   Meyer c.'s
>   Morgagni c.
>   Seiler c.
>   semilunar c.
>   sesamoid c. of larynx
>   sternal c.
>   supra-arytenoid c.
>   thyroid c.

NOTES

cartilage *(continued)*
    tracheal c.'s
    triangular c.
    triquetrous c.
    triticeal c.
    uniting c.
    Weitbrecht c.
    Wrisberg c.
    xiphoid c.
    Y c.
cartilaginous
    c. growth plate disorder
    c. loose body
    c. part of skeletal system
    c. septum
    c. tissue
cartilago, pl. **cartilagines**
    c. articularis
    c. auriculae
    c. costalis
    c. cricoidea
    cartilagines laryngis
    c. sesamoidea laryngis
    c. thyroidea
    cartilagines tracheales
    c. triticea
cartridge
    anesthesia c.
cartwheel fracture
caruncle
    Morgagni c.
    Santorini major c.
    Santorini minor c.
    urethral c.
caryothecae
    cisterna c.
Casanellas lacrimal operation
caseated tissue
caseating granulomatous inflammation
caseation
    c. necrosis
    tuberculous c.
case-by-case approach
caseous
    c. abscess
    c. inflammation
Casey operation
CaSki cell line
Caspar
    C. anterior plate fixation
    C. ring
Caspari repair
CASS
    coronary artery surgery study
Casselberry
    C. position
    C. sphenoid tube

Casser
    C. fontanel
    C. perforated muscle
cast
    c. application
    c. buccal tube
    c. immobilization
    c. removal
    c. wedge
Castaneda procedure
Castellani point
Castelli-Paparella collar button tube
casting ring
Castle procedure
Castle-Schneider resection interposition arthroplasty
cast-like tube
castrate
castration
    female c.
    functional c.
    male c.
    parasitic c.
Castroviejo
    C. capsulotomy
    C. iridectomy
    C. iridotomy
    C. keratectomy
    C. minikeratoplasty
    C. operation
    C. radial iridotomy
Castroviejo-Scheie cyclodiathermy operation
Catalano intubation set
cataract
    c. aspiration
    extracapsular extraction of c.
    c. extraction
    extraction of extracapsular c.
    extraction of intracapsular c.
    c. extraction operation
    flap operation c.
    c. formation
    hard c.
    intracapsular extraction of c.
    c. irradiation
    irradiation c.
    c. mask ring
    radiation c.
    reduplication c.
    ring-form congenital c.
    ring-shaped c.
    Soemmerring ring c.
    soft c.
    c. surgery
catarrhal
    c. inflammation
    c. marginal ulceration

caterpillar flap
catgut suture
catheter
    c. ablation
    c. dilation
    c. drainage
    c. embolectomy
    c. embolism
    c. entrapment
    c. exchange
    c. fixation
    c. fragment
    c. insertion
    c. instability
    c. introduction method
    c. kinking
    c. knotting
    c. malposition
    c. manipulation
    c. mapping
    c. obstruction
    c. patency
    peripherally inserted central c. (PICC)
    c. position
    c. specimen
    c. toe
    c. tunnel
    c. tunnel infection
catheter-deflecting bridge
catheter-directed
    c.-d. fenestration
    c.-d. interventional procedure
catheter-guided
    c.-g. biopsy
    c.-g. endoscopic intubation
catheter-induced
    c.-i. pulmonary artery hemorrhage
catheterization
    antegrade c.
    bladder c.
    bypass graft c.
    cardiac c.
    central venous c.
    chronic c.
    clean intermittent c.
    combined heart c.
    coronary sinus c.
    cystic duct c.
    diagnostic cardiac c.
    femoral artery c.
    hepatic vein c.

    in-and-out c.
    intermittent c.
    interventional cardiac c.
    Judkins-Sones technique of cardiac c.
    c. of lacrimal duct
    c. of lacrimonasal duct
    left heart c.
    long-term epidural c.
    percutaneous transhepatic cardiac c.
    pulmonary artery c.
    retrograde c.
    right heart c.
    Seldinger cystic duct c.
    selective c.
    subclavian vein c.
    c. technique
    thoracic epidural c.
    transfemoral venous c.
    transnasal bile duct c.
    transpapillary c.
    transseptal left heart c.
    transvaginal fallopian tube c.
    transvaginal tubal c.
    umbilical artery c.
    umbilical vein c.
    ureteral c.
    urinary c.
catheterize
catheter-related infection
catheter-securing technique
catholysis
Cath-Strip catheter fastener
cation
    c. exchange
    c. exchanger
cat's eye calculus
Cattell forked-type T tube
Catterall classification
cauda, pl. **caudae**
    c. epididymidis
    c. epididymis
    c. equina compression
    c. equina lesion
    c. equina syndrome
    c. pancreatis
caudad
caudal
    c. anesthesia
    c. angulation
    c. block
    c. canal

NOTES

caudal *(continued)*
    c. direction
    c. epidural anesthetic technique
    c. lamina resection
    c. ligament
    c. pancreatic artery
    c. pancreaticojejunostomy
    c. retinaculum
    c. sac
    c. translation
    c. transtentorial herniation
    c. transverse fissure
    c. vertebrae
caudalis
caudate
    c. body
    c. branches
    c. process
caudocephalad
causalgia
cause-effect relationship
cauterant
cauterization
    bipolar c.
    Bovie c.
    phenol c.
    unipolar c.
cauterize
cautery
    c. conization
    c. operation
cava (*pl. of* cavum)
caval
    c. insertion
cave
    C. hip approach
    C. knee approach
    trigeminal c.
Caverject injection
cavern
    c.'s of corpora cavernosa
    c.'s of corpus spongiosum
caverna, pl. **cavernae**
    cavernae corporis spongiosi
    cavernae corporum cavernosorum
cavernosal alpha blockade technique
cavernous
    c. body of clitoris
    c. body of penis
    c. groove
    c. malformation
    c. nerve of clitoris
    c. nerve of penis
    c. nerve-sparing prostatectomy
    c. part of internal carotid artery
    c. plexus of clitoris
    c. plexus of penis
    c. respiration

    c. sinus
    c. sinus fistula
    c. transformation of the portal vein
    c. veins of penis
Cave-Rowe shoulder dislocation technique
cavitary
    c. lung lesion
    c. small bowel lesion
cavitas, pl. **cavitates**
    c. abdominalis
    c. articularis
    c. laryngis
    c. medullaris
    c. pelvis
    c. peritonealis
    c. pharyngis
    c. pleuralis
    c. thoracis
    c. uteri
cavitating
    c. inflammation
    c. metastasis
cavitation
    collapse c.
    pulmonary c.
    stable c.
    transient c.
Cavitron ultrasonic surgical aspirator for laparoscopy
cavity
    abdominal c.
    abdominopelvic c.
    access c.
    c. access
    acetabular c.
    alveolar c.
    amniotic c.
    articular c.
    artificial classification c.
    axial surface c.
    body c.
    buccal c.
    chorionic c.
    c. classification
    complex c.
    compound c.
    c.'s of corpora cavernosa
    c.'s of corpus spongiosum
    cotyloid c.
    cranial c.
    c. débridement
    dental c.
    distal c.
    DO c.
    endodontic c.
    endometrial c.
    epidural c.

exocelomic c.
fissure c.
gingival c.
glenoid c.
greater peritoneal c.
idiopathic bone c.
incisal c.
inferior laryngeal c.
inflammatory c.
intermediate laryngeal c.
intracranial c.
intraperitoneal c.
joint c.
labial c.
c. of larynx
laser c.
lesser peritoneal c.
c. line angle
lingual c.
c. lining
c. lining agent
lung c.
c. margin
marrow c.
mastoid c.
Meckel c.
medullary c.
miniature uterine c.
MO c.
MOD c.
nasal c.
nephrotomic c.
nonseptate c.
occlusal c.
open c.
opening of orbital c.
optic papilla c.
oral c.
orbital c.
pelvic c.
peritoneal c.
pharyngonasal c.
c. of pharynx
pit and fissure c.
pleural c.
c. preparation
c. preparation base
prepared c.
c. primer
proximal c.
pulmonary c.
pulp c.

retroperitoneal c.
Retzius c.
saclike c.
c. seal
sinonasal c.
sinus c.
smooth surface c.
Stafne idiopathic bone c.
subarachnoid c.
subdural c.
superior laryngeal c.
synovial c.
syringohydromyelic c.
c. test
thoracic c.
c. toilet
toilet of c.
trigeminal c.
tympanic c.
uterine c.
vitreous c.
c. wall
cavo
    c. abducto varus deformity
    c. calcaneo valgus deformity
cavopulmonary anastomosis
cavotomy
    infrahepatic c.
cavovarus deformity
cavum, pl. cava
    c. abdominis
    c. articulare
    c. douglasi
    inferior vena cava (IVC)
    infrahepatic inferior vena cava
    c. laryngis
    c. mediastinale
    c. medullare
    c. pelvis
    c. peritonei
    c. pharyngis
    c. pleurae
    c. retzii
    Spencer plication of vena cava
    c. subdurale
    suprahepatic inferior vena cava
    c. thoracis
    c. trigeminale
    c. uteri
    c. vesicouterinum
cavus deformity

NOTES

Cawthorne
   C. destruction
   C. operation
Cawthorne-Day procedure
CBD
   common bile duct
CBP
   cardiac bypass
CCD
   central core disease
CCM
   critical care medicine
C-D
   C-D instrumentation fixation
      strength
   C-D instrumentation rigidity
   C-D rod insertion
   C-D screw modification
CDBR
   computerized diaphragmatic breathing
   retraining
      RFB System-I for CDBR
Cdyn
   dynamic compliance
ceanothus extract
ceca (*pl. of* cecum)
cecal
   c. arteries
   c. carcinoma
   c. colonoscopy
   c. deformity
   c. folds
   c. foramen of frontal bone
   c. foramen of the tongue
   c. hernia
   c. imbrication procedure
   c. recess
   c. volvulus
cecectomy
Cecil
   C. procedure
   C. urethroplasty
cecocolostomy
cecocystoplasty
cecofixation
cecoileostomy
cecopexy
cecoplication
cecoproctostomy
cecorrhaphy
cecosigmoidostomy
cecostomy
      percutaneous catheter c.
      tube c.
cecotomy
cecoureterocele
cecum, pl. **ceca**

Cedar anesthesia face rest
Cedars-Sinai classification
Celermajer method
Celestin
   C. endoesophageal tube
   C. esophageal tube
   C. latex rubber tube
celiac
   c. artery
   c. axis
   c. branches of vagus nerve
   c. ganglia
   c. glands
   c. (lymphatic) plexus
   c. lymph node metastasis
   c. lymph nodes
   c. (nervous) plexus
   c. plexus block
   c. plexus block anesthetic
      technique
   c. plexus reflex
   c. trunk
   c. tumor
celiectomy
celiocentesis
celioenterotomy
celiogastrostomy
celiogastrotomy
celiohysterectomy
celiohysterotomy
celioma
celiomyomectomy
celiomyomotomy
celioparacentesis
celiorrhaphy
celiosalpingectomy
celiosalpingotomy
celioscopy
celiotomy
      exploratory c.
      c. incision
      vaginal c.
celite-activated clotting time (CACT)
cell
   c. collection
   c. line
   c. membrane
   c. migration
   c. oxygenation
   packed red blood c.'s (PRBC)
   c. salvage system
   C. Saver 4 cardiopulmonary bypass
      blood centrifuge and washing
      equipment
   c. separation technique
   c. web
cell-extracellular matrix adhesion

cellophane tape method
cellula, pl. cellulae
    cellulae coli
cellular
    c. cooperation
    c. infiltration
    c. migration
    c. periosteal osteocartilaginous mass
cellulocutaneous flap
celluloid linen suture
cellulose-based membrane
celotomy
Celsite implanted port
Celsus-Hotz operation
Celsus spasmodic entropion operation
cement
    c. base
    c. disease
    c. interface
    c. line
    c. removal
    c. substance
    c. technique
cemental
    c. fracture
    c. lesion
    c. line
    c. repair
cementation
    final c.
    trial c.
cement-bone interface
cemented total hip arthroplasty
cementification
cementing line
cementless
    c. technique
    c. total hip arthroplasty
cementoid tissue
cementoma
cementophyte
cementum fracture
CEM/HIV-1 cell line
center
    c. of axial rotation
    c. of mass
centering ring
Centers for Disease Control classification for HIV infection
centesis
centra (pl. of centrum)

central
    c. anesthetic technique
    c. anticholinergic syndrome
    c. approach
    c. block
    c. bone
    c. canal of spinal cord
    c. carbon dioxide ventilatory response
    c. chemoreflex loop
    c. cord syndrome
    c. core disease (CCD)
    c. dislocation
    c. excitatory state
    c. extensor mechanism
    c. fibrous body
    c. fixation
    c. fracture
    c. fusion
    c. group of axillary lymph nodes
    c. heel pad syndrome
    c. herniation
    c. illumination
    c. iridectomy
    c. lesion
    c. mesenteric lymph nodes
    c. nervous system disease
    c. nervous system malformation
    c. nervous system tuberculosis
    c. pain
    c. palmar space
    c. physiolysis
    c. pontine myelinolysis
    c. posterior-anterior pressure
    c. ray amputation
    c. respiration
    c. slip sparing technique
    c. stellate laceration
    c. sulcal artery
    c. tegmental tract
    c. tendon of diaphragm
    c. tendon of perineum
    c. veins of liver
    c. vein of suprarenal gland
    c. venous alimentation
    c. venous cannulation anesthetic technique
    c. venous catheterization
    c. venous pressure (CVP)
    c. venous pressure line
    c. venous pressure monitoring

NOTES

central (*continued*)
    c. yellow point
    c. zone inflammation
central hemangioma
central-bearing point
centralization
    Bayne-Klug c.
    Bora c.
    Manske-McCarroll-Swanson c.
    tendon c.
centration
centric
    c. fusion
    c. jaw relation
    c. occluding relation
    c. occluding relation record
    point c.
    c. position
    c. relation occlusion
centriciput
Centriflo filter
centrifugal
    c. nerve
centrifugalization
centrilobular
    c. lesion
centriole
    distal c.
    proximal c.
centripetal nerve
centrocentral coaptation
centromedullary nail
centroneuroaxis anesthesia
Centronic 200 MGA respiratory mass spectrometer
centrum, pl. centra
    c. tendineum diaphragmatis
    c. tendincum perinei
    c. of a vertebra
    Willis c. nervosum
cephalad
    c. direction
    c. translation
cephalic
    c. arterial rami
    c. index
    c. tetanus
    c. triangle
    c. vein
    c. vein graft
cephalin-cholesterol flocculation
cephalization
cephalocaudal
    c. axis
cephalocele
    occipital c.
    oral c.
cephalocentesis

cephalodactyly
cephalomedullary nail fracture
cephalometric
    c. correction
    c. landmark
cephalo-orbital index
cephalopharyngeus
cephalorrhachidian
    c. index
cephaloscapular projection
cephalothoracic
cephalotrigonal technique
ceramic restoration
ceramometal
    c. implant bridge
    c. restoration
ceratectomy
ceratocricoid
    c. ligament
    c. muscle
cerclage
    c. operation
    c. wire fixation
cerebellar
    c. arteries
    c. ectopia
    c. hematoma
    c. hemisphere
    c. hemorrhage
    c. veins
cerebellomedullaris
    cisterna c.
cerebellomedullary
    c. cistern
    c. malformation syndrome
cerebellopontine
    c. angle approach
    c. angle cistern
    c. angle syndrome
cerebellorubral tract
cerebellothalamic tract
cerebra (*pl. of* cerebrum)
cerebral
    c. angioma
    c. aqueduct compression
    c. arteries
    c. arteriovenous malformation
    c. calculus
    c. circulation
    c. circulation time
    c. decompression
    c. decortication
    c. edema
    c. hemicorticectomy
    c. hemisphere
    c. hemorrhage
    c. hernia
    c. herniation

c. index
c. metastasis
c. palsy pathological fracture
c. part of arachnoid
c. part of dura mater
c. part of internal carotid artery
c. perfusion
c. perfusion pressure
c. protection
c. protective therapy
c. respiration
c. revascularization
c. sinuses
c. vascular malformation
c. veins
cerebral-sacral loop
cerebration
cerebri
    cisterna fossae lateralis c.
    cisterna venae magnae c.
    epiphysis c.
    hypophysis c.
cerebriform
cerebrospinal
c. fluid (CSF)
c. fluid-brain barrier
c. fluid fistula
c. fluid pressure (CSFP)
c. index
cerebrotomy
cerebrovascular
c. complication
c. disease
c. malformation
cerebrum, pl. cerebra
    cistern of great vein of c.
    cistern of lateral fossa of c.
cerecloth
Ceredase injection
certified registered nurse anesthetist
  (CRNA)
cervical
c. acceleration-deceleration
  syndrome
c. adenocarcinoma
c. amputation
c. anesthesia
c. anomaly
c. approach
c. branch of facial nerve
c. canal
c. carcinoma

c. carcinoma stimulation
c. compression syndrome
c. condyloma
c. cone biopsy
c. conization
c. corpectomy
c. decompression surgery
c. dilation
c. diskectomy
c. disk excision
c. disk surgery
c. esophagostomy
c. extension strength
c. fistula
c. flap
c. fusion syndrome
c. general rotation
c. glands
c. glands of uterus
c. iliocostal muscle
c. incision
c. infection
c. inflammation
c. insemination
c. interbody fusion
c. interspinales muscles
c. interspinal muscle
c. laceration
c. lesion
c. ligament of uterus
c. line
c. longissimus muscle
c. loop
c. manipulation
c. metastasis
c. midline disk herniation
c. nerve root injection
c. osteotomy
c. part of esophagus
c. part of internal carotid artery
c. part of spinal cord
c. part of thoracic duct
c. perivascular sympathectomy
c. pleura
c. plexus
c. plexus block anesthetic
  technique
c. position
c. rib
c. rotation in extension
c. rotator muscles
c. screw insertion technique

NOTES

115

cervical *(continued)*
    c. segments of spinal cord
    c. soft tissue
    c. spine fracture
    c. spine internal fixation
    c. spine kyphotic deformity
    c. spine laminectomy
    c. spine posterior fusion
    c. spine screw-plate fixation
    c. spine stabilization
    c. spine stabilization procedure
    c. splanchnic nerve
    c. spondylotic myclopathy fusion technique
    c. spondylotic myelopathy vertebrectomy
    c. suture
    c. transformation zone
    c. triangle
    c. tumor
    c. vein
    c. vertebrae
    c. vessel compression
    c. zone of tooth
cervicalis
    c. ascendens
cervicectomy
cervices (*pl. of* cervix)
cervicoaxillary canal
cervicobrachial
cervicofacial
cervicomedullary
    c. deformity
    c. junction compression
cervico-occipital
cervicoplasty
cervicothoracic
    c. ganglion
    c. junction stabilization
    c. junction surgery
    c. pedicle anatomy
    c. sympathectomy
    c. transition
cervicotomy
cervicotrochanteric displaced fracture
cervicovaginal
    c. artery
    c. fistula
    c. infection
cervicovesical
cervix, pl. cervices
    carcinoma of c.
    cone biopsy of c.
    conization of c.
    dilation of c.
    epidermidization of c.
    implant c.
    malignant tumor of c.

    c. uteri
    c. of uterus
    c. vesicae urinariae
cesarean
    c. hysterectomy
    c. operation
    c. resection
    c. section
cesium irradiation
Cetacaine
    C. topical anesthetic
C-form osteotomy
Chadwick-Bentley classification
chain
    obturator lymphatic c.
    c. suture
    c. suture technique
chain-of-lakes deformity
Chalet frame
challenge
    methacholine bronchoprovocation c.
Chamberlain
    C. mediastinoscopy
    C. palato-occipital line
    C. procedure
chamber rupture
Chambers
    C. osteotomy
    C. procedure
chamfer preparation
Chance
    C. fracture thoracolumbar spine
    C. vertebral fracture
chancre
    hard c.
    mixed c.
    monorecidive c.
    c. redux
    soft c.
chancriform
chancroid
Chandler
    C. hip fusion
    C. iridectomy
    C. vitreous operation
Chandler-Verhoeff
    C.-V. lens extraction
    C.-V. operation
Chang aniline-acid fuchsin method
change
    fractional area c. (FAC)
    nail c.
    c. point
    postthoracotomy c.
changer
    tracheal tube c.
    tube c.
Chang-Miltner incision

channel
    c. and core biopsy
    c. shoulder pin technique
Chaput
    C. anal operation
    C. fracture
characteristic radiation
charcoal filter
Charcot triad
Charest head frame
CHARGE association
charged-particle irradiation
Charles
    C. lensectomy
    C. procedure
Charnley
    C. compression
    C. compression arthrodesis
    C. compression-type knee fusion
    C. drain tube
    C. incision
    C. total hip arthroplasty
Charrière scale
Charters
    C. method
    C. technique
Chassaignac
    C. space
    C. tubercle
Chassar
    C. Moir-Sims procedure
    C. Moir sling procedure
Chauffard point
Chauffen-Pratt tube
chauffeur fracture
Chaussier
    C. line
    C. tube
Chaves-Rapp muscle transfer technique
Chayes method
CHCT
    caffeine and halothane contracture test
Cheatle
    C. slit
    C. syndrome
Cheatle-Henry hernia
check
    c. ligaments of eyeball, medial and
      lateral
    c. ligaments of odontoid

checkrein
    c. deformity
    c. procedure
cheek
    c. advancement flap
    c. bone
    c. muscle
    c. rotation flap
cheilectomy
    Garceau c.
    Mann-Coughlin-DuVries c.
    Sage-Clark c.
cheilion
cheiloangioscopy
cheiloplasty
cheilorrhaphy
cheilostomatoplasty
cheilotomy
cheiroplasty
chemexfoliation
chemical
    c. exchange
    c. exposure
    c. hemostasis
    c. litholysis
    c. matrixectomy
    c. shift misregistration
    c. splanchnicectomy
    c. sympathectomy
    c. thrombectomy
    c. vapor sterilization
chemicocautery
chemise
chemoactivation
chemocautery
chemocoagulation
chemolysis
    intrarenal c.
chemoneurolysis
    glycerol c.
    percutaneous retrogasserian
      glycerol c.
chemonucleolysis
    chymopapain c.
    double-needle c.
chemopallidectomy
chemopallidothalamectomy
chemopallidotomy
chemoreflex
chemostimulation
chemosurgery
chemosurgical gingivectomy

NOTES

chemothalamectomy
chemothalamotomy
cheoplasty
Cherney
    C. incision
    C. suture technique
Chernez incision
cherry angioma
Cherry-Crandall procedure
cherry-picking procedure
chessboard grafts
chest
    c. compression
    c. examination
    flat c.
    c. index
    c. physical therapy
    pneumonectomy c.
    c. port
    c. tube
    c. tube drainage (CTD)
    c. tube scar
    c. wall
    c. wall compliance
Chester-Winter procedure
Chevalier Jackson tracheal tube
chevron
    c. bunionectomy
    c. hallux valgus correction
    c. incision
    c. laceration
    c. osteotomy
    c. technique
chewing method
chew-in technique
Cheyne-Stokes respiration
Chiari
    C. anomaly
    C. I–III malformation
    C. II syndrome
    C. innominate osteotomy
    C. technique
Chiari-Salter-Steel pelvic osteotomy
chiasm
    Camper c.
    cistern of c.
    tendinous c. of the digital tendons
chiasma, pl. chiasmata
    c. formation
    c. tendinum
chiasmal
    c. compression
    c. lesion
    c. metastasis
chiasmapexy
chiasmata (pl. of chiasma)
chiasmatic
    c. cistern

    c. cisterna
    c. groove
chiasmatis
    cisterna c.
Chicago classification
Chick
    C. CLT frame
    C. nail
chief artery of thumb
Chiene incision
Chiffelle and Putt method
Child
    C. classification of liver disease
    C. esophageal varices classification
    C. hepatic dysfunction classification
    C. liver disease classification
    C. pancreaticoduodenostomy
    C. radical pancreatectomy
childbirth
    Bradley method of prepared c.
    Kitzinger method of c.
Child-Phillips bowel plication
Child-Pugh classification
children's coma scale
Childress ankle fixation technique
Child-Turcotte classification
chiloplasty
chilorrhaphy
chilostomatoplasty
chilotomy
chimera
    radiation c.
chin
    c. augmentation
    double c.
    c. elevation
    c. muscle
    c. position
Chinese
    C. fingertrap suture
    C. twisted silk suture
chip
    bone c.
    c. fracture
    c. graft
chiroplasty
chiropractic treatment of fracture
chisel fracture
chlamydial infection
Chlamydia trachomatis infection
chloramine
    c. B, T
    c. catgut suture
chloramine-T technique
chloranilate method
chlorazene
chlorbutol
chlordiazepoxide

Chloresium solution
chloride
    alcuronium c.
    benzocaine, butyl aminobenzoate,
        tetracaine, and benzalkonium c.
    doxacurium c.
    ethyl c.
    methyl c.
    mivacurium c.
    succinylcholine c.
    tubocurarine c.
chlormerodrin accumulation test
chloroazodin
chlorobutanol
chloroethane
chloroform
    acetone c.
chloromethane
chloropercha method
chloroprocaine
    c. hydrochloride
Chlorphed-LA Nasal solution
Chlor-Pro injection
Chlor-Trimeton injection
Cho
    C. anterior cruciate ligament
        reconstruction
    C. tendon technique
cholangiectasis
cholangiocarcinoma
cholangioenterostomy
cholangiofibroma
cholangiofibrosis
cholangiogastrostomy
cholangiogram
    intraoperative c. (IOC)
cholangiole
cholangioma
cholangiopancreatography
    endoscopic retrograde c. (ERCP)
cholangiopancreatoscopy
    peroral c.
cholangioplasty
cholangioscopy
    intraductal c.
    percutaneous transhepatic c.
    peroral c.
cholangiostomy
cholangiotomy
cholangitis
cholecyst
cholecystectasia

cholecystectomy
    laparoscopic c. (LC)
    lesser omentectomy with c.
    minilaparoscope c.
    percutaneous c.
    prophylactic c.
    surgical c.
    c. treatment
cholecystenteric fistula
cholecystenterostomy
cholecystenterotomy
cholecystic
cholecystis
cholecystitis
    acalculous c.
    acute calculous c.
cholecystocholedochal fistula
cholecystocholedocholithiasis
cholecystocolic fistula
cholecystocolonic fistula
cholecystocolostomy
cholecystoduodenal fistula
cholecystoduodenocolic fistula
cholecystoduodenostomy
    Jenckel c.
cholecystoendoprosthesis
    endoscopic retrograde c.
cholecystoenterostomy
cholecystogastrostomy
cholecystoileostomy
cholecystojejunostomy
cholecystolithiasis
cholecystolithotomy
    percutaneous c.
cholecystolithotripsy
cholecystomy
cholecystopaque
cholecystopexy
cholecystorrhaphy
cholecystoscopy
    percutaneous transhepatic c.
cholecystostomy
    laparoscopy-guided subhepatic c.
    percutaneous c.
    surgical c.
cholecystotomy
    laparoscopic c.
    transpapillary endoscopic c.
choledoch
    c. duct
choledochal
    c. basal pressure

C

NOTES

choledochal *(continued)*
    c. cyst disease
    c. sphincter
choledochectomy
choledochendysis
choledochocele
choledochocholedochostomy
choledochocolonic fistula
choledochoduodenal
    c. fistula
    c. fistulotomy
    c. junction
choledochoduodenostomy
choledochoenteric fistula
choledochoenterostomy
choledochofiberoscopic approach
choledochofiberoscopy
    T-tube tract c.
choledochojejunostomy
    end-to-side c.
    loop c.
    retrocolic end-to-side c.
    Roux-en-Y c.
choledocholith
choledocholithiasis
choledocholithotomy
choledocholithotripsy
choledocholithotrity
choledochoplasty
choledochorrhaphy
choledochoscopy
    Berci-Shore c.
    cystic duct c.
    jejunostomy tract c.
    operative c.
    postoperative c.
    T-tube tract c.
choledochostomy
choledochotomy
    c. incision
    longitudinal c.
choledochous
choledochus
choledococaval anastomosis
cholelith
cholelithiasis
cholelitholysis
cholelithotomy
cholelithotripsy
cholelithotrity
cholesteatoma
    c. pearl
cholesterol-cholesteroloxidase-phenol 4-
    aminophenazone method
cholesterol saturation index
cholicele
cholinergic
    c. blockade

    c. mechanism
    c. tract
cholinomimetic drug
chondral
    c. edge
    c. fracture
    c. fragment
chondrectomy
chondrification
chondrocostal
chondroepiphysis
chondroglossus muscle
chondrolysis
    posttraumatic c.
chondromalacia
chondromyofibroma
chondromyxofibroma
chondromyxoma
chondromyxosaroma
chondro-osseous
chondro-osteodystrophy
chondrophyte
chondroplasty
    abrasion c.
    arthroscopic abrasion c.
chondroporosis
chondrosarcoma
chondrosteoma
chondrosternal
chondrosternoplasty
chondrotomy
chondroxiphoid
    c. ligament
chop amputation
Chopart
    C. amputation
    C. ankle dislocation
    C. articulation
chopstick retention suture
chorda, pl. chordae
    c. obliqua
    c. spermatica
    chordae tendineae
    chordae tendineae rupture
    c. umbilicalis
    c. vocalis
    chordae willisii
chordablastoma
chordal rupture
chordee
chord incision
chordoblastoma
chordoma
    c. of sacrum
chordoplasty
chordotomy
chorioadenoma
chorioallantoic membrane

chorioamnionic infection
chorioangioma
chorioblastoma
choriocarcinoma
choriocele
chorioepithelioma
chorioma
chorionic
    c. cavity
    c. sac
    c. villus biopsy
chorioretinitis
choristoblastoma
choristoma
    c. nest
choroid
    c. plexus
    c. point
    c. vein
choroidal
    c. hemorrhage
    c. infiltration
    c. lesion
    c. metastasis
    c. neovascularization
    c. neovascular membrane
    c. ring
    c. rupture
choroidectomy
choroiditis
Chow technique
Chrisman-Snook
    C.-S. ankle technique
    C.-S. procedure
    C.-S. reconstruction
chromaffin
    c. body
    c. tissue
chromated catgut suture
chromate method
chromatic lens aberration
chromatin condensation
chromatinic body
chromatography
    gas c.
chrome alum hematoxylin-phloxine
  method
chromic
    c. blue-dyed suture
    c. catgut suture
    c. collagen suture

    c. gut pelviscopic loop ligature
    c. gut suture
chromicized catgut suture
chromocystoscopy
chromogenic method
chromohydrotubation
chromolytic method
chromopertubation
chromoscopy
chromotubation
chronic
    c. abscess
    c. allograft rejection
    c. anoplasty treatment
    c. atrial fibrillation
    c. catheterization
    c. Epstein-Barr virus infection
    c. extrinsic alveolitis
    c. graft-versus-host disease
    c. hyperventilation syndrome
    c. jejunal inflammation
    c. nonmalignant
    c. pain
    c. subcutaneous infusion
    c. subdural hematoma
    c. transplant rejection
Chuinard-Peterson ankle fusion
chylangioma
chyle
    c. cistern
    c. fistula
    c. vessel
chyliform ascites
chylocyst
chyloma
chyloperitoneum
chylous
    c. ascites
    c. leakage
chyme
chymopapain chemonucleolysis
Ciaccio method
Ciba-Corning 2500 co-oximeter
Cibis
    C. liquid silicone procedure
    C. operation
cicatrectomy
cicatrices (pl. of cicatrix)
cicatriceum
    ectropion c.

NOTES

cicatricial
   c. mass
   c. tissue
cicatricotomy
cicatrizant
cicatrization
Cicero anesthetic ventilator
Cidex
   C. activated dialdehyde solution
   C. Plus solution
Cierny-Mader technique
cilia ectopia
ciliarotomy
ciliary
   c. body
   c. body band
   c. canal
   c. ganglion
   c. injection
   c. ligament
   c. procedure
   c. ring
   c. zone
   c. zonule
ciliectomy
ciliodestructive surgery
ciliotomy
ciliovitrectomy
   c. block
Cimino-Brescia arteriovenous fistula
Cimino fistula
cinching operation
Cincinnati
   C. incision
   C. technique
cine-esophagoscopy
cinefluoroscopic method
cinefluoroscopy
   valve c.
cinegastroscopy
cingula (*pl. of* cingulum)
cingulate
   c. herniation
cingulectomy
cingulotomy
   rostral c.
cingulum, pl. cingula
   c. bundle
   c. membri inferioris
   c. membri superioris
cingulumotomy
Cipro injection
circinate exudate
circle
   c. absorption anesthesia
   articular vascular c.
   Bain c.
   closed c.

   c. dissipation
   Huguier c.
   c. loop biliary drainage
   Pagenstecher c.
   pediatric c.
   semiclosed c.
   c. system
   vascular c.
   venous c. of mammary gland
   c. of Willis
   c. wire nephrostomy
CircOlectric frame
circuit
   c. adapter
   anesthesia c.
   anesthetic c.
   Bentley Duraflo II extracorporeal perfusion c.
   breathing c.
   Carmeda BioActive surface extracorporeal c.
   extracorporeal cardiopulmonary c.
   feedback reduction c.
   Intertech anesthesia breathing c.
   Jackson-Rees c.
   low-flow c.
   Mapleson D type of T-piece c.
   multipurpose breathing c.
   ventilation c.
circular
   c. anastomosis
   c. folds
   c. griseotomy
   c. layer of muscular coat
   c. myotomy
   c. open amputation
   c. sinus
   c. suture
circulation
   airway, breathing, and c. (ABC)
   allantoic c.
   arterial c.
   assisted c.
   carotid c.
   cerebral c.
   collateral abdominal c.
   collateral mesenteric c.
   compensatory c.
   conjunctival c.
   coronary collateral c.
   cutaneous collateral c.
   derivative c.
   ductal-dependent pulmonary c.
   enterohepatic c.
   episcleral c.
   extracorporeal c. (ECC)
   extracranial carotid c.
   femoral c.

fetal c.
fetoplacental c.
hepatic c.
herpkinetic c.
hyperdynamic c.
hypophyseal portal c.
hypothalamic-hypophyseal portal c.
intracranial c.
left dominant coronary c.
mesenteric c.
perichondral c.
peripheral c.
persistent fetal c.
placental c.
portal-collateral c.
portal-hypophysial c.
portosystemic collateral c.
posterior fossa c.
pulmonary c.
c. rate
retinal c.
sludging of c.
systemic venous c.
thalamic c.
thebesian c.
c. time
umbilical c.
uteroplacental c.
venous c.
c. volume

circulator
sequential c.

circulatory
c. arrest
c. arrest anesthetic technique

circulus, pl. circuli
c. arteriosus cerebri
c. articularis vasculosus

circumalveolar fixation

circumanal
c. glands

circumaxillary

circumbulbar

circumcise

circumcision

circumcisional suture

circumcorneal injection

circumduction maneuver

circumference
fetal head c.

circumferentia
c. articularis radii
c. articularis ulnae

circumferential
c. esophageal reconstruction
c. fibrocartilage
c. fracture
c. implantation
c. mucosal dissection
c. suture tie
c. venolysis
c. wire-loop fixation

circumflex
c. femoral arteries
c. humeral arteries
c. iliac arteries
c. nerve
c. scapular artery
c. veins

circumintestinal

circumlental space

circummandibular fixation

circummesencephalic cistern

circumocular

circumorbital

circumrenal

circumscribed
c. inflammation
c. mass

circum-umbilical incision

circumvascular

circumzygomatic fixation

cirrhosis

CIS
carcinoma in situ

cis-acting

cisatracurium besylate

cistern
ambient wing of the quadrigeminal c.
basal c.
cerebellomedullary c.
cerebellopontine angle c.
c. of chiasm
chiasmatic c.
chyle c.
circummesencephalic c.
c. of great vein of cerebrum
interpeduncular c.
c. of lateral fossa of cerebrum
lumbar c.
mesencephalic c.

C

NOTES

cistern *(continued)*
  c. of nuclear envelope
  Pecquet c.
  perimesencephalic c.
  pontine c.
  prepontine c.
  quadrigeminal c.
  subarachnoid c.
  suprasellar subarachnoid c.
  sylvian c.
cisterna, pl. **cisternae**
  c. ambiens
  ambient c.
  c. basalis
  c. caryothecae
  c. cerebellomedullaris
  chiasmatic c.
  c. chiasmatis
  c. cruralis
  cylindrical confronting c.
  c. fossae lateralis cerebri
  c. interpeduncularis
  c. magna
  c. perilymphatica
  perinuclear c.
  c. pontis
  subsarcolemma c.
  c. superioris
  terminal c.
  c. venae magnae
  c. venae magnae cerebri
cisternal
  c. herniation
  c. puncture
Citanest
  C. Forte
  C. Plain
citrate
  carbetapentane c.
  fentanyl c.
  oral transmucosal fentanyl c.
   (OTFC)
  sufentanil c.
Civinini
  C. ligament
  C. process
2C-L
  two-chamber longitudinal
  2C-L image
Clado
  C. anastomosis
  C. band
  C. ligament
  C. point
Clagett
  C. Barrett esophagogastroscopy
  C. Barrett esophagogastrostomy
  C. closure

clam
  c. enterocystoplasty
  c. ileocystoplasty
clamshell
  c. closure
  c. technique
Clancy
  C. cruciate ligament reconstruction
  C. ligament technique
  C. patellar tendon graft
CLAP
  contact laser ablation of prostate
Clapton line
Clark
  C. level
  C. transfer technique
Clark-Collip method
Clark-Southwick-Odgen modification
clasped thumb deformity
classic abdominal Semm hysterectomy
classical transverse incision
classification
  Ackerman-Proffitt c. of
   malocclusion
  Acosta c.
  acromioclavicular injury c.
  Aitken epiphyseal fracture c.
  AJCC TNM tumor c.
  Allman acromioclavicular injury c.
  Alonso-Lej c.
  American Heart Association c.
  American Society of
   Anesthesiologists c.
  Anderson-D'Alonzo odontoid
   fracture c.
  Anderson modification of Berndt-
   Harty c.
  Angle c. of malocclusion
  Ann Arbor c.
  AO c.
  Arneth c.
  Ashhurst-Bromer c. of ankle
   fractures
  Astler-Coller A, B1, B2, C1,
   C2 c.
  Astler-Coller modification of
   Dukes c.
  Bado c.
  Bailyn c.
  Banff c.
  Bauer-Jackson c.
  Baume c.
  Bennett c.
  Bergey c.
  Berndt-Harty c.
  Bethesda Pap smear c.
  Binet system of c.
  Bishop c.

bismuth benign bile duct
stricture c.
Black c.
Borrmann gastric cancer c.
Bosniak c.
Boyd c.
Boyd-Griffin trochanteric fracture c.
Broders c.
Butchart staging c.
Caldwell-Moloy c.
Callender cell type c.
Cambridge c.
Canadian Cardiovascular Society c.
caries c.
Carnesale-Stewart-Barnes c. of hip
dislocation
Caroli-Sarles c.
Catterall c.
cavity c.
Cedars-Sinai c.
Centers for Disease Control c. for
HIV infection
Chadwick-Bentley c.
Chicago c.
Child esophageal varices c.
Child hepatic dysfunction c.
Child liver disease c.
Child c. of liver disease
Child-Pugh c.
Child-Turcotte c.
cleft palate c.
c. of cleft palate
Codman c.
Cohen-Rentrop c.
Colonna hip fracture c.
Colton c.
Cori c.
Correa c.
Couinaud c.
Croften c.
Crowe c.
Cummer c.
Dagradi esophageal variceal c.
Danis-Weber c. of ankle injuries
DeBakey c.
de Groot c.
Delbert hip fracture c.
DeLee c.
Denis Browne c. of sacral fracture
Denis Browne spinal fracture c.
denture c.
Denver c.

Dexter-Grossman c.
Diamond c.
Dias-Tachdijian c. of physeal
injury
dichotomous c.
Dickhaut-DeLee discoid meniscus c.
Dripps c.
Duane c.
Dubin-Amelar varicocele c.
Dukes c.
Dyck-Lambert c.
Eckert-Davis c.
Edmondson-Steiner c.
Efron jackknife c.
El-Ahwany c. of humeral
supracondylar fracture
Ellis c.
Enna c.
Enneking c.
Epstein hip dislocation c.
Epstein-Thomas c.
Essex-Lopresti calcaneal fracture c.
Evans intertrochanteric fracture c.
FAB c.
Federation of Gynecology and
Obstetrics c.
Fielding femoral fracture c.
Fielding-Magliato c. of
subtrochanteric fracture
Flatt c.
Foucher c. of epiphyseal injury
fracture c.
Fränkel neurologic deficit c.
Franz-O'Rahilly c.
Fredrickson hyperlipoproteinemia c.
Fredrickson, Levy and Lees c.
Freeman calcaneal fracture c.
French/American/British c.
Frykman distal radius fracture c.
Frykman radial fracture c.
Fukunaga-Hayes unbiased
jackknife c.
functional capacity c.
Garden femoral neck fracture c.
Gartland c. of humeral
supracondylar fracture
Gartland Universal radial
fracture c.
gastric mucosal pattern c.
Gell and Coombs c.
Goldman c.
Grantham c. of femoral fracture

C

NOTES

classification *(continued)*

Grantham femur fracture c.
Greenfield spinocerebellar ataxia c.
Gustilo-Anderson open fracture c.
Gustilo puncture wound c.
Gustilo c. of puncture wound
Haggitt c.
Hannover c.
Hansen c. of fracture
Hara c. of gallbladder inflammation
Hardcastle c. of tarsometatarsal
   joint injury
Hawkins c. of talar fracture
Hawkins talar fracture c.
Henderson c.
Herring lateral pillar c.
Hinchey c.
HIV c.
Hoaglund-States c.
Hohl-Luck tibial plateau fracture c.
Hohl-Moore c.
Hohl tibial condylar fracture c.
Holdsworth spinal fracture c.
House-Brackmann c.
Hughston c.
Hunt and Kosnik c.
Ideberg glenoid fracture c.
immunologic c.
Ingram-Bachynski c. of hip fracture
Insall patellar injury c.
International c. of cancer of cervix
International C. of Diseases,
   Adapted for Use in the United
   States (ICDA)
International Federation of
   Gynecology and Obstetrics c.
Jansky c.
Japanese cancer c.
Jeffery c. of radial fracture
Jensen c.
Jewett and Whitmore c.
Johner-Wruhs tibial fracture c.
Jones-Barnes-Lloyd-Roberts c.
Kajava c.
Kalamchi c.
Kasugai c.
Kauffman-White c.
Keil tumor cell c.
Keith-Wagener c.
Keith-Wagener-Barker c.
Kelami c.
Kellam-Waddel c.
Kennedy c.
Kernohan system of glioma c.
Key-Conwell c. of pelvic fracture
Kiel c.
Kilfoyle c. of humeral medial
   condylar fracture

Killip-Kimball heart failure c.
Kocher c.
KWB c.
Kyle-Gustilo c.
Kyle-Gustilo-Premer c.
Lagrange c. of humeral
   supracondylar fracture
Lancefield c.
Lauge-Hansen c.
Lauge-Hansen c. of ankle fracture
Lauren gastric carcinoma c.
Le Fort c.
Leishman c.
Lennert c.
Letournel-Judet acetabular
   fracture c.
Leung thumb loss c.
Lev c.
Levine-Harvey c.
Lindell c.
Linell-Ljungberg c.
Lloyd-Roberts-Catteral-Salamon c.
Loesche c.
Lown c.
Lukes and Butler c. of Hodgkin
   disease
Lukes-Collins c.
MacCallan c.
Macewen c.
MacNichol-Voutsinas c.
Mallampati oropharyngeal c.
Mallampati pharyngeal visibility c.
Marseille pancreatitis c.
Mason radial head fracture c.
Mast-Spieghel-Pappas c.
Mathews c. of olecranon fracture
Mayo carpal instability c.
Mayo c. of rheumatoid elbow
McNeer c.
Melone distal radius fracture c.
Meyers-McKeever c. of tibial
   fracture
microinvasive carcinoma c.
Milch condylar fracture c.
Milch elbow fracture c.
Milch c. of humeral fracture
Ming gastric carcinoma c.
Minnesota EKG c.
Moore tibial plateau fracture c.
morphologic c.
Moss c.
Mueller femoral supracondylar
   fracture c.
Mueller tibial fracture c.
multiaxial c.
Munro and Parker c. for
   laparoscopic hysterectomy
Nalebuff c.

Neer femur fracture c.
Neer-Horowitz c. of humeral fracture
Neer shoulder fracture c.
Newman c. of radial neck and head fracture
New York Heart Association c. of heart disease
Nicoll c.
O'Brien c. of radial fracture
O'Brien radial fracture c.
Ogden c. of epiphyseal fracture
Ogden knee dislocation c.
O'Rahilly limb deficiency c.
ordinal c.
Orthopaedic Trauma Association c.
Outerbridge c.
Paley c.
Papavasiliou c. of olecranon fracture
Paris c.
Pauwels femoral neck fracture c.
Pell and Gregory c.
Pennal c.
Pipkin c. of femoral fracture
Pipkin posterior hip dislocation c.
Pipkin subclassification of Epstein-Thomas c.
Poland c. of epiphyseal fracture
Poland c. of physeal injury
Potter c.
Pugh c.
Pulec and Freedman c.
Quénu-Küss tarsometatarsal injury c.
Quinby c. of pelvic fracture
Rai c.
Ranawat c.
Ranson acute pancreatitis c.
Rappaport c.
Rentrop c.
Riseborough-Radin c. of intercondylar fracture
Rockwood c. of acromioclavicular injury
Rockwood c. of clavicular fracture
Rosenthal c. of nail injuries
round-robin c.
Rowe calcaneal fracture c.
Rowe-Lowell hip dislocation c.
Rowe and Lowell c. system for fracture-dislocation

Ruedi-Allgower c.
Runyon c.
Russe c.
Russell-Taylor c.
Rüter c.
Rutledge c. of extended hysterectomy
Rye c. of Hodgkin disease
Sage-Salvatore c. of acromioclavicular joint injury
Saha shoulder muscle c.
Sakellarides c. of calcaneal fracture
Salter epiphyseal fracture c.
Salter-Harris c. of epiphyseal fracture
Santiani-Stone c.
Sassouni c.
scalar c.
Schatzker tibial plateau fracture c.
Scheie c.
Schuknecht c.
Schwarz c.
Seattle c.
Seddon c.
Seinsheimer c. of femoral fracture
sentence c.
Severin c.
Shaffer-Weiss c.
Shaher-Puddu c.
Shelton femoral fracture c.
Singh osteoporosis c.
Siurala c.
Skinner c.
Snyder c.
Solcia c.
Sonnenberg c.
Sorbie c. of calcaneal fracture
Spaulding c.
Speed radial head fracture c.
Spetzler-Martin c.
Stark c.
Steinbrocker c.
Suda type I, II, III c. of papilla
Sunderland c. of nerve injury
Swanson c.
Sydney system gastritis c.
Tachdjian c.
Tessier c.
Thomas c.
Thompson-Epstein c. of femoral fracture
Three Color Concept of wound c.

NOTES

classification *(continued)*
    Tile c.
    TIMI c.
    TNM c. of carcinoma
    TNM carcinoma c.
    tongue thrust c.
    Torg c.
    Torode-Zieg c.
    Toronto pelvic fracture c.
    Tronzo c. of intertrochanteric
      fracture
    Tscherne c.
    Tscherne-Gotzcn tibial fracture c.
    tumor, node, metastasis c.
    UICC tumor c.
    Universal distal radius fracture c.
    Vaughan Williams antiarrhythmic
      drug c.
    Veau c.
    Venn-Watson c.
    Visick dysphagia c.
    Vostal radial fracture c.
    Vostal c. of radial fractures
    Wagener-Clay-Gipner c.
    Wagner c.
    Walter Reed c.
    Walter Reed c. for HIV infection
    Warren-Marshall c.
    Wassel thumb duplication c.
    Watanabe discoid meniscus c.
    Watson-Jones tibial fracture c.
    Watson-Jones c. of tibial tubercle
      avulsion fracture
    Weber c.
    Weber-Danis ankle injury c.
    Weber c. of physeal injury
    Weiland c.
    Weissman c.
    White c.
    Whitehead c.
    WHO gastric carcinoma c.
    Wiberg patellar c.
    Wiley-Galey c.
    Wilkins c. of radial fracture
    Winquist femoral shaft fracture c.
    Winquist-Hansen femoral fracture c.
    Winter c.
    Wolfe c. of breast carcinoma
    Wolfe breast carcinoma c.
    Woofry-Chandler c. of Osgood-
      Schlatter lesion
    World Health Organization c.
    Yacoub and Radley-Smith c.
    Young pelvic fracture c.
    Zickel c.
    Zlotsky-Ballard c. of
      acromioclavicular injury

Class V Multiple Step Build-up
    technique
claudication
Claudius fossa
Clausen method
Claussen fragment stabilizer
claustral
claustrum, pl. **claustra**
clavicectomy
clavicle
    c. excision
clavicula, pl. **claviculae**
clavicular
    c. birth fracture
    c. branch of thoracoacromial artery
    c. epiphysis
    c. facet
    c. fracture aneurysm
    c. notch of sternum
    c. part of pectoralis major muscle
claviculectomy
clavipectoral fascia
clawfoot deformity
clawhand deformity
clawing deformity
clawtoe deformity
claw-type basic frame
clay-shoveler fracture
Clayton
    C. forefoot arthroplasty
    C. procedure
    C. procedure with panmetatarsal
      head resection
Clayton-Fowler technique
clean
    c. intermittent catheterization
    c. intermittent self-catheterization
clean-catch collcction method
cleaning solution
clear
    c. cell carcinoma of kidney
    c. cell hidradenoma
clearance technique
Cleartrace electrodes
Cleasby iridectomy operation
cleavage
    c. fracture
    c. lesion
    c. line
    c. plane
cleft
    anal c.
    c. closure
    corneal c.
    facial c.
    c. hand deformity
    Larrey c.
    c. lip

c. lip deformity
natal c.
c. nose
oblique facial c.
c. palate
c. palate classification
pudendal c.
residual c.
soft palate c.
subdural c.
urogenital c.
cleidocostal
cleidocranial
cleidotomy
cleidotripsy
Clerf laryngectomy tube
Cleveland
C. Clinic weighted scale of
endoscopic procedure
C. procedure
Cleveland-Bosworth-Thompson technique
clidal
clidocostal
clidocranial
clinch knot
clindamycin phosphate topical solution
clinical
c. correlation
c. examination
c. manifestation
c. spectroscopy
clinicopathologic
c. correlation
c. feature
Clinitron air-fluidized therapy
clinoid
c. process
clinoidectomy
anterior extradural c.
extradural c.
clinoparietal line
clip
c. application
c. graft
c. placement
c. technique
clitoral recession
clitoridectomy
clitoris
clitoroplasty
clitorovaginoplasty
clival

clivus
Blumenbach c.
c. canal line
c. metastasis
c. torcula line
CLO
C. biopsy
C. test
cloaca, pl. **cloacae**
ectopia cloacae
cloacal
c. formation
c. malformation
c. membrane
clockwise rotation
clomiphene fetal malformation
clonal expansion
C-loop intraocular lens
Cloquet
C. canal
C. canal remnant
C. hernia
C. septum
closed
c. anesthesia
c. anesthesia system
c. chest commissurotomy
c. chest thoracostomy
c. circle
c. circuit method
c. dislocation
c. drainage
c. flap amputation
c. head injury
c. hemorrhoidectomy
c. intramedullary osteotomy
c. irrigation
c. laparoscopy
c. manipulative maneuver
c. nail
c. patch test
c. pinning
c. reduction
c. reduction/chemical splinting
c. skull fracture
c. soft tissue injury
c. suction tube
c. surgery
c. surgery on eye
c. transventricular mitral
commissurotomy
c. tubule fixation technique

NOTES

closed *(continued)*
    c. water-seal suction tube
    c. wedge osteotomy
closed-break fracture
closed-circuit
    c.-c. anesthesia
    c.-c. anesthetic technique
closed-end ostomy pouch
closed-eye surgery
closed-loop
    c.-l. automated delivery
    c.-l. device
    c.-l. intestinal obstruction
closed-space infection
closed-system pars plana vitrectomy
closing
    c. abductory wedge osteotomy
    c. base wedge
    c. base wedge osteotomy
    c. pressure
    c. ring of Winkler-Waldeyer
    c. wedge manipulation and
      reapplication of plaster
clostridial
    c. infection
    c. myonecrosis
closure
    abdominal wall c.
    auditory c.
    Barsky cleft c.
    Beta-Cap II catheter c.
    Brandy scalp stretcher I, front c.
    Brandy scalp stretcher II, rear c.
    Clagett c.
    clamshell c.
    cleft c.
    compression skull cap c.
    crow-foot c.
    delayed primary c.
    double-umbrella c.
    epiphyseal c.
    exstrophy c.
    fascial c.
    flask c.
    floor-of-mouth c.
    Fontan fenestration c.
    forced-eye c.
    general c.
    glottic c.
    Graham c. with omental pouch
    ileostomy c.
    incision c.
    King ASD umbrella c.
    layered c.
    maxillary antrum c.
    muscularis tunnel c.
    nonoperative c.

    palatopharyngeal c.
    percutaneous patent ductus
      arteriosus c.
    premature airway c.
    premature ductus arteriosis c.
    c. pressure
    primary c.
    c. principle
    retainer c.
    scalloped c.
    scalp c.
    secondary c.
    shoelace fasciotomy c.
    single-layer c.
    sinus c.
    skin c.
    Smead-Jones c.
    Steri-Strip skin c.
    Steritapes c.
    Sureclosure c.
    sutureless colostomy c.
    SutureStrip Plus wound c.
    Tom Jones c.
    transcatheter c.
    umbrella c.
    Velcro c.
    velopharyngeal c.
    ventricular septal defect c.
    visual c.
    Von Langenbeck palatal c.
    watertight c.
    wound c.
clot
    exogenous fibrin c.
    Schede c.
clothespin
    c. H spinal fusion
    c. spinal fusion graft
clot-induced urinary tract obstruction
cloven hoof fracture of finger
cloverleaf
    c. condylar-plate fixation
    c. skull
    c. skull deformity
    c. skull syndrome
Cloward
    C. anterior spinal fusion
    C. back fusion
    C. cervical disk approach
    C. fusion diskectomy
    C. operation
    C. procedure
    C. technique
CLS stem insertion
clubbed
    c. nail
    c. penis

clubbing
    c. of nail
    nail c.
clubfoot deformity
cluneal
clunes
cluster reduction
CMAP
    compound muscle action potential
CML oxygenator
CMV
    controlled mechanical ventilation
        CMV infection
CMV-associated ulceration
CMV-induced esophageal ulceration
cnemial
cnemis
CO
    carbon monoxide
    cardiac output
CO_2
    carbon dioxide
    arterial partial pressure of CO_2
    CO_2 elimination
    CO_2 inhalation test
    CO_2 pneumoperitoneum
coagula (*pl. of* coagulum)
coagulate
coagulation
    argon beam c.
    BICAP c.
    bipolar c.
    Bipolar Circumactive Probe c.
    blood c.
    Bovie c.
    cold c.
    diffuse intravascular c.
    c. disorder
    disseminated intravascular c. (DIC)
    endoscopic microwave c.
    exogenous anticoagulant c.
    c. factor transfusion
    fibrinolysin c.
    free-beam c.
    heater probe c.
    c. and hemostatic resection of the prostate
    infrared c.
    laser c.
    light c.
    low current monopolar c.
    Meyer-Schwickerath light c.
    microwave c.
    monopolar c.
    multipolar c.
    c. necrosis
    c. pathway
    plasmin c.
    c. profile
    c. screen
    sepsis-induced disseminated intravascular c.
    tissue c.
coagulative
    c. laser therapy
    c. myocytolysis
coagulopathy
coagulum, pl. **coagula**
    c. formation
    c. pyelolithotomy
Coakley wash tube
coal-mining lensectomy
coapt
coaptation
    centrocentral c.
    c. suture
    urethral c.
coarct
coarctate
coarctation
    c. of aorta
    c. of pulmonary artery
    c. syndrome
coarctectomy
coarctotomy
coarticulation
    anticipatory c.
    backward c.
    forward c.
coat
    circular layer of muscular c.
    longitudinal layer of muscular c.
    muscular c. of bronchi
    muscular c. of colon
    muscular c. of ductus deferens
    muscular c. of esophagus
    muscular c. of female urethra
    muscular c. of gallbladder
    muscular c. of pharynx
    muscular c. of rectum
    muscular c. of small intestine
    muscular c. of stomach
    muscular c. of trachea
    muscular c. of ureter

NOTES

coat *(continued)*
    muscular c. of urinary bladder
    muscular c. of uterine tube
    muscular c. of uterus
    muscular c. of vagina
coated
    c. polyester suture
    c. Vicryl suture
Coats white ring
coaxial
    c. illumination
    c. pressure
cobalt-60 moving strip technique
cobalt blue filter
cobaltinitrite method
cobbler suture
Cobb scoliosis measuring technique
Cobe
    C. CML oxygenator
    C. Optima hollow-fiber membrane oxygenator
    C. Stöckert heart lung console
cobra-head anastomosis
cocaine
    c. anesthesia
    c. hydrochloride
    c. methylphenidate
cocaine-induced respiratory failure
coccidian body
Coccidioides **infection**
coccygeal
    c. body
    c. cornua
    c. dimple
    c. fistula
    c. foveola
    c. ganglion
    c. gland
    c. horn
    c. joint
    c. muscle
    c. nerve
    c. part of spinal cord
    c. plexus
    c. segments of spinal cord
    c. vertebrae
    c. whorl
coccygectomy
    Lougheed-White c.
coccygeus
    c. muscle
coccygotomy
coccyx
    c. fracture
cochlear lesion
cochleosacculotomy
cochleostomy

cochleovestibular
    c. approach
    c. neurectomy
cocked-half flap
Cocke maxillectomy
Cockett procedure
Cockroft method
cock-up deformity
cocoon thread suture
codfish deformity
Codivilla
    C. bone graft
    C. tendon lengthening technique
Codman
    C. classification
    C. frame
    C. ICP monitoring line
    C. incision
    C. saber-cut shoulder approach
coefficient
    c. of correlation
    octanol/water c.
    Spearman rank correlation c.
co-eluted
Coe-Soft
Coffey
    C. incision
    C. suspension
    C. technique
    C. ureterointestinal anastomosis
Coffey-Witzel jejunostomy technique
Cofield technique
cogwheel respiration
Cohen
    C. antireflux procedure
    C. cross-trigonal reimplantation
    C. cross-trigonal technique
Cohen-Rentrop classification
coherent bundle
coiled pressure algesimeter
coin
    c. biopsy
    fracture en c.
    c. lesion
    c. lesion of lung
coincidence correction
co-induction
    c.-i. of anesthesia
Coiter muscle
Colcher-Sussman method
cold
    c. abscess
    c. application
    c. coagulation
    c. conization
    c. cup biopsy
    c. exposure
    c. forceps ablation

c. knife endoureterotomy
c. knife method
c. lesion
c. pressor test (CPT)
c. pressor testing maneuver
c. saline-induced paresthesia technique
c. snare ablation
c. snare excision
c. soak solution
c. sterilization
cold-cup resection
cold-knife conization
Cole
C. endotracheal tube
C. hyperextension fracture frame
C. intubation procedure
C. orotracheal tube
C. osteotomy
C. osteotomy for midfoot deformity
C. pediatric tube
C. technique
C. tendon fixation
C. uncuffed endotracheal tube
colectasia
colectomy
abdominal c.
laparoscopic c.
open c.
prophylactic c.
subtotal c. (SC)
total c. (TC)
total abdominal c.
transverse c.
Coleman
C. flatfoot technique
C. plasty
coleocele
coleoptosis
coleotomy
colic
c. arteries
c. impression
c. lymph nodes
c. patch
c. patch esophagoplasty
c. sphincter
c. surface of spleen
c. teniae
ureteral c.
c. veins
colica

coliform urinary infection
coliplication
colipuncture
colitis
c. perineal complication
radiation-induced c.
ulcerative c.
colla (*pl. of* collum)
collagen
c. injection
c. staining method
c. suture
collagen-impregnated knitted Dacron velour graft
collagenolytic trabecular ring
collagenous
c. tissue
c. trabecular ring
Collagraft bone graft matrix
collapse
bone graft c.
c. cavitation
collar
c. bone
c. button tube
c. incision
collar-button ulceration
collared Press-Fit femoral stem implantation
collateral
c. abdominal circulation
c. digital artery
c. ligament
c. ligament rupture
c. mesenteric circulation
c. pulp canal
c. respiration
collateralization
ventilation c.
collection
abdominal air c.
air c.
arterial blood c.
cell c.
duodenal fluid c.
encysted intra-abdominal c.
expired air c.
extra-axial fluid c.
extracerebral fluid c.
fluid c.
gas c.
globular c.

NOTES

C

collection *(continued)*
    gravitational particle c.
    24-hour urine c.
    isokinetic c.
    pancreatic fluid c.
    periarticular fluid c.
    pericholecystic fluid c.
    perinephric fluid c.
    pleural fluid c.
    posttraumatic subcapsular hepatic
        fluid c.
    pus c.
    quantitative stool c.
    saccular c.
    urine specimen c.
Colles
    C. external fixation frame
    C. fascia
    C. fracture
    C. ligament
    C. space
colliculectomy
colliculi (*pl. of* colliculus)
colliculitis
colliculocentral point
colliculus, pl. **colliculi**
    facial c.
    seminal c.
Collier tract
Collin-Beard operation
Collins
    C. indigo carmine solution
    C. intracellular electrolyte solution
Collis
    C. antireflux operation
    C. broken femoral stem technique
    C. gastroplasty
    C. repair
Collis-Dubrul femoral stem removal
Collis-Nissen
    C.-N. fundoplication
    C.-N. fundoplication method
    C.-N. fundoplication procedure
    C.-N. fundoplication technique
collodion
    c. filter
    flexible c.
    hemostatic c.
    c. membrane
    styptic c.
collodium
colloid
    c. body
    c. osmotic pressure (COP)
    c. solution
    styptic c.
colloidal osmotic pressure
collum, pl. **colla**

    c. anatomicum humeri
    c. chirurgicum humeri
    c. costae
    c. femoris
    c. glandis penis
    c. humeri
    c. mallei
    c. ossis femoris
    c. radii
    c. scapulae
    c. tali
    c. vesicae biliaris
    c. vesicae felleae
coloanal
    c. anastomosis
    c. resection
coloboma
    c. anomalies
    c. of fundus
    c. of lens
    c. lobuli
    c. of optic nerve
    c. of retina
    c. retinae
colobronchial fistula
colocentesis
colocholecystostomy
colocolic
colocolonic anastomosis
colocolostomy
colocutaneous fistula
colocystoplasty
    seromuscular c.
coloendoanal anastomosis
cologastrocutaneous fistula
colohepatopexy
coloileal fistula
cololysis
colon
    ascending c.
    bands of c.
    c. carcinoma
    c. conduit
    descending c.
    c. flexure
    giant c.
    iliac c.
    c. incarceration
    lateral reflection of c.
    lead-pipe c.
    mucosa of c.
    pelvic peritonectomy with resection
        of sigmoid c.
    perforation of c.
    c. perforation
    c. procedure
    c. and rectal surgery
    c. resection

sigmoid c.
spastic c.
spike burst on electromyogram
   of c.
toxic dilation of c.
transverse c.
c. tumor
Colon-A-Sun colonic irrigation
colonic
   c. adenocarcinoma
   c. adenoma
   c. carcinoma
   c. dilation
   c. diverticular hemorrhage
   c. explosion
   c. fistula
   c. foreign body
   c. infiltration
   c. J-pouch
   c. lavage solution
   c. lesion identification
   c. loop
   c. mass
   c. metastasis
   c. mucosal line
   c. patch
   c. perforation
   c. vascular lesion
colonization infection
Colonna
   C. hip fracture classification
   C. trochanteric arthroplasty
Colonna-Ralston
   C.-R. ankle approach
   C.-R. incision
   C.-R. medial approach
colonoscopic
   c. appendectomy
   c. biopsy
   c. polypectomy
   c. removal
colonoscopy
   cecal c.
   c. complication
   diagnostic c.
   emergency c.
   high-magnification c.
   pediatric c.
   c. screening
   splenic flexure c.
   tandem c.
   therapeutic c.

total c.
upper endoscopy and c.
colonoscopy-related
   c.-r. emphysema
   c.-r. incarceration
colonostomy
colony formation
colopexostomy
colopexotomy
colopexy
Coloplast
   C. Flange pouch
   C. mini pouch
coloplasty pouch
coloplication
coloproctostomy
coloptosis
colopuncture
color
   c. aberration
   c. fusion
   c. saturation
colorectal
   c. adenocarcinoma
   c. adenoma
   c. anastomosis
   c. biopsy
   c. cancer endoscopy
   c. carcinoma
   c. distention pain
   c. hemorrhage
   c. surgery
   c. tumor
colorectostomy
colorrhaphy
colosigmoidostomy
colosigmoid resection
colostomy
   c. bridge
   continent c.
   decompression c.
   descending loop c.
   Devine c.
   diverting loop c.
   divided-stoma c.
   double-barrel c.
   dry c.
   end c.
   end-loop c.
   end-sigmoid c.
   exteriorization c.
   fecal diversion c.

C

NOTES

135

colostomy *(continued)*
Hartmann c.
ileoascending c.
ileosigmoid c.
ileotransverse c.
irrigation of c.
juxta-anal c.
loop transverse c.
Mikulicz c.
permanent end c.
c. pyloric autotransplantation
resective c.
sigmoid-end c.
sigmoid-loop rod c.
c. soiling
c. takedown
takedown of c.
temporary diverting c.
temporary end c.
terminal c.
transverse-loop rod c.
Turnbull c.
wet c.
colotomy
colovaginal fistula
colovesical fistula
colpectomy
skinning c.
colpocleisis
Latzko partial c.
Le Fort partial c.
colpocystoplasty
colpocystotomy
colpocystoureterotomy
colpocystourethropexy
colpohysterectomy
colpohysteropexy
colpohysterotomy
colpomicroscopy
colpomyomectomy
colpoperineoplasty
colpoperineorrhaphy
colpopexy
colpoplasty
colpopoiesis
colporectopexy
colporrhaphy
Goffe c.
colposcopy
digital imaging c.
estrogen-assisted c.
colpostenotomy
colposuspension
laparoscopic needle c.
laparoscopic retropubic c.
colpotomy
c. incision
colpoureterotomy

colpourethrocystopexy
retropubic c.
colpourethropexy
Burch c.
Coltart
C. calcaneotibial fusion
C. fracture technique
Colton
C. classification
C. empyema tube
columellar
c. reconstruction
c. repair
column
anal c.
anterior c.
Bertin c.'s
lateral c.
Morgagni c.'s
posterior c.
rectal c.'s
renal c.'s
rugal c.'s of vagina
spinal c.
vaginal c.'s
variceal c.
vertebral c.
coma
c. aberration
acute hepatic c.
alcoholic c.
apoplectic c.
barbiturate c.
c. dé passé
diabetic c.
electrolyte imbalance c.
Harvard criteria of irreversible c.
hepatic c.
hyperosmolar diabetic c.
hyperosmolar hyperglycemic
 nonketotic c.
irreversible c.
Kussmaul c.
metabolic c.
c. scale
thyrotoxic c.
trance c.
uremic c.
c. vigil
Comberg foreign body operation
combination
c. calculus
c. of isotonics technique
c. restoration
c. skin
c. surgery
combined
c. analysis

c. anterior and posterior approach
c. cavus deformity
c. chemoradiation therapy
c. epidural/general anesthesia
c. flexion-distraction injury and burst fracture
c. heart catheterization
c. hiatal hernia
c. low cervical and transthoracic approach
c. method
c. organ resection
c. presigmoid-transtransversarium intradural approach
c. radial-ulnar-humeral fracture
c. spinal/epidural anesthesia (CSE)
c. spinal/epidural anesthetic technique
c. system disease
c. transsylvian and middle fossa approach
c. ureterolysis

Combitube
C. endotracheal tube
C. esophageal tracheal tube

comblike septum
come-and-go anesthesia
comedocarcinoma
comedo extraction
Comfit endotracheal tube
Comfort
C. and sedation scoring system
C. Tears solution

commando
c. operation
c. procedure
C. radical glossectomy

commercial dialysis solution
comminuted
c. intra-articular fracture
c. orbital fracture
c. skull fracture

comminution
commissura, pl. **commissurae**
c. labiorum anterior
c. labiorum posterior

commissural
c. bundle
c. fusion
c. myelorrhaphy
c. myelotomy

commissure
anterior labial c.
c. of lips
posterior labial c.

commissurotomy
balloon mitral c.
Brockenbrough transseptal c.
closed chest c.
closed transventricular mitral c.
mitral balloon c.
percutaneous mitral balloon c.
percutaneous transatrial mitral c.
percutaneous transvenous mitral c.
transventricular mitral valve c.

common
c. basal vein
c. bile duct (CBD)
c. bile duct exploration
c. canal
c. carotid plexus
c. cavity phenomenon
c. dural sac
c. extensor tendon
c. facial vein
c. flexor sheath
c. hepatic artery
c. hepatic duct
c. iliac artery
c. iliac lymph nodes
c. interosseous artery
c. mode rejection ratio
c. palmar digital artery
c. peroneal artery
c. peroneal nerve
c. peroneal nerve syndrome
c. plantar digital artery
c. tendinous ring

commune
integumentum c.

communicating
c. artery
c. branches of spinal nerves
c. branches of sympathetic trunk
c. fistula
c. hematoma
c. rami of spinal nerves
c. rami of sympathetic trunk

communis
extensor digitorum c.

community-acquired infection
commutator

NOTES

137

compact
    c. bone
    c. substance
compages thoracis
companion
    c. artery to sciatic nerve
    c. lymph nodes of accessory nerve
comparative radiographic examination
comparison operation
compartment
    c. compression syndrome
    extra-axial c.
    extracellular c.
    extravascular c.
    c. procedure
    c. syndrome
compartmental
    c. pressure
    c. radioimmunoglobulin therapy
    c. volume
compartmentalization
Compat feeding tube
Compazine
    C. injection
    C. Oral
compensation
    c. reaction
    c. technique
compensatory
    c. basilar osteotomy
    c. circulation
    c. deformity
    c. head posture
    c. regeneration
    c. wedge
competing messages integration
compilation autogenous vein graft
complementary balloon angioplasty
complement fixation
complete
    c. anterior dislocation
    c. atrioventricular dissociation
    c. A-V dissociation
    c. bilateral deformity
    c. common peroneal nerve lesion
    c. duplication
    c. fistula
    c. fracture
    c. hernia
    c. inferior dislocation
    c. internal hemipelvectomy
    c. iridectomy
    c. lateral hemilaminectomy
    c. left bundle-branch block
    c. posterior dislocation
    c. pulpectomy
    c. pulpotomy
    c. right bundle-branch block

    c. superior dislocation
    c. surgical exploration
completion thyroidectomy
complex
    c. adrenal endocrine disorder
    c. anorectal fistula
    areolar c.
    c. cavity
    c. chest mass
    c. dissection
    c. endocrine disorder
    epispadias-exstrophy c.
    exstrophy-epispadias c.
    c. fracture
    fusion c.
    Ghon c.
    c. gonadal endocrine disorder
    growth plate c.
    juxtaglomerular c.
    limb-body wall c.
    c. pituitary endocrine disorder
    sling-ring c.
    c. thyroid endocrine disorder
    vertebral subluxation c.
compliance
    chest wall c.
    dynamic c. (Cdyn)
    pulmonary c.
    c., rate, oxygenation, and pressure
    c., rate, oxygenation, and pressure
      index
    c. of the total respiratory system
complicated fracture
complication
    bacterial c.
    benign pneumatic colonoscopy c.
    cardiopulmonary c.
    cardiorespiratory c.
    cardiovascular c.
    cerebrovascular c.
    colitis perineal c.
    colonoscopy c.
    delayed c.
    endoscopy c.
    extraintestinal c.
    feeding c.
    gastrointestinal c.
    gonadal c.
    hematologic c.
    hepatic c.
    immunologic c.
    infectious c.
    intraoperative c.
    metabolic c.
    neurologic c.
    neurovascular c.
    nonimmunologic c.
    obstetrical c.

operative site c.
opportunistic c.
oral c.
postbiopsy vascular c.
postoperative c.
pregnancy c.
pulmonary c.
c. rate
renal c.
respiratory c.
sclerotherapy c.
urologic c.
vascular c.

component of mastication

composite
c. addition technique
c. flap
c. free tissue transfer
c. joint
c. pelvic resection
c. pelvic resection method
c. pelvic resection procedure
c. pelvic resection technique
c. resin restoration
c. rib graft
c. skin graft
c. tissue transfer

compound
c. aneurysm
c. cavity
c. comminuted fracture
c. dislocation
c. flap
c. joint
c. muscle action potential (CMAP)
c. restoration
c. skull fracture
c. suture

compressed
c. body
c. fracture
c. Ivalon patch graft

compressible cavernous bodies

compression
c. anesthesia
anterior cord c.
anterior-posterior c.
anteroposterior c.
AO c.
c. arthrodesis
axial c.
barrel-hooping c.

c. bone conduction
c. of brain
brainstem c.
c. of breast
c. button gastrojejunostomy
cardiac c.
carotid artery c.
cauda equina c.
cerebral aqueduct c.
cervical vessel c.
cervicomedullary junction c.
Charnley c.
chest c.
chiasmal c.
cord c.
c. cough
c. cyanosis
disk c.
duodenal c.
duplex-guided c.
dynamic c.
elastic c.
esophageal c.
c. extension
external pneumatic calf c.
extrinsic bladder c.
c. fracture
gastric c.
c. girdle
head c.
image c.
c. injury
c. instrumentation posterior
  construct
interfragmentary c.
intermittent pneumatic c.
intrinsic c.
ischemic c.
lateral c.
limbal c.
mechanical variceal c.
median nerve c.
c. molding
napkin-ring c.
nerve root c.
neurovascular cross c.
optic chiasm c.
optic tract c.
c. overload
c. paralysis
c. plate fixation
c. plating

C

NOTES

compression *(continued)*
 pneumatic c.
 prechiasmal c.
 c. rod treatment
 root c.
 c. skull cap closure
 spinal cord c.
 spot c.
 static c.
 c. stocking
 c. strain
 suprascapular nerve c.
 c. suture
 c. switch
 c. syndrome
 c. technique
 c. test
 c. testing
 thecal sac c.
 tissue c.
 tracheal c.
 uterine c.
 variable release c.
 venous c.
 vertebral c.
 vertical c.
 c. wiring
compressor muscle of lips
compromise
 airway c.
compromised
computed
 c. tomography
 c. tomography scan (CT scan)
computer-assisted
 c.-a. anesthesia
 c.-a. continuous infusion anesthetic technique
 c.-a. design-controlled alignment method
 c.-a. stereotactic surgery
computer-controlled
 c.-c. drug administration anesthetic technique
 c.-c. infusion anesthetic technique
 c.-c. infusion pump
computerized
 c. diaphragmatic breathing retraining (CDBR)
 c. electronic endoscopy
3-D computer reconstruction
concatenation
concealed
 c. bypass tract
 c. hemorrhage
 c. hernia
 c. penis
 c. umbilical stoma

concentrates
 platelet c.
concentration
 ambient oxygen c.
 approximate lethal c.
 bactericidal c.
 blood alcohol c.
 carbon dioxide c.
 end-tidal nitrogen c.
 hazardous c.
 inspiratory vapor c.
 lethal c.
 mass c.
 maximal drug c.
 maximum permissible c.
 minimal anesthetic c. (MAC)
 minimal bactericidal c.
 minimum alveolar c. (MAC)
 1-minimum alveolar c. (1-MAC)
 minimum alveolar anesthetic c. (MAC)
 minimum bactericidal c.
 minimum detectable c.
 minimum effective c. (MEC)
 minimum effective analgesic c.
 minimum lethal c.
 minimum local analgesic c. (MLAC)
 c. performance test
 plasma gastrin c.
 plasma iron c.
 plasma norepinephrine c.
 plasma renin c.
 plasma urea c.
 predialysis plasma phosphate c.
 prick test c.
 c. procedure
 radioactive c.
 renal vein renin c.
 serum bactericidal c.
 serum bilirubin c.
 serum calcium c.
 serum lithium c.
 sodium butyrate c.
 steroid c.
 subanesthetic c.
 substance c.
 thyroid hormone serum c.
 time of maximum c.
 c. times time
 total L-chain c.
 total protein c.
concentration-effect relation
concentric
 c. hernia
 c. lesion
 c. reduction

concept
  c. formation
  C. nerve stimulator
  C. traction tower
concha, pl. conchae
  c. auriculae
  c. of ear
  sphenoidal conchae
  conchae sphenoidales
conchal crest of palatine bone
conchoidal
concomitant
  c. antireflux surgery
  c. medication
  c. therapy
Concord/Portex airway
concurrent hepatic laceration
concussion
  brain c.
  spinal c.
  spinal cord c.
condensation
  amalgam c.
  chromatin c.
  filling material c.
  gold foil c.
  heavy c.
  lateral c.
  porcelain c.
  pressure c.
  resin c.
  spatulation c.
  vibration c.
  warm c.
  whipping c.
condenser point
condition
  tumor-like bone c.
conditioning
  c. program
  c. therapy
conductance
  skin c.
conduction
  c. analgesia
  c. anesthesia
  compression bone c.
  osteotympanic bone c.
conductivity
  tissue c.
conduit
  antirefluxing colonic c.

colon c.
cutaneous appendiceal c.
ileal c.
ileocolic c.
intestinal c.
Mitrofanoff c.
Rastelli c.
respiratory syncytial virus c.
urinary c.
condylar
  c. articulation
  c. canal
  c. emissary vein
  c. femoral fracture
  c. guidance inclination
  c. guide inclination
  c. hinge position
  c. implant arthroplasty
  c. process
  c. process fracture
  c. screw fixation
condylarthrosis
condyle
  c. cord
  c. dissection
  c. head
  c. of humerus
  lateral c.
  medial c.
  occipital c.
  c. resection
condylectomy
  DuVries plantar c.
  mandibular c.
  plantar c.
condylion
condylocephalic nail
condyloid process
condyloma, pl. condylomata
  c. acuminatum
  anal c.
  cervical c.
  flat c.
  giant c.
  perianal c.
  c. planus
  pointed c.
condylomatous
condylotomy
condylus
  c. humeri
  c. lateralis

NOTES

141

condylus *(continued)*
   c. lateralis femoris
   c. lateralis tibiae
   c. medialis
   c. medialis femoris
   c. medialis tibiae
   c. occipitalis
cone
   c. biopsy
   c. biopsy of cervix
   C. suction tube
Cone-Bucy suction tube
conexus
   c. intertendineus
confirmation
   tissue c.
confluence
   venous c.
confluent inflammation
conformal radiation therapy
confrontation
   c. method
   c. testing
   c. visual field test
congenital
   c. above-elbow amputation
   c. arteriovenous fistula
   c. aspiration pneumonia
   c. below-elbow amputation
   c. brain malformation
   c. central hypoventilation syndrome
   c. cerebral aneurysm
   c. conotruncal anomaly
   c. cystic adenomatoid malformation
   c. cystic dilatation
   c. cystic dilatation of bile duct
   c. depigmentation
   c. diaphragmatic hernia
   c. dislocation of hip
   c. duplication
   c. elevation of the scapula
   c. fracture
   c. heart malformation
   c. hip dislocation
   c. HIV infection
   c. infection
   c. lens dislocation
   c. malrotation of the gut
   c. nasal mass
   c. postural deformity
   c. pulmonary arteriovenous fistula
   c. pyloric membrane
   c. renal mass
   c. ring
   c. ring syndrome
   c. scapular elevation
   c. stippled epiphysis
   c. tracheobiliary fistula

   c. urethroperineal fistula
   c. vascular malformation
   c. vertical talus foot deformity
congenitally altered anatomy
congestion
   brain c.
   flap c.
congestive
conglomerate mass
conglutinant
conglutination
coni (*pl. of* conus)
coniotomy
conization
   cautery c.
   cervical c.
   c. of cervix
   cold c.
   cold-knife c.
   hot-knife c.
   Hyam c.
   laser cervical c.
   LEEP c.
   loop diathermy cervical c.
conjoined
   c. anastomosis
   c. nerve-root anomaly
   c. tendon
conjoint tendon
conjugate
   c. axis
   c. foramen
   c. point
conjugation bridge
conjunctiva-associated lymphoid tissue
conjunctival
   c. angioma
   c. circulation
   c. cul-de-sac
   c. exudate
   c. flap
   c. fornix
   c. hemorrhage
   c. incision
   c. injection
   c. laceration
   c. melanotic lesion
   c. membrane
   c. patch graft
   c. ring
   c. sac
conjunctiva-Müller muscle excision
conjunctiviplasty
conjunctivitis
conjunctivodacryocystorhinostomy
conjunctivodacryocystostomy
conjunctivoplasty
conjunctivorhinostomy

conjunctivo-Tenon flap
Conley incision
Con-Lish polishing method
connecting cartilage
connection
    Luer c.
connective
    c. tissue
    c. tissue activating peptide
    c. tissue augmentation
    c. tissue disease
    c. tissue disorder
    c. tissue graft
    c. tissue massage
    c. tissue membrane
    c. tissue plasticity
connector
    Humid-Vent Port 1 elbow c.
    Luer c.
    Luer-Lok jet ventilator c.
    quick c.
    Saf-T-Flo T-tube c.
    SidePort AutoControl airway c.
    c. with lock washer
Connell
    C. incision
    C. stitch
    C. suture
Connolly
    C. procedure
    C. technique
Conn operation
conoid
    c. process
    c. tubercle
conotruncal anomaly
Conradi line
Conrad orbital blowout fracture operation
consciousness
conscious sedation
consecutive
    c. amputation
    c. aneurysm
    c. dislocation
consent
    informed c.
conservation surgery
conservative
    c. resection
    c. surgery
    c. therapy

console
    Cobe Stöckert heart lung c.
consolidation
    c. of lung
consonant-injection method
consonant position
consortial approach
constant
    c. flow insufflation
    c. infusion pump
constipation
constitutive heterochromatin method
constrained
    c. ankle arthroplasty
    c. reconstruction
    c. shoulder arthroplasty
constricting lesion
constriction
    esophageal c.'s
    pyloric c.
    c. ring
    c.'s of ureter
construct
    AO dynamic compression plate c.
    compression instrumentation posterior c.
    double-rod c.
    Edwards modular system bridging sleeve c.
    Edwards modular system compression c.
    Edwards modular system distraction-lordosis c.
    Edwards modular system kyphoreduction c.
    Edwards modular system neutralization c.
    Edwards modular system rod-sleeve c.
    Edwards modular system scoliosis c.
    Edwards modular system spondylo c.
    Edwards modular system standard sleeve c.
    hook-to-screw L4-S1 compression c.
    iliosacral and iliac fixation c.
    pedicle screw c.
    rod-hook c.
    screw-to-screw compression c.
    segmental compression c.
    single-rod c.

C

NOTES

construct *(continued)*
  TSRH double-rod c.
  TSRH pedicle screw-laminar
    claw c.
  Wiltse system double-rod c.
  Wiltse system H c.
  Wiltse system single-rod c.
construction
  Abbé vaginal c.
  absolute c.
  endocentric c.
  exocentric c.
  ileal reservoir c.
  McIndoe-Hayes c.
  pelvic ileal reservoir c.
  single denture c.
  sphincteric c.
  stent c.
  tandem c.
  Thiersch-Duplay urethral c.
  U pouch c.
  vaginal c.
consumption
  oxygen c.
  peak exercise oxygen c.
contact
  c. activation product
  c. area point
  c. dissolution therapy
  c. illumination
  c. laser ablation of prostate
    (CLAP)
  C. Laser vaporization
  c. manipulation
  c. metastasis
  c. method
contamination
  bacterial c.
  fecal c.
  gas c.
  hub c.
  metastatic c.
  post-autoclave c.
content
  aspiration of gastric c.'s
  evacuation of uterine c.'s
  mixed venous oxygen c.
  tissue water c.
Contigen tube
contiguous loop
contiguum
  per c.
continence
  sphincteric c.
continent
  c. colostomy
  c. cutaneous appendicocystostomy
  c. ileal pouch

  c. ileostomy
  c. urinary pouch
continuous
  c. albuterol nebulization
  c. anesthetic technique
  c. arteriovenous hemofiltration
  c. arteriovenous ultrafiltration
  c. atrial fibrillation
  c. bladder irrigation
  c. catheter drainage
  c. distending airway pressure
  c. endothelium
  c. epidural anesthesia
  c. gum technique
  c. hyperthermic peritoneal perfusion
  c. infusion anesthetic technique
  c. intramucosal PCO_2 measurement
  c. loop wiring
  c. lumbar peridural anesthesia
  c. mandatory ventilation
  c. negative airway pressure
  c. NG suction
  c. on-line recording
  c. positive airway pressure (CPAP)
  c. positive pressure breathing
    (CPPB)
  c. positive pressure ventilation
    (CPPV)
  c. postoperative closed lavage
  c. pull-through technique
  c. renal replacement therapy
  c. running horizontal mattress
    suture
  c. running monofilament suture
  c. sling suture
  c. spinal anesthesia
  c. spinal anesthetic technique
  c. subcutaneous insulin injection
  c. suction tube
  c. suture technique
  c. venovenous hemofiltration
continuous-flow ventilation
continuous-wave
  c.-w. laser ablation
  c.-w. technique
continuum
  per c.
contour
  corneal c.
  intonation c.
  c. line
  c. line of Owen
  c. restoration
  restoration c.
contoured
  c. adduction trochanteric-controlled
    alignment method
  c. anterior spinal plate technique

contra-angle
contra-aperture
contraceptive
    c. method
    c. technique
contracted
    c. kidney
    c. pelvis
contractile
    c. motility
    c. ring
    c. ring dysphagia
contraction
    c. of cyclitic membrane
    c. fasciculation
contract relax technique
contraindication
contralateral
    c. axillary metastasis
    c. groin exploration
contrast
    blood oxygenation level-
      dependent c.
    c. enema
    c. injection
    c. material instillation
    c. visualization
contrecoup
    c. fracture
    c. injury of brain
control
    endoscopic c.
    exsanguination tourniquet c.
    hemorrhage c.
    monitored anesthesia c.
    Pringle vascular c.
    pronation c.
    c. release suture
    tourniquet c.
    c. of ventilation
controlled
    c. diaphragmatic respiration
    c. expansion
    c. mechanical ventilation (CMV)
    c. release anesthetic technique
    c. rotational osteotomy
    c. ventilation
    c. water added technique
controller
    Asahi pressure c.
    Bronkhorst High Tec c.

    IVAC 831 drip c.
    mass flow c.
control-mode ventilation
contusion
    brain c.
    corneal c.
    myocardial c.
conus, pl. coni
    c. arteriosus
    c. elasticus
    coni epididymidis
    coni vasculosi
ConvaTec
    C. colostomy pouch
    C. Durahesive Wafer ostomy
    C. Little One Sur-Fit pouch
    C. ostomy pouch
    C. Sur-Fit two-piece pouch
    C. urostomy pouch
convenience
    c. jaw relation
    c. point
conventional
    c. method
    c. technique
    c. thoracoplasty
Conventry proximal tibial osteotomy
convergence
    c. facilitation
    c. point
    c. position
    c. projection
convergent beam irradiation
Converse
    scalping flap of C.
conversion
    above-knee amputation c.
    extraglandular c.
    pressure c.
converter
    SRR-5 digital-analogue c.
convex
    c. condylar implant arthroplasty
    c. fusion
    c. nail
convoluted
    c. part of kidney lobule
    c. seminiferous tubule
convulsion
    ether c.
convulsive therapy
Conyers technique

C

NOTES

Cook County tracheal suction tube
cooled-knife method
Cooley
> C. aortic sump tube
> C. graft suction tube
> C. intracardiac suction tube
> C. intrapericardial anastomosis
> C. modification of Waterston anastomosis
> C. sump suction tube
> C. vascular suction tube
> C. woven Dacron graft

Cooley-Anthony suction tube
Coolidge tube
cooling
> active core c.
> external c.
> passive tissue c.
> whole body c.

Coomassie brilliant blue technique
Coonrad-Morrey total elbow arthroplasty
Coonrad total elbow arthroplasty
Coonse-Adams
> C.-A. knee approach
> C.-A. technique

Cooper
> C. endotracheal stylet
> C. fascia
> C. hernia
> C. ligaments
> C. operation
> C. reduction
> C. syndrome

cooperation
> cellular c.

CooperVision balanced salt solution
co-oximeter
> Ciba-Corning 2500 c.-o.
> IL-282 c.-o.

co-oximetry
COP
> colloid osmotic pressure

Cope
> C. loop nephrostomy tube
> C. method
> C. technique

Copeland
> C. retinoscopy
> C. technique

Copeland-Howard scapulothoracic fusion
Cophene-B injection
copious irrigation
copper sulfate method
copper-wire
> c.-w. arteriole
> c.-w. artery
> c.-w. reflex

copular point
copulating pouch
coracoacromial
> c. ligament

coracobrachial
> c. bursa
> c. muscle

coracobrachialis
> c. muscle

coracoclavicular
> c. articulation
> c. ligament
> c. screw fixation
> c. space
> c. suture fixation
> c. technique

coracohumeral
> c. ligament

coracoid
> c. fracture
> c. process

coral calculus
Corbin technique
cord
> c. compression
> condyle c.
> false knot of umbilical c.
> false vocal c.
> Ferrein c.'s
> gangliated c.
> genital c.
> germinal c.'s
> gonadal c.'s
> lateral c. of brachial plexus
> lipoma of c.
> marginal insertion of umbilical c.
> medial c. of brachial plexus
> nephrogenic c.
> oblique c.
> posterior c. of brachial plexus
> presentation of c.
> punch resection of vocal c.
> rete c.'s
> space available for the c.
> spermatic c.
> c. structures
> subacute combined degeneration of the spinal c.
> tendinous c.'s
> testicular c.
> testis c.'s
> c. traction syndrome
> true vocal c.
> umbilical c.
> velamentous insertion of c.
> vocal c.
> Weitbrecht c.
> Willis c.'s

cordate pelvis
cordectomy
cordis
    scrobiculus c.
cordopexy
cordotomy
    anterolateral c.
    open c.
    percutaneous c.
    posterior column c.
    spinothalamic c.
    stereotactic c.
core
    c. drilling procedure
    c. hypothermia
    c. needle biopsy
    c. suture
    c. vitrectomy
corectomy
coreoplasty
corepexy
Coretemp deep tissue thermometer
coretomy
Cori classification
corkscrew maneuver
corn
    hard c.
    soft c.
    web c.
cornea, pl. corneae
    calcareous degeneration of c.
    degeneration of c.
    ectatic marginal degeneration of c.
    endothelial cell surface of c.
    endothelial dystrophy of c.
    fistula of c.
    c. guttate lesion
    lead incrustation of c.
    marginal degeneration of c.
    marginal ring ulcer of c.
    pigmented line of c.
    ring ulcer of c.
    rust ring of c.
    superficial line of c.
    transplantation of c.
    trepanation of c.
    ulceration of c.
    white ring of c.
corneal
    c. abrasion
    c. abscess
    c. abscission

    c. alkali burn
    c. anesthesia
    c. apex
    c. arcus
    c. astigmatism
    c. blood staining
    c. cap
    c. cleft
    c. contour
    c. contusion
    c. curvature
    c. dendrite
    c. diameter
    c. distortion
    c. dystrophy
    c. ectasia
    c. edema
    c. endothelium
    c. epithelium
    c. erosion
    c. erysiphake
    c. facet
    c. filament
    c. fissure
    c. fistula
    c. foreign body
    c. full-thickness
    c. graft
    c. graft operation
    c. graft step
    c. guttering
    c. incision
    c. inferior limbal
    c. inlays
    c. iron line
    c. laceration
    c. lamella
    c. lamellar groove
    c. leakage
    c. lens
    c. light reflex
    c. limbus
    c. luster
    c. marginal furrow
    c. meridian
    c. mushroom
    c. nebula
    c. neovascularization
    c. nerve
    c. perforation
    c. protrusion
    c. punctate lesion

C

NOTES

corneal *(continued)*
    c. reflection
    c. scar
    c. scarring
    c. spot
    c. staining test
    c. stria
    c. substance
    c. surgery
    c. thinning
    c. transplant
    c. transplantation
    c. transplant centering ring
    c. trauma
    c. trepanation
    c. tube
    c. ulceration
    c. velum
corneoscleral
    c. incision
    c. laceration
corner
    c. fracture
    4-c. midcarpal fusion
    c. suture
    C. tampon
corniculate tubercle
corniculum
    c. laryngis
cornification
    c. disorder
Corning
    C. 170 blood gas analyzer
    C. method
Cornoy solution
cornu, pl. **cornua**
    coccygeal cornua
    cornua coccygealia
    cornua of falciform margin of
      saphenous opening
    cornua of hyoid bone
    c. inferius
    c. inferius cartilaginis thyroideae
    c. inferius marginalis falciformis
      hiatus sapheni
    cornua of lateral ventricle
    c. majus ossis hyoidei
    c. minus ossis hyoidei
    sacral cornua
    cornua sacralia
    styloid c.
    c. superius cartilaginis thyroideae
    c. superius marginalis falciformis
    cornua of thyroid cartilage
    c. uteri
cornual anastomosis

cornucopia
    sinusoidal endothelium c.
corona, pl. **coronae**
    c. capitis
    c. glandis
    c. of glans penis
coronal
    c. angulation
    c. oblique projection
    c. plane
    c. plane correction
    c. plane deformity
    c. plane deformity sagittal
      translation
    c. pulp tissue
    c. reconstruction
    c. section
    c. split fracture
    c. suture
    c. suture line of skull
coronary
    c. angioplasty versus excisional
      atherectomy
    c. artery angioplasty
    c. artery anomaly
    c. artery bypass graft (CABG)
    c. artery bypass grafting (CABG)
    c. artery bypass grafting surgery
    c. artery dissection
    c. artery ectasia
    c. artery fistula (CAF)
    c. artery lesion
    c. artery revascularization procedure
    c. artery-right ventricular fistula
    c. artery surgery study (CASS)
    c. balloon angioplasty
    c. bifurcation
    c. collateral circulation
    c. endarterectomy
    c. flow reserve technique
    c. ligament of knee
    c. ligament of liver
    c. node
    c. perfusion pressure
    c. plexus
    c. revascularization
    c. ring
    c. rotational ablation
    c. rotational atherectomy
    c. sinus catheterization
    c. sulcus
    c. thrombolysis
    c. vein
    c. venous pressure
    c. vessel anatomy
coronoid
    c. fossa of humerus
    c. line

c. process
c. process fracture
coronoidectomy
coronoradicular stabilization
coroplasty
coroscopy
corotomy
Corpak
C. feeding tube
C. weighted-tip, self-lubricating
tube
corpectomy
anterior c.
cervical c.
median c.
c. model
vertebral c.
vertebral body c.
corpora (*pl. of* corpus)
corporal biopsy
corporeal
c. aspiration
c. reconstruction
c. rotation procedure
corporectomy amputation
corporoplasty
incisional c.
modified Essed-Schroeder c.
corporotomy
corpus, pl. corpora
c. adiposum fossae ischiorectalis
c. adiposum infrapatellare
c. adiposum orbitae
c. aorticum
c. arantii
corpora arenacea
c. callosotomy
c. cavernosum clitoridis
c. cavernosum penis
c. cavernosum urethrae
c. claviculae
c. clitoridis
c. coccygeum
c. costae
c. epididymidis
c. epididymis
c. femoris
c. gastricum [ventriculi]
c. geniculatum externum
c. glandulae sudoriferae
c. highmori
c. humeri

c. linguae
c. luteum hematoma
c. mammae
c. ossis femoris
c. ossis hyoidei
c. ossis ilii
c. ossis ischii
c. ossis pubis
c. ossis sphenoidalis
c. pampiniforme
c. pancreatis
corpora para-aortica
c. penis
c. phalangis
c. radii
c. spongiosum penis
c. sterni
c. tali
c. tibiae
c. triticeum
c. ulnae
c. uteri
c. vertebrae
c. vesicae biliaris
c. vesicae felleae
c. vesicae urinariae
Correa classification
correction
adaptive c.
Allen c.
anterior c.
anteroposterior c.
aphakic c.
astigmatism c.
attenuation c.
Beckenbaugh c.
Bonferroni c.
Byron Smith lazy-T c.
cephalometric c.
chevron hallux valgus c.
coincidence c.
coronal plane c.
cubitus varus c.
dioptric c.
epicanthal c.
frontal plane c.
hallux varus c.
heparinase c.
Johnson-Spiegl hallux varus c.
Kilsyn-Evans principle of frontal
plane c.
King type IV curve posterior c.

NOTES

C

correction *(continued)*
    Küstner uterine inversion c.
    kyphosis c.
    mechanism of c.
    occlusal c.
    oligosegmental c.
    optical c.
    phalangeal malunion c.
    protamine c.
    rotational c.
    Ruiz-Mora c.
    scatter c.
    scoliosis c.
    secondary ptosis c.
    skeletal c.
    spectacle c.
    speech c.
    Steel c.
    surgical c.
    Tukey post-hoc c.
    with c.
    without c.
    Yates c.
corrective therapy
correlation
    canonical c.
    clinical c.
    clinicopathologic c.
    coefficient of c.
    Kendall rank c.
    negative c.
    Pearson product-moment coefficient of c.
    positive c.
    semilinear canonical c.
    Spearman nonparametric univariate c.
    Spearman rank c.
    Spearman rank-order c.
    c. time
correlational method
Correra line
corresponding point
corridor
    c. incision
    c. procedure
Corrigan respiration
corrin ring
corrosion preparation
corrugator
    c. cutis muscle of anus
    c. supercilii muscle
corset suspension
cortex, pl. **cortices**
    adrenal c.
    aspiration of c.
    association c.
    c. glandulae suprarenalis

    c. of lymph node
    c. nodi lymphatici
    c. ovarii
    c. of ovary
    renal c.
    c. renis
    suprarenal c.
    c. of thymus
    vertebral body anterior c.
Corticaine
    C. cream
cortical
    c. arches of kidney
    c. bone
    c. bone graft
    c. bone primary canal
    c. destruction
    c. fracture
    c. fragment
    c. implantation
    c. lateralization
    c. lobules of kidney
    c. mass
    c. part
    c. part of middle cerebral artery
    c. perforation
    c. respiration
    c. strut graft
    c. substance
corticalosteotomy
corticectomy
cortices (*pl. of* cortex)
corticoadenoma
corticobulbar tract
corticocancellous bone graft
corticomedullary demarcation
corticopontine tract
corticospinal tract
corticosteroid
    depot c.
corticotomy
    DeBastiani c.
    percutaneous c.
    c. of proximal tibia
Cortone Acetate injection
Cortrosyn
    C. injection
    C. stimulation test
Corvert injection
Cosgrove mitral valve replacement
cosmesis
cosmetic
    c. surgery
costa, pl. **costae**
    c. cervicalis
    costae fluctuantes
    costae fluitantes

costae spuriae
costae verae
costal
  c. angle
  c. cartilage
  c. cartilage graft
  c. facets
  c. groove for subclavian artery
  c. notch
  c. part of diaphragm
  c. pit of transverse process
  c. pleura
  c. process
  c. respiration
  c. surface
  c. surface of scapula
  c. tuberosity
costectomy
Costen suction tube
costicartilage
costiform
costoaxillary vein
costocentral
costocervical
  c. artery
  c. trunk
costochondral
  c. joint
  c. junction
costoclavicular
  c. ligament
  c. line
  c. maneuver
  c. space
costocolic ligament
costocoracoid
costodiaphragmatic recess
costoinferior
costomediastinal
  c. recess
  c. sinus
costophrenic septal lines
costoscapular
costoscapularis
costosternal
costosternoplasty
costosuperior
costotomy
costotransverse
  c. foramen
  c. joint
  c. ligament

costotransversectomy
  Seddon dorsal spine c.
  c. technique
costoversion thoracoplasty
costovertebral
  c. joints
costoxiphoid
  c. ligament
Cotrel
  C. pedicle screw fixation strength
  C. pedicle screw rigidity
Cotrel-Dubousset fixation
Cotte
  C. operation
  C. presacral neurectomy
Cotting toenail operation
Cottle suction tube
cotton
  C. ankle fracture
  C. cartilage graft
  c. Duknatel suture
  c. nonabsorbable suture
  C. reduction of elbow dislocation
cottonloader position
cotton-wool
  c.-w. exudate
  c.-w. patch
Cottony Dacron suture
Cotunnius
  C. aqueduct
  C. canal
  C. space
cotyle
cotyloid
  c. cavity
  c. joint
  c. ligament
couch-mounted head frame
cough
  compression c.
  c. CPR technique
  extrapulmonary c.
  c. fracture
coughing
  expulsive c.
cough-pressure transmission ratio
Couinaud classification
coulometric titration
Coulter MD 16 hemocytometer
coumadinization
coumarin green tunable dye laser lithotripsy

NOTES

Councilman lesion
Counsellor-Davis artificial vagina
    operation
Counsellor-Flor modification of McIndoe
    technique
count
        posttetanic c.
counterclockwise rotation
countercurrent
        c. extraction
        c. heat exchanger
        c. mechanism
counterincision
counterirritation
counteropening
counterpulsation
        balloon c.
        enhanced external c.
        intra-aortic balloon c.
        intra-arterial c.
        percutaneous intra-aortic balloon c.
counterpuncture
countersinking osteotomy
countersink screw head
counterstimulation
coup injury of brain
Coupland nasal suction tube
coupling head
Courvoisier
        C. gastroenterostomy
        C. incision
Couvelaire
        C. ileourethral anastomosis
        C. incision
Coventry
        C. distal femoral osteotomy
        C. femoral osteotomy
        C. vagal osteotomy
cove plane
covered stent-graft
Cowen-Loftus toe-phalanx
    transplantation
cow face
cowl muscle
Cowper
        C. gland
        C. ligament
coxa, pl. coxae
coxal bone
Cox Maze III procedure
coxofemoral
        c. articulation
Coxsackievirus
        C. A virus
        C. B virus
Cozen-Brockway
        C.-B. technique
        C.-B. Z-plasty

CPAP
        continuous positive airway pressure
C-plasty
CPPB
        continuous positive pressure breathing
CPPV
        continuous positive pressure ventilation
CPR
        cardiopulmonary resuscitation
            simultaneous compression-ventilation
            CPR
CPT
        cold pressor test
        current perception threshold
Cracchiolo
        C. forefoot arthroplasty
        C. procedure
Cragg endoluminal graft
Craigie tube method
Crampton
        C. line
        C. test
crania (pl. of cranium)
craniad
cranial
        c. base
        c. bones
        c. cavity
        c. duplication
        c. epidural space
        c. extension
        c. fontanels
        c. fracture
        c. index
        c. insufflation
        c. irradiation
        c. nerve
        c. nerve dissection
        c. nerve manipulation
        c. nerve rhizotomy
        c. osteopetrosis
        c. osteosynthesis
        c. pins
        c. sinuses
        c. suture
        c. synchondroses
        c. vault
cranialis
craniamphitomy
craniectomy
        keyhole-shaped c.
        linear c.
        partial-thickness c.
        retromastoid suboccipital c.
cranio-aural
craniocele
craniocerebral

craniofacial ·
- c. anomaly
- c. axis
- c. deformity
- c. fixation
- c. malformation
- c. notch
- c. osteotomy
- c. reconstruction
- c. resection
- c. surgery
- c. suspension wiring

craniomeningocele
craniometric points
cranio-orbital surgery
craniopathy
craniopharyngeal
- c. duct

craniopharyngioma
- ectopic c.

cranioplasty
- aluminum c.
- metallic c.
- tantalum c.

craniopuncture
craniorrhachidian
craniosacral
cranioscopy
craniosinus fistula
craniospinal
- c. irradiation
- c. space

craniotomy
- attached c.
- awake c.
- bifrontal c.
- c. defect
- detached c.
- frontal c.
- frontotemporal c.
- open stereotactic c.
- osteoplastic c.
- pterional c.
- right frontotemporal c.
- right temporoparietal c.
- stereotactic c.
- supratentorial c.
- Yasargil c.

craniotonoscopy
craniotrypesis
craniotympanic
cranium, pl. **crania**

- c. cerebrale
- c. viscerale

crash technique
crater formation
Crawford
- C. graft inclusion technique
- C. head frame
- C. incision
- C. method
- C. sling operation
- C. suture ring
- C. tube

Crawford-Adams cup arthroplasty
Crawford-Marxen-Osterfeld technique
craze line
cream
- Corticaine c.
- EMLA c.
- lidocaine-prilocaine c.

crease
- digital flexion c.
- flexion c.
- inframammary c.
- palmar c.
- c. wound

creation
- kyphosis c.
- lordosis c.
- McIndoe vaginal c.
- Politano-Leadbetter tunnel c.
- tunnel c.

Credé
- C. maneuver
- C. method

Creech
- C. aortoiliac graft
- C. technique

Crego
- C. femoral osteotomy
- C. tendon transfer technique

cremaster
- c. muscle

cremasteric
- c. fascia
- c. reflex

crena, pl. **crenae**
- c. ani
- c. clunium

crenation of tongue
Creola body
crescent
- articular c.

C

NOTES

153

crescent *(continued)*
    c. body
    C. corneal graft
    glomerular c.
    c. operation
    sublingual c.
crescentic
    c. calcaneal osteotomy
    c. rupture
Crespo operation
crest
    articular c.'s
    buccinator c.
    conchal c. of palatine bone
    deltoid c.
    endoalveolar c.
    ethmoidal c.
    ethmoidal c. of maxilla
    ethmoidal c. of palatine bone
    external occipital c.
    falciform c.
    frontal c.
    c. of greater tubercle
    c. of head of rib
    iliac c.
    infratemporal c.
    inguinal c.
    intermediate sacral c.'s
    internal occipital c.
    interosseous c.
    intertrochanteric c.
    lateral epicondylar c.
    lateral sacral c.'s
    lateral supracondylar c.
    c. of lesser tubercle
    medial epicondylar c.
    medial supracondylar c.
    median sacral c.
    c.'s of nail bed
    c. of neck of rib
    obturator c.
    c. of palatine bone
    palpation of iliac c.
    c. of petrous part of temporal bone
    pubic c.
    sacral c.
    c. of scapular spine
    supinator c.
    supraventricular c.
    terminal c.
    tibial c.
    trochanteric c.
    urethral c. of female
    urethral c. of male
    vestibular c.
Cribier method
cribra (*pl. of* cribrum)

cribriform
    c. area of the renal papilla
    c. fascia
    c. plate of alveolar process
cribrous lamina
cribrum, pl. **cribra**
cricohyoidepiglottopexy
cricoid
    c. myotomy
    c. pressure
    c. pressure anesthetic technique
    c. ring
    c. yoke
cricomyotomy
cricopharyngeal
    c. myotomy
cricopharyngeus muscle
cricothyroid
    c. artery
    c. articular capsule
    c. articulation
    c. joint
    c. ligament
    c. membrane
    c. muscle
cricothyroideus
cricothyroidotomy
cricothyrotomy
    c. trocar tube
cricotracheal
    c. ligament
    c. membrane
cricotracheotomy
cricovocal membrane
Crippa lead tetraacetate method
crista, pl. **cristae**
    c. capitis costae
    c. colli costae
    c. ethmoidalis
    c. ethmoidalis maxillae
    c. ethmoidalis ossis palatini
    c. frontalis
    c. galli
    c. iliaca
    c. infratemporalis
    c. intertrochanterica
    c. musculi supinatoris
    c. obturatoria
    c. occipitalis externa
    c. occipitalis interna
    c. palatina
    c. phallica
    c. pubica
    cristae sacrales intermediae
    cristae sacrales laterales
    c. sacralis
    c. sacralis mediana
    c. supracondylaris lateralis

c. supracondylaris medialis
c. supraventricularis
c. terminalis
c. tuberculi majoris
c. tuberculi minoris
c. urethralis
c. urethralis femininae
c. urethralis masculinae
Critchett operation
critical
c. care anesthesiology
c. care medicine (CCM)
c. closing pressure
c. illumination
c. mass
Criticare HN-Isocal tube feeding set
Critikon automated blood pressure cuff
CRNA
certified registered nurse anesthetist
Crock encircling operation
Croften classification
Crolom Ophthalmic solution
Crookes-Hittorf tube
Crosby
C. capsule
C. reduction
Crosby-Kugler
C.-K. biopsy capsule
C.-K. capsule for biopsy
cross
c. flap
c. infection
c. section
cross-arch fulcrum line
cross-arm flap
crossbar deformity
cross-bracing
spinal rod c.-b.
Wiltse system c.-b.
cross-clamping
infrarenal aortic c.-c.
thoracic aortic c.-c. (TACC)
cross-consonant injection method
crossed
c. anesthesia
c. extension reflex
c. extensor reflex
c. fixation
c. pyramidal tract
cross-facial
c.-f. nerve graft

c.-f. nerve graft anastomosis
c.-f. technique
cross-finger flap
crosshatch incision
cross-leg flap
crosslink plate size
crossover toe deformity
cross-pin
cross-polarization photography
cross-section
c.-s. technique
cross-sectional
c.-s. method
c.-s. projection
cross-table lateral projection
cross-tolerance
cross-trigonal repair
cross-vector A-scan
crotaphion
croupous
c. inflammation
c. membrane
Crouzon
C. disease
C. syndrome
Crowe
C. classification
C. pilot point
crow-foot closure
crowing inspiration
crown
c. fracture
c. of head
c. inclination
c. restoration
C. suture technique
crown-contouring method
crown-root fracture
Crozat therapy
crucial incision
cruciate
c. anastomosis
c. eminence
c. incision
c. ligament of the atlas
c. ligament reconstruction
c. muscle
cruciform
c. eminence
c. ligament of atlas
crunch-stick anastomosis
cruor

NOTES

crura (*pl. of* crus)
crural
- c. arch
- c. fascia
- c. fossa
- c. hernia
- c. ring
- c. septum
- c. sheath

cruralis
- cisterna c.

crurotomy
crus, pl. **crura**
- ampullary crura of semicircular ducts
- anterior c. of stapes
- c. of antihelix
- c. clitoridis
- c. of clitoris
- c. corporis cavernosi penis
- c. dextrum diaphragmatis
- c. laterale anuli inguinalis superficialis
- lateral c. of facial canal
- lateral c. of the superficial inguinal ring
- left c. of diaphragm
- c. mediale annuli inguinalis superficialis
- medial c. of facial canal
- medial c. of the superficial inguinal ring
- c. of penis
- posterior c. of stapes
- right c. of diaphragm
- c. sinistrum diaphragmatis

crush
- c. fracture
- c. injury
- c. preparation
- c. syndrome

crushed
- c. eggshell fracture
- c. tissue

crusotomy
Crutchfield reduction technique
Cruveilhier
- C. fascia
- C. fossa
- C. plexus

Cruveilhier-Baumgarten anomaly
cryoablation
- encircling c.
- laparoscopically guided c.

cryoanalgesia
cryoanesthesia
cryoapplication
cryocautery

cryocoagulation
cryoconization
cryoelectron microscopy
cryoextraction operation
cryogenic ablation
cryohypophysectomy
Cryolife
- C. Single Step dilution method
- C. valve graft

cryolysis
cryopallidectomy
cryopexy
- barrage c.
- double freeze-stalk c.
- double freeze-thaw c.

cryopreserved
- c. aortic homograft
- c. heart valve allograft
- c. tissue banking

cryoprostatectomy
cryopulvinectomy
cryoretinopexy
cryoscopy
cryostat
- c. section
- c. tissue

cryosurgery
cryosurgical
- c. ablation
- c. technique

cryothalamectomy
cryotherapy
- c. operation

Cryotube
crypt
- c. abscesses
- anal c.
- Lieberkühn c.'s
- Morgagni c.'s
- tonsillar c.

crypta, pl. **cryptae**
- c. tonsillaris

cryptectomy
cryptococcal infection
Cryptococcus infection
cryptogenic infection
cryptorchid
- c. testis

cryptorchidectomy
cryptorchidopexy
cryptorchism
cryptosporidial infection
Crystaline indicator
crystalline lens equator
crystallized trypsin
crystalloid
- c. cardioplegic solution
- Reinke c.'s

Crysticillin A.S. injection
Csapody orbital repair operation
CSE
 combined spinal/epidural anesthesia
C-section
  lower uterine segment
   transverse C.-s.
  LUST C.-s.
CSF
 cerebrospinal fluid
  blood-tinged CSF
  CSF pressure
CSFP
 cerebrospinal fluid pressure
C-shaped
  C.-s. canal
  C.-s. scalp flap
4C-T
  four-chamber transverse
   4C-T image
5C-T
  five-chamber transverse
   5C-T image
CTD
 chest tube drainage
  mediastinal CTD
CT-guided
  C.-g. fine-needle aspiration
  C.-g. liver biopsy
  C.-g. needle-aspiration biopsy
  C.-g. stereotactic evacuation
CT scan
Cubbins
  C. arthroplasty
  C. incision
  C. open reduction
  C. shoulder approach
  C. shoulder dislocation technique
cubital lymph nodes
cubitus
  c. valgus deformity
  c. varus correction
cuboid bone
cue exposure
cuff
  aortic c.
  blood pressure c.
  Critikon automated blood
   pressure c.
  denuded rectal c.
  Dynamap blood pressure c.
  endotracheal tube c.

  inflatable tracheal tube c.
  Kendall endotracheal tube c.
  LMA c.
  c. malfunction
  oscillometric blood pressure c.
  Polmedco endotracheal tube c.
  Portex SS endotracheal tube c.
  Portex XL endotracheal tube c.
  c. resection
  rotator c.
  Rusch endotracheal tube c.
  Safe-Cuff blood pressure c.
  Sheridan endotracheal tube c.
  c. suspension
  c. tear arthroplasty
  Temp-Kuff blood pressure c.
  tracheal tube c.
  tracheostomy c.
  V-Lok disposable blood pressure c.
cuffed
  c. endotracheal tube
  c. tracheostomy tube
Cuignet method
CUI myringotomy tube
cuirass
  c. ventilation
Culcher-Sussman technique
cul-de-sac
  c.-d.-s. of Bruger
  conjunctival c.-d.-s.
  Douglas c.-d.-s.
  c.-d.-s. of Douglas
  c.-d.-s. fluid
  glaucomatous c.-d.-s.
  greater c.-d.-s.
  Gruber c.-d.-s.
  lesser c.-d.-s.
  c.-d.-s. mass
  ocular c.-d.-s.
  ophthalmic c.-d.-s.
  optic c.-d.-s.
  rectouterine c.-d.-s.
culdoplasty
  Halban c.
  Marion-Moschcowitz c.
  McCall c.
culdoscopy
culdotomy
culprit
  c. lesion
  c. lesion angioplasty
Culp spiral flap pyeloplasty

NOTES

cultured epithelial autograft
culturing technique
Cummer classification
cuneiform
    c. bone
    c. cartilage
    c. osteotomy
    c. tubercle
cuneocerebellar tract
cunnus
cup
    c. arthroplasty
    c. and cone method
    c. insemination
    c. pessary
cup-and-ball osteotomy
cup-cement interface
cup-patch technique
cupped
Cupper-Faden operation
Cüppers method of pleoptics
Cupper suture technique
cuprophane membrane
cup-shaped
cup-to-disk ratio
cupula
    c. pleurae
    pleural c.
cupular blind sac
curage
curare
curarization
curative
    c. intent
    c. operation
    c. resection
curb tenotomy
curetment
curettage
    dilatation and c. (D&C)
    dilation and c. (D&C)
    endocervical c.
    endometrial c.
    fractional dilation and c.
    periapical c.
    soft tissue c.
    suction c.
curettement
curlicue ureter
current
    amplitude-summation interferential c.
    demarcation c.
    c. of injury
    Limoge c.
    membrane c.
    c. perception threshold (CPT)
    pulsing c. for nonunion of fracture

    c. regulator
    saturation c.
curtain
    Allander air c.
Curth-Maklin cornification disorder
Curtin
    C. incision
    C. plantar fibromatosis excision
Curtis
    C. PIP joint capsulotomy
    C. technique
Curtis-Fisher knee technique
curvatura, pl. curvaturae
    c. ventriculi major
    c. ventriculi minor
curvature
    c. aberration
    anterior corneal c.
    canal c.
    corneal c.
    greater c. of stomach
    lesser c. of stomach
curve
    accommodation c.
    articulation c.
    calibration c.
    carbon dioxide dissociation c.
    discrimination c.
    displacement c.
    dissociation c.
    dose-effect c.
    dose-response c.
    elimination c.
    hemoglobin-oxygen dissociation c.
    indicator-dilution c.
    intracardiac pressure c.
    left ventricular pressure-volume c.
    load-deflection c.
    load-deformation c.
    load-displacement c.
    oxygen dissociation c.
    oxygen-hemoglobin dissociation c.
    oxyhemoglobin dissociation c.
    pressure-natriuresis c.
    pressure-volume c.
    strength-duration c.
    time/concentration c.
    Traube-Hering c.'s
    V-P c.
    whole-body titration c.
curved
    c. approach
    c. canal
    c. end-to-end anastomosis
    c. flank position
    c. radiolucent line
    c. scleral-limbal incision of Flieringa

curved-needle surgeon knot
curvilinear incision
Cushieri maneuver
Cushing
    C. pressure response
    C. reflex
    C. suture
Cusick operation
Cusick-Sarrail ptosis operation
cusp
    c. fenestration
    c. plane
    c. restoration
    valve c.'s
cusp-fossa relation
cuspid-molar position
Custodis
    C. nondraining procedure
    C. operation
cut
    c. point
    semi-lunate c.
cutaneobiliary fistula
cutaneomucosal
cutaneomucous muscle
cutaneomucouveal syndrome
cutaneous
    c. appendiceal conduit
    c. bacterial infection
    c. cervical nerve
    c. collateral circulation
    c. forearm flap
    c. glands
    c. graft-versus-host disease
    c. graft-versus-host reaction
    c. heat loss
    c. hemorrhoid
    c. ileocystostomy
    c. lesion
    c. loop ureterostomy
    c. malformation
    c. manifestation
    c. metastasis
    c. muscle
    c. tissue
    c. vesicostomy
    c. viral infection
cutback
    c. anoplasty
cutback-type vaginoplasty
cutdown
    c. access

    c. incision
    c. technique
    venous c.
cuticularization
cuticular stitch
cutin
cutis graft
Cutler-Beard
    C.-B. bridge flap
    C.-B. operation
Cutler-Ederer method
Cutler operation
cutoff
    anesthetic c.
cuts
    sector c.
cutting
    section c.
Cuvier
    canal of C.
C-valve
CVP
    central venous pressure
    CVP line
cyanoacrylate retinopexy
cyanocobalamin injection
cyanogen bromide method
cyanosis
    compression c.
    shunt c.
cyanotic induration
cyclarthrodial
cyclarthrosis
cyclectomy
cyclicotomy
cyclic respiration
cyclitic membrane
cyclocryopexy
cyclodestructive procedure
cyclodiathermy operation
cycloelectrolysis
cyclophotocoagulation
    Nd:YAG c.
    transpupillary c.
cyclopropane
Cyclops
    C. formation
    C. procedure
cycloscopy
cyclotomy
Cygnus transdermal fentanyl device
Cyklokapron injection

NOTES

cylicotomy
cylinder
    gas c.
    c. retinoscopy
    suction c.
cylindrical
    c. confronting cisterna
    c. osteotomy
cylindroadenoma
cylindroid aneurysm
cylindroma
cylindromatous lesion
cylindrosarcoma
cyma line
Cymed Micro Skin one-piece drainage pouch
Cyprane inhaler
cyst
    c. aspiration
    c. fenestration
cystadenocarcinoma
cystadenofibroma
cystadenoma
cystauchenotomy
cystectomy
    Bartholin c.
    ovarian c.
    partial c.
    pilonidal c.
    radical c.
    salvage c.
    total c.
    vulvovaginal c.
cysteic acid method
cystenterostomy
    direct c.
    endoscopic c.
cystgastrostomy
    endoscopic c.
    surgical c.
cystic
    c. acute inflammation
    c. adenocarcinoma
    c. adenomatoid malformation
    c. adnexal mass
    c. adrenal mass
    c. artery
    c. bone lesion
    c. chest mass
    c. chronic inflammation
    c. dilatation
    c. dilation
    c. disease of renal medulla
    c. duct
    c. duct catheterization
    c. duct choledochoscopy
    c. fibrosis transmembrane conductance regulator

c. granulomatous inflammation
c. hidradenoma
c. kidney
c. lymph node
c. lymphoepithelial AIDS-related lesion
c. medial necrosis
c. metastasis
c. node
c. pelvic mass
c. puncture
cysticercal infection
cystides (*pl. of* cystis)
cystidoceliotomy
cystidolaparotomy
cystidotrachelotomy
cystifelleotomy
cystine calculus
cystis, pl. cystides
    c. fellea
    c. urinaria
cystitis
cystjejunostomy
cystoadenoma
cystocarcinoma
cystocele
    c. repair
cystochromoscopy
cystocolostomy
cystodiaphanoscopy
cystoduodenal ligament
cystoduodenostomy
    endoscopic c.
    pancreatic c.
cystoenterocele
cystoenterostomy
cystoepithelioma
cystofibroma
cystogastric fistula
cystogastrostomy
    endoscopic c.
cystoid body
cystojejunostomy
cystolateral pancreatojejunostomy
cystolith
cystolithectomy
cystolithiasis
cystolithic
cystolitholapaxy
cystolithotomy
cystolysis
cystoma
cystopanendoscopy
cystopericystectomy
cystopexy
cystoplasty
    augmentation c.
    Gil-Vernet ileocecal c.

human lyophilized dura c.
ileocecal c.
nonsecretory sigmoid c.
sigmoid c.
cystoproctostomy
cystoprostatectomy
cystoprostatourethrectomy
cystoprostatovesiculectomy
cystorectostomy
cystorrhaphy
cystosarcoma
cystoscopic electrohydraulic lithotripsy
cystoscopy
percutaneous fetal c.
steerable c.
cystostomy
trocar c.
c. tube
cystotomy
suprapubic c.
cystotrachelotomy
cystourethrocele
cystourethropexy
obturator shelf c.
Pereyra-Raz c.
vaginal c.
cystourethroplasty
Kropp c.
Leadbetter c.

cystourethroscopy
dynamic c.
cytobrush biopsy
cytoid body
cytologic
c. biopsy
c. examination
cytology
aspiration biopsy c.
endometrial c.
endoscopic brush c.
endoscopic fine-needle aspiration c.
c. examination
exfoliative c.
fine-needle aspiration c.
guided-needle aspiration c.
needle aspiration c.
nipple aspiration c.
oral cavity c.
peritoneal c.
cytomegalovirus infection
cytoplasmic membrane
cytopreparation
cytoreductive surgery
cytospin collection fluid
Cytoxan injection
Czermak pterygium operation
Czerny-Lembert suture
Czerny suture

C

NOTES

D

D chromosome ring syndrome
D line
D point
Dacron
D. aortic bifurcation graft
D. aortobifemoral graft
D. bolstered suture
D. interposition graft
D. intracardiac patch
D. knitted graft
D. onlay patch-graft
D. preclotted graft
D. Sauvage graft
D. tightly-woven graft
D. traction suture
D. tube graft
D. velour graft
D. Weave Knit graft
dacryoadenectomy operation
dacryocyst
dacryocystectomy operation
dacryocystocele
dacryocystoethmoidostomy
dacryocystorhinostomy
dacryocystorhinotomy operation
dacryocystostomy operation
dacryocystotomy operation
dacryon
dacryorhinocystostomy
dacryorhinocystotomy
dacryostomy
Arroyo d.
Arruga d.
Dupuy-Dutemps d.
Kuhnt d.
Rowinski d.
dactylomegaly
dactyloscopy
dacuronium
Dagradi esophageal variceal classification
Dahlman diverticulum excision
Dailey operation
Daines-Hodgson anastomosis
Dakin-Carrel treatment
Dakin solution
Dakrina ophthalmic solution
Dalcaine
Dale-Laidlaw clotting time method
Dale ventilator tubing support
Dalgleish operation
damage
anterior cervical surgery vocal cord d.

endothelial d.
irradiation d.
obturator nerve d.
projection fiber d.
radiation d.
soft-tissue d.
sun and chemical combination d.
Damian graft procedure
Damus-Kaye-Stancel (DKS)
D.-K.-S. operation
D.-K.-S. procedure
D.-K.-S. procedure for single ventricle physiology
Damus-Stancel-Kaye procedure
DANA
designed after natural anatomy
Dana
D. operation
D. posterior rhizotomy
Dandy
D. maneuver
D. operation
D. suction tube
Dandy-Walker
D.-W. deformity
D.-W. malformation
D.-W. syndrome
Dane method
Danforth fetal operation
Dangel slip knot
danger space
Daniel iliac bone graft
Danielson method
Danis-Weber
D.-W. classification of ankle injuries
D.-W. fracture
Dansac
D. Karaya Seal one-piece drainage pouch
D. Standard Ileo pouch
dantrolene
d. sodium
Danus-Fontan procedure
Danus-Stanzel repair
Dardik umbilical graft
dark-field
d.-f. examination
d.-f. illumination
d.-f. microscopy
dark-ground illumination
Darling capsulotomy
Darrach
D. procedure
D. resection

D

163

Darrach-McLaughlin shoulder technique
darting incision
dartos
- d. fascia
- d. muliebris
- d. muscle
- d. pouch procedure

Das Gupta
- D. G. procedure
- D. G. scapular excision
- D. G. scapulectomy

dashboard
- d. dislocation
- d. fracture

data
- on-line d.

Datascope system 90 intra-aortic balloon pump
Datex
- D. As/3 anesthesia system
- D. model CH-S-23 pulse oximeter

Datta procedure
datum plane
Daubenton
- D. angle
- D. line
- D. plane

d'Aubigne
- d. femoral reconstruction
- d. resection reconstruction

Davey-Rorabeck-Fowler decompression technique
David pharyngolaryngectomy tube
Daviel operation
Davis
- D. drainage technique
- D. fusion
- D. intubated ureterostomy
- D. intubated ureterotomy
- D. muscle-pedicle graft

Davis-Geck blepharoplasty
Davis-Kitlowski procedure
Davol tube
Davydov procedure
DAWG procedure
Dawson-Yuhl suction tube
day
- 20-d. chromic catgut suture
- 40-d. chromic catgut suture

day care surgical unit (DCSU)
DBP
- diastolic blood pressure

D&C
- dilatation and curettage
- dilation and curettage

DCI hemolyte solution
DCSU
- day care surgical unit

DDAVP injection
D-dimer
D&E
- dilatation and evacuation
- dilation and evacuation

de
- d. Grandmont operation
- d. Groot classification
- d. Lapersonne operation
- d. Mussy point
- d. novo lesion
- d. novo needle knife technique
- d. Quervain fracture
- d. Quervain stenosing tenosynovitis release
- d. Quervain syndrome
- d. Vincentiis operation

dead
- d. space
- d. space:tidal volume ratio
- d. tract

deadspace
deafferentation
- d. pain
- d. pain syndrome

de-airing procedure
Dean
- D. wash tube
- D. and Webb titration

Deane tube
dearterialization
- hepatic d.

Deaver
- D. incision
- D. tube

DeBakey
- D. classification
- D. graft
- D. heart pump oxygenator
- D. suction tube

DeBakey-Adson suction tube
DeBakey-Creech aneurysm repair
DeBakey-type aortic dissection
DeBastiani corticotomy
Debeyre-Patte-Elmelik rotator cuff technique
debility
debouch
débouchement
Debove
- D. membrane
- D. tube

débridement
- autolytic d.
- canal d.
- cavity d.
- diagnostic arthroscopy and d.
- enzymatic d.

exploration and d.
operative d.
root canal d.
debris
valve d.
Debrun latex balloon preparation
debubbling procedure
debulking
d. operation
ovarian carcinoma d.
d. procedure
d. surgery
d. of tumor
decalcification
decamethonium bromide
decannulation
decapsulation of kidney
decayed, extracted, and filled
deceleration time
decentration
d. of contact lens
deceration
decerebration
bloodless d.
decerebrize
dechondrification
decidual
d. membrane
deciduous
decimal reduction time
declamping
d. phenomenon
d. shock
declination
d. angle
decompensation injury
decompression
anterior retroperitoneal d.
bone graft d.
cardiac d.
cerebral d.
d. colostomy
endoscopic biliary d.
extensive posterior d.
d. fasciotomy
gastric d.
internal d.
d. laminectomy
nerve d.
orbital d.
d. of orbit operation
paraclavicular thoracic outlet d.

pericardial d.
retroperitoneal d.
d. rhachotomy
Rowbotham orbital d.
spinal d.
suboccipital d.
subtemporal d.
surgical d.
d. technique
transduodenal endoscopic d.
trigeminal d.
d. tube
tube d.
variceal d.
vein d.
vertebral body d.
decompressive
d. laminectomy
d. surgery
deconditioned exercise response
deconvolution
decortication
arterial d.
cerebral d.
d. of heart
d. of lung
renal cyst d.
reversible d.
d. technique
decrease
hypoxic ventilatory d.
decreased respiration
decubitus position
decuspation
decussation
dorsal tegmental d.
Forel d.
fountain d.
Held d.
Meynert d.
motor d.
oculomotor d.
optic d.
pyramidal d.
rubrospinal d.
tectospinal d.
d. of trochlear nerve
ventral tegmental d.
Wernekinck d.
dedolation
de-endothelialization

D

NOTES

deep

d. artery of clitoris
d. artery of penis
d. artery of thigh
d. artery of tongue
d. articulation test
d. brachial artery
d. branch of the lateral plantar nerve
d. branch of the medial femoral circumflex artery
d. branch of the medial plantar artery
d. branch of the radial nerve
d. branch of the transverse cervical artery
d. branch of the ulnar nerve
d. cardiac plexus
d. cervical artery
d. cervical fascia
d. cervical vein
d. chest therapy
d. crural arch
d. delayed infection
d. Doppler velocity interrogation
d. dorsal sacrococcygeal ligament
d. dorsal vein of clitoris
d. dorsal vein of penis
d. epigastric artery
d. epigastric vein
d. facial vein
d. fascia of arm
d. fascia of forearm
d. fascia of leg
d. fascia of neck
d. fascia of penis
d. fascia of thigh
d. head of flexor pollicis brevis
d. hypothermic circulatory arrest
d. iliac dissection
d. infrapatellar bursa
d. inguinal lymph nodes
d. inguinal ring
d. lamina
d. layer of levator palpebrae superioris muscle
d. layer of temporalis fascia
d. lingual vein
d. lymphatic vessel
d. muscles of back
d. palmar branch of ulnar artery
d. parotid lymph nodes
d. part of external anal sphincter
d. part of flexor retinaculum
d. part of masseter muscle
d. part of parotid gland
d. perineal pouch
d. perineal space

d. peroneal nerve
d. plantar branch of dorsalis pedis artery
d. postanal anorectal space
d. posterior sacrococcygeal ligament
d. temporal artery
d. temporal nerve
d. temporal vcins
d. transverse muscle of perineum
d. transverse perineal muscle
d. tumor
d. vein of penis
d. veins of clitoris
d. wound infection

deep-gastric

d.-g. longitudinal (DG-L)
d.-g. transverse (DG-T)

de-epicardialization
de-epithelialization
de-epithelialized flap
deep-seated fungal infection
defalcated root canal
Defares rebreathing method
defect

atrioventricular canal d.
craniotomy d.
mass d.
napkin-ring d.
neural tube d.
oromandibular d.
osteoarticular d.
osteochondral d.
perineal d.
peritoneal d.
postresection d.
surgical d.
tumor d.
ventilation d.
ventilation/perfusion d.

deferent

d. canal
d. duct

deferentectomy
deferential

d. artery
d. plexus

deferred shock
defibrillation

cardiac d.
d. patch
d. shock
d. threshold

defined sterilization
definitive

d. method
d. stabilization

deflation
deformation

deformity
  abduction d.
  acetabular protrusio d.
  acquired d.
  adduction d.
  adduction-internal rotation d.
  adductovarus d.
  Åkerlund d.
  d. analysis
  Andy Gump d.
  angel-wing d.
  d. angle
  angular d.
  angulation d.
  Arnold-Chiari d.
  back-knee d.
  bell clapper d.
  bifid thumb d.
  bird-beak d.
  bony d.
  boutonnière d.
  bowing d.
  bowleg d.
  bulb d.
  bunion d.
  burn boutonnière d.
  buttonhole d.
  calcaneocavovarus d.
  calcaneocavus d.
  calcaneovalgus d.
  calcaneovarus d.
  cavo abducto varus d.
  cavo calcaneo valgus d.
  cavovarus d.
  cavus d.
  cecal d.
  cervical spine kyphotic d.
  cervicomedullary d.
  chain-of-lakes d.
  checkrein d.
  clasped thumb d.
  clawfoot d.
  clawhand d.
  clawing d.
  clawtoe d.
  cleft hand d.
  cleft lip d.
  cloverleaf skull d.
  clubfoot d.
  cock-up d.
  codfish d.
  combined cavus d.

  compensatory d.
  complete bilateral d.
  congenital postural d.
  congenital vertical talus foot d.
  coronal plane d.
  craniofacial d.
  crossbar d.
  crossover toe d.
  cubitus valgus d.
  Dandy-Walker d.
  dentofacial d.
  duodenal bulb d.
  elevatus d.
  equinovalgus d.
  equinovarus d.
  equinus d.
  Erlenmeyer flask d.
  eversion-external rotation d.
  extension d.
  facial d.
  finger d.
  fishtail d.
  fixed d.
  flat back d.
  flexion d.
  flexion-internal rotational d.
  foot d.
  funnel chest d.
  garden spade d.
  genu valgum d.
  genu varum d.
  gibbous d.
  gingival d.
  gooseneck d.
  gross d.
  Haglund d.
  hallux valgus d.
  hammertoe d.
  hand d.
  hatchet-head d.
  Hill-Sachs d.
  hindbrain d.
  hindfoot d.
  hip d.
  hockey-stick d.
  hook-nail d.
  hourglass d.
  humpback d.
  hyperextension d.
  internal rotation d.
  intrinsic minus d.
  intrinsic plus d.

D

NOTES

deformity *(continued)*
    joint d.
    J-sella d.
    keyhole d.
    Kirner d.
    kleeblatschädel d.
    Klippel-Feil d.
    knock-knee d.
    kyphotic d.
    lanceolate d.
    limb d.
    lobster-claw d.
    lumbar spine kyphotic d.
    Madelung d.
    mallet finger d.
    mallet toe d.
    Michel d.
    Mondini d.
    nasal d.
    one-plane d.
    opera-glass d.
    parachute d.
    pectus carinatum d.
    pectus excavatum d.
    pencil-in-cup d.
    penile d.
    pes planus d.
    phrygian cap d.
    pigeon-breast d.
    ping-pong ball d.
    plantar flexion-inversion d.
    posttraumatic spinal d.
    postural d.
    protrusio d.
    pseudoboutonnière d.
    rat-tail d.
    recurvatum angulation d.
    rotational d.
    rotoscoliotic d.
    round back d.
    round shoulder d.
    sabre-shin d.
    saddle-nose d.
    sagittal d.
    shepherd's-crook d.
    silver-fork d.
    skeletal d.
    spastic thumb-in-palm d.
    spinal coronal plane d.
    spine d.
    spinning-top d.
    splayfoot d.
    split-hand d.
    split-nail d.
    spondylitic d.
    Sprengel d.
    S-shaped d.
    subcondylar d.
    supination d.
    swan-neck finger d.
    talipes cavus d.
    thoracic spine kyphotic d.
    thoracic spine scoliotic d.
    three-plane d.
    thumb d.
    thumb-in-palm d.
    trefoil d.
    triphalangeal thumb d.
    turned-up pulp d.
    two-plane d.
    ulnar deviation d.
    ulnar drift d.
    valgus d.
    varus hindfoot d.
    Velpeau d.
    volar angulation d.
    Volkmann clawhand d.
    whistling d.
    Whitehead d.
    windblown d.
    windswept d.
    wrist d.
    Zancolli procedure for clawhand d.
    zig-zag compensatory d.
    Z-type d.
deformity/instability
    spinal d.
DEFT
    driven equilibrium Fourier transform
        DEFT technique
defunctionalization
Dega pelvic osteotomy
degenerated fibroadenolipoma
degeneration
    d. of cornea
degenerative
    d. discogenic end-plate disease
    d. inflammation
degloving procedure
Degnon suture
degradation
    d. of image
    d. product
degrade
degree
    d. of inspiration
    270-d. laparoscopic posterior
        fundoplasty
dehiscence
    abdominal incision d.
    staple line d.
    suture line d.
    wound d.
dehiscent mandibular canal
Dehist injection
dehydration fever

dehydrogenation
Deisting prostatic dilation technique
Deiter operation
deiterospinal tract
Dejerine-Roussy syndrome
dekalon suture
DeKlair operation
Deklene polypropylene suture
Deknatel silk suture
delayed
    d. complication
    d. expansion
    d. femoral osteotomy
    d. flap
    d. fracture union
    d. graft
    d. hyperacute transplant rejection
    d. open reduction
    d. primary closure
    d. primary repair
    d. suture
delay line
Delbert hip fracture classification
Delbet splint for heel fracture
DeLee
    D. classification
    D. maneuver
Delflex peritoneal dialysis solution
deliberate hypotension anesthetic
  technique
delimiting keratotomy
delivery
    buccal transmucosal d.
    closed-loop automated d.
    epidural d.
    spinal d.
    transmucosal d.
    vacuum extractor d.
Dellepiane hysterectomy
Deller modification
Delorme
    D. rectal prolapse operation
    D. thoracoplasty
delta
    D. external fixation frame
    d. tibial nail
Deltatrac metabolic unit
deltoid
    d. branch
    d. crest
    d. eminence
    d. flap

    d. insertion over joint
    d. muscle
deltoid-splitting
    d.-s. incision
    d.-s. shoulder approach
deltopectoral
    d. approach
    d. flap
Del Toro operation
deltoscapular flap
Demadex injection
demand-adapted administration
  anesthetic technique
demand flow machine
demarcation
    corticomedullary d.
    d. current
    line of d.
    d. line
    d. line of retina
    d. potential
Demerol
    D. injection
    D. Oral
demineralization
    bony d.
demineralized bone graft
Demours membrane
demucosalized augmentation with gastric
  segment
demyelinating lesion
demyelination
    autoimmune d.
    axonal d.
    intramedullary d.
DeMyer system of cerebral
  malformation
dendriform
dendrite
    corneal d.
dendritic
    d. calculus
    d. lesion
dendrocytoma
denervate
denervation
    d. disease
    d. hypersensitivity
    Krause d.
    law of d.
    d. potential

D

NOTES

denervation *(continued)*
    preganglionic sympathetic d.
    sinoaortic d.
dengue hemorrhagic fever infection
Denham external fixation
Denhardt solution
Denis
    D. Browne classification of sacral fracture
    D. Browne pouch
    D. Browne spinal fracture classification
    D. Browne urethroplasty technique
Denker
    D. sinus operation
    D. tube
Dennie line
Dennie-Morgan line
Dennis
    D. intestinal tube
    D. technique
    D. tube
Dennis-Brooke ileostomy
Dennis-Varco pancreaticoduodenostomy
Denonvilliers
    D. aponeurosis
    D. fascia
    D. ligament
dens
    d. anterior screw fixation
    d. fracture
dense
    d. body
    d. brain mass
density-dependent repair
dental
    d. anatomy
    d. anesthesia
    d. anomaly
    d. arch expansion
    d. articulation
    d. canal
    d. cavity
    d. fenestration
    d. fistula
    d. index
    d. infection
    d. nerve
    d. prosthetic laboratory procedure
    d. psychosedation
    d. pulp extirpation
    d. puncture
    d. restoration
    d. sac
    d. sinus tract
    d. surgery
    d. trepanation

    d. trephination
    d. wedge
DentaScan multiplanar reformation
dentate
    d. fracture
    d. line
    d. suture
dentatectomy
dentatothalamic tract
denticulate ligament
dentinal canal
dentin crystal alteration
dentinoenamel membrane
dentoalveolar
    d. joint
dentofacial
    d. anomaly
    d. deformity
    d. surgery
denture
    d. classification
    d. foundation
    d. foundation area
    d. foundation surface
    d. space
denudation
    endothelial d.
    interdental d.
denude
denuded
    d. connective tissue
    d. furcation
    d. rectal cuff
Denver classification
Depage-Janeway gastrostomy
DePalma modified patellar technique
DePaul tube
dependency
    ventilator d.
dependent drainage
depigmentation
    congenital d.
depilation
deplasmolysis
deployment
    stent d.
depMedalone injection
Depoject injection
depolarization block
depolarizing
    d. block
    d. relaxant
Depo-Medrol injection
Depopred injection
Depo-Provera injection
depot
    d. corticosteroid
    d. injection

depressant
depressed skull fracture
depression
    d. fracture
    d. of fragment
    inspiratory rib cage d.
    respiratory d.
    twitch d.
    ventilatory d.
depressor
    d. anguli oris muscle
    d. labii inferioris muscle
    d. muscle of epiglottis
    d. muscle of eyebrow
    d. muscle of lower lip
    d. muscle of septum
    d. septi muscle
    d. supercilii muscle
deprivation amblyopia
depth
    d. of anesthesia
    d. of anesthesia monitoring
    anesthetic d.
    d. caliper-meter stick method
    d. of insertion (DOI)
    d. pulse technique
DePuy hip prosthesis with Scuderi
  head
derby
    d. hat fracture
    D. operation
derivative circulation
dermabrasion
Dermagraft graft
dermal
    d. fasciectomy
    d. fat-free flap
    d. fat-free tissue transfer
    d. fat pedicle flap
    d. graft
    d. lesion
    d. pouch
    d. pouch reconstruction
    d. sinus tract
    d. suture
Dermalene polyethylene suture
dermal-fat graft
Dermalon cuticular suture
dermatoalloplasty
dermatoautoplasty
dermatocele
dermatofibroma

dermatofibrosarcoma
dermatoheteroplasty
dermatohomoplasty
dermatolysis
dermatomal level of analgesia
dermatome
    d. mapping
    trigeminal d.
    T7, T9, T11 d.
dermatomyoma
dermatophyte fungal infection
dermatoplasty
dermatoscopy
dermatosis
dermatoxenoplasty
dermis
    d. patch graft
dermodesis
    resection d.
dermoid
dermoidectomy
dermolipoma
dermolysis
dermoplasty
dermovascular
Derosa-Graziano step-cut osteotomy
derotation
derotational osteotomy
DES
    diethylstilbestrol
    DES exposure
desaturation
    arterial oxygen d.
    oxygen d.
    red d.
Desault wrist dislocation
Descemet
    D. membrane
    D. membrane detachment
descendens
    d. cervicalis
    d. hypoglossi
descending
    d. anterior branch
    d. artery of knee
    d. branch of occipital artery
    d. colon
    d. genicular artery
    d. loop colostomy
    d. palatine artery
    d. part of duodenum
    d. part of facial canal

D

NOTES

descending *(continued)*
d. posterior branch
d. scapular artery
d. technique
d. tract of trigeminal nerve
Descot fracture
desflurane
desiccation
electrosurgical d.
mucous d.
designated blood donation
designed after natural anatomy (DANA)
Desjardins point
Desmarres operation
desmocytoma
desmoid lesion
desmoplastic
d. medulloblastoma
d. trichilemmoma
desmopressin
desmotomy
destruction
bone d.
bony element d.
bony necrosis and d.
Cawthorne d.
cortical d.
moth-eaten bone d.
mucosal d.
destructive
d. bone lesion
d. interference technique
desyndactylization
Weinstock d.
detached
d. cranial section
d. craniotomy
detachment
Descemet membrane d.
exudative retinal d.
traction d.
detection threshold
detector response
detritus
tissue d.
detrusor
d. areflexia
d. instability
d. muscle of urinary bladder
d. pressure
d. stability
devascularization
paraesophagogastric d.
DeVega tricuspid valve annuloplasty
developer solution
developmental
d. coordination disorder
d. landmark

d. line
d. retardation
Deventer pelvis
Devereux-Reichek method
Deverle fixation
deviant articulation
deviation
d. to the right
device
Accutracker blood pressure d.
agent-specific filling d.
A-mode echo-tracking d.
Arrow emergency infusion d.
ATL Ultramark 7
echocardiographic d.
Bair Hugger fluid-warming d.
Bard Ambulatory PCA d.
Bassett electrical stimulation d.
CADD PCA d.
Camino intracranial pressure
monitoring d.
closed-loop d.
Cygnus transdermal fentanyl d.
Dinamap automated blood
pressure d.
Dinamap 1846SX oscillometric
blood pressure d.
emergency infusion d. (EID)
esophageal detector d.
fail-safe d.
Flotem IIe fluid-warming d.
forced-air active cooling d.
Grass pressure-recording d.
HOTLINE fluid-warming d.
In-Exsufflator respiratory d.
intracranial pressure monitoring d.
keyed filling d.
manual ventilation d.
Mosher Life Saver antichoke
suction d.
Neurometer d.
nitrous oxide-oxygen
proportioning d.
patient self-administration d.
PCA-plus infusion d.
Polar Bair forced-air active
cooling d.
POMS 20/50 oxygen
conservation d.
Provider 5500 patient-controlled
analgesia d.
Sullivan III nasal continuous
positive air pressure d.
Telectronic electrical stimulation d.
d. therapy
Throat-E-Vac suction d.
transdermal fentanyl d. (TFD)
VAMP d.

DeVilbiss
> D. suction pump
> D. suction tube

Devine
> D. colostomy
> D. exclusion
> D. hypospadias repair

Devine-Devine procedure
Devine-Millard-Frazier fiberoptic suction tube
devitalization
> pulp d.

devitalized
> d. bone graft
> d. tissue

devolvulization
> endoscopic d.

Devonshire technique
Dewar
> D. posterior cervical fixation procedure
> D. posterior cervical fusion
> D. posterior cervical fusion technique

Dewar-Barrington
> D.-B. arthroplasty
> D.-B. clavicular dislocation technique

Dewar-Harris shoulder technique
DeWecker
> D. anterior sclerotomy
> D. operation

dexamethasone
> d. solution

dexmedetomidine
> d. infusion

Dexon
> D. absorbable synthetic polyglycolic acid suture
> D. II suture
> D. Plus suture

Dexter-Grossman classification
dextrocardia
dextrogyration
dextromethorphan
dextrorotation
dextrose
> d. solution
> tetracaine with d.

dextrotorsion
dextroversion
DEY albuterol inhalation aerosol

Dey-Drop Ophthalmic solution
Deyerle femoral fracture technique
Dezocine
DG-L
> deep-gastric longitudinal
> DG-L image

DG Softgut suture
D&G suture
DG-T
> deep-gastric transverse
> DG-T image

D.H.E. 45 injection
diabetic
> d. coma
> d. puncture

diacele
diacetylcholine
diacondylar fracture
diagastric line
diagnosis
diagnostic
> d. anesthesia
> d. arthroscopy and débridement
> d. arthroscopy, operative arthroscopy, and possible operative arthrotomy
> d. articulation test
> d. cardiac catheterization
> d. colonoscopy
> d. fiberoptic stomatoscopy
> d. imaging evaluation
> d. and operative arthroscopy
> d. peritoneal lavage
> d. procedure
> d. program
> d. radiation
> d. surgical therapy
> d. tube

diagonal section
dial
> d. pelvic osteotomy
> d. periacetabular osteotomy

dialysate preparation module
dialysis
> d. access surgery
> arteriovenous d.
> d. disequilibrium syndrome
> d. encephalopathy syndrome
> extracorporeal d.
> d. fistula
> peritoneal d.

dialytic ultrafiltration

D

dialyzer membrane
diameter
    biparietal d.
    corneal d.
    end-diastolic d. (EDD)
    end-systolic d. (ESD)
diametric pelvic fracture
3,3-diaminobenzidine tetrahydrochloride
  solution
diamond
    D. classification
    d. ejection murmur
    d. inlay bone graft
Diamond-Gould
    D.-G. reduction syndactyly
    D.-G. syndactyly operation
Dianeal
    D. dialysis solution
    D. K-141
Dianoux operation
Diaphane solution
diaphragm
    eventration of the d.
    d. eventration
    excursion of the d.
    pelvic d.
    d. of sella
    traumatic rupture of the d.
    urogenital d.
diaphragma, pl. diaphragmata
    d. pelvis
    d. sellae
    d. urogenitale
diaphragmatic
    d. crural repair
    d. elevation
    d. eventration
    d. hernia
    d. nodes
    d. pleura
    d. respiration
    d. rupture
diaphragmatic-abdominal respiration
diaphyseal
    d. fracture
    d. osteotomy
diaphysial
diaphysis
    femoral d.
diarthric
diarthrodial
    d. cartilage
    d. joint
diarthrosis
diarticular
Dias-Giegerich
    D.-G. fracture technique
    D.-G. open reduction

Dias-Tachdijian classification of physeal
  injury
diastasis
    ankle mortise d.
    d. fibula
    iris d.
    palpable rib d.
    pubic d.
    d. recti
    d. recti abdominis
    rectus d.
    sutural d.
    symphysis pubis d.
    tibiofibular d.
diastatic skull fracture
Diastat vascular access graft
diastolic
    d. blood pressure (DBP)
    d. filling pressure
    d. pressure-time index
    d. pressure-volume relation
    d. relaxation
    d. suction
diathermic
    d. fistulotomy
    d. loop biopsy
    d. resection
    d. therapy
diathermocoagulation
diathermy
    electrocoagulation d.
    d. hemorrhoidectomy
    medical d.
    d. operation
    d. puncture
    short-wave d.
    surgical d.
diatomaceous earth
diazepam
    d. emulsified injection
diazo staining method
Dibbell cleft lip-nasal reconstruction
dibucaine
    d. hydrochloride
dibutyrate
    phorbol d.
DIC
    disseminated intravascular coagulation
    DIC tracheostomy tube
dichlorodifluoromethane and
  trichloromonofluoromethane
dichlorotetrafluoroethane
    ethyl chloride and d.
dichotomization
dichotomous classification
dichotomy
Dickey-Fox operation
Dickey operation

Dickhaut-DeLee
>D.-D. classification of discoid meniscus
>D.-D. discoid meniscus classification

Dickinson
>D. approach
>D. calcaneal bursitis technique

Dickinson-Coutts-Woodward-Handler osteotomy

Dick method

Dickson
>D. geometric osteotomy
>D. transplant technique

Dickson-Diveley procedure

Dickson-Wright operation

diclofenac analgesic therapy

dicondylar fracture

Didiee projection

Diebold-Bejjani osteotomy

Dieffenbach
>D. method
>D. operation

Dieffenbach-Duplay hypospadias technique

die punch fracture

dieresis

dieretic

Dieterle method

5,5-diethylbarbituric acid

diethyl ether

diethylstilbestrol (DES)

Dieulafoy
>D. lesion
>D. vascular malformation
>D. vascular malformation of the stomach

Dieulafoy-like lesion

difference
>alveolar-arterial pressure d.
>alveolar end-capillary d.
>field-echo d.

differential
>d. blood pressure
>d. force technique
>d. nerve block
>d. relaxation
>d. spinal anesthesia
>d. spinal block
>d. spinal block anesthetic technique
>d. ureteral catheterization test

differentiation failure

difficult ventilation

diffuse
>d. abscess
>d. acute inflammation
>d. air space disease
>d. aneurysm
>d. chronic inflammation
>d. fatty infiltration
>d. fibroma of gingiva
>d. fusiform dilatation
>d. illumination
>d. intravascular coagulation
>d. lymphatic tissue
>d. metastasis
>d. plane
>d. pulmonary alveolar hemorrhage
>d. reflection
>d. ulceration
>d. ulcerative lesion

diffusion
>d. anoxia
>exchange d.
>d. hypoxia
>d. respiration
>d. root canal filling method

Diflucan injection

digastric
>d. branch of facial nerve
>d. fossa
>d. groove
>d. muscle
>d. muscle flap
>d. space
>d. triangle

digastricus

digestive
>d. apparatus
>d. system vascular disease
>d. tract
>d. tube

Digi-Dyne cardiopulmonary bypass oxygenator

digit
>D. Symbol Substitution Test

digital
>d. artery protection
>d. beam attenuation
>d. block anesthesia
>d. collateral artery
>d. extensor mechanism
>d. extensor tendon
>d. flexion crease

D

NOTES

digital · dilation

digital *(continued)*
- d. furrow
- d. imaging colposcopy
- d. manipulation
- d. nail
- d. pad
- d. pressure
- d. pulp
- d. rectal evacuation
- d. rectal examination
- d. subtraction technique
- d. veins

digitalis effect
digitalization
digitally-guided biopsy
digitate impressions
digitation
digiti (*pl. of* digitus)
digitization
digitonin method
digitorum
- extensor d.

digitus, pl. **digiti**
- d. annularis
- d. auricularis
- d. manus
- d. medius
- d. minimus
- d. pedis
- d. primus
- d. quintus
- d. secundus
- d. tertius

digoxin effect
dihydrocodeine tartrate
dihydrocodeinone
dihydromorphinone hydrochloride
dihydropyridine calcium channel blocker
2,6-diisopropyl phenol
dilacerated canal
dilaceration
- sharp d.

dilatable lesion
dilatation
- aneurysmal d.
- balloon d.
- bile duct d.
- cardiac d.
- congenital cystic d.
- d. and curettage (D&C)
- cystic d.
- diffuse fusiform d.
- ductal d.
- esophageal d.
- d. and evacuation (D&E)
- ex vacuo d.
- fusiform d.
- gaseous d.

homatropine d.
junctional d.
pancreatic duct d.
pneumatic d.
poststenotic d.
prestenotic d.
pupillary d.
segmental d.
transurethral balloon d.
Virchow-Robin space d.

dilate
dilation
- achalasia balloon d.
- anal d.
- aneurysmal d.
- balloon d.
- biliary d.
- bootstrap d.
- bowel d.
- Brown-McHardy pneumatic mercury bougie d.
- capillary d.
- cardiac d.
- catheter d.
- cervical d.
- d. of cervix
- colonic d.
- d. and curettage (D&C)
- cystic d.
- ductal d.
- ectatic d.
- Eder-Puestow d.
- endoscopic papillary balloon d.
- episcleral vascular d.
- esophageal d.
- d. of esophagus
- d. and evacuation (D&E)
- extrahepatic biliary cystic d.
- finger d.
- Frank technique of d.
- gastric d.
- Grüntzig balloon d.
- d. of heart
- d. of hemorrhoid
- hepatic web d.
- hydrostatic balloon d.
- idiopathic d.
- inadequate d.
- intrahepatic biliary cystic d.
- intrahepatic ductal d.
- junctional d.
- lag d.
- d. lag
- mechanical ureteral d.
- medical d.
- mucosal vascular d.
- percutaneous balloon d.
- periportal sinusoidal d.

peroral esophageal d.
pneumatic bag esophageal d.
pneumatic balloon catheter d.
pneumostatic d.
poststenotic d.
d. of punctum
d. of punctum operation
pupil d.
pyloric d.
reactive d.
rectal d.
serial d.
submucosal vascular d.
d. therapy
through-the-scope balloon d.
tract d.
transurethral balloon d.
TTS balloon d.
urethral d.
Uromat d.
d. of ventricle
ventricular d.
Wirsung d.

dilator
d. muscle of ileocecal sphincter
d. muscle of pupil
d. muscle of pylorus
d. naris
d. naris muscle
d. placement
d. placement failure
d. pupillae
d. and sheath technique

Dillwyn-Evans
D.-E. osteotomy
D.-E. resection

Dilocaine
diltiazem
dilution
tracer d.

dilution-filtration technique
3-dimensional reconstruction wand
dimethyl *d*-tubocurarine
Dimon-Hughston
D.-H. fracture fixation
D.-H. intertrochanteric osteotomy
D.-H. technique

dimple
coccygeal d.

Dinamap
D. automated blood pressure device

D. 1846SX oscillometric blood
pressure device

dinitrogen monoxide
diode
laser d.
Microlase transpupillary d.

dioptric
d. aberration
d. correction

dioxide
arterial carbon d.
carbon d. (CO_2)
end-tidal carbon d.
fraction of expired carbon d.
fraction in expired gas of
carbon d.
partial pressure of arterial
carbon d. ($PaCO_2$)
partial pressure of carbon d.
(PCO_2)
partial pressure of intramuscular
carbon d. ($PiCO_2$)
partial pressure of mesenteric
venous carbon d. ($PmvCO_2$)

DIP
distal interphalangeal
DIP fusion

diphosphate buffer solution
diphtheritic membrane
diploë
diploic
d. canals

dipole-dipole
d.-d. relaxation
d.-d. relaxation rate

Diprivan
D. injection
D. technique

direct
d. acrylic restoration
d. brain stimulation
d. cardiac puncture
d. cautery puncture
d. composite resin restoration
d. current electrocoagulation
d. cystenterostomy
d. electrical nerve stimulation
d. embolectomy
d. flap
d. Fourier transformation imaging
d. fracture
d. gold restoration

D

NOTES

direct *(continued)*
    d. illumination
    d. inguinal hernia
    d. insertion technique
    d. intraperitoneal insemination
    d. laryngoscopy
    d. manipulation
    d. mechanical ventricular actuation
    d. method
    d. method for making inlays
    d. needle puncture
    d. neural stimulation
    d. obturator nerve block
    d. ophthalmoscopy
    d. pyramidal tract
    d. resin restoration
    d. respiration
    d. suturing
    d. transfusion
    d. vision internal urethrotomy
    d. vision liver biopsy
direct-current shock ablation
direct/indirect technique
direction
    angle of d.
    caudal d.
    cephalad d.
    flow d.
    line of d.
    pelvic d.
    phase-encoding d.
    principal line of d.
    principal visual d.
    visual d.
    Z d.
directional coronary atherectomy
disarticular amputation
disarticulation
    Batch-Spittler-McFaddin knee d.
    Boyd hip d.
    Burger technique for
      scapulothoracic d.
    elbow d.
    hip d.
    joint d.
    Lisfranc d.
    metatarsophalangeal joint d.
    sacroiliac d.
    shoulder d.
    wrist d.
disassociation
disc *(var. of* disk)
discectomy *(var. of* diskectomy)
Dischler rectoscopic suction insert
disci *(pl. of* discus)
disciform degeneration of retina
discission
    d. of lens operation

disclosing solution
Discofix stopcock
discoid skin lesion
disconnection syndrome
disconnect wedge
discontinuous
    d. endothelium
    d. neck dissection
    d. sterilization
discotomy
discrete
    d. blood supply to a bone graft
    d. coronary lesion
    d. mass
discrimination
    d. curve
    d. loss
    d. score
discus, pl. disci
    d. articularis
    d. articularis acromioclavicularis
    d. articularis sternoclavicularis
    d. articularis temporomandibularis
    d. interpubicus
    d. intervertebralis
disease
    acute graft-vs-host d.
    adaptation d.
    adhesive d.
    adult familial hyaline membrane d.
    air space d.
    amyloid oral cavity d.
    antiglomerular basement membrane
      antibody d.
    aortic occlusive d. (AOD)
    aortic valve d.
    aortoiliac occlusive d.
    Berger d.
    biliary tract d.
    Bright d.
    carcinoid valve d.
    cement d.
    central core d. (CCD)
    central nervous system d.
    cerebrovascular d.
    choledochal cyst d.
    chronic graft-versus-host d.
    combined system d.
    connective tissue d.
    Crouzon d.
    cutaneous graft-versus-host d.
    cystic d. of renal medulla
    degenerative discogenic end-plate d.
    denervation d.
    diffuse air space d.
    digestive system vascular d.
    early-onset graft-vs-host d.
    echinococcal cyst d.

Economo d.
elevator d.
endogenous d.
endomyocardial d.
eosinophilic endomyocardial d.
exanthematous d.
exogenous d.
exophytic joint d.
extensive-stage d.
extra-abdominal d.
extracapsular d.
extracranial carotid artery d.
extracranial carotid occlusive d.
extracranial occlusive vascular d.
extramammary Paget d.
extraorbital d.
extrapyramidal d.
exudative papulosquamous d.
Fournier d.
fracture d.
glomerular basement membrane d.
graft-versus-host d.
hard metal d.
hard pad d.
hepatic venous web d.
heritable connective tissue d.
humeroperoneal neuromuscular d.
hyaline membrane d.
hyperacute graft-vs-host d.
idiopathic eczematous d.
inclusion body d.
inflammatory bowel d.
intraperitoneal endometrial
  metastatic d.
Jackson and Parker classification of
  Hodgkin d.
Killip classification of heart d.
Lafora body d.
Leri-Weill d.
lichenoid graft-versus-host d.
lupus-associated valve d.
lysosomal storage d.
Marion d.
microcystic d. of renal medulla
minimal-change d.
mixed connective-tissue d.
nil d.
node-negative d.
node-positive d.
occlusive d.
Ormond d.
osteoarthritis d.

Paget extramammary d.
pelvic adhesive d.
peripheral arterial aneurysmal d.
Peyronie d.
popliteal artery occlusive d.
  (PAOD)
preeclamptic liver d.
pulmonary valve d.
radiation-induced d.
radiation lung d.
Recklinghausen d. type I
Reiter d.
sclerodermoid graft-versus-host d.
sixth venereal d.
space-occupying d.
Steinert d.
Takayasu d.
thin basement membrane d.
tricuspid valve d.
undifferentiated connective tissue d.
upper tract d.
urinary tract d.
van Buren d.
venous stasis d.
venous web d.
vibration d.
von Economo d.
Winiwarter-Buerger d.
dish face
dishpan fracture
disinfectant
  Endospore d.
disinfecting solution
disinfection
  high level d.
  root canal d.
  spray-wipe-spray d.
  surface d.
  thermal d.
disintegration
  endoscopic stone d.
  d. rate
disinvagination
disjoined pyeloplasty
disk, disc
  acromioclavicular d.
  annulus fibrosus of intervertebral d.
  articular d. of temporomandibular
    joint
  d. compression
  d. diffusion method
  d. drusen hemorrhage

NOTES

D

disk *(continued)*
excavation of optic d.
d. excision
excision of intervertebral d.
extruded d.
d. extrusion
d. fragment
free fragment d.
herniated d.
d. herniation
intercalated d.
interpubic d.
intervertebral d.
Krupin valve with d.
d. lesion
mandibular d.
Marlen double-faced adhesive d.
neovascularization of d.
d. neovascularization
optic d.
d. oxygenation
d. oxygenator
d. plication
d. pressure
protruded d.
ruptured d.
sacrococcygeal d.
d. sensitivity method
d. space
d. space infection
d. space narrowing
d. space saline acceptance test
sternoclavicular d.
temporomandibular articular d.
Disk-Criminator sensory testing
diskectomy, discectomy
anterior d.
automated percutaneous d.
cervical d.
Cloward fusion d.
laminotomy and d.
lumbar d.
microlumbar d.
microsurgical d.
partial d.
percutaneous lumbar d.
Robinson anterior cervical d.
Smith-Robinson anterior cervical d.
thoracic d.
transthoracic d.
Williams d.
dislocation
acromioclavicular joint d.
antenatal d.
anterior complete d.
anterior hip d.
anterior-inferior d.
anterior shoulder d.

anterolateral d.
atlantoaxial d.
atlanto-occipital joint d.
atypical d.
Bankart shoulder d.
bayonet d.
Bell-Dally cervical d.
Bennett d.
bilateral interfacetal d.
bilateral intrafacetal d.
boutonnière hand d.
bursting d.
carpometacarpal joint d.
central d.
Chopart ankle d.
closed d.
complete anterior d.
complete inferior d.
complete posterior d.
complete superior d.
compound d.
congenital hip d.
congenital lens d.
consecutive d.
d. contour abnormality
dashboard d.
Desault wrist d.
divergent elbow d.
dorsal perilunate d.
dorsal transscaphoid perilunar d.
dysplasia d.
elbow d.
facet d.
fracture d.
d. fracture
frank d.
gamekeeper thumb d.
glenohumeral joint d.
habitual d.
Hill-Sachs shoulder d.
hip d.
incomplete d.
inferior complete closed d.
inferior complete compound d.
interphalangeal joint d.
intraocular lens d.
isolated d.
Kienböck d.
knee d.
d. of lens
lens d.
Lisfranc d.
lumbosacral d.
lunate d.
luxatio erecta shoulder d.
mandibular d.
medial swivel d.
metatarsophalangeal joint d.

midcarpal d.
milkmaid elbow d.
Monteggia d.
Nélaton ankle d.
occipitoatlantal d.
Otto pelvis d.
Palmer transscaphoid perilunar d.
panclavicular d.
parachute jumper d.
partial d.
patellar intra-articular d.
pathologic d.
perilunar transscaphoid d.
perilunate carpal d.
peroneal d.
phalangeal d.
posterior hip d.
posterior shoulder d.
posteromedial d.
prenatal d.
primitive d.
proximal tibiofibular joint d.
radial head d.
radiocarpal d.
recent d.
recurrent patellar d.
retrosternal d.
rotational d.
sacroiliac d.
scapholunate d.
shoulder d.
Smith d.
spontaneous hyperemic d.
sternoclavicular joint d.
subastragalar d.
subcoracoid shoulder d.
subglenoid shoulder d.
subtalar d.
superior d.
swivel d.
talar d.
tarsal d.
tarsometatarsal d.
temporomandibular joint d.
teratologic d.
tibialis posterior d.
tibiofibular joint d.
transscaphoid perilunate d.
traumatic d.
triquetrolunate d.
unilateral interfacetal d.
unilateral intrafacetal d.

unreduced d.
volar semilunar wrist d.
wrist d.

dismember
dismembered
    d. anastomosis
    d. pyeloplasty
    d. reimplanted appendicocystostomy
disobliteration
disorder
    accommodation d.
    acquired cornification d.
    articulation d.
    autoimmune connective tissue d.
    blood coagulation d.
    cartilaginous growth plate d.
    coagulation d.
    complex adrenal endocrine d.
    complex endocrine d.
    complex gonadal endocrine d.
    complex pituitary endocrine d.
    complex thyroid endocrine d.
    connective tissue d.
    cornification d.
    Curth-Maklin cornification d.
    developmental coordination d.
    ejaculation d.
    elimination d.
    endocrine d.
    endonasal d.
    evacuation d.
    experimental d.
    gamma-loop d.
    gonadal endocrine d.
    immune-mediated coagulation d.
    keratitis-deafness cornification d.
    lysosomal enzyme d.
    mastication d.
    mitral valve d.
    mixed connective tissue d.
    nail d.
    organic articulation d.
    pituitary endocrine d.
    posttransplantation
      lymphoproliferative d.
    thyroid endocrine d.
    unilateral hemidysplasia
      cornification d.
    urinary tract d.
disparate point
displaced fracture

D

NOTES

displacement
>d. analysis
>d. curve
>d. implantation
>d. osteotomy
>d. threshold

disposable Yankauer suction tube
disruption
dissect
dissected tissue arm
dissecting
>d. aneurysm
>d. intramural hematoma

dissection
>d. of aorta
>aortic d.
>arterial d.
>arterial wall d.
>axillary d.
>balloon d.
>bilateral neck d.
>blunt and sharp d.
>bone d.
>bone/ligament d.
>bony d.
>carotid artery d.
>circumferential mucosal d.
>complex d.
>condyle d.
>coronary artery d.
>cranial nerve d.
>DeBakey-type aortic d.
>deep iliac d.
>discontinuous neck d.
>elective lymph node d. (ELND)
>elective neck d.
>en bloc d.
>epiphenomena of d.
>extended obturator node and
> iliopsoas node d.
>extracapsular d.
>extraperitoneal endoscopic pelvic
> lymph node d.
>field of d.
>finger fracture d.
>flank d.
>functional neck d.
>gauze d.
>groin d.
>hard palate d.
>hydraulic d.
>incisural d.
>inguinal canal d.
>inguinal-femoral node d.
>intracapsular d.
>intradural d.
>intramural air d.
>jugular vein d.

>laparoscopic pelvic lymph node d.
>lateral d.
>limited obturator node d.
>lymph node d.
>d. margin
>medial d.
>mediastinal d.
>middle fossa floor/petrous d.
>modified radical neck d.
>muscle d.
>nasal d.
>neck d.
>nerve-sparing d.
>node d.
>Pack-Ehrlich deep iliac d.
>para-aortic lymph node d.
>parotid d.
>partial zonal d.
>pelvic lymph node d. (PLND)
>pelvic node d.
>perirectal pelvic d.
>plane of d.
>postradical neck d.
>preadventitial d.
>radical axillary d.
>radical lymph node d.
>radical neck d.
>retroperitoneal pelvic lymph
> node d. (RPLND)
>scissors d.
>selective inguinal node d.
>sharp d.
>in situ d.
>soft tissue d.
>spiral d.
>spontaneous coronary artery d.
>Stanford-type aortic d.
>subligamentous d.
>submucosal d.
>subperiosteal d.
>subtemporal d.
>suction d.
>suprahyoid neck d.
>supraomohyoid neck d.
>sylvian d.
>systemic d.
>Taussig-Morton node d.
>therapeutic d.
>thoracic aortic d.
>tongue-jaw-neck d.
>transthoracic d.
>d. tubercle
>two-team d.
>vertebral d.

disseminated
>d. asymptomatic unilateral
> neovascularization
>d. CMV infection

d. gonococcal infection
d. inflammation
d. intravascular coagulation (DIC)
dissemination
Disse space
dissipation
    circle d.
dissociated
    d. anesthesia
    d. position
dissociation
    atrial d.
    atrioventricular d.
    A-V d.
    complete atrioventricular d.
    complete A-V d.
    d. curve
    electromechanical d.
    electromyocardial d.
    hypnotic d.
    incomplete atrioventricular d.
    incomplete A-V d.
    interference d.
    intracavitary pressure-electrogram d.
    isorhythmic d.
    longitudinal d.
    lunotriquetral d.
    microbic d.
    d. movement
    radioulnar d.
    scapholunate d.
    scapulothoracic d.
    sleep d.
    syringomyelic d.
    tabetic d.
dissociative anesthesia
distal
    d. anastomosis
    d. biceps brachii tendon rupture
    d. catheter lengthening
    d. cavity
    d. centriole
    d. clavicular excision
    d. ectasia
    d. esophageal ring
    d. esophagectomy
    d. extension restoration
    d. femoral epiphyseal fracture
    d. fragment
    d. gastrectomy
    d. humeral epiphysis
    d. humeral fracture

d. interphalangeal (DIP)
d. interphalangeal joint approach
d. metaphysis
d. metastasis
d. metatarsal osteotomy
d. nail matrix
d. neurolysis
d. oblique sliding osteotomy
d. pancreatectomy
d. part of anterior lobe of hypophysis
d. perfusion
d. radial fracture
d. radioulnar joint stabilization
d. shave section
d. tibiofibular fusion
d. ureterectomy
distal-occlusal (DO)
distal-row carpectomy
distance
    interincisoral d.
    skin-to-tumor d.
    thyromental d.
    tube-carina d.
    tube-patient d.
    tube-to-film d.
distant
    d. flap
    d. metastasis
distantial aberration
distention
    gastric d.
distoangular position
distobuccal line angle
distobucco-occlusal point angle
distolabial line angle
distolabioincisal point angle
distolingual line angle
distolinguoincisal point angle
distolinguo-occlusal point angle
disto-occlusal (DO)
    d.-o. point angle
distortion
    d. aberration
    corneal d.
    pin-cushion d.
distract
distraction
    d. arthroplasty
    d. of fracture
    d. technique

NOTES

distraction/compression scoliosis treatment
distractive extension
distribution
    lesion d.
    loop d.
    pattern of d.
    ventilation/perfusion d.
diurnal
    d. enuresis
    d. intraocular pressure measurement
divergent
    d. elbow dislocation
    d. ray projection
diversion
    Camey enterocystoplasty urinary d.
    Duke pouch cutaneous urinary d.
    Gil-Vernet ileocecal cystoplasty urinary d.
    ileal conduit urinary d.
    ileocolonic pouch urinary d.
    Indiana continent reservoir urinary d.
    Khafagy modified ileocecal cystoplasty urinary d.
    Kock pouch cutaneous urinary d.
    Laparostat with fiber d.
    Mainz pouch cutaneous urinary d.
    Studer reservoir urinary d.
diversionary ileostomy
diverticula (*pl. of* diverticulum)
    d. of lacrimal sac
diverticular
    d. hemorrhage
diverticulation abnormality
diverticulectomy
    bladder d.
    endocavitary bladder d.
    Harrington esophageal d.
    pharyngoesophageal d.
    urethral d.
    vesical d.
    d. with myotomy
diverticulitis
diverticulopexy
diverticulum, pl. **diverticula**
    caliceal d.
diverting
    d. loop colostomy
    d. loop ileostomy
    d. stoma
divided respiration
divided-stoma colostomy
divinyl ether
division
    anterior primary d.
    d. I–IV lesion
    maturation d.

    posterior primary d.
    reduction d.
    vascular ring d.
divulse
divulsion
Dix-Hallpike maneuver
Dixon
    D. fat suppression method
    D. method opposed imaging
    D. technique
Dizac injection
DKS
    Damus-Kaye-Stancel
    DKS operation
D-loop transposition of the great arteries
D-Med injection
DO
    distal-occlusal
    disto-occlusal
    DO cavity
Dobbhoff
    D. feeding tube
    D. gastric decompression tube
    D. PEG tube
dobutamine
Dobutrex injection
DOC exchange technique
Docktor suture
documentation
Döderlein
    D. method
    D. method of vaginal hysterectomy
    D. roll-flap operation
Dodge area-length method
Doesel-Huzly bronchoscopic tube
dog ear of anastomosis
dog-ear repair
dog-leg fracture
DOI
    depth of insertion
Dolenc technique
dolichocephalic head
dolichoectatic artery
dolichopellic pelvis
Dollinger tendinous ring
doll's
    d. eye maneuver
    d. head maneuver
    d. head phenomenon
Doll trochanteric reattachment technique
dolorosa
    anesthesia d.
D'ombrain operation
dome
    d. excursion
    d. fracture
    d. osteotomy

Domeboro solution
dome-shaped osteotomy
dominant mass
domino procedure
Donald-Fothergill operation
Donald procedure
Donaldson
    D. eustachian tube
    D. eye patch
    D. tube
    D. ventilation tube
donation
    autologous blood d.
    blood d.
    designated blood d.
Donati suture
Donders
    D. line
    D. pressure
    D. procedure
    space of D.
donor
    d. hepatectomy
    d. iliac Y graft
    non-heart-beating d.
    d. tissue
Dooley nail
dopamine
    d. receptor
dopaminergic
    d. medication
    d. tract
Doppler
    D. auto-correlation technique
    D. color flow
    D. color flow imaging
    endoscopic color D.
    D. interrogation
    D. pressure gradient
    D. pulse evaluation
    D. tissue imaging
    transcranial D. (TCD)
    D. ultrasound segmental blood pressure testing
dopplergram
Dopram injection
Dor
    D. fundoplication
    D. fundoplication method
    D. fundoplication procedure
    D. fundoplication technique
Dorello canal

Dormia noose
Dornier
    D. extracorporeal shock wave lithotripsy
    D. MPL 9000 gallstone lithotripsy
Dorrance procedure
dorsa (*pl. of* dorsum)
dorsabdominal
Dorsacaine
dorsal
    d. artery of clitoris
    d. artery of penis
    d. aspect
    d. birthing position
    d. branch of the lumbar artery
    d. branch of the posterior intercostal arteries 3–11
    d. branch of the posterior intercostal veins 4–11
    d. branch of the subcostal artery
    d. branch of the superior intercostal artery
    d. branch of the ulnar nerve
    d. closing wedge osteotomy
    d. column stimulation
    d. column stimulator
    d. cord stimulation
    d. cross-finger flap
    d. digital artery
    d. digital veins of toes
    d. enteric fistula
    d. finger approach
    d. horn
    d. induction
    d. interosseous artery
    d. interosseous muscles of foot
    d. interosseous muscles of hand
    d. interosseous nerve
    d. linear incision
    d. lingual branches of lingual artery
    d. lithotomy
    d. lithotomy position
    d. longitudinal incision
    d. lumbotomy incision
    d. midline approach
    d. nerve of clitoris
    d. nerve of penis
    d. nerve of scapula
    d. pancreatic artery
    d. perilunate dislocation
    d. plate of neural tube

NOTES

dorsal *(continued)*
    d. point
    d. primary ramus of spinal nerve
    d. proximal metatarsal osteotomy
    d. recumbent position
    d. rhizotomy
    d. root
    d. root entry zone (DREZ)
    d. root entry zone lesion
    d. root ganglion
    d. root ganglionectomy
    d. sacrococcygeal muscle
    d. sacrococcygeus muscle
    d. scapular artery
    d. scapular nerve
    d. scapular vein
    d. spine
    d. spinocerebellar tract
    d. surface of scapula
    d. synovectomy
    d. talonavicular bone
    d. tegmental decussation
    d. tenosynovectomy
    d. thoracic artery
    d. translation
    d. transscaphoid perilunar dislocation
    d. transverse capsulotomy
    d. transverse incision
    d. tubercle of radius
    d. vein patch graft
    d. veins of clitoris
    d. veins of penis
    d. vertebrae
    d. wire-loop fixation
dorsalis
    d. pedis artery
    d. pedis artery anatomy
    d. pedis flap
dorsal-V osteotomy
dorsalward approach
dorsiflexory wedge osteotomy
dorsiscapular
dorsispinal
    d. veins
dorsocephalad
dorsolateral
    d. approach
    d. and medial capsulotomy
    d. tract
dorsolumbar
dorsomedial
    d. approach
    d. incision
dorsoplantar
    d. approach
    d. projection
dorsoradial approach

dorsorostral approach
dorsosacral position
dorsoulnar approach
dorsoventrad
dorsum, pl. **dorsa**
    d. ephippii
    d. linguae
    d. manus
    d. pedis
    d. of penis
    d. penis
    d. scapulae
    d. sellae
    d. of tongue
dose
    epinephrine test d.
    d. escalation
    priming d.
    subparalyzing d.
    tissue tolerance d.
dose-effect curve
dose-related effect
dose-response curve
dot-and-blot hemorrhage
dot-blot
    d.-b. procedure
    d.-b. technique
dot hemorrhage
Dotter-Judkins technique
Dotter technique
Doubilet sphincterotomy
double
    d. antibody method
    d. burst stimulation
    d. burst transmission
    d. chin
    d. contrast enema
    d. decidual sac
    d. enterostomy
    d. exposure
    d. extra stimulus
    d. fracture
    d. freeze-stalk cryopexy
    d. freeze-thaw cryopexy
    d. incision
    d. jaw surgery
    d. loop hernia
    d. loop pouch
    d. Maddox rod test
    d. osteotomy
    d. papilla pedicle graft
    d. pedicle flap
    d. pyloroplasty
    d. right-angle suture
    d. ring
    d. setup endotracheal tube
    d. simultaneous stimulation
    d. velour knitted graft

double-balloon
    d.-b. technique
    d.-b. valvotomy
    d.-b. valvuloplasty
double-barrel
    d.-b. colostomy
    d.-b. ileostomy
double-cannula tracheostomy tube
double-contrast
    d.-c. barium enema examination
    d.-c. visualization
double-dummy technique
double-exposed rib
double-flanged valve sewing ring
double-focus tube
double-folded cup-patch technique
double-freeze technique
double-incision fasciotomy
double-inlet ventricle anomaly
double-looped
    d.-l. gracilis graft
    d.-l. semitendinosus technique
double-lumen
    d.-l. endobronchial tube
    d.-l. suction irrigation tube
double-needle chemonucleolysis
double-point threshold
double-puncture laparoscopy
double-rod
    d.-r. construct
    d.-r. technique
double-sealant technique
double-stapled
    d.-s. ileoanal reservoir method
    d.-s. ileoanal reservoir procedure
    d.-s. ileoanal reservoir technique
double-staple technique
double-stick technique
double-tube technique
double-umbrella closure
double-volume exchange transfusion
double-wire technique
doubly
    d. armed suture
    d. ligated
    d. sutured
doughnut
    d. ring
Douglas
    D. abscess
    D. bag collection method
    D. bag technique

    cul-de-sac of D.
    D. cul-de-sac
    D. fold
    D. graft
    D. line
    pouch of D.
    D. pouch
Dow
    D. Corning tube
    D. method
dowel
    d. bone graft
    d. spinal fusion
    d. technique
doweling spondylolisthesis technique
Downey-McGlamery procedure
downstream
    d. sampling method
    d. venous pressure
downward drainage
doxacurium chloride
doxapram hydrochloride
Doxychel injection
Doyen vaginal hysterectomy
Doyle operation
DR-70 tumor marker test
Drabkin solution
Dragendorff solution
Dräger
    D. Nrkomed II ventilator
    D. Vapor 19
dragon worm infection
Dragstedt graft
drainable ostomy pouch
drainage
    capillary d.
    catheter d.
    chest tube d. (CTD)
    circle loop biliary d.
    closed d.
    continuous catheter d.
    dependent d.
    downward d.
    endoscopic biliary d.
    endoscopic nasobiliary catheter d.
    endoscopic pancreatic d.
    endoscopic transpapillary cyst d.
    external ventricular d.
    extrapetrosal d.
    hematoma d.
    incision and d.
    internal d.

D

NOTES

drainage *(continued)*
  d. of lacrimal gland operation
  d. of lacrimal sac
  d. of lacrimal sac operation
  lymphocele d.
  Molteno d.
  nephrostomy d.
  open d.
  percutaneous abscess d. (PAD)
  percutaneous catheter d.
  postoperative irrigation-suction d.
  postural d.
  sclerotomy with d.
  stereotactic catheter d.
  suction d.
  Thora-Drain III chest d.
  thorascopic d.
  through d.
  tidal d.
  T-tube d.
  d. tube
  Wangensteen d.
  wound d.
drain-to-wall suction tube
drain-trap stomach
drain volume
Drake tandem clipping technique
draw-over vaporizer
Dreiling tube
dresser
dressing therapy
Dreulofoy lesion
DREZ
  dorsal root entry zone
  DREZ lesion
  DREZ modification of Eriksson
    technique
  DREZ procedure
  DREZ surgery
drilling technique
drip
  intravenous d.
  d. transfusion
Dripps-American Surgical Association
  score
Dripps classification
drip-tube feeding
drive
  exploratory d.
  hypercapnic d.
driven
  d. equilibrium Fourier transform
    (DEFT)
  d. equilibrium Fourier transform
    technique
drop
  flow-dependent pressure d.
  d. metastasis

droperidol
  d. and fentanyl
droplet infection
drop-lock ring
Dr. Twiss duodenal tube
Drualt
  D. bundle
  bundle of D.
drug
  d. administration
  β-adrenergic blocking d.
  antifibrinolytic d.
  calcium entry blocking d.
  cholinomimetic d.
  hydrophilic d.
  lipophilic d.
  nonsteroidal anti-inflammatory d.
    (NSAID)
  opioid-sparing d.
  d. resistance
  second-line d.
  sympathomimetic d.
  d. synergy
  synthetic lysine analog
    antifibrinolytic d.
drum membrane
Drummond
  D. spinous wiring technique
  D. wire technique
drunken sailor effect
drusen
dry
  d. abscess
  d. amputation
  d. colostomy
  d. field technique
  d. heat oven sterilization
  d. hernia
  d. mucous membrane
2-D TEE system Ultra-Neb 99
dual
  d. compression scoliosis treatment
  d. impression technique
  d. onlay cortical bone graft
  d. percutaneous endoscopic
    gastrostomy
  d. percutaneous gastrostomy tube
dual-lumen sump nasogastric tube
Duane
  D. anomaly
  D. classification
Duane-Hunt relation
Dubin-Amelar varicocele classification
Dubowitz
  D. evaluation
  D. examination
Duckett procedure

duct
    aberrant bile d.'s
    accessory pancreatic d.
    Bartholin d.
    Bernard d.
    bifurcation of common bile d.
    bile d.
    biliary d.
    Blasius d.
    bucconeural d.
    d. of bulbourethral gland
    canalicular d.'s
    d. cannulation
    d. carcinoma
    catheterization of lacrimal d.
    catheterization of lacrimonasal d.
    d. cell adenocarcinoma
    choledoch d.
    common bile d. (CBD)
    common hepatic d.
    congenital cystic dilatation of
      bile d.
    craniopharyngeal d.
    cystic d.
    deferent d.
    efferent d.
    ejaculatory d.
    endolymphatic d.
    d. of epididymis
    excretory d. of seminal vesicle
    extrahepatic bile d.
    frontonasal d.
    galactophorous d.'s
    gall d.
    Gartner d.
    genital d.
    hemithoracic d.
    Hensen d.
    hepatic d.
    hepatocystic d.
    Hoffmann d.
    hypophysial d.
    incisive d.
    jugular d.
    lactiferous d.'s
    left d. of caudate lobe
    left hepatic d.
    longitudinal d. of epoöphoron
    lymphatic d.
    main pancreatic d. (MPD)
    mamillary d.'s
    mammary d.'s

    mesonephric d.
    metanephric d.
    middle extrahepatic bile d.
    milk d.'s
    minor sublingual d.'s
    Müller d.
    pancreatic d.
    papillary d.'s
    paramesonephric d.
    paraurethral d.'s
    parotid d.
    Pecquet d.
    percutaneous dilatation of biliary d.
    perilymphatic d.
    pronephric d.
    prostatic d.'s
    right d. of caudate lobe
    right hepatic d.
    right lymphatic d.
    Rivinus d.'s
    salivary d.
    Santorini d.
    Schüller d.'s
    secretory d.
    semicircular d.'s
    seminal d.
    d.'s of Skene glands
    spermatic d.
    Stensen d.
    striated d.
    subclavian d.
    submandibular d.
    submaxillary d.
    sudoriferous d.
    sweat d.
    d. of sweat glands
    testicular d.
    thoracic d.
    thyroglossal d.
    thyrolingual d.
    uniting d.
    utriculosaccular d.
    Walther d.'s
    Wharton d.
    Wirsung d.
    wolffian d.

ductal
    d. adenoma
    d. carcinoma
    d. dilatation
    d. dilation

D

NOTES

ductal *(continued)*
    d. ectasia
    d. system perforation
ductal-dependent
    d.-d. lesion
    d.-d. pulmonary circulation
ductless glands
ductopenic rejection
ductule
    aberrant d.'s
    biliary d.'s
    efferent d.'s of testis
    inferior aberrant d.
    interlobular d.'s
    prostatic d.'s
    superior aberrant d.
    transverse d.'s of epoöphoron
ductulus, pl. ductuli
    d. aberrans inferior
    d. aberrans superior
    ductuli aberrantes
    ductuli biliferi
    d. efferens testis
    ductuli interlobulares
    ductuli prostatici
    ductuli transversi epoöphori
ductus
    d. aberrantes
    d. biliferi
    d. choledochus
    d. cysticus
    d. deferens
    d. deferens vestigialis
    d. dorsopancreaticus
    d. ejaculatorius
    d. endolymphaticus
    d. epididymidis
    d. epoöphori longitudinalis
    d. excretorius
    d. excretorius vesiculae seminalis
    d. glandulae bulbourethralis
    d. hemithoracicus
    d. hepaticus communis
    d. hepaticus dexter
    d. hepaticus sinister
    d. lactiferi
    d. lobi caudati dexter
    d. lobi caudati sinister
    d. lymphaticus dexter
    d. mesonephricus
    d. pancreaticus
    d. pancreaticus accessorius
    d. paramesonephricus
    d. paraurethrales
    d. parotideus
    d. perilymphaticus
    d. prostatici
    d. reuniens

    d. sublinguales minores
    d. sublingualis major
    d. sudoriferus
    d. thoracicus
    d. thoracicus dexter
    d. utriculosaccularis
Duddell membrane
Duecollement
    D. hemicolectomy
    D. maneuver
Dufourmentel technique
Duhamel colon operation
Dührssen
    D. incision
    D. vaginofixation of uterus
Dujovny microsuction dissection set
Duke
    D. pouch
    D. pouch cutaneous urinary
      diversion
    D. tube
Duke-Elder operation
Dukes
    D. classification
    D. classification of carcinoma
    D. procedure
    D. stage
Dul45 cell line
Dulox suture
dumbbell
    d. mass
    d. tumor
dumping syndrome
Duncan-Lovell modification
Duncan position
Dundas-Grant tube
Dunn
    D. biopsy
    D. osteotomy
    D. technique
Dunn-Brittain foot stabilization
    technique
Dunnett test
Dunn-Hess trochanteric osteotomy
Dunnington operation
duodenal
    d. adenocarcinoma
    d. adenoma
    d. ampulla
    d. bulb
    d. bulb deformity
    d. cap
    d. compression
    d. contents examination
    d. duplication
    d. endoscopic polypectomy
    d. fistula
    d. fluid collection

d. foreign body
d. fossae
d. glands
d. hematoma
d. hernia
d. impression
d. lesion
d. loop
d. mass
d. metastasis
d. perforation
d. sphincter
d. tumor
d. ulceration
d. web
duodenectomy
duodenobiliary pressure gradient
duodenocaval fistula
duodenocholecystostomy
duodenocholedochotomy
duodenocolic fistula
duodenocystostomy
duodenoduodenostomy
duodenoenterocutaneous fistula
duodenoenterostomy
duodenogastroscopy
retrograde d.
duodenojejunal
d. angle
d. flexure
d. fold
d. fossa
d. hernia
d. junction
d. recess
d. sphincter
duodenojejunostomy
suprapapillary Roux-en-Y d.
duodenolysis
duodenomesocolic fold
duodenopancreaticocholedochal rupture
duodenorenal ligament
duodenorrhaphy
duodenoscopy
duodenostomy
Witzel d.
duodenotomy
transverse d.
duodenum
Duofilm solution
Duo-Trach
Duplay I, II technique

duplex-guided compression
duplication
alimentary tract d.
d. anomaly
complete d.
congenital d.
cranial d.
duodenal d.
esophageal d.
fetal d.
gallbladder d.
gastric d.
incomplete d.
partial d.
renal d.
symmetric thumb d.
thumb d.
trunk d.
tubular colonic d.
ureteral d.
Wassel type IV thumb d.
Dupuy-Dutemps
D.-D. dacryocystorhinostomy dye test
D.-D. dacryostomy
D.-D. operation
Dupuytren
D. canal
D. fracture
D. suture
dura
d. mater
d. mater of brain
d. mater cranialis
d. mater encephali
d. mater of spinal cord
d. mater spinalis
Duragesic
D. Transdermal
dural
d. arteriovenous fistula
d. arteriovenous malformation
d. cavernous sinus fistula
d. ectasia
d. incision
d. patch reconstruction
d. puncture
d. repair
d. ring
d. shunt syndrome
d. venous sinuses
Duralite tube

NOTES

Duralone injection
Duralon-UV nylon membrane
Duralutin injection
Duramorph injection
Duran
    D. annuloplasty ring
    D. approach
Duranest
    D. injection
duraplasty
DuraPrep surgical solution
duration
    d. of anesthesia
    d. of expiration
    d. of inspiration
    D. Nasal solution
    d. tetany
    d. time
    d. of treatment
Duret
    D. hemorrhage
    D. lesion
Durham
    D. flatfoot operation
    D. plasty
    D. tracheostomy tube
Durkan carpal compression test
Durr
    D. nonpenetrating keratoplasty
    D. operation
dusky stoma
Dutcher body
duToit-Roux
    d.-R. arthroplasty
    d.-R. staple capsulorrhaphy
Duval
    D. pancreaticojejunostomy
    D. procedure
Duverger-Velter operation
Duverney
    D. fissures
    D. fracture
    D. gland
    D. muscle
DuVries
    D. approach
    D. deltoid ligament reconstruction
      technique
    D. hammertoe repair
    D. incision
    D. plantar condylectomy
DuVries-Mann modified bunionectomy
Dwar-Barrington resection
dwarf pelvis
Dwelle Ophthalmic solution
Dwyer
    D. clawfoot operation
    D. incision

    D. osteotomy
    D. procedure
Dyban technique
Dyck-Lambert classification
dyclonine hydrochloride
dye
    d. dilution technique
    Evans blue d.
    d. exclusion test
    flashlamp excited pulsed d.
    d. injection
    methylene blue d.
    occlusal registration d.
    d. reduction spot test
    d. scattering method
    d. sham intrarenal lesion
dye-dilution method
dyed starch method
Dynamap blood pressure cuff
dynamic
    d. bolus tracking technique
    d. cardiomyoplasty
    d. closure pressure
    d. compliance (Cdyn)
    d. compression
    d. compression-plate fixation
    d. condylar-screw fixation
    d. cystourethroscopy
    d. end-tidal forcing
    d. fluorescence video endoscopy
    d. graciloplasty
    d. lumbar stabilization
    d. relation
    d. relaxation
    d. repair
    d. spatial reconstructor
    d. storage allocation
    d. supporting suture
    d. traction method
dynamometer
    Micro FET isometric force d.
dynamometry
    isometric force d.
dysarthric lesion
dyscrasic fracture
dysesthesia
    burning d.
dysfunction
    endothelial d.
    esophageal body motor d.
    extensor mechanism d.
    late graft d.
    pelvic floor d.
    postanesthetic central nervous
      system d.
    postgastrectomy d.
    sphincter of Oddi d.
dysgenesis

dysgnathic anomaly
dyskinesia
    extrapyramidal d.
    retrolisthesis positional d.
dysmenorrheal membrane
dysmyelination
dysosteogenesis
dysostosis
dyspepsia
    postcholecystectomy flatulent d.
dysphagia
    contractile ring d.
    postvagotomy d.
    soft food d.
dysphasia
    expressive d.
dyspigmentation
dysplasia
    asphyxiating thoracic d.
    bronchopulmonary d. (BPD)
    d. dislocation
    oculoauriculovertebral d. (OAV)

dysplasia-associated
    d.-a. lesion
    d.-a. mass
dyspnea
    exertional d.
    expiratory d.
    one-flight exertional d.
    d. on exertion
    two-flight exertional d.
dysraphic malformation
dysrhythmogenicity
dystonia
    muscle d.
dystopia transversa externa testis
dystrophic nail
dystrophy
    corneal d.
    reflex sympathetic d.
dysuria
dysuric

NOTES

D

E.
  E. Benson Hood Laboratories esophageal tube
  E. Benson Hood Laboratories salivary bypass tube
EA
  epidural anesthesia
Eagle-Barrett syndrome
Eames technique
ear
  e. anesthesia
  e. bones
  e. canal
  e. cartilage inflammation
  external e.
  e. lobe
  e. surgery
Earle solution
earlobe adipose tissue
early gastric cancer
early-onset graft-vs-host disease
earth
  diatomaceous e.
easily reducible hernia
Eastman suction tube
Eastwood technique
Eaton
  E. closed reduction
  E. implant arthroplasty
  E. volar plate arthroplasty
Eaton-Littler
  E.-L. ligament reconstruction
  E.-L. technique
Eaton-Malerich
  E.-M. fracture-dislocation operation
  E.-M. fracture-dislocation technique
  E.-M. reduction
Ebbehoj procedure
Eberle contracture release technique
Ebner
  imbrication lines of E.
  imbrication lines of von E.
  E. line
  E. reticulum
ebonation
ébranlement
Ebstein
  E. cardiac anomaly
  E. malformation
eburnation
EBV
  Epstein-Barr virus
  EBV infection
ECA
  external carotid artery

ECA-PCA bypass surgery
ECC
  extracorporeal circulation
ECCE
  extracapsular cataract extraction
eccentric
  e. fixation
  e. hypertrophy
  e. interocclusal record
  e. jaw position
  e. jaw relation
  e. ledge
  e. maxillomandibular record
  e. narrowing
  e. occlusion
eccentricity index
ecchondrosis
ecchymosed
ecchymosis, pl. ecchymoses
  e. of eyelid
ecchymotic
  e. mark
  e. mask
eccouchement forcé
eccrine sweat gland
ECF-A
  eosinophilic chemotactic factor of anaphylaxis
ECFV
  extracellular fluid volume
ECG
  electrocardiogram
  electrocardiography
  ECG signal-averaging technique
ecgonine
echinococcal
  e. cyst disease
  e. liver abscess
echo
  e. formation
  e. imaging
  magnetization prepared-rapid gradient e. (MP-RAGE)
  magnitude preparation-rapid acquisition gradient e. (MP-RAGE)
  e. rephasing
  e. reverberation
  e. score
  e. texture
  e. zone
echocardiographic assessment
echocardiography
  transesophageal e. (TEE)

E

echodense
  e. mass
  e. structure
echoduodenoscopy
echo-free space
echogenic
  e. liver
  e. plaque
  e. tissue
echographic layer
echolucent plaque
echopenic liver metastasis
echoplanar magnetic resonance imaging
echo-poor layer
echovirus infection
Ecker fissure
Ecker-Lotke-Glazer
  E.-L.-G. patellar tendon repair
  E.-L.-G. tendon reconstruction
    technique
Eckert-Davis classification
Eck fistula
Eckhout vertical gastroplasty
eclipse
  e. amblyopia
  e. phase
ECLS
  extracorporeal life support
ECMO
  extracorporeal membrane oxygenation
    ECMO pump
ECoG
  electrocorticography
    ECoG monitoring
    ECoG performance status scale
Economo disease
ECOR
  extracorporeal CO_2 removal
ECPL
  endocavitary pelvic lymphadenectomy
ECRB
  extensor carpi radialis brevis
ECRL
  extensor carpi radialis longus
ECS
  elective cosmetic surgery
  electrocerebral silence
  extracellular-like, calcium-free solution
    ECS cardioplegic solution
ECST
  European Carotid Surgery Trial
ectal origin
ectasia
  alveolar e.
  artery e.
  corneal e.
  coronary artery e.
  distal e.

ductal e.
dural e.
iris e.
mammary duct e.
papillary e.
scleral e.
senile e.
vascular e.
ectasis
ectatic
  e. aneurysm
  e. bronchus
  e. carotid artery
  c. dilation
  e. emphysema
  e. marginal degeneration of cornea
  e. vascular lesion
  e. vessel
ecthyma gangrenosum
ectoderm
ectodermal
ectopia
  cerebellar e.
  cilia e.
  e. cloacae
  gallbladder e.
  macular e.
  renal e.
  e. renis
  testicular e.
  e. testis
  ureteral e.
  e. vesica
ectopic
  e. ACTH syndrome
  e. anus
  e. atrial tachycardia
  e. bone
  e. craniopharyngioma
  e. cutaneous schistosomiasis
  e. endometrial tissue
  e. eruption
  e. eyelash
  e. focus
  e. gastric mucosa
  e. impulse
  e. kidney
  e. pancreas
  e. parathormone production
  e. rhythm
  e. sebaceous gland
  e. spleen
  e. testis
  e. ureter
  e. ureterocele
  e. varices
ectosteal
ectostosis

ectothrix infection
ECTR
>endoscopic carpal tunnel release

ectropion
>e. cicatriceum
>e. of eyelid
>e. luxurians
>e. sarcomatosum

ECU
>extensor carpi ulnaris

eczematoid pruritic plaque
eczematous
>e. lesion
>e. patch
>e. polymorphous light eruption
>e. reaction

EDA
>end-diastolic cross-sectional area

EDD
>end-diastolic diameter

edea
Edebohls
>E. incision
>E. position

Edecrin Sodium injection
edema
>brain e.
>bullous e.
>bullous e. vesicae
>cerebral e.
>corneal e.
>endothelial cell e.
>e. of lower eyelid
>nephrotic e.
>neurogenic pulmonary e. (NPE)
>peripheral extremity e.
>stasis e.

Eden-Hybbinette
>E.-H. arthroplasty
>E.-H. procedure

Eden-Lange procedure
Eden-Lawson hysterectomy
edentulous space
Eder-Puestow dilation
edge
>chondral e.
>spectral e.

edge-detection method
edgewise
>e. buccal tube
>e. technique

Edinburgh
>E. 2 Coma Scale
>E. suture

Edlan-Mejchar operation
Edlich gastric lavage tube
Edmondson grading system for hepatocellular carcinoma
Edmondson-Steiner classification
Edwards
>E. modular system bridging sleeve construct
>E. modular system compression construct
>E. modular system distraction-lordosis construct
>E. modular system kyphoreduction construct
>E. modular system neutralization construct
>E. modular system rod-sleeve construct
>E. modular system scoliosis construct
>E. modular system spondylo construct
>E. modular system standard sleeve construct
>E. procedure
>E. septectomy
>E. woven Teflon aortic bifurcation graft

Edwards-Tapp arterial graft
EEG
>electroencephalography

EELV
>end-expiratory lung volume

effect
>amnestic e.
>Bohr e.
>cardioprotective e.
>cardiotoxic e.
>cardiovascular adverse e.
>digitalis e.
>digoxin e.
>dose-related e.
>drunken sailor e.
>esophageal e.
>hypnotic e.
>hypothermic e.
>oxygen e.
>second gas e.
>sedative e.

E

NOTES

197

effective
  e. renal blood flow
  e. renal plasma flow
  e. setting expansion
effector
  e. operation
  e. organ
  e. pathway
efferent
  e. duct
  e. ductules of testis
  e. glomerular arteriole
  e. loop
  e. nerve activity
Effler-Groves mode of Allison procedure
Effler hiatal hernia repair
effluent
effusion
  exudative pleural e.
Efron jackknife classification
Eftekhar broken femoral stem technique
EG/BUS
  external genitalia/Bartholin, urethral, and Skene glands
EGD
  esophagogastroduodenoscopy
egg
  e. activation
  e. membrane
  e. shell nail
Egger line
Eggers
  E. neurectomy
  E. tendon transfer technique
Eggleston method
Eglis glands
Ehrenritter ganglion
Ehrlich
  E. inner body
  E. theory of antibody formation
Ehrlich-Türck line
Eicken method
EID
  emergency infusion device
  Arrow EID
eight-ball hemorrhage
eighth cranial nerve
Einhorn tube
Eisenberger technique
ejaculation
  e. disorder
ejaculatory
  e. duct
ejection
  e. murmur
  e. phase

  e. phase index
  e. rate
  e. shell image
  e. time
ejection-fraction image
Ejrup maneuver
Eklund technique
El-Ahwany classification of humeral supracondylar fracture
elastance
  airway e.
elastic
  e. band fixation
  e. band ligation
  e. barrier
  e. compression
  e. lamella
  e. laminae of arteries
  e. ligature
  e. O ring
  e. recoil pressure
  e. silicone membrane
  e. suture
  e. tissue
elastica
elastic-fiber fragmentation
elastofibroma
elastolysis
  generalized e.
Elaut triangle
elbow
  e. arthroplasty
  articular vascular network of e.
  e. disarticulation
  e. dislocation
  e. extensor tendon
  fat pad of e.
  e. fracture
elective
  e. cosmetic surgery (ECS)
  e. dilatational tracheostomy
  e. lymph node dissection (ELND)
  e. neck dissection
electric
  e. anesthesia
  e. aversion therapy
  e. differential therapy
  e. induction
  e. nerve stimulator
  e. stimulation
electrical
  e. activation abnormality
  e. alternation of heart
  e. catheter ablation
  e. fulguration
  e. heart position
  e. nerve stimulation
  e. stimulation therapy

e. stimulator waveform
e. surface stimulation
Electro-Acuscope stimulator
electroanalgesia
electroanesthesia
electrocardiogram (ECG)
electrocardiography (ECG)
electrocauterization
electrocautery resection
electrocerebral silence (ECS)
electrocholecystectomy
electrocholecystocausis
electrocoagulation
bipolar e.
e. diathermy
direct current e.
endoscopic e.
monopolar e.
multipolar e.
e. necrosis
pinpoint e.
RF e.
snare e.
transendoscopic e.
electroconvulsive therapy
electrocorticography (ECoG)
electrode
Cleartrace e.'s
e. impedance
e. migration
e. placement
e. potential
e. response time
electrodesiccated bleeding point
electrodesiccation
electrode-skin interface
electrodispersive skin patch
electroejaculation
rectal probe e.
electroencephalography (EEG)
electroepilation
electrofulguration
electrogalvanic
e. stimulation
e. stimulator
electrohemostasis
electrohydraulic
e. fragmentation
e. shock wave lithotripsy (ESWL)
electrolysis
Faraday law of e.
One-Touch e.

electrolyte
e. flush solution
e. imbalance coma
electrolyte-polyethylene glycol lavage solution
electrolytic solution
electromagnetic
e. radiation exposure
e. removal of foreign body
electromechanical dissociation
electromyocardial dissociation
electronarcosis
electroneurolysis
electronic
e. bone stimulation
e. magnification
electron microscopy
electroparacentesis
electrophrenic respiration
electrophysiologic
e. function
e. monitoring
electrophysiological stimulation
electrophysiology
flickering blockade e.
patch clamp e.
e. study
electropuncture
electroresection
electroscission
electrosection
electrosterilization
root canal e.
electrostimulation
e. for nonunion of fracture
electrosurgery
electrosurgical
e. desiccation
e. fulguration
e. snare polypectomy
electrotherapeutic sleep therapy
electrotomy
elementary
e. fracture
e. lesion
elevation
e. angle
blanched cutaneous e.
chin e.
congenital scapular e.
diaphragmatic e.
e. of extremity

E

NOTES

elevation *(continued)*
    fetus growth e.
    flap e.
    e. paresis
    periosteal e.
    scapular c.
    ST segment e.
    unilateral diaphragmatic e.
elevator
    e. disease
    e. esophagus
    e. extraction
    e. muscle
    e. muscle of anus
    e. muscle of prostate
    e. muscle of rib
    e. muscle of scapula
    e. muscle of soft palate
    e. muscle of thyroid gland
    e. muscle of upper eyelid
    e. muscle of upper lip
    e. muscle of upper lip and wing
      of nose
elevatus deformity
eleventh
    e. cranial nerve
    e. rib flank incision
    e. rib transperitoneal incision
elimination
    carbon dioxide e. (VECO$_2$)
    CO$_2$ e.
    e. curve
    e. disorder
    nonpulmonary route of e. (NPE)
    e. pocket
    e. procedure
    e. reaction
Elizabethtown osteotomy
Elliot
    E. B solution
    E. operation
    E. position
ellipsoidal joint
ellipsoid method
elliptical
    e. anastomosis
    e. biopsy
    e. excision technique
    e. uterine incision
Ellis
    E. classification
    E. skin traction technique
    E. technique for Barton fracture
Ellis-Jones peroneal tendon technique
Ellison
    E. lateral knee reconstruction
    E. technique
Elmed peristaltic irrigation pump

Elmslie
    E. procedure
    E. reconstruction
Elmslie-Cholmely procedure
Elmslie-Trillat
    E.-T. patellar proccdure
    E.-T. patellar realignment method
ELND
    elective lymph node dissection
Eloesser flap
Elschnig
    E. blepharorrhaphy
    E. body
    E. canthorrhaphy
    E. canthorrhaphy operation
    E. central iridectomy
    E. keratoplasty
eltanolone
Ely operation
embolectomy
    catheter e.
    direct e.
    femoral e.
    pulmonary e.
emboli (*pl. of* embolus)
emboliform
embolism
    air e.
    atheroma e.
    catheter e.
    gas e.
    paradoxical e.
    tumor e.
    venous air e. (VAE)
embolotherapy
embolus, pl. emboli
    e. migration
embouchement
embrasure space
embroscopy
embryectomy
embryo
    e. biopsy
    e. encapsulation
    preimplantation e.
    e. reduction
embryoma of the kidney
embryonic
    e. fixation syndrome
    e. neural tube
    e. sac
embryotomy
emedullate
emergence
    anesthetic e.
emergency
    e. airway management
    e. appendectomy

e. colonoscopy
e. infusion device (EID)
e. laparotomy
E. Medical Services (EMS)
surgical e.
e. tracheal intubation
e. ventilation
emergent
e. appendectomy
e. intubation
eminence
arcuate e.
articular e. of temporal bone
cruciate e.
cruciform e.
deltoid e.
frontal e.
genital e.
hypothenar e.
ileocecal e.
iliopectineal e.
iliopubic e.
intercondylar e.
orbital e. of zygomatic bone
parietal e.
radial e. of wrist
e. of scapha
thenar e.
thyroid e.
ulnar e. of wrist
eminentia, pl. eminentiae
e. arcuata
e. articularis ossis temporalis
c. carpi radialis
e. carpi ulnaris
e. fossae triangularis auricularis
e. frontalis
e. hypothena'ris
e. iliopubica
e. intercondylaris
e. intercondyloidea
e. orbitalis ossis zygomatici
e. parietalis
e. scaphae
e. symphysis
e. thenaris
EMI scan
emissarium
e. condyloideum
e. mastoideum
e. occipitale
e. parietale

emissary
e. sphenoidal foramen
e. vein
emission line
EMLA
eutectic mixture of local anesthetics
EMLA anesthetic
EMLA cream
EMLA Topical
EMMA
eye-movement measuring apparatus
Emmet
E. operation
E. suture technique
Emmon osteotomy
emphysema
colonoscopy-related e.
ectatic e.
endoscopy-related e.
nonbullous e.
subcutaneous e.
subgaleal e.
surgical e.
empty
e. gestational sac
e. sella
empyema
postpneumonectomy tuberculous e.
e. tube
empyemic
EMR
endoscopic mucosal resection
EMS
Emergency Medical Services
en
e. bloc
e. bloc dissection
e. bloc distal pancreatectomy
e. bloc excision
e. bloc, no-touch technique
e. bloc resection
e. face position
enalapril
enamel
e. excrescence
e. fracture
e. knot
e. membrane
e. projection
e. rod inclination
e. sac
enameloplasty

NOTES

enantiomer
enarthrodial
    e. joint
enarthrosis
encapsulation
    embryo e.
    peritoneal e.
    tumor e.
Encapsulon TFX-Medical bacterial filter
encatarrhaphy
encephalemia
encephalitis
encephalization
encephalocele
encephaloma
encephalomeningocele
encephalomyelitis
    experimental allergic e.
encephalomyelocele
encephalopathy
    traumatic progressive e.
encephaloscopy
encephalotomy
enchondral
enchondroma
    e. of bone
enchondrosarcoma
encircling
    e. cryoablation
    e. endocardial ventriculotomy
    e. explant
    e. of globe operation
    e. polyethylene tube
    e. of scleral buckle operation
encroachment
encrustation
    bile e.
encu method
encysted
    e. calculus
    e. intra-abdominal collection
end
    e. colostomy
    e. expiratory
    e. ileostomy
    e. point
    e. stoma
    e. tube
endarterectomy
    blunt eversion carotid e.
    carotid e.
    coronary e.
    e. and coronary artery bypass
      grafting
    femoral e.
    gas e.
    surgical e.

endaural
    e. incision
    e. mastoid incision
end-diastolic
    e.-d. cross-sectional area (EDA)
    e.-d. diameter (EDD)
    e.-d. left ventricular pressure
endemic fungal infection
Ender femoral fracture technique
end-exhalation
end-expiration
end-expiratory
    e.-e. intragastric pressure
    e.-e. lung volume (EELV)
    e.-e. phase
endgut
end-inhalation
end-inspiration
end-inspiratory volume
endless-loop tachycardia
end-loop
    e.-l. colostomy
    e.-l. ileocolostomy
    e.-l. ileostomy
    e.-l. stoma
endoabdominal
    e. fascia
endoalveolar crest
endoanal
    e. anastomosis
    e. mucosectomy
endoaneurysmoplasty
endoaneurysmorrhaphy
    ventricular e.
endoauscultation
Endo-Avitene
endobrachial double-lumen tube
endobrachyesophagus
endobronchial
    e. brachytherapy
    e. cancer
    e. fistula
    e. intubation
    e. intubation anesthetic technique
    e. tree
    e. tube
    e. tuberculosis
endocapsular
endocardiac
endocardial
    e. flow
    e. mapping
    e. mapping of ventricular
      tachycardia
    e. murmur
    e. resection
    e. stain

e. thickening
e. tube
endocarditic
endocarditis
endocardium
endocavitary
    e. bladder diverticulectomy
    e. pelvic lymphadenectomy (ECPL)
    e. radiation therapy
endoceliac
endocentric construction
endocervical
    e. canal
    e. curettage
    e. mucosa
    e. polyp
    e. sampling
endocervix
endochondral
    e. bone
endocolitis
endocolpitis
endocranial
endocranium
endocrine
    e. adenomatosis
    e. disorder
    e. fracture
    e. gland
    e. imaging
    e. part of pancreas
    e. screening
    e. toxicity
    e. tumor
endocrinopathy
    multiple e.
endocryopexy
endocryophotocoagulation
endocryoretinopexy
endocyst
endodermal sinus
endodiathermy
endodontia
endodontic
    e. armamentarium
    e. cavity
    e. irrigation
    e. stabilizer
    e. surgery
    e. technique
endodontics
    one-sitting e.

pedodontic e.
surgical e.
endodontist
endodontium
endodontologist
endodontology
endoesophageal tube
endofaradism
endofluoroscopic technique
endofluoroscopy
    flexible e.
    percutaneous e.
    rigid e.
endogalvanism
endogastric
endogenous
    e. algogenic agent
    e. aneurysm
    e. disease
    e. event-related potential
    e. fiber
    e. flora
    e. infection
    e. lipid pneumonia
    e. opiate receptor
    e. opioid
    e. opioid peptide
    e. pyrogen
    e. smile
    e. steroid
    e. uveitis
endoglobar
endoherniotomy
endoillumination
Endoknot suture
endolaryngeal
Endolav lavage pump
endoligature
endolith
Endoloop suture
endoluminal
    e. excision
    e. stenting
endolymph
endolymphatic
    e. duct
    e. sac
endolymphaticus
    ductus e.
endolymphic
endometria (*pl. of* endometrium)

NOTES

E

endometrial
  e. ablation
  e. adenocarcinoma
  e. atrophy
  e. biopsy
  e. cancer
  e. carcinoma
  e. cavity
  e. chemical shift imaging
  e. curettage
  e. cytology
  e. island
  e. jet washing
  e. morphology
  e. polyp
  e. receptor
  e. resection
  e. sampling
  e. shedding
  e. spiral artery
  e. thickness
  e. tuberculosis
endometrioid
endometrioma
endometriosis
endometriotic focus
endometritis
endometrium, pl. **endometria**
endometropic
endomyocardial
  e. biopsy
  e. disease
endonasal disorder
endoneural tube
endoneurial tube
endoneurolysis
end-on mattress suture
endo-osseous
endopelvic fascia
endophlebitis of retinal vein
endophotocoagulation
  argon laser e.
endophytic
endoplasmic recticulum
endoprosthetic flange
endopyelotomy
endopyeloureterotomy
  percutaneous e.
endorectal
  e. coil magnetic resonance imaging
  e. flap
  e. ileal pouch
  e. ileal pull-through
  e. ileoanal pull-through
  e. ileoanal pull-through method
  e. ileoanal pull-through procedure
  e. ileoanal pull-through technique
endoretinal

endoribonuclease
endorrhachis
endoscope-body position relationship
endoscope impaction
endoscopic
  e. anterior cruciate ligament
    reconstruction
  e. aspiration lumpectomy
  e. band ligation
  e. band ligation of varices
  e. biliary decompression
  e. biliary drainage
  e. biliary stent placement
  e. biopsy site
  e. bladder neck suspension
  e. brush cytology
  e. carpal tunnel release (ECTR)
  e. color Doppler
  e. color Doppler assessment
  e. control
  e. cystenterostomy
  e. cystgastrostomy
  e. cystoduodenostomy
  e. cystogastrostomy
  e. devolvulization
  e. electrocoagulation
  e. electrohydraulic lithotripsy
  e. esophagogastric variceal ligation
  e. ethmoidectomy
  e. examination
  e. extirpation cicatricial obliteration
  e. extraction pancreatic duct stone
  e. finding
  e. fine-needle aspiration cytology
  e. fine-needle puncture
  e. fistulotomy
  e. fulguration
  e. gastrostomy
  e. gastrostomy tube
  e. hemostasis
  e. hemostatic therapy
  e. incision
  e. India ink injection
  e. injection sclerotherapy
  e. injection therapy
  e. jejunostomy
  e. laser therapy
  e. light source
  e. management
  e. microwave
  e. microwave coagulation
  e. mucosal resection (EMR)
  e. mucosal resection method
  e. mucosal resection procedure
  e. mucosal resection technique
  e. nasobiliary catheter drainage
  e. optical urethrotomy
  e. pancreatic drainage

e. pancreatic duct sphincterotomy
e. pancreatic stenting
e. pancreatic therapy
e. papillary balloon dilation
e. papillotomy
e. papillotomy and stenting
e. photography
e. plantar fasciotomy
e. pulsed dye laser lithotripsy
e. reflectance
e. reflectance spectrophotometry
e. removal
e. retroflexion
e. retrograde biliary stenting
e. retrograde cannulation
e. retrograde cholangiopancreatography (ERCP)
e. retrograde cholecystoendoprosthesis
e. retrograde sclerotherapy
e. sessile polypectomy
e. sigmoidopexy
e. sinus surgery
e. small bowel biopsy
e. snare resection
e. sphenoidal biopsy
e. sphincterectomy
e. stent exchange
e. stigmata of hemorrhage
e. stone disintegration
e. stricturotomy
e. surveillance
e. technology
e. transesophageal fine-needle aspiration
e. transpapillary cannulation
e. transpapillary catheter of the gallbladder
e. transpapillary cyst drainage
e. treatment
e. tube
e. ultrasonographic imaging
e. ultrasound evaluation
e. variceal sclerotherapy
endoscopically
e. normal patient
endoscopic-controlled lithotripsy
endoscopist
endoscopy
advanced therapeutic e.
anal e.
biliary e.

colorectal cancer e.
e. complication
computerized electronic e.
dynamic fluorescence video e.
fiberoptic intraosseous e.
flexible fiberoptic e.
fluorescent electronic e.
gastrointestinal e.
high-altitude e.
high-magnification e.
intestinal e.
intragastric provocation under e.
intraoperative biliary e.
intraventricular e.
laser-assisted spinal e.
lumbar epidural e.
lung-imaging fluorescent e.
nasal e.
outpatient e.
pancreaticobiliary e.
pediatric e.
percutaneous e.
peripartum e.
peroral e.
postsurgical e.
primary diagnostic e.
e. procedure
e. suite
therapeutic upper e.
transesophageal e.
transnasal e.
UGI e.
ultra high-magnification e.
upper alimentary e.
upper gastrointestinal e.
video e.
endoscopy-related emphysema
endoskeleton
Endosoft reinforced cuffed tube
endosonography-guided drainage of pancreatic pseudocyst
endosonoscopy
Endospore disinfectant
endosseous
Endostat calibration pod insert
endosteal
e. implant arm
e. surface
e. vessel
endosteum
endostitis
endostoma

E

NOTES

endotenon
endothelia (*pl. of* endothelium)
endothelial
    e. barrier
    e. bleb
    e. cell basement membrane
    e. cell edema
    e. cell surface of cornea
    e. damage
    e. denudation
    e. dysfunction
    e. dystrophy of cornea
    e. injury
    e. lysis
    e. tube
endothelial-dependent relaxation
endothelin
    e. A, B receptor
    e. plasma level
endotheliochorial placenta
endothelio-endothelial placenta
endothelioma
endotheliosis
endothelium, pl. endothelia
    e. camerae anterioris bulbi
    capillary e.
    continuous e.
    corneal e.
    discontinuous e.
    fenestrated e.
    gastrointestinal e.
    e. oculi
    sinusoidal e.
    vascular e.
endothelium-dependent fibrinolysis
endothelium-mediated relaxation
endothoracic fascia
endothorax
    tension e.
endothrix infection
endotoxemia
    systemic e.
endotoxic
    e. shock
endotoxicosis
endotoxin
    bacterial e.
    e. shock
Endotrac endoscopic carpal tunnel release
endotracheal (ET)
    e. anesthesia
    e. aspirate
    e. insufflation
    e. intubation
    e. stylet
    e. suctioning
    e. tube (ETT)
    e. tube actuator/adaptor
    e. tube cuff
    e. tube placement
endotrachelitis
Endotrol
    e. endotracheal tube
    e. tracheal tube
ENDO-Tube nasal jejunal feeding tube
endoureterotomy
    cold knife e.
endourologic
endourological
    e. cold-knife incision
    e. therapy
endourology
endovaginal
    e. finding
    e. imaging
endovascular
    e. balloon occlusion
    e. graft
    e. graft insertion
    e. technique
    e. therapy
    e. treatment
endovasculitis
    hemorrhagic e.
endovenous
    e. septum
endoventricular circular patch plasty
endplate
    e. invagination
end-point
    e.-p. measurement
end-sigmoid colostomy
endstage lung
end-systolic
    e.-s. cross-sectional area
    e.-s. diameter (ESD)
    e.-s. left ventricular pressure
    e.-s. pressure-length relationship (ESPLR)
    e.-s. pressure-volume relation
    e.-s. stress-dimension relation
    e.-s. wall thickness (ESWT)
end-tidal
    e.-t. carbon dioxide
    e.-t. nitrogen concentration
end-to-end
    e.-t.-e. anastomosis
    e.-t.-e. enterostomy
    e.-t.-e. ileo-anal anastomosis without mucosal resection
    e.-t.-e. reconstruction
    e.-t.-e. reconstruction method
    e.-t.-e. reconstruction procedure
    e.-t.-e. reconstruction technique

e.-t.-e. suture
e.-t.-e. tendon repair
end-to-side
e.-t.-s. anastomosis
e.-t.-s. arteriotomy
e.-t.-s. choledochojejunostomy
e.-t.-s. reimplantation
e.-t.-s. repair
e.-t.-s. suture
e.-t.-s. vasoepididymostomy
technique
end-weave anastomosis
enema
air contrast barium e.
barium e.
contrast e.
double contrast e.
Hypaque e.
small bowel e.
energy expenditure
enervation
enflurane
e. anesthesia
engaged head
Englisch sinus
English
E. position
E. rhinoplasty
engorged
engorgement
Engstrom multigas monitor
enhanced external counterpulsation
enhancing
e. brain lesion
e. ring
Enlon injection
Enna classification
Enneking
E. classification
E. resection-arthrodesis
enoximone
ensiform
e. cartilage
e. process
ensisternum
ensu method
entangling technique
enteral
e. alimentation
e. feeding tube
enterelcosis

enteric
e. fistula
e. infection
e. plexus
enteritis
radiation e.
enteroanastomosis
enterocele sac
enterocentesis
enterocholecystostomy
enterocholecystotomy
enterocleisis
omental e.
enteroclysis tube
enterocolic fistula
enterocolostomy
enterocutaneous fistula
enterocystoplasty
Camey e.
clam e.
sigmoid e.
enteroenteral fistula
enteroenteric fistula
enteroenterostomy
Parker-Kerr e.
two-layer e.
enterogenital fistula
enterohepatic circulation
enterolith
enterolithiasis
enterolithotomy
enterolysis
enteropathy
radiation e.
enteroperitoneal abscess
enteropexy
enteroplasty
enterorenal
enterorrhagia
enterorrhaphy
enteroscopy
intraoperative e.
push e.
push-type e.
Roux-en-Y limb e.
small bone e.
small bowel e.
transgastrostomic e.
video small bowel e.
enterostomal therapy
enterostomy
double e.

E

NOTES

enterostomy *(continued)*
    end-to-end e.
    percutaneous e.
enterotomy
    antimesenteric e.
    inadvertent e.
    longitudinal e.
enterourethral fistula
enterourethrostomy
enterovaginal fistula
enterovesical fistula
enterovesicoplasty
enteroviral infection
entocranial
entocranium
entomion
Entonox
entoptoscopy
entrainment
    air e.
    e. with concealed fusion
entrapment
    catheter e.
    lateral canal e.
    peroneal nerve e.
EntriStar
    E. feeding tube
    E. polyethylene PEG tube
    E. polyurethane PEG tube
entropionize
entropy
    approximate e.
entry
    air e.
    implant e.
    e. phenomenon
    e. point
    e. site
    e. zone
    e. zone lesion
enucleate
enucleation
    eye e.
    e. of eyeball operation
    Foix e.
    leiomyoma e.
    e. method
    e. procedure
    surgical e.
    e. technique
enuresis
    diurnal e.
    nocturnal e.
envelope
    cistern of nuclear e.
    e. flap
    peritoneal e.
    soft tissue e.

environmental mycobacterial infection
environment modification
enzymatic
    e. débridement
    e. zonulolysis
enzyme induction
eosinophilic
    e. chemotactic factor of
      anaphylaxis (ECF-A)
    e. endomyocardial disease
    e. fibrohistiocytic lesion
    e. granuloma of bone
    e. granuloma of lung
epactal bones
eparterial
    e. bronchus
epaulet flap
epaxial
ependymoblastoma
ependymoma
epiaortic imaging technique
epicanthal
    e. correction
    e. fold
epicardial
    e. defibrillator patch
    e. fat pad
    e. monitoring
epicondylar avulsion fracture
epicondyle
    lateral e. of femur
    lateral e. of humerus
    medial e. of femur
    medial e. of humerus
epicondylectomy
    medial e.
epicondyli (*pl. of* epicondylus)
epicondylian
epicondylic
epicondylus, pl. **epicondyli**
    e. lateralis humeri
    e. lateralis ossis femoris
    e. medialis humeri
    e. medialis ossis femoris
epicoracoid
epicranial
    e. aponeurosis
    e. muscle
epicranium
epicranius muscle
epicystotomy
epidermal
    e. necrolysis
    e. ridges
epidermalization
epidermatoplasty
epidermic graft

epidermidization
    e. of cervix
epidermization
epidermoanal canal
epidermoidoma
    black e.
    incisural e.
    intradural e.
    prepontine white e.
epidermoid resection
epidermolysis
epididymal
    e. sperm aspiration
epididymectomy
epididymidectomy
epididymis, pl. epididymides
    caput e.
    cauda e.
    corpus e.
    e. lesion
    microsurgical extraction of sperm
      from e.
    postvasectomy change in e.
epididymisoplasty
epididymitis
epididymo-orchitis
epididymoplasty
epididymotomy
epididymovasectomy
epididymovasostomy
epidural
    e. abscess evacuation
    e. administration
    e. anesthesia (EA)
    e. anesthetic
    e. anesthetic technique
    e. block
    e. blood patch
    e. blood patch anesthetic technique
    e. cavity
    e. delivery
    e. extramedullary lesion
    e. hematoma
    e. hemorrhage
    e. infusion
    e. neural blockade
    e. opioid
    e. opioid infusion
    e. pressure waveform (EPWF)
    e. space
    e. space infection
    e. steroid injection
    e. top-up
    e. tumor evacuation
epidurography
epiduroscopic
epifascicular epineurotomy
epigastric
    e. angle
    e. fold
    e. fossa
    e. hernia
    e. incision
    e. region
    e. veins
epigastrium
epigastrius
epiglottic
    e. reconstruction
    e. vallecula
epiglottoplasty
epihyal ligament
epihyoid
epi-illumination
epikeratophakic keratoplasty
epikeratoplasty
    tectonic e.
epilans
epilation
epilepidoma
epilepsy surgery
epimorphic regeneration
epimysiotomy
epinephrine
    lidocaine with e.
    Nervocaine with e.
    Sensorcaine with e.
    e. test dose
    Xylocaine with e.
epinephrine-anesthetic mixture
epinephros
epineural
    e. repair
epineurectomy
    interfascicular e.
epineurial neurorrhaphy
epineurolysis
    volar e.
epineurotomy
    anterior e.
    epifascicular e.
    interfascicular e.
    local e.
epipapillary membrane

E

NOTES

epipharynx
epiphenomena of dissection
epiphrenic
epiphyseal
 e. bar resection
 c. closure
 e. growth plate fracture
 e. plate injury
 e. ring
 e. slip fracture
 e. tibial fracture
epiphyseal-metaphyseal osteotomy
epiphyseolysis
epiphyses (*pl. of* epiphysis)
epiphysial
 e. line
epiphysiodesis
 open bone graft e.
 screw e.
epiphysiolysis
 femoral e.
 proximal femoral e.
epiphysis, pl. epiphyses
 atavistic e.
 ball-and-socket e.
 balloon e.
 capital femoral e.
 capitular e.
 e. cerebri
 clavicular e.
 congenital stippled e.
 distal humeral e.
 femoral e.
 humeral e.
 iliac e.
 ossifying e.
 pressure e.
 ring e.
 slipped capital femoral e.
 stippled e.
 tibial e.
 traction e.
epiphyte
epiploic, pl. epiploicae
 e. appendage
 e. appendix
 e. branches
epiploon
epiplopexy
epipteric
 e. bone
epiretinal membrane
episcleral
 e. circulation
 e. explant
 e. space
 e. tissue
 e. vascular dilation

episioperineoplasty
episioperineorrhaphy
episioplasty
episiorrhaphy
episiotomy
 median e.
 mediolateral e.
 e. repair
 ruptured e.
 e. scar
epispadias
epispadias-exstrophy complex
epispinal
epistasis
epistaxis
episternal
 e. bone
episternum
epistropheus
epitarsus
epitenon suture
epithelial
 e. barrier
 e. basement membrane
 e. inlay
 e. invagination
 e. migration
epithelialization
 e. technique
epithelioplasty
epithelium
 corneal e.
 external dental e.
 external enamel e.
 germinal e.
 placoid pigmentation of e.
 proliferation of the gastric e.
 surface e.
 transitional e.
epithelization
epitrochlea
epitrochlear
epituberculous infiltration
épluchage
E point
epoophorectomy
epoöphoron
Eppendorf tube
Eppright dial osteotomy
EPS-410
 Venodyne external pneumatic
  compression System E.
epsilonaminocaproic acid
Epstein
 E. hip dislocation classification
 E. method

Epstein-Barr
  E.-B. viral infection
  E.-B. virus (EBV)
Epstein-Thomas classification
EPTFE
  expanded polytetrafluoroethylene
  E. graft
  E. vascular suture
epulofibroma
EPWF
  epidural pressure waveform
equal sagittal flap
equation
  alveolar gas e.
  Bohr e.
equator
  anatomic e.
  e. bulbi oculi
  crystalline lens e.
  eyeball e.
  geometric e.
  lens e.
equatorial plane
equilibrating operation
equilibration
  mandibular e.
  occlusal e.
equilibrium
  acid-base e.
  sedimentation e.
equinovalgus deformity
equinovarus deformity
equinus
  e. deformity
  e. position
equipment
  Acuson echocardiographic e.
  Cell Saver 4 cardiopulmonary
    bypass blood centrifuge and
    washing e.
  insertion e.
equipotential line
Equisetene suture
equivalence
  e. point
  e. relation
equivalent
  e. refracting plane
  ventilation e.
erasion
Erbakan inferior fornix operation

Erb point
ERCP
  endoscopic retrograde
    cholangiopancreatography
  ERCP cannulation
ERCP-guided biopsy
ERCP-induced splenic rupture
erect illumination
erection
  intraoperative penile e.
  penile e.
  pharmacologically induced e.
  reflex e.
  reflexogenic e.
erector
  e. muscle of spine
  e. spinae
  e. spinae muscles
erector-spinal reflex
ergolines
ergonovine provocation test
Erickson-Leider-Brown technique
Eriksson
  E. brachial block technique
  E. ligament technique
  E. reconstruction
Erlangen pull-type sphincterotomy
Erlenmeyer flask deformity
erosion
  corneal e.
  implant e.
  infraspinatus insertion e.
  limiting plate e.
  recurrent corneal e.
  tumor e.
  wedge-shaped e.
erosive inflammation
erroneous projection
eruption
  ectopic e.
  eczematous polymorphous light e.
  surgical e.
erysipelas
  surgical e.
erysipelas-like skin lesion
erysiphake
  corneal e.
  oval cup e.
  e. technique
erythema
erythroblastoma

E

NOTES

erythrocyte
    e. mass
    e. membrane
erythrocytolysis
erythrodermatous lesion
erythroid colony formation
erythrokeratolysis hiemalis
erythrolysis
escalation
    dose e.
Escapini cataract operation
eschar
escharectomy
escharotomy
Eschmann endotracheal tube introducer
escoloplasty
Escort II patient monitoring system
ESD
    end-systolic diameter
ESKA-Buess esophageal tube
Esmarch tube
esmolol
    e. HCl
esodic nerve
esophageal
    e. A, B ring
    e. adenocarcinoma
    e. arteries
    e. banding technique
    e. band ligation
    e. biopsy
    e. body motor dysfunction
    e. branches of the inferior thyroid artery
    e. branches of the left gastric artery
    e. branches of the thoracic aorta
    e. branches of the vagus nerve
    e. carcinoma
    e. compression
    e. constrictions
    e. contractile ring
    e. contraction ring
    e. detector device
    e. dilatation
    e. dilation
    e. dilation treatment
    e. duplication
    e. ectopic sebaceous gland
    e. effect
    e. fistula
    e. foreign body
    e. fungal infection
    e. hernia
    e. hiatus
    e. impression
    e. infection

    e. inflammation
    e. intramural hematoma
    e. intubation
    e. Lewy body
    e. mass
    e. measurement
    e. mucosal ring
    e. muscular ring
    e. myotomy
    e. obturator airway
    e. perforation
    e. peristaltic pressure
    e. pH
    e. pH monitoring
    e. photodynamic therapy
    e. plexus
    e. resection
    e. ring
    e. rupture
    e. sling procedure
    e. sphincter relaxation
    e. stethoscope
    e. transection
    e. tube
    e. tumor
    e. ulceration
    e. variceal bleeding
    e. variceal sclerotherapy
    e. veins
    e. web
esophagectasis
esophagectomy
    distal e.
    Ivor Lewis two-stage subtotal e.
    subtotal e.
    transhiatal blunt e.
    transthoracic e.
    e. with thoracotomy
esophagi (*pl. of* esophagus)
esophagitis
esophagobronchial fistula
esophagocardioplasty
esophagocolic anastomosis
esophagocutaneous fistula
esophagoduodenostomy
esophagoenterostomy
esophagogastrectomy
    Ivor Lewis e.
    thoracoabdominal e.
esophagogastric
    e. fat pad
    e. intubation
    e. junction
    e. orifice
    e. resection
    e. variceal bleeding
    e. vestibule

esophagogastroanastomosis
esophagogastroduodenoscopy (EGD)
    pediatric e.
esophagogastromyotomy
esophagogastroplasty
    Grondahl-Finney e.
esophagogastroscopy
    Abbott e.
    Clagett Barrett e.
    intrathoracic e.
    Johnson e.
    Thal e.
    Woodward e.
esophagogastrostomy
    Abbott e.
    Clagett Barrett e.
    intrathoracic e.
    Johnson e.
    Thal e.
    Woodward e.
esophagojejunostomy
    loop e.
    Roux-en-Y e.
esophagomediastinal fistula
esophagomyotomy
    Heller e.
esophagoplasty
    Belsey e.
    colic patch e.
    Grondahl e.
esophagoplication
esophagoproximal gastrectomy
esophagopulmonary fistula
esophagorespiratory fistula
esophago-Roux-en-Y-jejunostomy
esophagoscopy
    fiberoptic e.
    Lugol dye e.
    video e.
esophagostomy
    cervical e.
    palliative e.
esophagotomy
esophagotracheal fistula
esophagus, pl. **esophagi**
    A ring of e.
    Barrett e.
    B ring of e.
    brusque dilatation of e.
    dilation of e.
    elevator e.
    pneumatic bag dilation of e.

    e. temperature
    Torek resection of thoracic e.
    variceal sclerotherapy in e.
esotropia
ESPLR
    end-systolic pressure-length relationship
essential brown induration of lung
Esser
    E. graft
    E. inlay operation
Essex-Lopresti
    E.-L. axial fixation technique
    E.-L. calcaneal fracture
      classification
    E.-L. calcaneal fracture technique
    E.-L. joint depression fracture
    E.-L. open reduction
established cell line
esterase-metabolized opioid
Estersohn osteotomy
Estes
    E. operation
    E. procedure
esthetic
    e. restoration
    e. rhinoplasty
    e. septorhinoplasty
    e. surgery
esthetics
    gingival tissue e.
estimated
    e. Fick method
    e. time of ovulation (ETO)
Estlander
    E. flap
    E. operation
Estlander-Abbé flap
estradiol transderm patch
estrogen-assisted colposcopy
estrogen receptor localization
ESWL
    electrohydraulic shock wave lithotripsy
ESWT
    end-systolic wall thickness
ET
    endotracheal
      ET tube
etamsylate
Etch-Master electrolyte solution
Ethamolin injection
ethamsylate

E

NOTES

ethanol
    e. ablation
    e. injection
    e. injection therapy
ethanol-induced tumor necrosis
ether
    anesthetic e.
    e. convulsion
    diethyl e.
    divinyl e.
    ethyl e.
    methyl-*tert*-butyl e. (MTBE)
    solvent e.
    sulfuric e.
    vinyl e.
    xylostyptic e.
etherization
Ethibond polyester suture
Ethicon
    E. micropoint suture
    E. Sabreloc suture
    E. silk suture
Ethicon-Atraloc suture
Ethiflex retention suture
Ethilon nylon suture
ethinamate
ethinyl
    e. trichloride
Ethi-pack suture
ethmocranial
ethmofrontal
ethmoid
    e. bone
    e. canal
    e. exenteration
    e. fistula
    e. infundibulum
    e. registration point
    e. sinus carcinoma
ethmoidal
    e. crest
    e. crest of maxilla
    e. crest of palatine bone
    e. foramen
    e. groove
    e. infundibulum
    e. labyrinth
    e. lacrimal fistula
    e. notch
    e. osteotomy
    e. veins
ethmoidale
ethmoidectomy
    anterior e.
    endoscopic e.
    external e.
    internal e.
    intranasal e.

    partial e.
    total e.
    transantral e.
ethmoidomaxillary suture
ethmolacrimal
ethmomaxillary
ethmonasal
ethmopalatal
ethmosphenoid
ethmoturbinals
ethmovomerine
ethoxazene hydrochloride
ethoxysclerol
Ethrane
ethyl
    e. chloride
    e. chloride and
        dichlorotetrafluoroethane
    e. ether
    c. oxide
ethylene
    e. oxide sterilization
etidocaine
    e. hydrochloride
ETO
    estimated time of ovulation
    ETO sterilization
etomidate
    e. injection
etorphine
ETT
    endotracheal tube
eucaine
eucupine
eugnathic anomaly
euplastic
euprocin hydrochloride
Euro-Collins solution
European Carotid Surgery Trial (ECST)
euryon
eustachian
    e. tube
    e. tube orifice
eutectic mixture of local anesthetics (EMLA)
euthyroid sick syndrome
euthyscopy
evacuation
    CT-guided stereotactic e.
    digital rectal e.
    dilatation and e. (D&E)
    dilation and e. (D&E)
    e. disorder
    epidural abscess e.
    epidural tumor e.
    fimbrial e.
    fluid e.

hematobilia e.
hematoma e.
nail bed hematoma e.
e. procedure
e. proctography
rectal e.
stool e.
transsphenoidal e.
e. of uterine contents
evacuator tubing
evagination
optic e.
evaluation
acute physiologic assessment and
  chronic health e.
acute physiology and chronic
  health e.
anthropometric e.
audiological e.
baseline capacity e.
buccal smear for sex chromatin e.
diagnostic imaging e.
Doppler pulse e.
Dubowitz e.
endoscopic ultrasound e.
follow-up e.
functional capacity e.
genitourinary e.
hearing aid e.
hormonal e.
infertility e.
job capacity e.
manometric e.
medical care e.
mental status e.
metabolic e.
neurodiagnostic e.
neurologic e.
noninvasive e.
pedicle e.
physical capacity e.
preoperative e.
presurgical medical e.
pretransplant e.
pretreatment e.
quantitative e.
quantity not sufficient for e.
real-time acquisition and velocity e.
roentgenographic e.
sexual e.
Smith physical capacities e.
static e.

status e.
stent e.
urological e.
uterine e.
videourodynamic e.
visual function e.
wake-up e.
Wright-Giemsa e.
Evans
E. ankle reconstruction technique
E. anterior calcaneal osteotomy
E. blue dye
E. intertrochanteric fracture
  classification
E. procedure
E. reconstruction
Evans-Steptoe procedure
Eve method
even-echo rephasing
event
intra-anesthetic e.
soft e.
eventration
diaphragm e.
e. of the diaphragm
diaphragmatic e.
Everard Williams procedure
Eversbusch operation
eversion
e. operation
e. orchiopexy
e. osteotomy
eversion-external rotation deformity
evert
everting mattress suture
evidement
eviration
evisceration
e. of eyeball
e. operation
Ruedemann e.
total abdominal e.
evisceroneurotomy
EVM grading of Glasgow Coma Scale
evoked
e. external urethral sphincter
  potential monitoring
e. potential technique
e. twitch
evolution
lesion e.
evulsion

NOTES

215

Ewald
 E. capitellocondylar total elbow arthroplasty
 E. tube
Ewald-Walker kinematic knee arthroplasty
Ewing
 extraosseous E.
 E. operation
ex
 e. amblyopia
 e. situ
 e. situ in vivo procedure
 e. vacuo dilatation
 e. vivo
 e. vivo cannulation
 e. vivo fertilization
 e. vivo gene therapy
 e. vivo marrow treatment
 e. vivo perfusion
 e. vivo technique
exacerbated
exacerbation
 e. of pain
Exact skin product
exaggerated
 e. sniffing position
examination
 abdominal e.
 arthroscopic e.
 Ballard e.
 barium e.
 BB to MM e.
 belly button to medial malleolus e.
 bench e.
 bile fluid e.
 bimanual pelvic e.
 bone marrow e.
 cardiac e.
 chest e.
 clinical e.
 comparative radiographic e.
 cytologic e.
 cytology e.
 dark-field e.
 digital rectal e.
 double-contrast barium enema e.
 Dubowitz e.
 duodenal contents e.
 endoscopic e.
 e. of eye
 eye e.
 flashlight e.
 follow-up e.
 full-body cutaneous e.
 full-spine radiographic e.
 funduscopic e.
 gastric residue e.

 gray scale e.
 immunofluorescent e.
 KOH e.
 limited e.
 mediastinoscopic e.
 mental status e.
 motor e.
 neonate e.
 neurologic e.
 neurological nerve conduction velocity e.
 neuro-ophthalmologic e.
 neurotologic e.
 newborn e.
 ophthalmic e.
 oral peripheral e.
 palpatory e.
 parasternal e.
 pelvic e.
 pericardial fluid e.
 peritoneal fluid e.
 physical e.
 pleural fluid e.
 postmortem e.
 proctoscopic e.
 radiological e.
 rectal e.
 rectovaginal e.
 reflex e.
 retinal e.
 self-breast e.
 sensory e.
 serologic e.
 small bowel follow-through e.
 speculum e.
 sterile vaginal e.
 suboptimal e.
 supraclavicular e.
 suprasternal e.
 synovial fluid e.
 tangent screen e.
 thermographic e.
 vaginal e.
 Wood light e.
examnialis
 graviditas e.
exam under anesthesia
exanthemas
exanthematous
 e. disease
 e. fever
 e. inflammation
exanthesis
 e. arthrosia
excavatio
 e. disci
 e. papillae nervi optici
 e. rectouterina

e. rectovesicalis
e. vesicouterina
excavation
atrophic e.
glaucomatous e.
e. of optic disk
physiologic e.
retinal e.
excavatum
pectus e.
Excedrin IB
Excell polishing point
excementosis, pl. excementoses
extension e.
intraepithelial e.
pronglike e.
ultraterminal e.
excess
e. androgen
mandibular e.
marginal e.
maxillary e.
e. mucus
vertical maxillary e.
excessive
e. bleeding
e. blood loss
e. callus formation
e. fatigue
e. heat production
e. lacrimation
e. lip support
e. spacing
e. straining
e. tearing
e. weight loss
exchange
air e.
air-fluid e.
blood-gas e.
body-fluid e.
catheter e.
cation e.
chemical e.
e. diffusion
endoscopic stent e.
fetal-maternal e.
fluid-gas e.
gas e.
gas-fluid e.
lens e.
multiple inert gas e.

plasma e.
pulmonary-gas e.
respiratory e.
e. technique
e. transfusion
wire-guided balloon-assisted
   endoscopic biliary stent e.
exchangeable mass
exchanger
airway heat and moisture e.
cation e.
countercurrent heat e.
heat and moisture e. (HME)
HumidFilter heat and moisture e.
hygroscopic heat and moisture e.
moisture e.
Portex ThermoVent heat and
   moisture e.
ThermoVent heat and moisture e.
thymocyte NA+/H+ e.
excimer
e. laser coronary angioplasty
e. laser photorefractive keratectomy
e. vascular recanalization
excipient
excise
excision
abdominoperineal e.
alar wedge e.
Arlt-Jaesche e.
e. arthroplasty
Bartlett nail fold e.
bone cyst e.
Bose nail fold e.
C2-C3 cervical disk e.
cervical disk e.
clavicle e.
cold snare e.
conjunctiva-Müller muscle e.
Curtin plantar fibromatosis e.
Dahlman diverticulum e.
Das Gupta scapular e.
disk e.
distal clavicular e.
en bloc e.
endoluminal e.
extratemporal e.
Ferciot e.
Ferciot-Thomson e.
Flatt e.
funicular e.
fusiform e.

NOTES

excision *(continued)*
    hemivertebral e.
    interdental e.
    e. of intervertebral disk
    intralesional e.
    e. of lacrimal gland operation
    e. of lacrimal sac operation
    large loop e.
    laser hemorrhoid e.
    local e.
    marginal e.
    McKeever-Buck fragment e.
    meniscal e.
    mesorectal e.
    microlumbar disk e.
    pentagonal block e.
    radical compartmental e.
    retropulsed bone e.
    ruptured disk e.
    Stewart distal clavicular e.
    Thompson e.
    total mesorectal e. (TME)
    transanal e.
    ulnar head e.
    wedge e.
    wide local e.
    William microlumbar disk e.
excisional
    e. arthrodesis
    e. biopsy
    e. biopsy method
    e. biopsy procedure
    e. biopsy technique
    e. cardiac surgery
    e. removal
excision-curettage technique
excitability test
excitatory
    e. junction potential
    e. postsynaptic potential
    e. synapse
excited
    e. skin syndrome
    e. state
excitement phase
exciting eye
excitoreflex nerve
excitor nerve
exclave
exclusion
    Devine e.
    hepatic vascular e. (HVE)
    e. of pupil
    subtotal gastric e.
    vascular e.
excoriate
excoriated

excoriation
    neurotic e.
excrement
excrementitious
excrescence
    bony e.
    enamel e.
    Lambl e.'s
    wart-like e.
excreta
excrete
excretion
excretory
    e. duct of seminal vesicle
excursion
    e. of the diaphragm
    dome e.
    insertional e.
    lateral e.
    protrusive e.
    range of e.
    respiratory e.
    retrusive e.
    tendon e.
excystation
execute
execution
    e. time
executive
Exelderm topical
exemia
exencephalia
exencephalic
exencephalocele
exencephalous
exencephaly
exenteration
    anterior pelvic e.
    ethmoid e.
    Iliff e.
    orbital e.
    e. of orbital contents operation
    pelvic e.
    petrous pyramid e.
    posterior pelvic e.
    pyelonephritis in e.
    stress reaction in e.
    supralevator pelvic e.
    total pelvic e.
exenteratio orbitae
exercise
    e. capacity
    e. hyperemia blood flow
    e. imaging
    e. index
    e. ischemia
    e. physiology
    e. study

exercise-associated acute renal failure
exercise-induced
    e.-i. arrhythmia
    e.-i. asthma
    e.-i. bronchospasm
    e.-i. incontinence
    e.-i. silent myocardial ischemia
    e.-i. ventricular tachycardia
exeresis
    palliative e.
exergonic reaction
exertion
    dyspnea on e.
    perceived e.
    rated perceived e.
    rating of perceived e.
exertional
    e. amblyopia
    e. anterior compartment syndrome
    e. compartment syndrome
    e. deep posterior compartment
      syndrome
    e. dyspnea
    e. rhabdomyolysis
Exeter bone lavage
exfoliant
exfoliate
exfoliated
exfoliation
    lamellar e.
    e. of lens
    e. of lens capsule
    e. syndrome
    true e.
exfoliative
    e. cytology
exhalation
exhaustion
    e. atrophy
    nervous e.
    ovarian follicle e.
    postactivation e.
    e. state
exhilarant
exine
Exirel
existential pain
exit
    e. access
    e. block
    e. block murmur
    e. point

    e. pupil
    e. site
    e. site infection
    e. wound
Exna
Exner plexus
exocardia
exocardial murmur
exoccipital bone
exocelomic
    e. cavity
    e. membrane
exocentric construction
exocervix
exocranial orifice
exocrine
    e. insufficiency
    e. pancreatic insufficiency
    e. part of pancreas
exocrinopathic process
exodic nerve
exodontia
exodontics
exodontist
exodontology
exogamy
exogenous
    e. aneurysm
    e. anticoagulant coagulation
    e. disease
    e. fiber
    e. fibrin clot
    e. flora
    e. IGF-1
    e. infection
    e. PGE2
    e. reconstruction
    e. smile
    e. substance
exognathia
exognathion
exophoria
exophoric
exophthalmic
exophthalmica
    cachexia e.
    tachycardia traumosa e.
exophthalmogenic
exophthalmometric
exophthalmometry
exophthalmos
    e. due to pressure

E

NOTES

exophthalmos *(continued)*
    e. due to tower skull
    recurrent e.
exophthalmos-producing
    e.-p. substance
exophthalmus
exophytic
    e. growth
    e. gut mass
    e. joint disease
exoplant
    scleral e.
exopneumopexy
Exorcist technique
exoserosis
exoskeletal
exoskeleton
exosmosis
Exo-static
exostectomy
exostosectomy
exostosis, pl. exostoses
    hereditary multiple exostoses
    multiple exostoses
Exosurf
exothermic
exotropia
exotropic
expandable
expanded
    e. plasma
    e. polytetrafluoroethylene (EPTFE)
    e. polytetrafluoroethylene vascular
      graft
expanding
    e. retroperitoneal hematoma
expansible
expansile
    e. abdominal mass
    e. unilocular well-demarcated bone
      lesion
expansion
    e. and activator therapy
    e. of the arch
    clonal e.
    controlled e.
    delayed e.
    dental arch e.
    effective setting e.
    field e.
    hygroscopic e.
    infarct e.
    intravascular volume e.
    investment e.
    lateral extensor e.
    linear thermal e.
    maxillary e.
    medial extensor e.

    mercuroscopic e.
    mesangial matrix e.
    palatal e.
    perceptual e.
    plasma volume e.
    rapid maxillary e.
    repeated tissue e.
    secondary e.
    setting e.
    slow maxillary e.
    stent e.
    thermal coefficient e.
    tissue e.
    volume e.
    wax e.
expansive
    e. laminaplasty
expectancy
    life e.
expectant management
expectation
expectorate
expectoration
    prune-juice e.
Expedited Recovery Program
expenditure
    caloric e.
    energy e.
    resting energy e.
experimental
    e. allergic encephalomyelitis
    e. disorder
    e. method
    e. neurasthenia
    e. pain
    e. pathology
    e. threshold
    e. treatment
expiration
    duration of e.
    prolongation of e.
expiratory
    e. computed tomography
    e. dyspnea
    end e.
    e. flow rate
    e. grunt
    e. murmur
    e. positive airway pressure
    e. prolongation
    e. reserve volume
    e. residual volume
    e. retard
    e. rhonchi
    e. trapping of air
    e. valve
    e. wheezing
expired air collection

explanation
explant
    encircling e.
    episcleral e.
    Molteno episcleral e.
    posterior e.
    segmental e.
    silicone sponge e.
    sponge e.
explantation
explanted heart
explicit memory
explode
exploration
    common bile duct e.
    complete surgical e.
    contralateral groin e.
    e. and débridement
    groin e.
    laparoscopically guided
      transcystic e.
    laparoscopic transcystic common
      bile duct e. (LTCBDE)
    petrous pyramid air cell e.
    sclerotomy with e.
exploratory
    e. celiotomy
    e. drive
    e. insight-oriented
    e. laparotomy
    e. stroke
exploring
explosimeter
explosion
    colonic e.
    e. fracture
    e. injury
explosion-proof
explosive doubling time
exponential phase
expose
exposed
    e. pulp
exposure
    Abbott-Gill epiphyseal plate e.
    accidental pulp e.
    aerosolized pollutant e.
    allergen e.
    anesthetic gas e.
    anterior surgical e.
    bone e.
    bony e.

    carious pulp e.
    chemical e.
    cold e.
    cue e.
    DES e.
    double e.
    electromagnetic radiation e.
    extradural e.
    extrapharyngeal e.
    fast film e.
    graded e.
    half-and-half e.
    heat e.
    Henry posterior interosseous
      nerve e.
    imaginal e.
    incident e.
    industrial e.
    e. keratopathy
    Kocher-Langenbeck e.
    light e.
    limitation of e.
    log relative e.
    magnetic radiation e.
    maternal mercury e.
    mechanical pulp e.
    methamphetamine e.
    middle fossa e.
    midline e.
    noise e.
    occupational toxin e.
    operator e.
    prenatal diethylstilbestrol e.
    prior drug e.
    radiation e.
    repeated e.
    subperiosteal e.
    sun e.
    surgical pulp e.
    thoracolumbar junction surgical e.
    thoracolumbar spine anterior e.
    toxin e.
    transperitoneal e.
    upper cervical spine anterior e.
    in utero e.
    vertebral e.
    vinyl chloride e.
express
expressed
    e. skull fracture
expression
    facial e.

NOTES

E

expressive
    e. dysphasia
expressivity
expressor loop
expulsion
    graft e.
expulsive
    e. coughing
    e. hemorrhage
    e. pain
exquisite
    e. pain
exquisitely tender abdomen
exsanguinate
exsanguinated
exsanguinating hemorrhage
exsanguination
    fetal e.
    e. protocol
    c. tourniquct control
    e. transfusion
exsanguine
exsanguinotransfusion
exsect
exsection
Exsel
EXS femoropopliteal bypass graft
exsiccant
exsiccate
exsiccation
    e. fever
exstrophy
    e. of bladder
    e. closure
exstrophy-epispadias complex
extended
    e. field irradiation therapy
    e. iliofemoral approach
    e. jargon paraphasia
    e. left subcostal incision
    e. maxillotomy
    e. obturator node and iliopsoas
      node dissection
    e. pelvic lymphadenectomy
    e. pyelotomy
    e. radical mastectomy
    e. resection
    e. Ross procedure
    e. shoulder flap
    e. subfrontal approach
extending
Extendryl
extensibility
    penile e.
extensible
extensile approach
extension
    angle of greatest e.

atlanto-occipital e.
attached gingiva e.
e. base
e. block splinting method
e. bridge
caliceal e.
cervical rotation in e.
compression e.
cranial e.
e. deformity
distractive e.
e. excementosis
external rotation in e.
extranodal tumor e.
extrascleral e.
femoral-trunk e.
e. fiber
finger-like e.'s
flexion and e.
flexion, abduction, external
  rotation, e.
e. form
full e.
groove e.
hip e.
infarct e.
e. injury
e. injury posterior atlantoaxial
  arthrodesis
e. instability
internal rotation in e.
intrasellar e.
knee e.
local tumor e.
lumbar e.
e. malposition
orbital e.
e. osteotomy
paraplegia in e.
e. for prevention
radiolucent operating room table e.
e. restriction
ridge e.
e. ridge
subependymal e.
e. teardrop fracture
thrombus e.
e. tube
extension-type cervical spine injury
extensive
    e. bilateral pneumonia
    e. posterior decompression
extensive-stage disease
extensometer
extensor
    e. carpi radialis brevis (ECRB)
    e. carpi radialis brevis muscle
    e. carpi radialis brevis tendon

e. carpi radialis longus (ECRL)
e. carpi radialis longus muscle
e. carpi radialis longus tendon
e. carpi ulnaris (ECU)
e. carpi ulnaris muscle
e. carpi ulnaris tendon
e. comminicus muscle
e. digiti minimi
e. digiti minimi muscle
e. digiti minimi tendon
e. digiti quinti
e. digiti quinti muscle
e. digiti quinti tendon
e. digitorum
e. digitorum brevis
e. digitorum brevis muscle
e. digitorum brevis tendon
e. digitorum communis
e. digitorum communis muscle
e. digitorum communis tendon
e. digitorum longus
e. digitorum longus muscle
e. digitorum longus tendon
e. hallucis
e. hallucis brevis muscle
e. hallucis longus
e. hallucis longus muscle
e. hallucis longus strength
e. hallucis longus tendon
e. hood mechanism
e. indicis
e. indicis proprius
e. indicis proprius muscle
e. indicis proprius musculus
e. indicis proprius tendon
knee e.
e. lengthening
long e.
e. mechanism dysfunction
e. pollicis brevis
e. pollicis brevis muscle
e. pollicis brevis tendon
e. pollicis longus
e. pollicis longus muscle
e. pollicis longus tendon
e. quinti tendon
radial wrist e.
e. retinaculum
e. surface
e. tendon injury
e. tendon repair
e. tenodesis

e. tenotomy
e. tensor pollicis brevis
e. tetanus
e. thrust reflex
toe e.
wrist e.'s
extensus
hallux e.
Extenzyme
exteriorization
e. colostomy
exteriorize
exteriorized
e. stuttering
e. uterine repair
externae
fibrae arcuatae e.
external
e. absorption
c. acoustic foramen
e. anal sphincter
e. anal sphincter muscle
e. arcuate fiber
e. auditory canal
e. auditory larynx
e. auditory meatus
e. axis of eye
e. base of skull
e. beam irradiation
e. beam radiation therapy
e. bevel incision
e. biliary fistula
e. biliary lavage
c. bracing
e. branch of accessory nerve
e. branch of superior laryngeal nerve
e. canthotomy
e. canthus
e. capsule
e. cardiac massage
e. carotid
e. carotid artery (ECA)
e. carotid plexus
e. cooling
e. cuneate nucleus
e. dental epithelium
e. ear
e. elastic lamina
e. elastic strap
e. enamel epithelium
e. ethmoidectomy

NOTES

external *(continued)*
e. female genital organs
e. fetal monitoring
e. fistula
e. fixator frame
e. geniculate body
e. genitalia
e. genitalia/Bartholin, urethral, and Skene glands (EG/BUS)
e. grid
e. hemipelvectomy
e. hemorrhage
e. hemorrhoid
e. hordeolum
e. iliac artery
e. iliac lymph nodes
e. iliac plexus
e. ilium
e. ilium movement
c. inguinal ring
e. intercostal membrane
e. intercostal muscle
e. intercostal muscles
e. jugular vein
e. ligament
e. ligament of mandibular articulation
e. ligament of temporomandibular articulation
e. limiting membrane
e. lock suture
e. male genital organs
e. mammary artery
e. maxillary artery
e. maxillary plexus
e. nasal nerve
e. nose
e. oblique
e. oblique aponeurosis
e. oblique fascia
e. oblique line
e. oblique muscle
e. oblique reflex
e. oblique ridge
e. obturator muscle
e. occipital crest
e. occipital protuberance
e. opening of urethra
e. orbital fracture
e. orthovoltage irradiation
e. os
e. os of uterus
e. pin fixation
e. pneumatic calf compression
posteroinferior e.
e. pterygoid muscle
e. pudendal arteries
e. pudendal veins

e. rectal sphincter
e. respiration
e. rotation
e. rotation-abduction stress test
e. rotation in extension
e. rotation-recurvatum test
e. rotator
e. route
e. saphenous nerve
e. scanning
e. shock wave lithotripsy
e. spermatic artery
e. spermatic fascia
e. spermatic nerve
e. spermatic vein
e. sphincter muscle of anus
e. sphincterotomy
e. spinal fixation
e. stimulus
e. support
e. surface
e. surface of frontal bone
e. surface of parietal bone
e. swelling
e. trauma
e. urethral orifice
e. urethral sphincter
e. urethrotomy
e. vacuum therapy
e. ventricular drainage
e. x-ray therapy
external-coil electrical stimulation
external/internal
e. rotation
e. rotation ratio
externalization
externally
e. releasable knot
e. rotated
externum
corpus geniculatum e.
hordeolum e.
os tibiale e.
pericardium e.
externus
axis bulbi e.
obturator e.
plexus maxillaris e.
extinction
c. phenomenon
sensory e.
visual e.
extinguish
extinguishing
extirpate
extirpated
extirpation
Amreich vaginal e.

dental pulp e.
nodal e.
pulp e.
Rubbrecht e.
surgical e.
extorsion
extortor
extra
e. octave fracture of finger
e. toe
extra-abdominal disease
extra-alveolar
extra-anatomic
e.-a. bypass
e.-a. bypass method
e.-a. bypass procedure
e.-a. bypass technique
extra-anatomical renal revascularization technique
extra-arachnoid
e.-a. injection
extra-articular
e.-a. ankylosis
e.-a. arthrodesis
e.-a. augmentation
e.-a. graft
e.-a. hip fusion
e.-a. knee ligament
e.-a. pain syndrome
e.-a. procedure
e.-a. reconstruction
e.-a. resection
e.-a. structure
e.-a. subtalar fusion
e.-a. subtalar joint
e.-a. technique
e.-a. tissue
e.-a. tuberculosis
extra-axial
e.-a. compartment
e.-a. fluid collection
extrabuccal
extrabursal approach
extracaliceal
extracanthic
extracapillary crescent formation
extracapsular
e. ankylosis
e. aphakia
e. arterial ring
e. cataract extraction (ECCE)
e. cataract extraction operation

e. disease
e. dissection
e. extraction
e. extraction of cataract
e. fracture
e. ligaments
e. metastasis
e. tissue
extracardiac
e. mass
e. murmur
extracellular
e. compartment
e. fluid
e. fluid volume (ECFV)
e. granule
e. ground substance
e. matrix
e. matrix remodeling
e. plasma
e. space
e. toxin
extracellular-like, calcium-free solution (ECS)
extracerebral
e. fluid collection
extrachorial placenta
extrachromic suture
extrachromosomal
extraciliary fiber
extracolonic
extraconal fat reticulum
extracoronal
e. retention
e. splinting
extracoronary
extracorporeal
e. cardiopulmonary circuit
e. circulation (ECC)
e. CO_2 removal (ECOR)
e. dialysis
e. exchange hypothermia
e. heart
e. irradiation
e. life support (ECLS)
e. liver perfusion
e. membrane oxygenation (ECMO)
e. membrane oxygenator
e. method
e. partial nephrectomy
e. piezoelectric shock wave lithotripsy

E

NOTES

extracorporeal *(continued)*
    e. procedure
    e. pump
    e. pump oxygenator
    e. renal preservation
    e. repair
    e. surgery
    e. technique
    e. ultrafiltration
    e. venous bypass
extracranial
    e. carotid artery disease
    e. carotid circulation
    e. carotid occlusive disease
    e. cerebral vasculature
    e. mass lesion
    e. occlusive vascular disease
    e. vasculature
extracraniale
    ganglion e.
extracranial-intracranial
    e.-i. bypass
    e.-i. bypass surgery
extract
    adipose tissue e.
    adrenocortical e.
    anterior pituitary e.
    aqueous e.
    bovine dialyzable leukocyte e.
    calf lung surfactant e.
    ceanothus e.
    glycerinated e.
    lyophilized e.
    pancreatic e.
    parathyroid e.
    phenol-preserved e.
    Rauwolfia e.
    venom e.
    whole-body e.
extraction
    Arroyo cataract e.
    Arruga cataract e.
    Baker pyridine e.
    e. balloon technique
    e. bile duct stone
    breech e.
    cataract e.
    Chandler-Verhoeff lens e.
    comedo e.
    countercurrent e.
    elevator e.
    extracapsular e.
    extracapsular cataract e. (ECCE)
    e. of extracapsular cataract
    first-pass e.
    e. flap
    forceps e.
    foreign body e.

    harpoon e.
    e. of intracapsular cataract
    intracapsular cataract e.
    intraocular cataract e.
    lactate e.
    liquid e.
    magnetic e.
    Marshall-Taylor vacuum e.
    menstrual e.
    micro liquid e.
    e. pancreatic stone
    partial breech e.
    planned extracapsular cataract e.
    podalic e.
    progressive e.
    rubber-band e.
    serial e.
    solid phase e.
    solvent e.
    e. space
    spontaneous breech e.
    stone e.
    tooth e.
    total breech e.
    vacuum e.
extracystic
extradental
    e. projection
extradomain A positive
extradural
    e. abscess
    e. anesthesia
    e. anesthetic technique
    e. block
    e. clinoidectomy
    e. exposure
    e. granulation
    e. hematoma
    e. hematorrhachis
    e. hemorrhage
    e. phase
    e. space
    e. vertebral artery
extraembryonic
    e. fetal membrane
    e. mesoderm
extraepiphysial
extrafascial hysterectomy
extrafective
extragenital
extraglandular conversion
extraglomerular mesangium
extragonadal
extrahepatic
    e. bile duct
    e. bile duct cancer
    e. bile duct obstruction
    e. biliary atresia

e. biliary cystic dilation
e. biliary obstruction
e. binary obstruction
e. lesion
e. metastasis
e. portal vein
e. portal vein obstruction
e. portal venous hypertension
e. stone

extraintestinal
e. complication

extrajection
extralaryngeal approach
extraligamentous
extralobar
extraluminal
e. gas
e. hemorrhage

extralymphatic metastasis
extramammary Paget disease
extramaxillary anchorage
extramedullary
e. alignment
e. alignment arch
e. involvement
e. myelopoiesis
e. segment
e. toxicity

extramucosal mass
extramural
e. lesion
e. upper airway obstruction

extraneous
e. movement

extranodal
e. site
e. tumor extension

extraoctave fracture
extraocular
e. movements
e. muscle involvement
e. muscles
e. muscles of Tillaux

extraoral
e. anchorage
e. radiographic examination profile

extraorbital disease
extraosseous
e. Ewing

extraovular
extrapancreatic
e. nerve plexus

extrapapillary
extraperineal
extraperiosteal
extraperitoneal
e. approach
e. carbon dioxide insufflation
e. cesarean section
e. CO_2 insufflation
e. endoscopic hernia repair
e. endoscopic pelvic lymph node dissection
e. fascia
e. laparoscopic bladder neck suspension
e. laparoscopic herniorrhaphy
e. laparoscopic nephrectomy
e. tissue

extrapetrosal drainage
extrapharyngeal
c. approach
e. exposure

extraplacental
extrapleural
e. air
e. apicolysis
e. pneumothorax
e. space

extrapolate
extrapolated end-tidal carbon dioxide tension ($PETCO_2$)
extrapolation
extraprostatic
extrapsychic
extrapulmonary
e. cough
e. *Pneumocystis carinii* infection
e. site
e. tuberculosis

extrapyramidal
e. disease
e. dyskinesia
e. function assessment
e. nucleus
e. pathway
e. reaction
e. syndrome
e. tract

extrarectus
extrarenal
e. mass
e. renal pelvis

extraretinal

E

NOTES

extrasaccular hernia
extrascleral
  e. extension
extrasensory
extraskeletal
extrasphincteric anal fistula
extrastimulus test
extratemporal excision
extratesticular
  e. lesion
extrathoracic
  e. metastasis
  e. tuberculosis
extratracheal
extrauterine
  e. pelvic mass
extravaginal
  e. testicular torsion
extravasate
extravasated
extravasation
  e. extremity
  e. extrusion
  e. feces
  e. gas
  e. injury
  e. irrigation solution
  e. phenomenon
extravascular
  e. compartment
  e. granulomatous feature
  e. lung water
  e. mass
  e. space
extraventricular
extraversion
  urinary e.
extravesical
  e. anastomosis
  e. infrasphincteric ectopic ureter
  e. ureteral reimplantation technique
  e. ureterolysis
extrema
  capsula e.
extreme
  e. capsule
  e. hearing loss
  e. lateral transcondylar approach
  e. somatosensory evoked potential
extremital
extremitas
  e. acromialis claviculae
  e. anterior
  e. inferior
  e. inferior renis
  e. inferior testis
  e. posterior
  e. sternalis claviculae

  e. superior
  e. superior renis
  e. superior testis
  e. tubaria ovarii
  e. uterina ovarii
extremity
  e. abnormality
  acromial e. of clavicle
  e. amputation
  anterior e.
  elevation of e.
  extravasation e.
  flaccid e.
  e. ischemia
  left lower e.
  left upper e.
  lower e.
  e. malformation
  e. mobilization technique
  e. preservation
  right lower e.
  right upper e.
  sternal e. of clavicle
  upper e.
extrinsic
  e. allergic alveolitis
  e. asthma
  e. bladder compression
  e. entrapment test
  e. environmental staining
  e. esophageal impression
  e. mass
  e. mechanism
  e. muscles
  e. muscles of the larynx
  e. muscles of the tongue
  e. muscle strength
  e. pathway
  e. rearfoot post
  e. semiconductor
  e. sphincter
extrodactyly
extrospection
extroversion
extrude
extruded
  e. disk
  e. disk fragment
  e. teeth
extrudoclusion
extrusion
  bone graft e.
  disk e.
  extravasation e.
  implant e.
  oocyte e.
  placental e.
  sealer e.

tube e.
wire e.
extubate
extubation
    e. anesthetic technique
    postoperative e.
exuberant granulation tissue
exudate
    acute inflammatory e.
    circinate e.
    conjunctival e.
    cotton-wool e.
    fatty e.
    fibrinous e.
    fluffy cotton-wool e.
    foaming e.
    gingival e.
    hard e.
    inflammatory e.
    mucopurulent e.
    pharyngeal e.
    purulent e.
    retinal e.
    sanguineous e.
    serous e.
    soft e.
    suppurative e.
    waxy e.
exudation
    fibrinous e.
    gingival e.
    proteinaceous aqueous e.
    purulent e.
exudative
    e. ascites
    e. eye
    e. granulomatous inflammation
    e. papulosquamous disease
    e. pleural effusion
    e. retinal detachment
    e. tuberculosis
    e. vitreoretinopathy
    e. zone
exude
exulcerans
exumbilication
eye
    accommodation of e.
    appendage of e.
    closed surgery on e.
    e. enucleation
    examination of e.

e. examination
exciting e.
external axis of e.
exudative e.
e. irrigating solution
e. muscle surgery
e. patch
pineal e.
e. point
e. restored to normotensive
  pressure
e. rotation
stony-hard e.
e. tumor
tumor of interior of e.
e. tumor localization
web e.
eyeball
    e. compression reflex
    e. equator
    evisceration of e.
    luxation of e.
eyebrow
    e. fixation
    e. laceration
eye-closure reflex
eye-ear plane
eyelash
    ectopic e.
    e. reflex
eyelid
    basal cell carcinoma of e.
    capillary hemangioma of e.
    carcinoma of e.
    ecchymosis of e.
    ectropion of e.
    edema of lower e.
    fusion of e.'s
    e. fusion
    incision into e.
    inflammation of e.
    levator muscle of upper e.
    lower e.
    melanoma of e.
    e. molluscum contagiosum infcction
    plastic repair of e.
    reconstruction of e.
    squamous cell carcinoma of e.
    e. surgery
    tumor of e.
    e. tumor
    upper e.

E

NOTES

eyelid-closure reflex
Eye-Lube-A solution
eye-movement measuring apparatus (EMMA)
Eye-Sed solution
Eye-Sine solution
Eye-Stream solution
Eye Wash solution
Eyler flexorplasty

F2 focal point
FA
   fluorescent antibody
      FA technique
FAB
   French/American/British
      FAB classification
      FAB staging of carcinoma
Fabricius ship
FAC
   fractional area change
face
   cow f.
   dish f.
   f. form
   f. line
   f. mask
face-a-face venacavaplasty
face-down position
face-lift
facet
   f. anomaly
   articular f.
   f. of atlas for dens
   clavicular f.
   corneal f.
   costal f.'s
   f. dislocation
   f. excision technique
   f. fracture stabilization wiring
   f. fusion
   fusion f.
   inferior articular f. of atlas
   inferior costal f.
   f. joint injection
   f. joint preparation
   f. joints
   f. plane
   f. rhizotomy
   f. subluxation stabilization wiring
   superior articular f. of atlas
   superior costal f.
   transverse costal f.
facetectomy
   O'Donoghue f.
   partial f.
face-to-pubes position
facetted corneal scar
facial
   f. angle
   f. artery
   f. axis
   f. bones
   f. butt joint preparation
   f. canal

f. cleft
f. colliculus
f. deformity
f. excursion measurement
f. expression
f. foundation
f. fracture
f. height
f. hematoma
f. index
f. lymph nodes
f. muscles
f. nerve
f. nerve-preserving parotidectomy
f. osteosynthesis
f. plane
f. plexus
f. profile
f. reanimation
f. restoration
f. root
f. triangle
f. vein
facialis
facies
   acromial articular f. of clavicle
   f. anterior corneae
   f. anterior corporis maxillae
   f. anterior glandulae suprarenalis
   f. anterior palpebrarum
   f. anterior pancreatis
   f. anterior prostatae
   f. anterior renis
   f. anterior ulnae
   f. articularis acromialis claviculae
   f. articularis acromii
   f. articularis anterior dentis
   f. articularis capitis costae
   f. articularis cartilaginis
      arytenoideae
   f. articularis inferior atlantis
   f. articularis sternalis claviculae
   f. articularis superior atlantis
   f. articularis talaris media calcanei
   f. articularis talaris posterior
      calcanei
   f. articularis thyroidea cricoideae
   f. articularis tuberculi costae
   f. bovina
   f. colica splenis
   f. costalis
   f. costalis scapulae
   f. dorsalis scapulae
   f. externa
   f. externa ossis frontalis

F

facies *(continued)*
 f. externa ossis parietalis
 f. inferior partis petrosae ossis
  temporalis
 f. inferolateralis prostatae
 f. infratemporalis maxillae
 f. interlobares pulmonis
 f. interna
 f. interna ossis frontalis
 f. interna ossis parietalis
 f. intestinalis uteri
 f. lateralis ossis zygomatici
 f. lateralis testis
 f. maxillaris alae majoris
 f. maxillaris ossis palatini
 f. medialis ovarii
 f. medialis testis
 f. nasalis maxillae
 f. nasalis ossis palatini
 f. orbitalis
 f. posterior cartilaginis arytenoideae
 f. posterior corneae
 f. posterior glandulae suprarenalis
 f. posterior pancreatis
 f. posterior partis petrosae ossis
  temporalis
 f. posterior prostatae
 f. posterior renis
 Potter f.
 f. pulmonalis cordis
 f. renalis glandulae suprarenalis
 f. renalis lienis
 f. renalis splenis
 f. sacropelvina ossis ilii
 f. scaphoidea
 f. sternocostalis cordis
 f. symphysialis
 f. temporalis
 f. urethralis penis
 f. vesicalis uteri
 f. visceralis hepatis
 f. visceralis splenis
facilitated angioplasty
facilitating restoration
facilitation
 convergence f.
 neuromuscular f.
 postactivation f.
 posttetanic f.
 proprioceptive neuromuscular f.
  (PNF)
 Wedensky f.
facioplasty
faciotelencephalic malformation
F.A.C.S.
 Fellow of American College of Surgeons

factor
 eosinophilic chemotactic f. of
  anaphylaxis (ECF-A)
 f. replacement therapy
faculty
 fusion f.
 f. fusion
fade
 tetanic f.
Faden
 F. operation
 F. procedure
 F. suture
Fahey
 F. approach
 F. technique
Fahey-O'Brien technique
Fahraeus method
failed
 f. anesthesia
 f. back surgery syndrome
 f. femoral osteotomy
 f. intubation
 f. procedure
 f. spinal
 f. surgery
fail-safe device
failure
 anastomotic f.
 f. to awaken
 cocaine-induced respiratory f.
 differentiation f.
 dilator placement f.
 exercise-associated acute renal f.
 f. of fixation suppression
 graft f.
 Harrington rod instrumentation f.
 implant f.
 implantation f.
 instrumentation f.
 intubation f.
 irradiation f.
 multiorgan system f.
 multiple organ f. (MOF)
 multiple system organ f.
 pacemaker f.
 spinal implant load to f.
 wound f.
Fairbanks
 F. technique
 F. technique with Sever
  modification
Fairbanks-Sever procedure
falcate
falces (*pl. of* falx)
falciform
 f. cartilage
 f. crest

f. ligament of liver
f. process
Falconer lobectomy
Falk-Shukuris operation
Falk vesicovaginal fistula technique
Fallat-Buckholz method
fallopian
f. canal
f. hiatus
f. ligament
f. tube
f. tube carcinoma
f. tube mass
f. tube metastasis
Fallot
tetralogy of F.
Falope tubal sterilization ring
false
f. aneurysm
f. channel formation
f. cord carcinoma
f. knot
f. knot of umbilical cord
f. membrane
f. pelvis
f. projection
f. ribs
f. suture
f. vertebrae
f. vocal cord
falx, pl. falces
f. aponeurotica
f. inguinalis
f. laceration
familial
f. aortic ectasia syndrome
f. atypical multiple mole melanoma syndrome
f. cardiac myxoma syndrome
f. cholestasis syndrome
f. cxudative vitreoretinopathy
f. osteochondrodystrophy
f. paroxysmal rhabdomyolysis
famotidine
fan beam projection
Fanta cataract operation
far
f. lateral inferior suboccipital approach
f. point

Farabeuf
F. ischiopubiotomy
F. triangle
Faraday
F. law of electrolysis
F. law of induction
far-and-near suture
Farmer
F. operation
F. technique
Farre white line
Fasanella operation
Fasanella-Servat
F.-S. procedure
F.-S. ptosis operation
fascia, pl. fascias, fasciae
Abernethy f.
f. adherens
anal f.
antebrachial f.
f. antebrachii
f. axillaris
axillary f.
brachial f.
f. brachii
broad f.
f. buccopharyngea
buccopharyngeal f.
Buck f.
Camper f.
f. cervicalis
f. cervicalis profunda
clavipectoral f.
f. clavipectoralis
f. clitoridis
f. of clitoris
Colles f.
Cooper f.
cremasteric f.
f. cremasterica
cribriform f.
f. cribrosa
crural f.
f. cruris
Cruveilhier f.
dartos f.
deep f. of arm
deep cervical f.
deep f. of forearm
deep layer of temporalis f.
deep f. of leg
deep f. of neck

F

NOTES

fascia *(continued)*
    deep f. of penis
    deep f. of thigh
    Denonvilliers f.
    f. diaphragmatis pelvis inferior
    f. diaphragmatis pelvis superior
    f. diaphragmatis urogenitalis inferior
    f. diaphragmatis urogenitalis
      superior
    endoabdominal f.
    endopelvic f.
    endothoracic f.
    f. endothoracica
    external oblique f.
    external spermatic f.
    f. of extraocular muscles
    extraperitoneal f.
    fatty layer of superficial f.
    f. of forearm
    fusion f.
    Gerota f.
    Godman f.
    Hesselbach f.
    iliac f.
    f. iliaca
    iliopectineal f.
    inferior f. of pelvic diaphragm
    inferior f. of urogenital diaphragm
    infundibuliform f.
    intercolumnar fasciae
    internal spermatic f.
    investing f.
    investing layer of deep cervical f.
    lacrimal f.
    f. lata
    f. lata freeze-thawed graft
    f. lata sling for ptosis operation
    f. of leg
    lumbodorsal f.
    masseteric f.
    f. masseterica
    membranous layer of superficial f.
    middle cervical f.
    muscular f. of extraocular muscle
    f. muscularis musculorum bulbi
    f. nuchae
    nuchal f.
    obturator f.
    f. obturatoria
    orbital fasciae
    fasciae orbitales
    parietal pelvic f.
    parotid f.
    f. parotidea
    parotideomasseteric f.
    f. parotideomasseterica
    pectoral f.
    f. pectoralis

    pelvic f.
    f. pelvis
    f. pelvis parietalis
    f. pelvis visceralis
    f. of penis
    f. penis profunda
    f. penis superficialis
    f. perinei superficialis
    perirenal f.
    pharyngobasilar f.
    f. pharyngobasilaris
    phrenicopleural f.
    f. phrenicopleuralis
    poplitcal f.
    Porter f.
    presacral f.
    pretracheal f.
    prevertebral f.
    f. profunda
    f. prostatae
    f. of prostate
    rectovesical f.
    renal f.
    f. renalis
    retrosacral f.
    Scarpa f.
    Sibson f.
    f. spermatica externa
    f. spermatica interna
    subperitoneal f.
    f. subperitonealis
    superficial f.
    f. superficialis
    superficial f. of penis
    superficial f. of perineum
    superior f. of pelvic diaphragm
    superior f. of urogenital diaphragm
    temporal f.
    f. temporalis
    f. thoracolumbalis
    thoracolumbar f.
    Toldt f.
    f. transversalis
    transversalis f.
    Treitz f.
    triangular f.
    f. triangularis abdominis
    Tyrrell f.
    umbilical prevesical f.
    umbilicovesical f.
    visceral pelvic f.
    Zuckerkandl f.

fascial
    f. arthroplasty
    f. closure
    f. graft
    f. hernia
    f. plane

f. sheaths of extraocular muscles
f. sling approach
f. sling procedure
f. space
f. space infection
f. suture
fasciaplasty
fascias (*pl. of* fascia)
fascia-splitting incision
fascicular
f. graft
f. repair
fasciculation
benign f.
contraction f.
malignant f.
f. potential
tongue f.
fasciculus, pl. fasciculi
f. atrioventricularis
wedge-shaped f.
fasciectomy
dermal f.
limited f.
partial f.
radical palmar f.
fasciitis
fasciocutaneous free flap
fasciodesis
fasciola
fascioplasty
fasciorrhaphy
fasclotomy
decompression f.
double-incision f.
endoscopic plantar f.
Fronet f.
percutaneous plantar f.
plantar f.
prophylactic f.
Rorabeck f.
single-incision f.
Skoog f.
subcutaneous f.
Yount f.
fashion
Z f.
fast
f. exposure technique
f. film exposure

f. Fourier transformation spectrum analyzer
f. neutron radiation therapy
fast-flush test
fastigiobulbar tract
fasting
preoperative f.
Fast-Patch
fast-pathway radiofrequency ablation
fat
body f.
f. body of cheek
f. body of ischiorectal fossa
f. cell space
f. flap
f. graft
herniated preperitoneal f.
f. herniation
f. line
f. pad
f. pad of elbow
f. plane
preperitoneal f.
properitoneal f.
total body f.
fat-density line
fat-free mass
fatigue
excessive f.
f. fracture
implant f.
suture f.
fat-patch graft
fat-suppression technique
fatty
f. ascites
f. degeneration of heart
f. exudate
f. hernia
f. infiltration
f. infiltration of liver
f. layer of superficial fascia
f. prostatic tissue
f. renal capsule
fauces
faucial
f. branches of lingual nerve
faulty
f. contact point
f. restoration
Favaloro saphenous vein bypass graft
Fay suction tube

F

NOTES

235

F body
FDA
    Food and Drug Administration
        FDA Anesthesia Apparatus
          Checkout Recommendations
FDPCA
    fixed-dose patient-controlled analgesia
Feagin shoulder dislocation test
feather-edged proximal finishing line
featural surgery
feature
    clinicopathologic f.
    extravascular granulomatous f.
fecal
    f. abscess
    f. contamination
    f. diversion colostomy
    f. fistula
    f. impaction
    f. incontinence
fecalith
    appendiceal f.
fecaloma
fecaluria
feces
    extravasation f.
Federation of Gynecology and
Obstetrics classification
feedback reduction circuit
feeder-frond technique
feeding
    f. complication
    drip-tube f.
    f. gastrostomy
    gastrostomy f.
    f. gastrostomy tube
    jejunostomy elemental diet f.
    jejunostomy tube f.
    postoperative regimen for oral
      early f. (PROEF)
    tube f.
    f. tube placement
Fehling solution
Feiss line
Feist-Mankin position
Feldman buffer solution
Fellow of American College of
Surgeons (F.A.C.S.)
felodipine
felon infection
Felson
    silhouette sign of F.
felt pad
feltwork
felypressin
female
    f. castration
    f. gonad

    f. prostate
    f. urethra
    f. urethral syndrome
feminization syndrome
feminizing genitoplasty
femoral
    f. arch
    f. artery
    f. artery approach
    f. artery catheterization
    f. branch of genitofemoral nerve
    f. canal
    f. circulation
    f. cortical ring allograft
    f. diaphysis
    f. embolectomy
    f. endarterectomy
    f. epiphysiolysis
    f. epiphysis
    f. fossa
    f. head
    f. head line
    f. hernia
    f. intertrochanteric fracture
    f. metaphysis
    f. muscle
    f. neck fracture
    f. neck fracture reduction
    f. nerve
    f. nerve block
    f. nerve traction test
    f. osteotomy
    f. plexus
    f. prosthesis fixation
    f. puncture
    f. region
    f. resection
    f. ring
    f. septum
    f. shaft fracture
    f. sheath
    f. supracondylar fracture
    f. 3-in-1 technique
    f. triangle
femoral-tibial-peroneal bypass
femoral-trunk extension
femoroischial transplantation
femoropopliteal
    f. bypass
    f. bypass graft
femorotibial
femur
    f. graft
    lateral condyle of f.
    medial condyle of f.
fender fracture
fenestra, pl. **fenestrae**
    f. of the cochlea

f. cochleae
f. ovalis
f. rotunda
f. of the vestibule
f. vestibuli

fenestrated
f. endothelium
f. Fontan operation
f. membrane
f. sheath
f. tracheostomy tube
f. tube

fenestration
alveolar plate f.
f. of alveolar process
aortopulmonary f.
apical f.
atrophic f.
baffle f.
catheter-directed f.
cusp f.
cyst f.
dental f.
intercellular f.
laparoscopic f.
Lempert f.
f. operation
tracheal f.

fenoldopam

fentanyl
f. citrate
droperidol and f.
intraoperative f. (IOF)
f. lollipop
F. Oralet

fentanyl-neostigmine analgesia
Fenton vaginoplasty
FEP-ringed Gore-Tex vascular graft
Ferciot excision
Ferciot-Thomson excision
Ferguson
F. scoliosis measuring method
F. suction

Ferguson-Frazier suction tube
Ferguson-Thompson-King two-stage osteotomy
Fergus operation
Fergusson incision
Ferkel torticollis technique
fermentation
mannitol f.
mixed acid f.

Fernandez
F. extensile anterior approach
F. osteotomy
ferning technique
Ferrein
F. canal
F. cords
F. foramen
F. ligament
F. pyramid
ferromagnetic microembolization treatment
Ferry line
fertility
fertilization
f. age
ex vivo f.
in vitro f.
in vivo f.
festination
fetal
f. acoustic stimulation test
f. aspiration syndrome
f. body movement
f. bone fracture
f. cardiac anomaly
f. chest anomaly
f. circulation
f. cystic adenomatoid malformation
f. drug therapy
f. duplication
f. exsanguination
f. gastrointestinal anomaly
f. growth acceleration
f. growth retardation
f. head
f. head:abdominal circumference ratio
f. head circumference
f. head position
f. heart rate acceleration
f. hemorrhage
f. infection
f. intracranial anatomy
f. liver biopsy
f. liver transplantation
f. lymphoid tissue
f. malpresentation
f. membrane
f. reduction
f. rejection
f. scalp oxygenation

F

NOTES

fetal *(continued)*
    f. skin biopsy
    f. surgery
    f. thymus transplantation
    f. tissue sampling
    f. tissue transplant
    f. urogenital tract
    f. vascular anomaly
fetal-maternal
    f.-m. exchange
    f.-m. hemorrhage
fetation
fetomaternal hemorrhage
fetoplacental circulation
fetoscopy
fetus
    asynclitic position of f.
    f. growth elevation
    presentation of f.
    retroperitoneal f.
Feuerstein
    F. drainage tube
    F. split ventilation tube
fever
    f. caused by infection
    dehydration f.
    exanthematous f.
    exsiccation f.
    fracture f.
    inundation f.
    Mediterranean exanthematous f.
    syphilitic f.
fiber
    accelerator f.
    association f.
    bundle f.
    f. bundle
    f. bundle volume
    endogenous f.
    exogenous f.
    extension f.
    external arcuate f.
    extraciliary f.
    Gerdy f.'s
    intercolumnar f.'s
    intercrural f.'s
    Myer loop f.
    Nélaton f.'s
    oblique f.'s of stomach
    osteogenetic f.'s
    projection f.
    rod f.
    Rosenthal f.
    Sappey f.'s
    skinned muscle f.
    f. tip modification
    zonular f.'s
fiberglass graft

fiberoptic
    f. bronchoscopy
    f. bronchoscopy anesthetic
      technique
    f. bundle
    f. endoscopy anesthetic technique
    f. esophagoscopy
    f. injection sclerotherapy
    f. intraosseous endoscopy
    f. intubation
    f. intubation anesthetic technique
    f. intubation method
    f. intubation procedure
    f. panendoscopy
    f. partial pressure of carbon
      dioxide sensor
    f. PCO_2 sensor
    f. sigmoidoscopy
    f. suction tube
    f. tracheal intubation anesthetic
      technique
fiberoptics
fiberotomy
fiberscope
    superfine f.
fiber-splitting incision
fibra, pl. **fibrae**
    fibrae arcuatae externae
    fibrae intercrurales
    fibrae obliquae gastrici
    fibrae zonulares
fibrillary astrocyte
fibrillation
    atrial f.
    auricular f.
    cardiac f.
    chronic atrial f.
    continuous atrial f.
    idiopathic ventricular f.
    lone atrial f.
    paroxysmal atrial f. (PAF)
    f. potential
    f. rhythm
    synchronized f.
    f. threshold
    ventricular tachycardia/ventricular f.
fibrillation-flutter
    atrial f.-f.
fibrillogranuloma
fibrin
    f. calculus
    f. degradation product
    f. glue
    f. plate method
    postvitrectomy f.
fibrinogen
    f. degradation product
    f. method

fibrinogen-fibrin degradation product
fibrinogenolysis
fibrinoid necrotizing inflammation
fibrinolysin coagulation
fibrinolysis
    endothelium-dependent f.
    primary f.
fibrinopeptide A
fibrinopurulent inflammation
fibrinoscopy
fibrinous
    f. adhesion
    f. exudate
    f. exudation
    f. inflammation
fibroadenolipoma
    degenerated f.
fibroadenoma
    f. of breast
fibroadipose tissue
fibroangioma
fibroblastic tissue
fibroblastoma
fibrocalcification
fibrocalcific lesion
fibrocarcinoma
fibrocartilage
    basilar f.
    circumferential f.
    interarticular f.
    semilunar f.
    stratiform f.
fibrocartilago
    f. basalis
    f. interarticularis
    f. intervertebralis
fibrocaseous inflammation
fibrocementoma
fibrochondroma
fibrocystoma
fibrodentinoma
fibroelastic
    f. membrane of larynx
    f. tissue
fibroelastoma
fibroenchondroma
fibroepithelioma
fibrofascial compartment syndrome
fibrofatty breast tissue
fibrofolliculoma
fibrogliosis
fibrogranuloma

fibrohemangioma
fibrohistiocytic lesion
fibrohistiocytoma
fibroid
    f. adenoma
    f. inflammation
fibroidectomy
fibrokeratoma
fibroleiomyoma
fibrolipoma
fibroliposarcoma
fibroma
    f. pendulum
    f. sarcomatosum
fibromectomy
fibromuscular
fibromusculoelastic lesion
fibromyalgia trigger point
fibromyectomy
fibromyoma
    uterine f.
fibroneuroma
fibro-osseous
    f.-o. lesion
    f.-o. ring of Lacroix
fibroplate
fibroproliferative membrane
fibrosarcoma
fibroscopy
fibrosis
    idiopathic pulmonary f. (IPF)
    interstitial pulmonary f. (IPF)
fibrosis
fibrotic nub
fibrotomy
fibrous
    f. adhesion
    f. appendix of liver
    f. articular capsule
    f. bone lesion
    f. capsule of kidney
    f. capsule of liver
    f. capsule of parotid gland
    f. capsule of spleen
    f. capsule of thyroid gland
    f. connective tissue
    f. joint
    f. loose body
    f. obliteration
    f. polypoid lesion
    f. repair
    f. ring

NOTES

F

fibrous *(continued)*
  f. ring of heart
  f. ring of intervertebral disk
  f. scar tissue
  f. skeleton of heart
  f. tendon sheath
  f. trigones of heart
  f. tunic of corpus spongiosum
  f. union
fibula
  diastasis f.
fibular
  f. flap
  f. fracture
  f. head
  f. lymph node
  f. metaphysis
  f. ostectomy
  f. sesamoidectomy
  f. strut graft
fibularis
fibulectomy
  partial f.
fibulocalcaneal
  f. ligament
Ficat procedure
Fick
  F. cardiac output measurement
  F. oxygen extraction method
  F. oxygen method
  F. position
  F. principle
  F. technique
Ficoll-Hypaque technique
field
  f. block
  f. block anesthesia
  f. cancerization
  f. of dissection
  f. expansion
  f. of fixation
  f. method
  pulsed electromagnetic f. (PEMF)
field-echo
  f.-e. difference
  f.-e. image
  f.-e. imaging
Fielding
  F. femoral fracture classification
  F. membrane
  F. modification of Gallie technique
Fielding-Magliato classification of subtrochanteric fracture
fifth
  f. cranial nerve
  f. metatarsal base fracture
fighter fracture

FIGO
  International Federation of Gynecology
    and Obstetrics
      FIGO classification staging
figure-eight
  f.-e. preparation
  f.-e. stitch
figure-four position
figure-of-eight suture
fila (*pl. of* filum)
filament
  corneal f.
  f. suture
filar mass
Filatov
  F. flap
  F. keratoplasty
  F. operation
Filatov-Gillies
  F.-G. flap
  F.-G. tubed pedicle
Filatov-Marzinkowsky operation
Filcard vena cava filter
fil d'Arion silicone tube
filled
  decayed, extracted, and f.
filler graft
filleted graft
fillet local flap graft
filling
  bead technique f.
  brush technique f.
  f. canal
  f. first technique
  flow technique f.
  f. material condensation
  nature root canal f.
  postresection f.
  pressure technique f.
  root canal f.
film
  f. identification
  f. oxygenation
filopressure
filter
  Adams kidney stone f.
  air f.
  aluminum f.
  anesthesia circuit f.
  antimicrobial f.
  arterial line f.
  bacterial f.
  bird's nest vena cava f.
  BTF-37 arterial blood f.
  Centriflo f.
  charcoal f.
  cobalt blue f.
  collodion f.

Encapsulon TFX-Medical
bacterial f.
Filcard vena cava f.
Gianturco bird's nest f.
Gianturco-Roehm bird's nest vena
cava f.
Greenfield IVC f.
Greenfield titanium inferior vena
cava f.
Jostra arterial blood f.
Kim-Ray Greenfield antiembolus f.
Kim-Ray Greenfield vena cava f.
K-37 pediatric arterial blood f.
Mobin-Uddin umbrella f.
Mobin-Uddin vena cava f.
Nitinol inferior vena cava f.
Pall Biomedical heat- and
moisture-exchanging f.
Pall ELD-series f.
Pall ELD-96 Set Saver f.
Pall leukocyte removal f.
Pall PL-series f.
Pall RC-series f.
Pall SP 3840 arterial line f.
Pall transfusion f.
Portex bacterial f.
Simon Nitinol inferior vena
cava f.
Simon Nitinol IVC f.
Steriflex-Braun bacterial f.
f. straw
superior vena cava f.
Swank high-flow arterial blood f.
titanium Greenfield vena cava f.
vena cava f.
Vena Tech dual vena cava f.
Vena Tech-LGM vena cava f.
William Harvey arterial blood f.
filtered-back projection
filtering
f. operation
f. procedure
filtration
f. angle
gel f.
glass-wool f.
glomerular f.
rate of fluid f.
spontaneous ascites f.
f. surgery
filtration-slit membrane

filtrum
Merkel f. ventriculi
f. ventriculi
filum, pl. fila
f. durae matris spinalis
fila olfactoria
fila radicularia
f. of spinal dura mater
terminal f.
f. terminale
fimbria, pl. fimbriae
ovarian f.
f. ovarica
fimbriae tubae uterinae
fimbriae of uterine tube
fimbrial evacuation
fimbriated end of fallopian tube
fimbriectomy
fimbrioplasty
Bruhat laser f.
final
f. cementation
f. cone position
f. consonant position
finding
endoscopic f.
endovaginal f.
ultrasonic endovaginal f.
fine
f. chromic suture
f. manipulation
f. silk suture
fine-needle
f.-n. aspiration (FNA)
f.-n. aspiration biopsy
f.-n. aspiration cytology
finger
cloven hoof fracture of f.
f. deformity
f. dilation
extra octave fracture of f.
f. flap
f. fracture
f. fracture dissection
f. fracture technique
f. indicator
f. joint arthroplasty
F. Oscillation Test
ring f.
f. web
finger-like extensions
fingernail

NOTES

fingerprint line
fingertip
    f. amputation
    f. lesion
fingertrap
    f. suspension
    f. suture
finish line
Fink
    F. operation
    F. valve
Finkelstein maneuver
Finney
    F. gastroenterostomy
    F. operation
    F. pyloroplasty
    F. stricturoplasty
Finochietto-Billroth I gastrectomy
  technique
Finsterer
    F. myringotomy split tube
    F. suction tube
Fired-Hendel procedure
firm lesion
first
    f. arch syndrome
    f. carpometacarpal joint fracture
    f. cone position
    f. cranial nerve
    f. cuneiform bone
    f. degree burn
    f. degree radiation injury
    f. duodenal sphincter
    f. echelon lymph node
    f. parallel pelvic plane
    f. ray surgery
    F. Response manual resuscitator
    f. rib resection via subclavicular
      approach technique
    f. twitch height (T1)
    f. web space
first-grade fusion
first-line screening technique
first-pass
    f.-p. extraction
    f.-p. technique
first-set graft rejection
first-stage repair
FirstTemp thermometer
Fischer
    F. projection
    F. ring
Fish cuneiform osteotomy technique
Fisher advancement flap
Fisher-Paykel RD1000 resuscitator
Fishgold line
fish-mouth
    f.-m. amputation

    f.-m. anastomosis
    f.-m. end-to-end suture
    f.-m. fracture
    f.-m. incision
fishtail deformity
Fisk and Subbarow method
fissura, pl. fissurae
    f. choroidea
    f. horizontalis pulmonis dextri
    f. ligamenti teretis
    f. ligamenti venosi
    f. obliqua pulmonis
    f. orbitalis inferior
    f. orbitalis superior
    f. petro-occipitalis
    f. petrosquamosa
    f. petrotympanica
    f. pterygoidea
    f. pterygomaxillaris
    f. pterygopalatina
    f. pudendi
    f. sphenopetrosa
    f. tympanomastoidea
    f. tympanosquamosa
fissure
    auricular f.
    azygos f.
    caudal transverse f.
    f. cavity
    corneal f.
    Duverney f.'s
    Ecker f.
    glaserian f.
    horizontal f. of right lung
    inferior accessory f.
    inferior orbital f.
    left sagittal f.
    f. for ligamentum teres
    f. of ligamentum venosum
    f.'s of liver
    f.'s of lung
    major f.
    minor f.
    oblique f. of lung
    oral f.
    palpebral f.
    petro-occipital f.
    petrosquamous f.
    petrotympanic f.
    portal f.
    pterygoid f.
    pterygomaxillary f.
    right sagittal f.
    f. of round ligament of liver
    sphenoidal f.
    sphenomaxillary f.
    sphenopetrosal f.
    squamotympanic f.

superior orbital f.
transverse f. of the lung
tympanomastoid f.
tympanosquamous f.
umbilical f.
f. of venous ligament
vestibular f. of cochlea
fissured fracture
fistula, pl. **fistulae**
abdominal f.
alveolar f.
amphibolic f.
amphibolous f.
anal f.
f. in ano
anorectal f.
antecubital arteriovenous f.
aortocaval f.
aortoduodenal f.
aortoenteric f.
aortoesophageal f.
aortogastric f.
aortograft duodenal f.
aortosigmoid f.
arterial-arterial f.
arterial-enteric f.
arterial-portal f.
arteriobiliary f.
arterioportal f.
arterioportobiliary f.
arteriosinusoidal penile f.
arteriovenous f. (AVF)
aural f.
AV Gore-Tex f.
benign duodenocolic f.
biliary f.
biliary-bronchial f.
biliary-cutaneous f.
biliary-duodenal f.
biliary-enteric f.
f. bimucosa
bladder f.
blind f.
Blom-Singer tracheoesophageal f.
bowl f.
BP f.
brachioaxillary bridge graft f.
brachiosubclavian bridge graft f.
branchial f.
Brescia-Cimino AV f.
bronchobiliary f.
bronchoesophageal f.

bronchopleural f.
bronchopleurocutaneous f. (BPCF)
bronchopulmonary f.
calyceal f.
cameral f.
carotid-cavernous sinus f.
carotid-dural f.
cavernous sinus f.
cerebrospinal fluid f.
cervical f.
cervicovaginal f.
cholecystenteric f.
cholecystocholedochal f.
cholecystocolic f.
cholecystocolonic f.
cholecystoduodenal f.
cholecystoduodenocolic f.
choledochocolonic f.
choledochoduodenal f.
choledochoenteric f.
chyle f.
Cimino f.
Cimino-Brescia arteriovenous f.
coccygeal f.
colobronchial f.
colocutaneous f.
cologastrocutaneous f.
coloileal f.
colonic f.
colovaginal f.
colovesical f.
communicating f.
complete f.
complex anorectal f.
congenital arteriovenous f.
congenital pulmonary
  arteriovenous f.
congenital tracheobiliary f.
congenital urethroperineal f.
f. of cornea
corneal f.
coronary artery f. (CAF)
coronary artery-right ventricular f.
craniosinus f.
cutaneobiliary f.
cystogastric f.
dental f.
dialysis f.
dorsal enteric f.
duodenal f.
duodenocaval f.
duodenocolic f.

F

NOTES

243

fistula *(continued)*
    duodenoenterocutaneous f.
    dural arteriovenous f.
    dural cavernous sinus f.
    Eck f.
    endobronchial f.
    enteric f.
    enterocolic f.
    entcrocutancous f.
    enteroenteral f.
    enteroenteric f.
    enterogenital f.
    enterourethral f.
    enterovaginal f.
    enterovesical f.
    esophageal f.
    esophagobronchial f.
    esophagocutaneous f.
    esophagomediastinal f.
    esophagopulmonary f.
    esophagorespiratory f.
    esophagotracheal f.
    ethmoid f.
    ethmoidal lacrimal f.
    external f.
    external biliary f.
    extrasphincteric anal f.
    fecal f.
    forearm graft arteriovenous f.
    gastric f.
    gastrocolic f.
    gastrocutaneous f.
    gastroduodenal f.
    gastroenteric f.
    gastrointestinal f.
    gastrojejunocolic f.
    gastropleural f.
    genitourinary f.
    gingival f.
    Gore-Tex AF f.
    Gore-Tex aortofemoral f.
    graft-enteric f.
    Gross tracheoesophageal f.
    hepatic artery-portal vein f.
    hepatopleural f.
    hepatoportal biliary f.
    horseshoe f.
    H-type tracheoesophageal f.
    iatrogenic arteriovenous f.
    ileoduodenal f.
    ileosigmoid f.
    ileovesical f.
    incomplete f.
    inflammatory f.
    internal lacrimal f.
    intersphincteric anal f.
    intestinal f.
    intracranial arteriovenous f.

intrahepatic arterial-portal f.
intrahepatic AV f.
intrahepatic spontaneous
  arterioportal f.
intralabyrinthine f.
intraocular f.
jejunocolic f.
labyrinthine f.
lacrimal f.
lacteal f.
mammary f.
Mann-Bollman f.
mesenteric arteriovenous f.
metroperitoneal f.
mucous f.
oroantral f.
orocutaneous f.
orofacial f.
oronasal f.
pancreatic cutaneous f.
pancreaticopleural f.
pararectal f.
parietal f.
perianal f.
perilymph f.
perilymphatic f.
perineal urinary f.
perineovaginal f.
pharyngocutaneous f.
pilonidal f.
pleurobiliary f.
pleuroesophageal f.
postbiopsy renal AV f.
postoperative pleurobiliary f.
postradiation f.
posttraumatic pancreatic-cutaneous f.
preauricular f.
pseudocystobiliary f.
pulmonary arteriovenous f. (PAF)
radiculomedullary f.
rectal f.
rectolabial f.
rectourethral f.
rectourinary f.
rectovaginal f.
rectovesical f.
rectovestibular f.
rectovulvar f.
renal f.
renogastric f.
respiratory-esophageal f.
retroperitoneal f.
reverse Eck f.
salivary f.
scleral f.
sigmoid cutaneous f.
sigmoidovesical f.
solitary pulmonary arteriovenous f.

spermatic f.
spinal dural arteriovenous f.
splanchnic AV f.
splenic AV f.
splenobronchial f.
stercoral f.
subclavian arteriovenous f.
submental f.
suprasphincteric f.
sylvian f.
synovial f.
systemic arteriovenous f.
TE f.
f. test
thigh graft arteriovenous f.
Thiry f.
Thiry-Vella f.
thoracic duct f.
thromboembolic f.
thyroglossal f.
tracheobiliary f.
tracheobronchoesophageal f.
tracheocutaneous f.
tracheoesophageal f. (TEF)
transsphincteric anal f.
traumatic f.
ulcerogenic f.
umbilical f.
urachal f.
ureteral f.
ureterocolic f.
ureterocutaneous f.
ureteroperitoneal f.
ureterouterine f.
ureterovaginal f.
urethrocavernous f.
urethrorectal f.
urethrovaginal f.
urinary f.
urinary-umbilical f.
urinary-vaginal f.
urogenital f.
uteroperitoneal f.
vaginal f.
vasocutaneous f.
Vella f.
venobiliary f.
vesical f.
vesicoacetabular f.
vesicocolic f.
vesicocutaneous f.
vesicoenteric f.

vesicointestinal f.
vesico-ovarian f.
vesicorectal f.
vesicosalpingovaginal f.
vesicouterine f.
vesicovaginal f.
vesicovaginorectal f.
vitelline f.
fistular formation
fistulation
artificial f.
spreading f.
fistulectomy
fistulization
fistulizing surgery
fistuloenterostomy
fistulotomy
choledochoduodenal f.
diathermic f.
endoscopic f.
laying-open f.
Parks method of anal f.
Parks staged f.
fistulous
f. tract
Fite method
fitting
Shrader f.
Fitzpatrick suction tube
five-chamber transverse (5C-T)
five-incision procedure
five-one
f.-o. knee ligament repair
f.-o. reconstruction
five-port "fan" placement
fixate
fixation
adjunctive screw f.
alcohol f.
Allen-Ferguson Galveston pelvic f.
AMBI f.
angled blade plate f.
anomalous f.
f. anomaly
anterior internal f.
anterior metallic f.
anterior plate f.
anterior screw f.
anterior spinal f.
AO external f.
AO rigid f.
AO spinal internal f.

F

NOTES

fixation *(continued)*
  APR cement f.
  atlantoaxial rotatory f.
  autotrophic f.
  axial f.
  axis f.
  bar bolt f.
  Barr open reduction and internal f.
  Barr tibial fracture f.
  f. base
  bicortical screw f.
  bifocal f.
  bifoveal f.
  binocular f.
  biologic f.
  biphase pin f.
  blade plate f.
  bolt f.
  bone-ingrowth f.
  bridge plate f.
  brow f.
  buttressing in internal f.
  Calandruccio f.
  Campbell screw f.
  capsular f.
  carbon dioxide f.
  Caspar anterior plate f.
  catheter f.
  central f.
  cerclage wire f.
  cervical spine internal f.
  cervical spine screw-plate f.
  circumalveolar f.
  circumferential wire-loop f.
  circummandibular f.
  circumzygomatic f.
  cloverleaf condylar-plate f.
  Cole tendon f.
  complement f.
  compression plate f.
  condylar screw f.
  coracoclavicular screw f.
  coracoclavicular suture f.
  Cotrel-Dubousset f.
  craniofacial f.
  crossed f.
  Denham external f.
  dens anterior screw f.
  Deverle f.
  Dimon-Hughston fracture f.
  dorsal wire-loop f.
  dynamic compression-plate f.
  dynamic condylar-screw f.
  f. dysfunction of the lumbar spine
  eccentric f.
  elastic band f.
  external pin f.
  external spinal f.

  eyebrow f.
  femoral prosthesis f.
  field of f.
  four-point f.
  fracture f.
  Galveston pelvic f.
  Gouffon pin f.
  graft f.
  greenstick f.
  Guyton-Noyes f.
  Hackethal intramedullary bouquet f.
  half-pin f.
  Halifax clamp posterior cervical f.
  Harrington rod f.
  Herbert screw f.
  Hex-Fix external f.
  hook f.
  hook-plate f.
  iliac f.
  Ilizarov external f.
  ingrowth f.
  interference fit f.
  intermaxillary f.
  intermedullary rod f.
  internal spinal f.
  interosseous wire f.
  intestinal f.
  intramedullary rod f.
  intraosseous f.
  Kavanaugh-Brower-Mann f.
  Kirschner pin f.
  Kirschner wire f.
  Kristiansen-Kofoed external f.
  Kronner external f.
  Kyle internal f.
  lag screw f.
  line of f.
  loop f.
  lumbar pedicle f.
  lumbar spine segmental f.
  lumbar spine transpedicular f.
  Luque-Galveston f.
  Luque loop f.
  Luque rod f.
  Magerl posterior cervical screw f.
  mandibular f.
  mandibulomaxillary f.
  Matta-Saucedo f.
  maxillomandibular f.
  Mayfield head f.
  McKeever medullary clavicle f.
  medial malleolus f.
  medullary nail f.
  metallic rod f.
  Microplate f.
  microwave f.
  Modulock posterior spinal f.
  monocular f.

monofilament wire f.
multiple-point sacral f.
nail plate f.
nasomandibular f.
near f.
neutralization plate f.
Nichols sacrospinous f.
f. object
occipitocervical f.
odontoid fracture internal f.
open reduction and internal f.
OrthoFrame external f.
OrthoSorb pin f.
osseous f.
pedicle screw-rod f.
pedicular f.
f. peg
pelvic f.
percutaneous f.
phalangeal fracture f.
Phemister acromioclavicular pin f.
pigtail f.
pin and plaster f.
plate f.
plate-screw f.
f. point
point of f.
porous ingrowth f.
posterior cervical f.
posterior screw f.
posterior segmental f.
Press-Fit f.
prophylactic skeletal f.
provisional f.
pubic f.
ReFix noninvasive f.
f. reflex
restorative f.
rigid internal f.
rigid plate f.
f. ring
rod sleeve f.
Roger-Anderson pin f.
role f.
Roy-Camille posterior screw
  plate f.
sacral pedicle screw f.
sacral spine f.
sacroiliac extension f.
sacroiliac flexion f.
sacrospinous ligament vaginal f.
sacrum fusion screw f.

Schneider f.
Schuind external f.
scoliotic curve f.
screw f.
screw-and-plate f.
screw-and-wire f.
Searcy f.
secondary f.
segmental f.
SOF'WIRE spinal f.
spinal f.
split f.
spring f.
staple f.
static f.
Steinmann pin f.
strut plate f.
sublaminar f.
sulcus f.
suture f.
f. target
f. technique
tension band f.
three-pin Mayfield head f.
transarticular wire f.
transcapitellar wire f.
transiliac rod f.
transpedicular screw-rod f.
transverse f.
TSRH rod f.
tunnel and sling f.
visual f.
Volkov-Oganesian external f.
Ward-Tomasin-Vander-Griend f.
Warner-Farber ankle f.
Webb f.
white f.
Wilson-Jacobs tibial f.
wire loop f.
Zickel nail f.
Zickel subtrochanteric fracture f.

fixation/anchor ring
fixator
  f. frame
  f. interne
  f. muscle
fixed
  f. deformity
  f. drain pipe urethra
  f. maintainer space
  f. point
  f. sediment method

F

NOTES

fixed-dose
> f.-d. analysis
> f.-d. patient-controlled analgesia
> (FDPCA)

fixer solution

fixture
> implant f.

flaccid extremity

flag flap

Flajani operation

FLAK
> flow artifact killer
> FLAK technique

flame hemorrhage

flame-shaped hemorrhage

flammable
> f. anesthetic

Flamm technique

Flanagan-Burem apposing hemicylindric graft

flange
> endoprosthetic f.

flanged Teflon tube

flank
> f. approach
> f. bone
> f. dissection
> f. incision
> f. mass
> f. position

flap
> Abbé f.
> abdominal fasciocutaneous f.
> advancement of rectal f.
> anterior helical rim free f.
> apron f.
> arm f.
> arterial f.
> arterialized f.
> Atasoy triangular advancement f.
> Atasoy volar V-Y f.
> axial pattern scalp f.
> axillary f.
> Bakamjian f.
> base of f.
> bicoronal scalp f.
> bilateral V-Y Kutler f.
> bilobed skin f.
> bilobed transposition f.
> bipedicle dorsal f.
> bladder f.
> Blaskovics f.
> Boari bladder f.
> Boari-Ockerblad f.
> bone f.
> brachioradialis f.
> bridge pedicle f.
> buccal mucosal f.
> bulbocavernosus fat f.
> buried f.
> butterfly f.
> Byers f.
> caterpillar f.
> cellulocutaneous f.
> cervical f.
> cheek advancement f.
> cheek rotation f.
> cocked-half f.
> composite f.
> compound f.
> f. congestion
> conjunctival f.
> conjunctivo-Tenon f.
> cross f.
> cross-arm f.
> cross-finger f.
> cross-leg f.
> C-shaped scalp f.
> cutaneous forearm f.
> Cutler-Beard bridge f.
> de-epithelialized f.
> delayed f.
> deltoid f.
> deltopectoral f.
> deltoscapular f.
> dermal fat-free f.
> dermal fat pedicle f.
> digastric muscle f.
> direct f.
> distant f.
> dorsal cross-finger f.
> dorsalis pedis f.
> double pedicle f.
> f. elevation
> Eloesser f.
> endorectal f.
> envelope f.
> epaulet f.
> equal sagittal f.
> Estlander f.
> Estlander-Abbé f.
> extended shoulder f.
> extraction f.
> fasciocutaneous free f.
> fat f.
> fibular f.
> Filatov f.
> Filatov-Gillies f.
> finger f.
> Fisher advancement f.
> flag f.
> flat f.
> foot first web f.
> foramen ovale f.
> forearm f.
> forehead f.

foreskin f.
fornix-based f.
free bone f.
free microsurgical f.
free skin f.
French f.
full-thickness periodontal f.
fusiform f.
gastrocnemius f.
Gilbert scapular f.
gingival f.
glabellar bilobed f.
glabellar rotation f.
gluteus maximus f.
gracilis muscle f.
f. graft
groin f.
Gunderson conjunctival f.
hemipulp f.
hemitongue f.
hinged f.
horizontal f.
horseshoe-shaped f.
Hughes tarsoconjunctival f.
hypogastric f.
ideal f.
iliac crest free f.
iliac crest osseous f.
iliac crest osteocutaneous f.
iliac crest osteomuscular f.
iliofemoral pedicle f.
immediate f.
Imre sliding f.
Indian f.
intercostal f.
internal oblique osteomuscular f.
interpolated f.
interpolation f.
intimal f.
intraoral f.
inverted skin f.
I-shaped scalp f.
island pedicle scalp f.
island skin f.
Italian f.
jejunal free f.
jump f.
Karapandzic f.
Koerner f.
Kutler double lateral
  advancement f.
Kutler V-Y f.

lateral thigh f.
lateral thoracic f.
lateral trapezius f.
lateral upper arm f.
latissimus dorsi muscle f.
latissimus dorsi musculocutaneous f.
latissimus dorsi myocutaneous f.
latissimus/scapular muscle f.
latissimus/serratus muscle f.
limbal-based f.
Limberg f.
lined f.
lingual tongue f.
Linton f.
lip switch f.
liver f.
local muscle f.
local skin f.
long anterior f.
long posterior f.
lower trapezius f.
Martius bulbocavernosus fat f.
masseter muscle f.
Mathieu island onlay f.
McCraw gracilis myocutaneous f.
McFarlane skin f.
melolabial f.
f. meniscal tear
mesiolabial bilobed transposition f.
microvascular free f.
midline forchead f.
Moberg advancement f.
Morrison neurovascular free f.
mucoperichondrial f.
mucoperiosteal periodontal f.
mucoperiosteal sliding f.
mucosal periodontal f.
multistaged carrier f.
muscle f.
muscle-periosteal f.
musculocutaneous free f.
musculotendinous f.
Mustardé rotational cheek f.
myocutaneous f.
myodermal f.
myofascial f.
nape of neck f.
nasolabial rotation f.
neck f.
f. necrosis
neurovascular free f.
oblique f.

F

NOTES

flap *(continued)*
    Ochsenbein-Luebke f.
    Ockerblad-Boari f.
    omental f.
    omocervical f.
    onlay island f.
    open f.
    opening f.
    f. operation
    f. operation cataract
    osteocutaneous f.
    osteomusculocutaneous f.
    osteomyocutaneous f.
    osteoperiosteal f.
    osteoplastic bone f.
    palatal f.
    palmar advancement f.
    palmar cross-finger f.
    parabiotic f.
    para-exstrophy skin f.
    parascapular f.
    parasitic f.
    partial-thickness f.
    pectoralis major f.
    pectoralis major myocutaneous f.
    pectoralis myofascial f.
    pedicled myocutaneous f.
    pedicle groin f.
    peg f.
    penile island f.
    pericardial f.
    pericoronal f.
    pericranial temporalis f.
    perineal f.
    periodontal f.
    periosteal f.
    permanent pedicle f.
    pharyngeal f.
    platysma myocutaneous f.
    Pontén fasciocutaneous f.
    postangioplasty intimal f.
    posterior f.
    pulp f.
    racket-shaped f.
    radial-based f.
    radial forearm f.
    random cutaneous f.
    random pattern f.
    rectus abdominis free f.
    rectus abdominis muscle f.
    rectus abdominis
      musculocutaneous f.
    rectus abdominis myocutaneous f.
    rectus femoris f.
    regional f.
    remote pedicle f.
    retinal f.
    retroauricular free f.

    reversal pedicle f.
    reverse cross-finger f.
    reverse forearm island f.
    rhomboid transposition f.
    rope f.
    rotation f.
    rotational f.
    Rubens breast f.
    saphenous f.
    scalping f.
    scalp sickle f.
    scapular f.
    Scardino f.
    scleral f.
    semilunar f.
    serratus anterior muscle f.
    sickle f.
    simple periodontal f.
    skew f.
    skin f.
    sliding f.
    soft tissue f.
    split-thickness periodontal f.
    Steichen neurovascular free f.
    subcutaneous f.
    supramalleolar f.
    supraorbital pericranial f.
    supraperiosteal f.
    surgical f.
    tarsoconjunctival f.
    f. technique
    temporalis fascia f.
    temporalis muscle f.
    tensor fascia femoris f.
    tensor fascia lata muscle f.
    Tenzel rotational cheek f.
    thenar f.
    thoracoacromial f.
    thoracoepigastric f.
    tongue f.
    f. tracheostomy
    TRAM f.
    transposition f.
    transverse rectus abdominis
      muscle f.
    trapezius f.
    triangular advancement f.
    Truc f.
    tubed groin f.
    tubed pedicle f.
    tubularized cecal f.
    turnover f.
    tympanomeatal f.
    unipedicled f.
    unrepositioned f.
    upper trapezius f.
    Urbaniak neurovascular free f.
    Urbaniak scapular f.

U-shaped scalp f.
Van Lint f.
vascularized free f.
ventrum penis f.
vertical f.
visor f.
von Langenbeck bipedicle
  mucoperiosteal f.
von Langenbeck pedicle f.
V-Y advancement f.
V-Y Kutler f.
waltzed f.
Warren f.
web space f.
Widman f.
winged V double f.
wraparound neurovascular free f.
Zimany bilobed f.
flapping valve syndrome
flap-valve mechanism
flashlamp excited pulsed dye
flashlight examination
flash photolysis
flash-point temperature
flask closure
flat
  f. back deformity
  f. bone graft
  f. chest
  f. condyloma
  f. depressed lesion
  f. elevated lesion
  f. flap
  f. pelvis
  f. plate of abdomen
  f. substrate method
flatfoot
  peroneal spastic f.
Flatt
  F. classification
  F. excision
  F. technique
flatus tube insertion
flavoxate hydrochloride
Flaxedil
  F. suture
Flechsig tract
Fleischer keratoconus ring
Fleischer-Strumpell ring
Fleischmann bursa
Fleischner line
Fleish No. 2 pneumotachograph

Fletcher rule of irradiation tolerance
flexed position
flexibility
flexible
  f. collodion
  f. endofluoroscopy
  f. fiberoptic bronchoscopy
  f. fiberoptic endoscopy
  f. fiberoptic myeloscopy
  f. hinge suspension
  f. laparoscopy
  f. nephroscopy
  f. sigmoidoscopy
  f. ureteropyeloscopy
  f. wand
Flexiflo
  F. enteral feeding tube
  F. gastrostomy tube
  F. Inverta-Peg tube
  F. Sacks-Vine tube
  F. stoma creator tube
  F. Stomate gastrostomy tube
  F. suction feeding tube
  F. tap-fill enteral tube
  F. Taptainer tube
  F. tungsten-weighted feeding tube
  F. Versa-PEG tube
flexion
  f. in abduction and external
    rotation
  f., abduction, external rotation,
    extension
  f., adduction, internal rotation
  f. in adduction and internal
    rotation
  f. compression spine injury
    stabilization
  f. crease
  f. deformity
  f. and extension
  f. osteotomy
  f. teardrop fracture
flexion-extension
  f.-e. arc
  f.-e. axis
  f.-e. injury
  f.-e. maneuver
  f.-e. plane
  f.-e. reflex
flexion-internal rotational deformity
flexion-rotation-drawer
  f.-r.-d. knee instability test

NOTES

F

251

Flexi-Rod
Flexitone suture
Flexon steel suture
flexor
 f. pollicis longus abductor-plasty
 f. tendon anastomosis
 f. tendon graft
 f. tendon laceration
 f. tendon repair
 f. tendon rupture
 f. tenosynovectomy
flexorplasty
 Bunnell modification of Steindler f.
 Eyler f.
 Steindler f.
flexor-pronator
 f.-p. origin
 f.-p. origin release
flexura, pl. flexurae
 f. coli dextra
 f. coli sinistra
 f. duodeni inferior
 f. duodeni superior
 f. duodenojejunalis
 f. perinealis recti
 f. sacralis recti
 f. sigmoidea
flexural
flexure
 anorectal f.
 colon f.
 duodenojejunal f.
 hepatic f.
 inferior f. of duodenum
 left colic f.
 lumbar f.
 perineal f. of rectum
 right colic f.
 sacral f. of rectum
 sigmoid f.
 splenic f.
 superior f. of duodenum
flicker-fusion
 f.-f. frequency technique
 f.-f. stimulus
 f.-f. threshold
flickering
 f. blockade
 f. blockade electrophysiology
Flick-Gould technique
Flieringa
 curved scleral-limbal incision of F.
 F. fixation ring
 F. scleral ring
Flieringa-Kayser
 F.-K. copper ring
 F.-K. fixation ring

Flieringa-LeGrand
 F.-L. fixation ring
flip-flap
 Mathieu-Horton-Devine f.-f.
 f.-f. procedure
 f.-f. technique
floating
 f. forehead operation
 f. kidney
 f. organ
 f. ribs
 f. spleen
floccillation
floccular
 f. fossa
flocculation
 cephalin-cholesterol f.
 limit of f.
 Ramon f.
 thymol f.
flocculonodular arteriovenous malformation
Flolan injection
floor
 f. fracture
 f. of orbit
 f. of tympanic cavity
floor-of-mouth
 f.-o.-m. closure
 f.-o.-m. lesion
Flo-Pack
 Anectine F.-P.
floppy
 f. Nissen fundoplication
 f. Nissen fundoplication method
 f. Nissen fundoplication procedure
 f. Nissen fundoplication technique
 f. valve syndrome
flora
 endogenous f.
 exogenous f.
 GI tract f.
Florida urinary pouch
florid duct lesion
flotation rate
Flotem IIe fluid-warming device
flow
 f. artifact killer (FLAK)
 carotid arterial blood f.
 f. convergence method
 f. detection technique
 f. direction
 Doppler color f.
 effective renal blood f.
 effective renal plasma f.
 endocardial f.
 exercise hyperemia blood f.
 hepatofugal f.

hepatopetal f.
f. interruption technique
f. mapping technique
f. misregistration
peak expiratory f.
plug f.
f. regulated suction tube
f. technique filling
tricuspid valve f.
flow-dependent pressure drop
Flower
F. bone
F. dental index
flowmeter
infrared laser-Doppler f.
MBF3 infrared laser-Doppler f.
peak f.
flowmetry
laser-Doppler f.
Periflux 3 laser-Doppler f.
flow-on gradient-echo image
flow-over vaporizer
Flowtron DVT prophylactic deep venous thrombosis unit
Floxin injection
floxuridine in hepatic metastasis
flucrylate
fluctuans
myotonia f.
fluctuant mass
fluctuation test
fluffy cotton-wool exudate
fluffy-cuffed tube
fluid
f. aspiration
bloody peritoneal f.
body f.
cerebrospinal f. (CSF)
f. collection
cul-de-sac f.
cytospin collection f.
f. evacuation
extracellular f.
free peritoneal f.
LKB Optiphase 2 scintillation f.
f. loading anesthetic technique
loculation of f.
motor oil peritoneal f.
peritoneal cavity f.
pleural f.
prostatic f.
prune-juice peritoneal f.

Rees-Ecker f.
respiratory tract f.
f. resuscitation
seminal f.
synovial f.
turbid peritoneal f.
University of Wisconsin
preservation f.
f. warmer
fluid-filled sac
fluid-gas exchange
fluke
tissue f.
flumazenil
Fluomar
Fluoracaine
fluorescein
f. dye and stain solution
f. fundus angioscopy
f. instillation test
f. string test
fluorescence
f. microscopy
f. polarization method
fluorescent
f. antibody (FA)
f. electronic endoscopy
f. optode
f. optode technology
fluoride solution
Fluori-Methane Topical Spray
fluorinated ether anesthetic
Fluoroscan C-arm fluoroscopy
fluoroscopic
f. pushing technique
f. visualization
fluoroscopy
biplane f.
C-arm f.
Fluoroscan C-arm f.
kV f.
portable C-arm image intensifier f.
rapid scan f.
two-plane f.
video f.
Xi-scan f.
Fluosol
Fluothane
flurazepam hydrochloride
Fluro-Ethyl Aerosol
fluroxene

F

NOTES

flush
    f. and bathe technique
    f. method
flushing technique
Flynn
    F. femoral neck fracture reduction
    F. technique
FNA
    fine-needle aspiration
    FNA biopsy
foam
    human fibrin f.
foaming exudate
focal
    f. bleeding point
    f. fatty infiltration
    f. fatty infiltration of liver
    f. granulomatous inflammation
    f. illumination
    f. image point
    f. infection
    f. nonfatty infiltration of liver
    f. parenchymal brain lesion
    f. plane
    f. rupture of basement membrane
    f. splenic lesion
    f. tumor
focus, pl. foci
    ectopic f.
    endometriotic f.
    image-space f.
    object-space f.
    residual foci
focused radiation therapy
Föerster
    F. lacrimal sac
    F. operation
fogging retinoscopy
foil
    adhesive f.
Foix enucleation
fold
    alar f.'s
    anterior axillary f.
    aryepiglottic f.
    axillary f.
    Bartlett nail f.
    cecal f.'s
    f. of chorda tympani
    circular f.'s
    Douglas f.
    duodenojejunal f.
    duodenomesocolic f.
    epicanthal f.
    epigastric f.
    gastric f.'s
    gastropancreatic f.'s
    Guérin f.

Hasner f.
head and tail f.
Houston f.'s
ileocecal f.
incudal f.
inferior duodenal f.
inguinal aponeurotic f.
interureteric f.
Kerckring f.'s
labioscrotal f.'s
lacrimal f.
f. of laryngeal nerve
lateral glossoepiglottic f.
lateral nail f.
lateral umbilical f.
longitudinal f. of duodenum
malar f.
medial umbilical f.
median umbilical f.
middle transverse rectal f.
middle umbilical f.
mucobuccal f.
mucosal f.'s of gallbladder
nail f.
nasojugal f.
Nélaton f.
palmate f.'s
palpebronasal f.
pharyngoepiglottic f.
pleuroperitoneal f.
polypoid degeneration of the true f.
presplenic f.
rectal f.'s
rectouterine f.
rectovesical f.
retinal f.
sacrogenital f.'s
sacrouterine f.
sacrovaginal f.
sacrovesical f.
semilunar f. of colon
spiral f. of cystic duct
superior duodenal f.
f. of superior laryngeal nerve
synovial f.
tarsal f.
transverse palatine f.
transverse rectal f.'s
transverse vesical f.
Treves f.
urachal f.
ureteric f.
uterovesical f.
vascular f. of the cecum
Vater f.
ventricular f.
vestibular f.

folding larynx
Foley
    F. operation
    F. Y-plasty pyeloplasty
    F. Y-V plasty
Folin and Wu method
follicle
    f. maturation stimulation
follicular
    f. carcinomas
    f. hematoma
    f. inflammation
folliculoma
folliculus, pl. folliculi
    folliculi lymphatici aggregati
    folliculi lymphatici gastrici
    folliculi lymphatici recti
    folliculi lymphatici solitarii
    f. lymphaticus
follow-up
    f.-u. evaluation
    f.-u. examination
Fome-Cuf
    F.-C. endotracheal tube
    F.-C. tracheostomy tube
Fones
    F. method
    F. technique
Fonio solution
Fontan
    F. atriopulmonary anastomosis
    F. fenestration closure
    F. modification of Norwood procedure
    F. operation
    F. repair
Fontana
    F. canal
    F. space
    space of F.
Fontana-Masson staining method
Fontan-Baudet procedure
fontanel, fontanelle
    anterior f.
    anterolateral f.
    bregmatic f.
    Casser f.
    cranial f.'s
    frontal f.
    Gerdy f.
    mastoid f.
    occipital f.

    posterior f.
    posterolateral f.
    sagittal f.
    sphenoidal f.
Fontan-Kreutzer procedure
fonticulus, pl. fonticuli
    f. anterior
    f. anterolateralis
    fonticuli cranii
    f. mastoideus
    f. posterior
    f. posterolateralis
    f. sphenoidalis
Food and Drug Administration (FDA)
foot
    f. deformity
    f. first web flap
    f. puncture wound
    F. reticulin method
    f. rotation
forage
    f. core biopsy
    f. procedure
foramen, pl. foramina
    alveolar foramina
    foramina alveolaria
    anterior condyloid f.
    aortic f.
    f. of Arnold
    blind f. of frontal bone
    blind f. of the tongue
    f. bursae omentalis majoris
    carotid f.
    cecal f. of frontal bone
    cecal f. of the tongue
    f. cecum of frontal bone
    f. cecum ossis frontalis
    f. cecum of tongue
    f. compression test
    conjugate f.
    f. costotransversarium
    costotransverse f.
    f. diaphragmatis sellae
    emissary sphenoidal f.
    ethmoidal f.
    f. ethmoidale
    external acoustic f.
    Ferrein f.
    frontal f.
    f. frontale
    great f.
    Hyrtl f.

NOTES

foramen *(continued)*
    inferior dental f.
    internal auditory f.
    intervertebral f.
    f. ischiadicum
    jugular f.
    f. jugulare
    lacerated f.
    f. lacerum
    f. lacerum anterius
    f. lacerum medium
    f. lacerum posterius
    f. magnum
    f. magnum line
    malar f.
    f. mandibulae
    mandibular f.
    mastoid f.
    f. mastoideum
    mental f.
    f. mentale
    Morgagni f.
    nasal f.
    foramina nervosa
    f. nutricium
    nutrient f.
    obturator f.
    optic f.
    f. opticum
    f. ovale
    f. ovale flap
    foramina papillaria renis
    papillary foramina of kidney
    parietal f.
    f. parietale
    petrosal f.
    f. petrosum
    pleuroperitoneal f.
    posterior condyloid f.
    f. processus transversi
    f. quadratum
    f. rotundum
    round f.
    sacral f.
    f. sacrale
    Scarpa foramina
    f. singulare
    solitary f.
    sphenopalatine f.
    f. sphenopalatinum
    sphenotic f.
    f. spinosum
    stylomastoid f.
    f. stylomastoideum
    supraorbital f.
    f. supraorbitale
    f. transversarium
    transverse f.

    f. of transverse process
    f. of vena cava
    vena caval f.
    f. venae cavae
    f. venosum
    venous f.
    vertebral f.
    f. vertebrale
    vertebroarterial f.
    f. vertebroarterialis
    Vesalius f.
    zygomaticofacial f.
    f. zygomaticofaciale
    zygomatico-orbital f.
    f. zygomatico-orbitale
    zygomaticotemporal f.
    f. zygomaticotemporale
foraminal
    f. approach
    f. compression test
    f. herniation
    f. node
foraminotomy
Forane
Forbes
    F. modification of Phemister graft technique
    F. onlay bone graft
force
    f. application
    f. of mastication
    f. translation (FTR)
forcé
    eccouchement f.
    redressement f.
force-couple splint reduction
forced
    f. alimentation
    f. expiratory capacity
    f. expiratory spirogram
    f. expiratory time
    f. expiratory volume
    f. expiratory volume in 1 second to forced vital capacity ratio
    f. expiratory volume timed to forced vital capacity ratio
    f. generation test
    f. mandatory intermittent ventilation
    f. respiration
forced-air
    f.-a. active cooling device
    f.-a. patient warming system
    f.-a. warming
forced-eye closure
force-frequency relation
force-length relation
forceps
    f. extraction

f. maneuver
f. removal
f. rotation
force-velocity-length relation
force-velocity relation
force-velocity-volume relation
forcing
dynamic end-tidal f.
forcipate
forcipressure
Ford triangulation technique
forearm
f. amputation
f. flap
f. fracture
f. graft arteriovenous fistula
f. ischemic exercise test
f. plethysmography
f. supination test
forefoot arthroplasty
Foregger-Racine adapter
foregut malformation
forehead
f. flap
forehead-nose position
foreign
f. body
f. body aspiration
f. body carcinogenesis
f. body extraction
f. body loop
f. body management
f. body removal
f. body response
f. body sclerotomy
f. body trauma
f. body tumorigenesis
foreign-body reaction
forekidney
Forel decussation
forequarter amputation
foreskin
f. flap
f. restoration
Forest-Hastings technique
Forest I, II lesion
forestomach
form
extension f.
face f.

formal
f. hemipelvectomy
f. method
formaldehyde
f. catgut suture
melamine f.
f. solution
formaldehyde-induced fluorescence method
formalin-ether sedimentation method
formatio, pl. **formationes**
formation
abscess f.
adhesion f.
anterior synechia f.
antiantibody f.
aspergilloma f.
balloon cell f.
blood vessel f.
bone f.
branching tubule f.
bunion f.
calculous f.
callus f.
cataract f.
chiasma f.
cloacal f.
coagulum f.
colony f.
concept f.
crater f.
Cyclops f.
echo f.
erythroid colony f.
excessive callus f.
extracapillary crescent f.
false channel f.
fistular f.
gallstone f.
gender identity f.
germinal center f.
Gothic arch f.
heat of f.
hemostatic plug f.
heterotopic bone f.
identity f.
image f.
impulse f.
intramembranous f.
keloid f.
kerion f.
ketone body f.

F

NOTES

257

formation *(continued)*
    lappet f.
    localized plaque f.
    median bar f.
    mesencephalic reticular f.
    micelle f.
    midbrain reticular f.
    neointima f.
    osteophyte f.
    pannus f.
    paramedian pontine reticular f.
    periosteal new bone f.
    personality f.
    pontine paramedian reticular f.
    posterior synechia f.
    procallus f.
    pseudoaneurysm f.
    pseudopod f.
    reaction f.
    reticular f.
    root f.
    rouleaux f.
    sac f.
    scar f.
    somite f.
    spur f.
    standard enthalpy of f.
    star f.
    stone granuloma f.
    struvite crystal f.
    symptom f.
    trellis f.
    twin f.
    web f.
formocresol pulpotomy
formol ammonium bromide solution
fornix, pl. **fornices**
    f. approach
    body of f.
    caliceal f.
    f. conjunctivae
    conjunctival f.
    f. of the lacrimal sac
    pharyngeal f.
    f. pharyngis
    f. reformation
    f. sacci lacrimalis
fornix-based flap
Forte
    Citanest F.
fortification
fortified topical preparation
forward
    f. coarticulation
    f. head posture
    f. traction test
    f. triangle method
    f. triangle technique

Foscavir injection
Fosnaugh nail biopsy
fossa, pl. **fossae**
    anterior cranial f.
    articular f. of temporal bone
    f. axillaris
    axillary f.
    Bichat f.
    Biesiadecki f.
    Broesike f.
    f. canina
    canine f.
    Claudius f.
    f. condylaris
    coronoid f. of humerus
    f. cranii media
    f. cranii posterior
    crural f.
    Cruveilhier f.
    digastric f.
    f. digastrica
    f. ductus venosi
    f. of ductus venosus
    duodenal fossae
    duodenojejunal f.
    epigastric f.
    f. epigastrica
    femoral f.
    floccular f.
    gallbladder f.
    f. for gallbladder
    Gerdy hyoid f.
    f. glandulae lacrimalis
    glenoid f.
    greater supraclavicular f.
    Gruber-Landzert f.
    hypophysial f.
    f. hypophysialis
    iliac f.
    iliacosubfascial f.
    f. iliacosubfascialis
    iliopectineal f.
    inferior duodenal f.
    infraclavicular f.
    f. infraclavicularis
    infraduodenal f.
    f. infraspinata
    infraspinous f.
    infratemporal f.
    f. infratemporalis
    inguinal f.
    f. inguinalis lateralis
    f. inguinalis medialis
    intercondylar f.
    f. intercondylaris
    intercondyloid f.
    f. intermesocolica transversa
    intrabulbar f.

ischioanal f.
ischiorectal f.
f. ischiorectalis
Jobert de Lamballe f.
Jonnesco f.
jugular f.
f. jugularis
f. of lacrimal gland
lacrimal sac f.
f. of lacrimal sac
Landzert f.
lateral inguinal f.
lesser supraclavicular f.
Malgaigne f.
f. malleoli fibulae
f. malleoli lateralis
mandibular f.
f. mandibularis
mastoid f.
medial inguinal f.
meningioma of posterior f.
Merkel f.
mesentericoparietal f.
middle cranial f.
Mohrenheim f.
Morgagni f.
mylohyoid f.
f. navicularis Cruveilhier
f. navicularis urethrae
f. navicularis vestibulae vaginae
navicular f. of urethra
paraduodenal f.
parajejunal f.
f. parajejunalis
pararectal f.
paravesical f.
f. paravesicalis
peritoneal fossae
petrosal f.
piriform f.
pituitary f.
f. poplitea
popliteal f.
posterior cranial f.
f. provesicalis
pterygoid f.
f. pterygoidea
pterygomaxillary f.
f. pterygopalatina
pterygopalatine f.
radial f. of humerus
f. radialis humeri

retroduodenal f.
retromandibular f.
f. retromandibularis
retromolar f.
Rosenmüller f.
f. sacci lacrimalis
scaphoid f.
f. scaphoidea ossis sphenoidalis
scaphoid f. of sphenoid bone
sigmoid f.
sphenomaxillary f.
splenic f.
f. subarcuata
subarcuate f.
subcecal f.
subinguinal f.
sublingual f.
submandibular f.
f. submandibularis
submaxillary f.
subscapular f.
f. subscapularis
superior duodenal f.
f. supraclavicularis major
f. supraclavicularis minor
supramastoid f.
f. supraspinata
supraspinous f.
supravesical f.
f. supravesicalis
temporal f.
f. temporalis
f. terminalis urethrae
Treitz f.
trochlear f.
f. trochlearis
umbilical f.
Velpeau f.
f. venae umbilicalis
f. venosa
vermian f.
f. vesicae biliaris [felleae]
Waldeyer fossae
zygomatic f.
fossula
f. petrosa
petrosal f.
fossulate
Foster suture
Fothergill
F. operation
F. stitch

NOTES

Fothergill-Donald operation
Fothergill-Hunter operation
Foucher classification of epiphyseal
  injury
Fould entropion operation
foundation
  anhydrous facial f.
  denture f.
  facial f.
  level f.
  oil-based facial f.
  f. surface
  water-based facial f.
  water-free facial f.
fountain decussation
four-chamber transverse (4C-T)
four-flap Z-plasty
Fourier
  F. transformation spectrum analyzer
  F. transform infrared
    microspectroscopy
  F. transform infrared spectroscopy
four-incision procedure
four-limb Z-plasty
four-lumen tube
four-maximal breath preoxygenation
  technique
Fournier disease
four-part fracture
four-point
  f.-p. biopsy
  f.-p. fixation
four-port
  f.-p. "diamond" placement
  f.-p. method
  f.-p. procedure
  f.-p. technique
four-star exercise program
fourth
  f. carpometacarpal joint fracture
  f. cranial nerve
  f. degree radiation injury
  f. lumbar nerve
  f. parallel pelvic plane
four-wire trochanter reattachment
fovea
  f. articularis inferior atlantis
  f. articularis superior atlantis
  f. centralis retinae
  f. costalis inferior
  f. costalis processus transversi
  f. costalis superior
  f. dentis atlantis
  f. elliptica
  f. hemielliptica
  f. hemispherica
  f. inguinalis interna
  Morgagni f.

  pterygoid f.
  f. pterygoidea
  f. spherica
  f. sublingualis
  f. submandibularis
  f. submaxillaris
  f. supravesicalis
  trochlear f.
  f. trochlearis
foveola, pl. foveolae
  f. coccygea
  coccygeal f.
  f. gastrica
  foveolae granulares
  f. suprameatica
foveolar
Fowler
  F. central slip tenotomy
  F. maneuver
  F. osteotomy
  F. position
  F. procedure
  F. solution
  F. technique
  F. thoracoplasty
Fowler-Philip
  F.-P. approach
  F.-P. incision
Fowler-Stephens
  F.-S. maneuver
  F.-S. orchiopexy
  F.-S. procedure
Fowles
  F. dislocation technique
  F. open reduction
Fox-Blazina procedure
Fox operation
Fr
  French
fraction
  f. of expired carbon dioxide
  f. in expired gas of carbon
    dioxide
fractional
  f. area change (FAC)
  f. dilation and curettage
  f. epidural anesthesia
  f. excretion of lithium
  f. spinal anesthesia
  f. sterilization
fractionated
  f. external beam irradiation
  f. radiation therapy
fractionation
  indicator f.
  f. protocol
fracture
  abduction-external rotation f.

acetabular rim f.
acute f.
Aebi-Etter-Coscia fixation dens f.
agenetic f.
alveolar process f.
alveolar socket wall f.
anatomic f.
Anderson-Hutchins unstable tibial
  shaft f.
angulated f.
angulation f.
ankle mortise f.
anterior column f.
anterolateral compression f.
apex f.
apophyseal f.
arch f.
articular mass separation f.
articular pillar f.
Atkin epiphyseal f.
atlantal f.
atlas f.
atlas-axis combination f.
atrophic f.
avulsion stress f.
axial loading f.
axis f.
axis-atlas combination f.
backfire f.
banana f.
f. band
Bankart f.
Barton-Smith f.
basal neck f.
basal skull f.
baseball finger f.
basilar femoral neck f.
basilar skull f.
bayonet position of f.
beak f.
f. bed
bedroom f.
Bennett comminuted f.
bicondylar T-shaped f.
bicondylar Y-shaped f.
bicycle spoke f.
bimalleolar ankle f.
birth f.
f. blister
blow-in f.
blow-out f.
boot-top f.

Bosworth f.
both-bone f.
both-column f.
bowing f.
boxer f.
f. bracing
bronchial f.
bucket-handle f.
buckle f.
bumper f.
bunk-bed f.
burst f.
butterfly f.
buttonhole f.
calcaneal avulsion f.
calcaneal displaced f.
f. callus
capillary f.
capitate f.
capitellar f.
capitulum radiale humeri f.
carpal bone stress f.
carpometacarpal joint f.
cartwheel f.
cemental f.
cementum f.
central f.
cephalomedullary nail f.
cerebral palsy pathological f.
cervical spine f.
cervicotrochanteric displaced f.
Chance vertebral f.
Chaput f.
chauffeur f.
chip f.
chiropractic treatment of f.
chisel f.
chondral f.
circumferential f.
f. classification
clavicular birth f.
clay-shoveler f.
cleavage f.
closed-break f.
closed skull f.
coccyx f.
Colles f.
combined flexion-distraction injury
  and burst f.
combined radial-ulnar-humeral f.
comminuted intra-articular f.
comminuted orbital f.

F

NOTES

fracture *(continued)*

comminuted skull f.
complete f.
complex f.
complicated f.
compound comminuted f.
compound skull f.
compressed f.
compression f.
condylar femoral f.
condylar process f.
congenital f.
contrecoup f.
coracoid f.
corner f.
coronal split f.
coronoid process f.
cortical f.
Cotton ankle f.
cough f.
cranial f.
crown f.
crown-root f.
crush f.
crushed eggshell f.
Danis-Weber f.
dashboard f.
Delbet splint for heel f.
dens f.
dentate f.
depressed skull f.
depression f.
de Quervain f.
derby hat f.
Descot f.
diacondylar f.
diametric pelvic f.
diaphyseal f.
diastatic skull f.
dicondylar f.
die punch f.
direct f.
f. disease
dishpan f.
f. dislocation
dislocation f.
displaced f.
distal femoral epiphyseal f.
distal humeral f.
distal radial f.
distraction of f.
dog-leg f.
dome f.
double f.
Dupuytren f.
Duverney f.
dyscrasic f.
elbow f.

electrostimulation for nonunion
   of f.
elementary f.
enamel f.
f. en coin
endocrine f.
f. en rave
epicondylar avulsion f.
epiphyseal growth plate f.
epiphyseal slip f.
epiphyseal tibial f.
Essex-Lopresti joint depression f.
explosion f.
expressed skull f.
extension teardrop f.
external orbital f.
extracapsular f.
extraoctave f.
facial f.
fatigue f.
femoral intertrochanteric f.
femoral neck f.
femoral shaft f.
femoral supracondylar f.
fender f.
fetal bone f.
f. fever
fibular f.
fifth metatarsal base f.
fighter f.
finger f.
first carpometacarpal joint f.
fish-mouth f.
fissured f.
f. fixation
flexion teardrop f.
floor f.
forearm f.
four-part f.
fourth carpometacarpal joint f.
f. fragment
frontal sinus f.
Gaenslen f.
Galeazzi f.
f. gap
Garden femoral neck f.
glenoid rim f.
Gosselin f.
greater trochanteric femoral f.
greater tuberosity f.
greenstick f.
growing f.
Guérin f.
gunshot f.
Gustilo-Anderson open clavicular f.
gutter f.
Hahn-Steinthal f.
hairline f.

hamate tail f.
hangman f.
head-splitting humeral f.
healed f.
healing f.
f. healing
hemicondylar f.
Henderson f.
Hermodsson f.
hickory-stick f.
high-energy f.
Hill-Sachs f.
hip f.
hockey-stick f.
Hoffa f.
Holstein-Lewis f.
hook of the hamate f.
hoop stress f.
horizontal maxillary f.
humeral head-splitting f.
humeral physeal f.
humeral shaft f.
humeral supracondylar f.
Hutchinson f.
hyoid bone f.
ice skater f.
ileofemoral wing f.
impacted f.
implant f.
impression f.
incomplete compound f.
indirect f.
inflammatory f.
infraction f.
insufficiency f.
intercondylar femoral f.
intercondylar humeral f.
intercondylar tibial f.
internal fixation f.
interperiosteal f.
intertrochanteric femoral f.
intertrochanteric four-part f.
intra-articular proximal tibial f.
intracapsular f.
intraoperative f.
intrauterine f.
inverted-Y f.
ipsilateral femoral neck f.
ipsilateral femoral shaft f.
irreducible f.
Jefferson f.
joint depression f.

Jones f.
juxtacortical f.
knee f.
Kocher f.
laminar f.
lap seatbelt f.
laryngeal cartilage f.
lateral condylar humeral f.
lateral humeral condyle f.
lateral malleolar f.
lateral mass f.
lateral tibial plateau f.
Laugier f.
lead-pipe f.
Le Fort fibular f.
Le Fort I-III f.
Le Fort mandibular f.
Le Fort-Wagstaffe f.
lesser trochanter f.
f. line
linear skull f.
Lisfranc f.
long bone f.
longitudinal f.
long oblique f.
loose f.
lorry-driver f.
low-energy f.
low lumbar spine f.
lumbar spine burst f.
lumbosacral junction f.
Maisonneuve fibular f.
malar f.
Malgaigne pelvic f.
malleolar f.
mallet f.
malunited calcaneus f.
malunited forearm f.
malunited radial f.
mandibular body f.
mandibular condyle f.
mandibular ramus f.
mandibular symphysis f.
March f.
marginal ridge f.
maternal f.
maxillary f.
maxillofacial f.
medial epicondyle humeral f.
mesiodistal f.
metacarpal neck f.
metaphyseal tibial f.

F

NOTES

fracture *(continued)*

metatarsal f.
middle tibial shaft f.
midface f.
midfoot f.
midshaft f.
milkman f.
minimally displaced f.
minipilon f.
missed f.
Moberg-Gedda f.
molar tooth f.
monomalleolar ankle f.
Monteggia forearm f.
Montercaux f.
Moore f.
Mouchet f.
multangular ridge f.
multilevel f.
multiple f.
multiray f.
nasal f.
naso-orbital f.
navicular f.
naviculocapitate f.
f. of necessity
neck f.
neoplastic f.
neurogenic f.
neuropathic f.
nightstick f.
nonarticular distal radial f.
noncontiguous f.
nondisplaced f.
nonphyseal f.
nonrotational burst f.
nonunion f.
nonunited f.
nutcracker f.
oblique f.
obturator avulsion f.
occipital condyle f.
occult f.
odontoid condyle f.
olecranon f.
one-part f.
open-book f.
open-break f.
open skull f.
f. of orbit
orbital blow-out f.
orbital floor f.
orbital rim f.
orbital wall f.
osteochrondral slice f.
osteoporotic f.
outlet strut f.
pacemaker lead f.

Pais f.
paratrooper f.
pars interarticularis f.
patellar sleeve f.
pathologic f.
Pauwels f.
pedicle f.
pelvic avulsion f.
pelvic ring f.
pelvic straddle f.
penetrating f.
periarticular f.
periprosthetic f.
peritrochanteric f.
petrous pyramid f.
phalangeal diaphyseal f.
physeal f.
Piedmont f.
pillion f.
pillow f.
pilon ankle f.
ping-pong f.
pisiform f.
plafond f.
plaque f.
plastic bowing f.
pond f.
porcelain f.
Posada f.
posterior arch f.
posterior column f.
posterior element f.
posterior ring f.
posterior wall f.
postirradiation f.
postoperative f.
Pott ankle f.
profundus artery f.
pronation-abduction f.
pronation-eversion f.
proximal femoral f.
proximal humeral f.
proximal tibial metaphyseal f.
pyramidal f.
radial head f.
radial neck f.
radial styloid f.
reduction of f.
f. reduction
f. repair
reverse Barton f.
reverse Colles f.
reverse Monteggia f.
rib f.
ring f.
ring-disrupting f.
Rolando f.
roof f.

root f.
rotation f.
rotational burst f.
sacral f.
sacroiliac f.
sacrum f.
sagittal slice f.
Salter I-VI f.
scaphoid f.
scotty-dog f.
seatbelt f.
secondary f.
segmental f.
Segond f.
sentinel spinous process f.
SER-IV f.
shaft f.
shear f.
Shepherd f.
short oblique f.
sideswipe elbow f.
simple skull f.
single f.
f. site
skier f.
Skillern f.
skull f.
sleeve f.
slice f.
slot f.
Smith f.
spinal compression f.
spinous process f.
spiral oblique f.
splintered f.
split f.
split-heel f.
splitting f.
spontaneous f.
sprain f.
sprinter f.
stability of f.
f. stabilization
stable burst f.
stairstep f.
stellate skull f.
Stieda f.
straddle f.
stress f.
strut f.
subcapital f.
subperiosteal f.

subtrochanteric femoral f.
supination-adduction f.
supination-eversion f.
supination-external rotation IV f.
supracondylar humeral f.
supracondylar Y-shaped f.
surgical neck f.
T f.
talar avulsion f.
talar neck f.
talar osteochondral f.
tarsal bone f.
T-condylar f.
teacup f.
teardrop f.
temporal bone f.
tension f.
testis f.
thoracic spine f.
thoracolumbar burst f.
thoracolumbar spine f.
three-part f.
through-and-through f.
thrower f.
tibial bending f.
tibial condyle f.
tibial diaphyseal f.
tibial open f.
tibial plafond f.
tibial plateau f.
tibial shaft f.
tibial triplane f.
tibial tuberosity f.
Tillaux-Chaput f.
Tillaux-Kleiger f.
toddler f.
tongue f.
tooth f.
torsional f.
torus f.
trabecular bone f.
tracheal f.
traction f.
trampoline f.
transcaphoid f.
transcapitate f.
transcervical femoral f.
transchondral f.
transcondylar f.
transepiphyseal f.
transhamate f.
transiliac f.

F

NOTES

fracture *(continued)*
    translational f.
    transsacral f.
    transscaphoid dislocation f.
    transtriquetral f.
    transverse comminuted f.
    transverse facial f.
    transversely oriented endplate
      compression f.
    transverse maxillary f.
    transverse process f.
    trapezium f.
    traumatic f.
    trimalleolar ankle f.
    triplane tibial f.
    tripod f.
    triquetral f.
    trophic f.
    tuft f.
    two-part f.
    type C pelvic ring f.
    type I, II, III, IIIA, IIIB, IIIC
      open f.
    ulnar f.
    uncinate process f.
    undisplaced f.
    unicondylar f.
    unimalleolar f.
    unstable f.
    ununited f.
    vertebral body f.
    vertebral stable burst f.
    vertebral wedge compression f.
    vertebra plana f.
    vertical shear f.
    vertical tooth f.
    Volkmann f.
    wagon-wheel f.
    Wagstaffe f.
    Walther f.
    wedge compression f.
    wedge-shaped uncomminuted tibial
      plateau f.
    "western boot" in open f.
    willow f.
    Wilson f.
    Y f.
    Y-T f.
    zygomatic arch f.
    zygomatic maxillary complex f.
    zygomaticomaxillary f.
fracture-dislocation
    atlantoaxial f.-d.
    Bennett f.-d.
    carpometacarpal f.-d.
    Galeazzi f.-d.
    Lisfranc f.-d.
    pedicolaminar f.-d.

    perilunate f.-d.
    posterior f.-d.
    f.-d. reduction
    tarsometatarsal f.-d.
    thoracolumbar spine f.-d.
    tibial plateau f.-d.
    transcapitate f.-d.
    transhamate f.-d.
    transtriquetral f.-d.
    unstable f.-d.
    volar plate arthroplasty
      technique f.-d.
fragilis
    osteosclerosis f.
fragment
    alignment of fracture f.
    articular f.
    autotransplantation of splenic f.
    avascular f.
    avulsed f.
    bone f.
    bony f.
    butterfly fracture f.
    capital f.
    catheter f.
    chondral f.
    cortical f.
    depression of f.
    disk f.
    distal f.
    f. E
    extruded disk f.
    fracture f.
    free disk f.
    free-floating cartilaginous f.
    hinged f.
    Hoskins razor blade f.
    hypervascular f.
    loose f.
    metallic f.
    osteochondral f.
    overriding of fracture f.'s
    placental f.
    residual f.
    retained placental f.
    retropulsion of posterior f.
    trap-door f.
    tuberosity f.
    wedge-shaped uncomminuted f.
fragmentation
    elastic-fiber f.
    electrohydraulic f.
    graft f.
    laser-induced f.
    f. of myocardium
    stone f.
    ultrasonic f.
Fraley syndrome

frame
    Ace-Colles fracture f.
    Ace-Fischer fracture f.
    Ace-Fischer ring f.
    Alexian Brothers overhead
        fracture f.
    Andrews spinal f.
    anterior quadrilateral triplane f.
    f. application
    Balkan fracture f.
    bilateral f.
    Böhler-Braun fracture f.
    Böhler reducing fracture f.
    Bradford fracture f.
    Brooker f.
    Brown-Roberts-Wells head f.
    B-scan f.
    Buck extension f.
    Chalet f.
    Charest head f.
    Chick CLT f.
    CircOlectric f.
    claw-type basic f.
    Codman f.
    Cole hyperextension fracture f.
    Colles external fixation f.
    couch-mounted head f.
    Crawford head f.
    Delta external fixation f.
    external fixator f.
    fixator f.
    halo fracture f.
    halo head f.
    Hoffmann-Vidal-Adrey f.
    implant superstructure f.
    ramus f.
    xylonite f.
framework
    implant f.
Franceschetti
    F. coreoplasty operation
    F. corepraxy operation
    F. deviation operation
    F. keratoplasty operation
    F. pupil deviation operation
    F. syndrome
Franco triflange ventilation tube
Frangenheim-Goebell-Stoeckel operation
frank
    f. dislocation
    f. nonsurgical perineal autodilation
    f. permanent gastrotomy technique

    F. procedure
    F. technique of dilation
Fränkel
    F. head band
    F. neurologic deficit classification
    F. white line
Frankenhäuser ganglion
Frankfort
    F. horizontal light line
    F. horizontal plane
    F. mandibular incisor angle
    F. mandibular plane angle
Frank-Starling relation
Franz-O'Rahilly classification
frappage therapy
Fraser syndrome
Frater suture
Fraunfelder
    F. "no touch" technique
    F. technique
Fraunhofer line
Frazier
    F. aspirating tube
    F. Britetrac nasal suction tube
    F. incision
    F. nasal suction tube
    F. suction
Frazier-Paparella mastoid suction tube
Frazier-Spiller
    F.-S. operation
    F.-S. rhizotomy
FRC
    functional residual capacity
FreAmine amino acid solution
Frederick-Miller tube
Fredet-Ramstedt
    F.-R. operation
    F.-R. procedure
Fredrickson hyperlipoproteinemia
    classification
Fredrickson, Levy and Lees
    classification
free
    f. bone flap
    f. border of ovary
    f. disk fragment
    f. fat graft
    f. flap transfer
    f. fragment disk
    f. fragment herniation
    f. gingival graft
    f. hepatic venous pressure

F

NOTES

free *(continued)*
    f. jejunal graft
    f. margin of eyelids
    methylparaben f. (MPF)
    f. microsurgical flap
    f. muscle graft
    f. peritoneal fluid
    f. peritoneal graft
    f. skin flap
    f. skin graft
    f. tenia
    f. tenotomy
    f. tissue transfer
free-beam coagulation
Freebody-Bendall-Taylor fusion technique
free-floating cartilaginous fragment
free-hand
    f.-h. method
    f.-h. suturing technique
Freeman
    F. calcaneal fracture classification
    F. solution
freeway space
freeze-cleave method
freeze-dried graft
freeze-etch method
freeze-fracture-etch method
freeze-thawed graft
freezing
    gastric f.
    f. point
Freezone solution
frena (*pl. of* frenum)
frenal
French (Fr)
    F. flap
    F. fracture technique
    F. lateral closing wedge osteotomy
    F. method
    F. plane
    F. scale
    F. supracondylar fracture operation
French/American/British (FAB)
    FAB classification
frenectomy
frenoplasty
frenotomy
Frenta System II feeding pump
frenula (*pl. of* frenulum)
frenulectomy
frenuloplasty
frenulum, pl. **frenula**
    f. of ileocecal valve
    f. linguae
    lingual f.
    f. of lower lip
    f. of Morgagni

    f. of prepuce
    f. preputii
    synovial frenula
    f. of tongue
    f. valvae ileocecalis
frenum, pl. **frena**
    Morgagni f.
    synovial frena
Frenzel maneuver
frequency
    f. modulation
    spectral edge f. (SEF)
    wavelength f.
frequency-difference interferential current therapy
frequency-duration index
fresh tissue allocation
Fresnel membrane
fretum
Freund
    F. anomaly
    F. operation
Friberg microsurgical agglutination test
Fricke operation
friction knot
Friedenwald-Guyton operation
Friedenwald operation
Friede operation
Friedewald approximation
Fried-Green foot procedure
Fried-Hendel tendon technique
fringe
    Richard f.
    synovial f.
FRODO technique
frog-leg
    f.-l. lateral projection
    f.-l. position
Froimson
    F. procedure
    F. technique
Froimson-Oh repair
Fronet fasciotomy
frons
frontal
    f. angle of parietal bone
    f. arteriovenous malformation
    f. artery
    f. belly of occipitofrontalis muscle
    f. bone
    f. border
    f. border of parietal bone
    f. border of sphenoid bone
    f. branch of superficial temporal artery
    f. craniotomy
    f. crest
    f. eminence

f. fontanel
f. foramen
f. gyrectomy
f. lobotomy
f. margin
f. notch
f. plane
f. plane correction
f. process of zygomatic bone
f. projection
f. region of head
f. section
f. sinus
f. sinus fracture
f. sinus mucocele
f. sinus septoplasty
f. squama
f. suture
f. triangle
f. tuber
f. veins
frontalis
f. muscle
f. sling technique
frontoanterior position
frontoethmoidal
f. mucocele
f. suture
frontoethmoidectomy
frontolacrimal suture
frontolateral laryngectomy
frontomalar
frontomaxillary
f. suture
frontonasal
f. duct
f. suture
frontonasomaxillary osteotomy
fronto-occipital
fronto-orbital osteotomy
frontoparietal
f. arteriovenous malformation
frontopontine tract
frontoposterior position
frontosphenoidal process
frontotemporal
f. approach
f. craniotomy
f. tract
frontotemporale
frontotransverse position

frontozygomatic
f. suture
Froriep induration
Frost
F. procedure
F. stitch
F. suture
frosted liver
Frost-Lang operation
Frouin
quadrangulation of F.
frozen section method
Frumin valve
Frykman
F. distal radius fracture
classification
F. radial fracture classification
FTR
force translation
Fuchs
F. canthorrhaphy operation
F. iris bombe transfixation
operation
F. position
Fukala operation
**Fukunaga-Hayes unbiased jackknife
classification**
fulcrum line
Fulford procedure
fulgurant
fulgurating
fulguration
f. in bladder cancer
electrical f.
electrosurgical f.
endoscopic f.
nephroscopic f.
full
f. cast restoration
f. extension
f. flap in mucogingival surgery
f. shoulder preparation
full-body cutaneous examination
Fuller bivalve trach tube
full-spine radiographic examination
full-surface micro mesh teeth
full-thickness
f.-t. burn
corneal f.-t.
f.-t. corneal graft
f.-t. periodontal flap

F

NOTES

full-thickness *(continued)*
    f.-t. periodontal graft
    f.-t. skin graft
fulminant
    f. hepatitis
    f. hyperpyrexia
function
    atrioventricular nodal f.
    electrophysiologic f.
    neorectal f.
    proctocolectomy with preservation
      of anal sphincter f.
    sinoatrial nodal f.
    splinted in position of f.
functional
    f. activation PET scanning
    f. capacity classification
    f. capacity evaluation
    f. castration
    f. electrical stimulation
    f. endoscopic sinus surgery
    f. neck dissection
    f. neuromuscular stimulation
    f. neurosurgery
    f. orthodontic therapy
    f. prepubertal castration syndrome
    f. repair
    f. residual capacity (FRC)
    f. sphincter
    f. technique
    f. veloplasty
fundal plication
fundament
fundectomy
fundi *(pl. of* fundus)
fundiform ligament of penis
fundoplasty
    270-degree laparoscopic posterior f.
    Gomez f.
    posterior f.
    Thal f.
fundoplication
    Belsey Mark II, IV f.
    Belsey Mark IV 240-degree f.
    Belsey partial f.
    Belsey two-thirds wrap f.
    Collis-Nissen f.
    Dor f.
    floppy Nissen f.
    Heller myotomy with Dor f.
    intrathoracic Nissen f.
    laparoscopic Nissen f.
    modified Belsey f.
    f. of Nissen
    Nissen 360-degree wrap f.
    Nissen-Rosseti f.
    Rossetti modification of Nissen f.
    slipped Nissen f.

    Thal f.
    total f.
    Toupet f.
    uncut Collis-Nissen f.
fundus, pl. fundi
    coloboma of f.
    f. of gallbladder
    f. gastricus
    f. glands
    f. microscopy
    f. rotation gastroplasty
    f. tympani
    f. uteri
    f. ventriculi
    f. vesicae biliaris (felleae)
    f. vesicae urinariae
funduscopic examination
fundusectomy
fungal infection
fungating
    f. mass
    f. sore
    f. tumor
Fungoid Topical solution
fungous infection
funic reduction
funicular
    f. excision
    f. graft
    f. inguinal hernia
    f. process
funiculopexy
funiculus, pl. funiculi
    f. spermaticus
    f. umbilicalis
funis
funnel
    f. chest deformity
    f. stitch
funnelization of metaphysis
funnel-shaped pelvis
furcal nerve
furcation
    f. canal
    denuded f.
    invaded f.
    root f.
**Furlow-Fisher modification of Virag 1
   operation**
Furnas-Haq-Somers technique
furrier suture
furrow
    corneal marginal f.
    digital f.
    mentolabial f.
fusiform
    f. aneurysm
    f. dilatation

f. excision
f. flap
fusing point
fusion
    Adkins spinal f.
    Albee spinal f.
    amplitude of f.
    Anderson ankle f.
    ankle f.
    anterior cervical diskectomy and f.
    anterior lumbar vertebral
      interbody f.
    anterior spinal f.
    f. area
    atlantoaxial f.
    atlanto-occipital f.
    Bailey-Badgley cervical spine f.
    binaural f.
    binocular f.
    Blair f.
    Bosworth spinal f.
    Bradford f.
    Brooks type f.
    calcaneotibial f.
    central f.
    centric f.
    cervical interbody f.
    cervical spine posterior f.
    Chandler hip f.
    Charnley compression-type knee f.
    Chuinard-Peterson ankle f.
    clothespin H spinal f.
    Cloward anterior spinal f.
    Cloward back f.
    color f.
    Coltart calcaneotibial f.
    commissural f.
    f. complex
    convex f.
    Copeland-Howard scapulothoracic f.
    4-corner midcarpal f.
    Davis f.
    Dewar posterior cervical f.
    DIP f.
    distal tibiofibular f.
    dowel spinal f.
    entrainment with concealed f.
    extra-articular hip f.
    extra-articular subtalar f.
    eyelid f.
    f. of eyelids
    f. facet

facet f.
f. faculty
faculty f.
f. fascia
first-grade f.
Gallie spinal f.
Gallie subtalar ankle f.
Glissane ankle f.
f. grade
Hall facet f.
Harris-Smith cervical f.
Henry-Geist spinal f.
H-graft f.
Hibbs-Jones spinal f.
Horwitz-Adams ankle f.
f. implantation
interbody spinal f.
interfacet wiring and f.
intertransverse f.
intra-articular knee f.
joint f.
Kellogg-Speed lumbar spinal f.
King intra-articular hip f.
knee f.
labial f.
Langenskiöld f.
lateral f.
long segment spinal f.
lower cervical spine f.
lumbar spinal f.
lumbar spine f.
lumbar vertebral interbody f.
lumbosacral f.
lunotriquetral f.
motor f.
müllerian duct f.
naviculocuneiform f.
f. nonunion rate
occipitocervical f.
pantalar f.
f. peptide
peripheral f.
posterior cervical f.
posterior-interbody lumbar spinal f.
posterior-lateral lumbar spinal f.
posterior lumbar interbody f.
  (PLIF)
posterior spinal f.
posterolateral interbody f.
posterolateral lumbosacral f.
radiolunate f.
radioscaphoid f.

F

NOTES

fusion *(continued)*
    f. reflex
    robertsonian f.
    Robinson cervical spine f.
    root f.
    sacral spine f.
    scaphocapitate f.
    scapulothoracic f.
    second-grade f.
    selective thoracic spine f.
    sensory f.
    short segment spinal f.
    Simmons cervical spine f.
    single-level spinal f.
    f. in situ
    in situ spinal f.
    Smith-Petersen sacroiliac joint f.
    Smith-Robinson anterior f.
    Smith-Robinson cervical f.
    Smith-Robinson interbody f.
    Soren ankle f.
    spinal f.
    splenogonadal f.
    Stamm procedure for intra-articular
      hip f.
    f. stiffness
    symmetric vertebral f.
    talocalcaneal f.

    talonavicular f.
    f. technique
    third-grade f.
    thoracic facet f.
    thoracic spinal f.
    tibiofibular f.
    tibiotalar f.
    tibiotalocalcaneal f.
    tissue f.
    trapeziometacarpal f.
    triscaphe f.
    f. tube
    two-stage hip f.
    upper cervical spine f.
    urethrohymenal f.
    vertebral f.
    Watkins f.
    Watson scaphotrapeziotrapezoidal f.
    f. welding
    White posterior ankle f.
    whole-arm f.
    Wilson ankle f.
    Wiltberger f.
    Wiltse bilateral lateral f.
    Winter convex f.
fusion-free position
Futcher line

GA
   general anesthesia
Gabastou hydraulic method
Gabriel Tucker tube
Gaenslen
   G. fracture
   G. split-heel incision
   G. split-heel technique
Gailliard-Arlt suture
galactocele
galactophorous
   g. canals
   g. ducts
Galanti-Giusti colorimetric method
Galbiati bilateral fetal ischiopubiotomy
galea
   g. aponeurotica
Galeati glands
galeatomy
Galeazzi
   G. fracture
   G. fracture-dislocation
   G. patellar operation
Galen
   G. anastomosis
   G. nerve
galenic
   g. preparation
   g. venous malformation
gall
   g. bladder
   g. duct
gallamine triethiodide
gallbladder, gall bladder
   adenomyoma of g.
   g. carcinoma
   g. duplication
   g. ectopia
   g. ejection rate
   endoscopic transpapillary catheter of
     the g.
   g. fossa
   mucocele of g.
   nonvisualization of g.
   g. perforation
   perforation of g.
   porcelain g.
   stasis g.
gallbladder-vena cava line
Gallego differentiating solution
Gallie
   G. atlantoaxial fusion technique
   G. procedure
   G. spinal fusion
   G. subtalar ankle fusion

   G. transplant
   G. wiring technique
gallstone
   g. formation
   g. migration
   silent g.'s
GALT
   gut-associated lymphoid tissue
galvanic stimulation
galvanocautery
galvanosurgery
Galveston
   G. pelvic fixation
   G. technique
Gambee suture
Gambro oxygenator
gamekeeper thumb dislocation
gamete
   g. manipulation
   g. micromanipulation
Gamgee tissue
gamma
   g. irradiation
   g. thalamotomy
gamma-loop disorder
Gamna-Gandy body
ganglia (*pl. of* ganglion)
gangliated
   g. cord
   g. nerve
gangliectomy
gangliocytoma
ganglioglioma
gangliolysis
   percutaneous radiofrequency g.
ganglioma
   intracerebral g.
ganglion, pl. ganglia
   aberrant g.
   Acrel g.
   Andersch g.
   aorticorenal ganglia
   ganglia aorticorenalia
   Arnold g.
   Auerbach ganglia
   auricular g.
   ganglia of autonomic plexuses
   g. blockage
   g. blocker
   Bock g.
   carotid g.
   celiac ganglia
   ganglia celiaca
   g. cervicale inferius
   g. cervicale medium

G

ganglion *(continued)*
  g. cervicale superius
  cervicothoracic g.
  g. cervicothoracicum
  g. ciliare
  ciliary g.
  coccygeal g.
  dorsal root g.
  Ehrenritter g.
  g. extracraniale
  g. of facial nerve
  Frankenhäuser g.
  gasserian g.
  geniculate g.
  g. geniculi
  hypogastric ganglia
  g. impar
  inferior cervical g.
  inferior mesenteric g.
  inferior g. of vagus nerve
  g. inferius nervi glossopharyngei
  g. inferius nervi vagi
  ganglia intermedia
  intermediate ganglia
  g. of intermediate nerve
  intervertebral g.
  intracranial g.
  jugular g.
  Laumonier g.
  Lee g.
  Lobstein g.
  Ludwig g.
  ganglia lumbalia
  lumbar ganglia
  Meckel g.
  g. mesentericum inferius
  g. mesentericum superius
  middle cervical g.
  g. of nervus intermedius
  nodose g.
  otic g.
  g. oticum
  parasympathetic ganglia
  paravertebral ganglia
  pelvic ganglia
  ganglia pelvica
  petrosal g.
  phrenic ganglia
  ganglia phrenica
  ganglia plexuum autonomicorum
  prevertebral ganglia
  pterygopalatine g.
  g. pterygopalatinum
  Remak ganglia
  renal ganglia
  ganglia renalia
  Ribes g.
  sacral ganglia

  ganglia sacralia
  Scarpa g.
  Schacher g.
  semilunar g.
  solar ganglia
  sphenopalatine g.
  spinal g.
  g. spinale
  splanchnic g.
  g. splanchnicum
  stellate g.
  g. stellatum
  sublingual g.
  g. sublinguale
  superior cervical g.
  superior g. of glossopharyngeal
    nerve
  superior mesenteric g.
  superior g. of vagus nerve
  g. superius nervi glossopharyngei
  g. superius nervi vagi
  ganglia of sympathetic trunk
  terminal g.
  g. terminale
  thoracic ganglia
  ganglia thoracica
  trigeminal g.
  g. trigeminale
  ganglia trunci sympathici
  g. of trunk of vagus
  vertebral g.
  g. vertebrale
  vestibular g.
  g. vestibulare
  Vieussens ganglia
  Walther g.
ganglionated
ganglionectomy
  dorsal root g.
  Meckel sphenopalatine g.
  sphenopalatine g.
  superior cervical g.
ganglioneuroblastoma
ganglioneuroma
ganglionic
  g. blockade
  g. branches of lingual nerve
  g. branches of maxillary nerve
  g. branch of internal carotid artery
ganglionostomy
gangrene
  Meleney g.
  pressure g.
gangrenosum
  ecthyma g.
gangrenous granulomatous inflammation
Ganley technique
Gant osteotomy

gantry rotation
Ganzfeld stimulation
gap
Bochdalek g.
fracture g.
interincisor g.
Garamycin injection
Garceau
G. cheilectomy
G. tendon technique
garden
G. femoral neck fracture
G. femoral neck fracture
classification
g. spade deformity
Gardner
G. meningocele repair
G. operation
Garré
sclerosing osteomyelitis of G.
Garrett orientation line
Gartland
G. classification of humeral
supracondylar fracture
G. procedure
G. Universal radial fracture
classification
Gartner
G. canal
G. duct
Gärtner method
gas
g. abscess
anesthetic g.
g. anesthetic
arterial blood g.
G. Check blood analyzer
g. chromatography
g. chromatography-mass
spectrometry
g. clearance method
g. collection
g. contamination
g. cylinder
g. density line
g. embolism
g. endarterectomy
g. exchange
extraluminal g.
extravasation g.
inspired g.
g. insufflation

g. isotope ratio mass spectrometry
laughing g.
nonanesthetic g.
partial pressure of CO_2 g.
g. sterilization
venous blood g.
volume of expired g.
xenon g.
gaseous
g. dilatation
g. laparoscopy
g. laparoscopy method
g. laparoscopy procedure
g. laparoscopy technique
gas-fluid exchange
gas-forming pyogenic liver infection
Gaskell bridge
gasless
g. laparoscopic approach
g. laparoscopy
g. laparoscopy method
g. laparoscopy procedure
g. laparoscopy technique
gas-producing streptococcal infection
gasserian
g. ganglion
g. ganglion blockade
gaster
gastrectasis
gastrectomy
Billroth I, II g.
Billroth I partial g.
distal g.
esophagoproximal g.
high subtotal g.
Hofmeister g.
Horsley g.
palliative total g.
partial g.
Pólya g.
proximal g.
radical g.
subtotal g.
total g.
gastric
g. accommodation test
g. adenocarcinoma
g. angioma
g. area
g. arteries
g. arteriovenous malformation
g. augment and single pedicle tube

G

NOTES

gastric *(continued)*
- g. balloon implantation
- g. branches of anterior vagal trunk
- g. branches of posterior vagal trunk
- g. bypass
- g. bypass procedure
- g. bypass surgery
- g. calculus
- g. canal
- g. carcinoma
- g. cardia
- g. coin removal
- g. compression
- g. decompression
- g. dilation
- g. distention
- g. duplication
- g. electrical stimulation
- g. emptying procedure (GEP)
- g. epithelial cell infiltration
- g. fistula
- g. fluid aspiration
- g. folds
- g. foreign body
- g. freezing
- g. fundus wrap
- g. glands
- g. hemorrhage
- g. hernia
- g. impression
- g. insufflation
- g. lesion
- g. mass
- g. mucosa
- g. mucosal barrier
- g. mucosal pattern classification
- g. pacemaker region
- g. perforation
- g. pit
- g. plexuses of autonomic system
- g. polypectomy
- g. pouch
- g. pressure
- g. pull-through procedure
- g. reduction surgery
- g. residue examination
- g. rupture
- g. stapling
- g. tonometry
- g. ulceration
- g. valve tightening
- g. valve tightening method
- g. valve tightening procedure
- g. valve tightening technique
- g. variceal bleeding
- g. veins
- g. volvulus

gastricus
gastrinoma
gastroanastomosis
gastrocardiac
gastrocele
gastrocnemius
- g. flap
- lateral head of g.

gastrocolic
- g. fistula
- g. ligament
- g. omentum

gastrocolostomy
gastrocplasty
- V-Y g.

gastrocutaneous fistula
gastrocystoplasty
gastrodiaphragmatic ligament
gastroduodenal
- g. artery
- g. fistula
- g. lymph nodes
- g. mucosal protection
- g. orifice

gastroduodenopancreatectomy
gastroduodenoscopy
gastroduodenostomy
- Billroth I g.
- Jaboulay g.
- vagotomy and antrectomy with g.

gastroenteric
- g. fistula

gastroenteroanastomosis
gastroenterocolostomy
gastroenteroplasty
gastroenteroptosis
gastroenterostomy
- Balfour g.
- Billroth I, II g.
- Braun-Jaboulay g.
- Courvoisier g.
- Finney g.
- Heineke-Mikulicz g.
- Hofmeister g.
- percutaneous g.
- Pólya g.
- Roux-en-Y g.
- Schoemaker g.
- g. stoma
- truncal vagotomy and g.
- Von Haberer g.
- Wölfler g.

gastroenterotomy
gastroepiploic
- g. artery (GEA)
- g. veins

gastroesophageal
- g. hernia

g. variceal plexus
g. vestibule
gastroesophagostomy
gastrogastrostomy
gastrogavage
gastrohepatic
g. omentum
gastroileac augmentation
gastroileostomy
gastrointestinal (GI)
g. anastomosis
g. carcinoma
g. complication
g. complication of radiation therapy
g. endoscopy
g. endothelium
g. fistula
g. infection
g. lesion
g. metastasis
g. stoma
g. surgical gut suture
g. surgical linen suture
g. surgical silk suture
g. tract
g. tract adenocarcinoma
g. tract hemorrhage
g. tract obstruction
g. tube
g. ulceration
gastrointestinal-associated lymphoid tissue
gastrojejunal loop obstruction syndrome
gastrojejunocolic
g. fistula
gastrojejunostomy
antecolic long-loop isoperistaltic g.
Billroth II g.
compression button g.
loop g.
partial inferior retrocolic end-to-side g.
partial superior retrocolic end-to-side g.
retrocolic end-to-side g.
Roux-en-Y g.
total retrocolic end-to-side g.
gastrokinesograph
gastrolavage
gastrolienal
g. ligament
gastrolith

gastrolithiasis
gastrolysis
Gastrolyte oral solution
gastromelus
gastronesteostomy
gastro-omental arteries
gastropancreatic folds
gastroparesis
postvagotomy g.
gastropexy
Boerema anterior g.
Hill posterior g.
gastrophrenic
g. ligament
gastroplasty
Collis g.
Eckhout vertical g.
fundus rotation g.
Gomez horizontal g.
greater curvature banded g.
horizontal g.
Laws g.
Mason vertical banded g.
O'Leary lesser curvature g.
silicone elastomer ring vertical g.
Stamm g.
tubular vertical g.
unbanded g.
vertical banded g. (VBG)
vertical Silastic ring g.
gastropleural fistula
gastroplication
gastropneumonic
gastroptosis
gastroptyxis
gastropulmonary
gastropylorectomy
gastropyloric
gastrorrhagia
gastrorrhaphy
gastrorrhexis
gastroschisis
gastroscopic
gastroscopy
high-magnification g.
infrared transillumination g.
gastrosphincteric pressure gradient
gastrosplenic
g. ligament
g. omentum
gastrostaxis
gastrostenosis

G

NOTES

gastrostogavage
gastrostolavage
gastrostomy
    Beck g.
    button one-step g.
    Depage-Janeway g.
    dual percutaneous endoscopic g.
    endoscopic g.
    g. feeding
    feeding g.
    g. feeding tube
    Glassman g.
    Kader g.
    Olympus g.
    palliative g.
    Partipilo g.
    percutaneous endoscopic g. (PEG)
    Russell percutaneous endoscopic g.
    g. scarring
    Ssabanejew-Frank g.
    Stamm g.
    Surgitek One-Step percutaneous
      endoscopic g.
    g. tube migration
    ultrasound-assisted percutaneous
      endoscopic g.
    venting percutaneous g.
    Witzel g.
gastrotomy
gastrulation
gate
    spinal g.
gated technique
Gatellier-Chastang
    G.-C. ankle approach
    G.-C. incision
    G.-C. posterolateral approach
Gatron nerve stimulator
Gauderer-Ponsky PEG operation
gauge
    Bourdon tube pressure g.
Gaur balloon distension technique
gaussian line
gauze dissection
gavage
Gavard muscle
Gavriliu gastric tube
gay
    g. bowel infection
    G. glands
Gayet operation
Gaynor-Hart position
GBH bypass tube
GEA
    gastroepiploic artery
    GEA graft
Geenen sphincterotomy

gelatin
    g. compression body
    glycerinated g.
    g. Hank buffered solution
gelatinous
    g. acute inflammation
    g. ascites
    g. infiltration
gelatin-resorcin-formalin glue
gelation
gel filtration
Gelfoam particles transarterial
    embolization treatment
Gell and Coombs classification
Gelman
    G. procedure
    G. technique
gelotripsy
Gelpi-Lowry hysterectomy
Gély suture
gemination
gemistocyte
gemistocytoma
GEM nonlatex medical bag
gena
genal
gender identity formation
gene
    g. induction
    g. replacement therapy
general
    g. adaptation reaction
    g. anesthesia (GA)
    g. anesthetic
    g. anesthetic technique
    g. bloodletting
    g. closure
    g. closure suture
    g. endotracheal anesthesia
    g. radiation
    g. thrust manipulation
generalized
    g. cortical hyperostosis
    g. elastolysis
genetic
    g. anomaly
    g. approach
    g. lesion
gene-transfer therapy
genial
genicula (*pl. of* geniculum)
genicular arteries
geniculate
    g. body
    g. ganglion
geniculocalcarine
    g. radiation
    g. tract

geniculotemporal tract
geniculum, pl. genicula
    g. canalis facialis
    g. of facial canal
    g. of facial nerve
    g. nervi facialis
genioglossal muscle
genioglossus
    g. muscle
geniohyoid
    g. muscle
    g. space
geniohyoideus
genion
genioplasty
    augmentation g.
genital
    g. branch of genitofemoral nerve
    g. branch of iliohypogastric nerve
    g. carcinoma
    g. cord
    g. duct
    g. eminence
    g. gland
    g. infection
    g. organs
    g. papulosquamous lesion
    g. reconstruction
    g. swellings
    g. tract
    g. tract trauma
    g. tract tumor
    g. tubercle
    g. ulceration
genitalia
    ambiguous external g.
    external g.
    indifferent g.
genitals
genitocrural
    g. nerve
genitofemoral
    g. nerve
genitoinguinal ligament
genitoplasty
    feminizing g.
    masculinizing g.
genitourinary (GU)
    g. anomaly
    g. apparatus
    g. evaluation
    g. fistula

    g. infection
    g. lesion
    g. tract
Gennari
    line of G.
genu
    g. of facial canal
    g. valgum deformity
    g. varum deformity
genual
genucubital position
genupectoral position
geographic stippling of nail
geometric
    g. equator
    g. supracondylar extension
      osteotomy
Georgariou cyclodialysis operation
George
    G. Lewis technique
    G. line
Georgia valve
GEP
    gastric emptying procedure
Gepfert procedure
Gerbert-Mellilo method
Gerbert osteotomy
Gerbode annuloplasty
Gerdy
    G. fibers
    G. fontanel
    G. hyoid fossa
    G. tubercle
geriatric anesthesia
Gerlach valvula
germ
    g. line
    g. tube
    g. tube test
German method
germinal
    g. center formation
    g. cords
    g. epithelium
    g. matrix hemorrhage
    g. membrane
germinoma
Gerota
    G. capsule
    G. fascia
Ger technique
Gesell test with Knobloch modification

G

NOTES

gestant anomaly
gestational sac
Gesterol injection
Getty decompression technique
Gey solution
Ghon
> G. complex
> G. primary lesion

GI
> gastrointestinal
> GI pop-off silk suture
> GI tract
> GI tract flora

Giannestras
> G. modification of Lapidus technique
> G. oblique metatarsal osteotomy

giant
> g. cell carcinoma of thyroid gland
> g. cell lesion
> g. cell tumor of bone
> g. cell tumor of lung
> g. cell tumor of tendon sheath
> g. colon
> g. condyloma

Gianturco bird's nest filter
Gianturco-Roehm bird's nest vena cava filter
gibbous
> g. deformity
> g. deformity of the spine

Gibson
> G. approach
> G. incision

Gibson-Piggott osteotomy
Gibson-type incision
Gierke respiratory bundle
Gifford delimiting keratotomy operation
Gigli operation
Gilbert scapular flap
Gilbert-Tamai-Weiland technique
Gilchrist procedure
Giliberty bipolar femoral head
Gill
> G. laminectomy
> G. lesion
> G. massive sliding graft
> G. procedure
> G. sliding graft technique

Gilles operation
Gilliam-Doleris
> G.-D. operation
> G.-D. uterine suspension

Gilliam operation
Gillies
> G. bone graft
> G. scar correction operation

Gillies-Millard cocked-hat technique

Gillis suture
Gill-Jonas modification of Norwood procedure
Gill-Manning-White spondylolisthesis technique
Gillquist
> G. procedure
> G. suction tube

Gillquist-Stille arthroplasty suction tube
Gills-Welsh guillotine port
Gilquist arthroscopy
Gil-Vernet
> G.-V. ileocecal cystoplasty
> G.-V. ileocecal cystoplasty urinary diversion
> G.-V. operation
> G.-V. procedure
> G.-V. technique

Gimbernat ligament
gingiva
> diffuse fibroma of g.

gingival
> g. anatomy
> g. augmentation
> g. cavity
> g. cavity wall
> g. deformity
> g. exudate
> g. exudation
> g. finishing line
> g. fistula
> g. flap
> g. hemorrhage
> g. inflammation
> g. onlay graft
> g. point
> g. position
> g. space
> g. stimulation
> g. tissue
> g. tissue esthetics
> g. zone

gingivectomy
> chemosurgical g.
> Ochsenbein g.

gingivolabial groove
gingivoplasty
ginglymoarthrodial
ginglymoid
> g. joint

ginglymus
> helicoid g.
> lateral g.

Giordano operation
Girard
> G. keratoprosthesis operation
> G. procedure
> G. scleral ring

girdle
    g. anesthesia
    compression g.
    Neptune g.
    pelvic g.
    shoulder g.
    thoracic g.
Girdlestone
    G. hip procedure
    G. laminectomy
    G. resection
    G. resection arthroplasty
Girdlestone-Taylor procedure
Gironcoli hernia
Gittes
    G. operation
    G. procedure
    G. technique
    G. urethropexy
Gittes-Loughlin
    G.-L. bladder neck suspension
    G.-L. procedure
glabella
glabellad
glabellar
    g. bilobed flap
    g. exposure osteotomy
    g. rotation flap
    g. tapping
gladiate
gladiolus
glancing wound
gland
    accessory parotid g.
    accessory suprarenal g.'s
    accessory thyroid g.
    acid g.
    acinic cell tumor of salivary g.
    acinous g.
    admaxillary g.
    adrenal g.
    aggregate g.'s
    agminate g.'s
    Albarran g.'s
    anterior lingual g.
    apical g.
    apocrine g.
    areolar g.'s
    arteriococcygeal g.
    arytenoid g.'s
    axillary sweat g.'s
    Bartholin g.

Bauhin g.
g.'s of biliary mucosa
Blandin g.
Boerhaave g.'s
Bowman g.
brachial g.
bronchial g.'s
Brunner g.'s
bulbourethral g.
cardiac g.'s of esophagus
celiac g.'s
cervical g.'s
cervical g.'s of uterus
circumanal g.'s
coccygeal g.
Cowper g.
cutaneous g.'s
ductless g.'s
duodenal g.'s
Duverney g.
eccrine sweat g.
ectopic sebaceous g.
Eglis g.'s
endocrine g.
esophageal ectopic sebaceous g.
external genitalia/Bartholin, urethral, and Skene g.'s (EG/BUS)
g.'s of the female urethra
fundus g.'s
Galeati g.'s
gastric g.'s
Gay g.'s
genital g.
giant cell carcinoma of thyroid g.
Gley g.'s
greater vestibular g.
Guérin g.'s
Havers g.'s
hematopoietic g.
inguinal g.'s
g.'s of internal secretion
intestinal g.'s
Knoll g.'s
labial g.'s
lactiferous g.
laryngeal g.'s
lesser vestibular g.'s
Lieberkühn g.'s
Littré g.'s
Luschka g.
lymph g.
g.'s of the male urethra

NOTES

G

gland *(continued)*
  mammary g.
  master g.
  meibomian g.'s
  Méry g.
  mesenteric g.'s
  milk g.
  mixed tumor of salivary g.
  Montgomery g.'s
  mucilaginous g.
  muciparous g.
  mucous g.
  Nuhn g.
  odoriferous g.
  oil g.'s
  parathyroid g.
  paraurethral g.'s
  parotid g.
  peptic g.
  perspiratory g.'s
  Peyer g.'s
  pharyngeal g.'s
  pineal g.
  pituitary g.
  Poirier g.
  prehyoid g.
  preputial g.'s
  prostate g.
  pyloric g.'s
  Rivinus g.
  Rosenmüller g.
  seminal g.
  seromucous g.
  serous g.
  sexual g.
  Skene g.'s
  solitary g.'s
  sublingual g.
  sudoriferous g.'s
  suprahyoid g.
  suprarenal g.
  sweat g.'s
  synovial g.'s
  target g.
  thymus g.
  thyroid g.
  tracheal g.'s
  trachoma g.
  Tyson g.'s
  urethral g.'s
  uterine g.'s
  vaginal g.
  vesical g.
  vestibular g.'s
  vulvovaginal g.
  Waldeyer g.'s
  Wasmann g.'s
  Wepfer g.'s

  Wölfler g.
  Zeis g.'s
glandes (*pl. of* glans)
glandula, pl. **glandulae**
  glandulae areolares
  g. atrabiliaris
  g. basilaris
  glandulae bronchiales
  g. bulbourethralis
  glandulae cervicales uteri
  glandulae circumanales
  glandulae cutis
  glandulae duodenales
  glandulae endocrinae
  glandulae esophageae
  glandulae gastricae
  glandulae intestinales
  glandulae labiales
  glandulae laryngeae
  g. lingualis anterior
  g. mammaria
  g. mucosa
  g. parathyroidea
  g. parotidea
  g. parotidea accessoria
  g. parotis
  g. parotis accessoria
  glandulae pharyngeae
  g. pituitaria
  glandulae preputiales
  glandulae propriae
  g. prostatica
  glandulae pyloricae
  glandulae sebaceae
  g. seminalis
  g. seromucosa
  g. serosa
  glandulae sine ductibus
  g. sublingualis
  glandulae sudoriferae
  glandulae suprarenales accessoriae
  g. suprarenalis
  g. thyroidea
  g. thyroidea accessoria
  glandulae tracheales
  glandulae tubariae
  glandulae urethrales femininae
  glandulae urethrales masculinae
  glandulae uterinae
  glandulae vestibulares minores
  g. vestibularis major
glandular
  g. branches
  g. branches of facial artery
  g. branches of inferior thyroid artery
  g. branches of submandibular ganglion

g. carcinoma
g. substance of prostate
g. tissue
glandulectomy
glandulopexy
glans, pl. **glandes**
g. clitoridis
g. of clitoris
g. penis
glansplasty
meatal advancement and g.
glanuloplasty
glaserian fissure
Glasgow
G. Coma Scale
G. Coma Score
glass
Worst corneal contact g.
glass-bead retention method
Glasser gastrostomy tube
Glassman gastrostomy
glass-rod
g.-r. negative phenomenon
g.-r. positive phenomenon
glass-wool filtration
glassy membrane
glaucoma surgery
glaucomatous
g. cul-de-sac
g. excavation
g. ring
Gleason score
Gledhill technique
Gleich
G. osteotomy
G. osteotomy for pes valgo planus
Glen
G. Anderson technique
G. Anderson ureteroneocystostomy
Glenn
G. anastomosis
G. operation
G. procedure
glenohumeral
g. adhesive capsulitis
g. articulation
g. dislocation repair
g. joint dislocation
glenoid
g. cavity
g. fossa
g. osteotomy

g. point
g. rim fracture
g. surface
glenoplasty
posterior g.
Scott posterior g.
Gley glands
glial ring
gliding-hole-first technique
gliding joint
glioblastoma
glioma
g. of retina
g. sarcomatosum
glioma-polyposis
gliomatous
glioneuroma
gliosarcoma
gliosis
gliotic membrane
Glissane ankle fusion
Glisson
G. capsule
G. sphincter
globe
globular collection
globus, pl. **globi**
g. major
g. minor
glomangioma
glomangiomatous osseous malformation syndrome
glomangiosarcoma
glomangiosis
pulmonary g.
glomectomy
glomera aortica
glomerular
g. basement membrane
g. basement membrane disease
g. capillary pressure
g. capsule
g. crescent
g. extracellular matrix
g. filtration
g. filtration rate
g. hyperfiltration
g. macrophage infiltration
g. neutrophil infiltration
g. tip lesion
g. ultrafiltration
glomerulation

G

NOTES

glomeruli (*pl. of* glomerulus)
glomerulitis
glomerulonephritis
glomerulus, pl. **glomeruli**
    g. of mesonephros
    g. of pronephros
glomus
    g. arteriovenous malformation
    g. body
    g. coccygeum
    g. intravagale
    g. jugulare
glossectomy
    Commando radical g.
    partial g.
    subtotal g.
    total g.
glossocinesthetic
glossopharyngeal
    g. nerve
glossopharyngeus
glossoplasty
glossorrhaphy
glossoscopy
glossotomy
    labiomandibular g.
    median labiomandibular g.
glottic
    g. carcinoma
    g. closure
glove anesthesia
gloved-fist technique
glover
    G. suction tube
    g. suture
    G. suture technique
glow modulator tube
glucagonoma syndrome
glucose oxidase method
glucuronidation
glue
    fibrin g.
    gelatin-resorcin-formalin g.
    g. patch
    g. patch leak
    tissue g.
glue-in suture
glutaraldehyde sterilization
glutaraldehyde-tanned
    g.-t. bovine collagen tube
    g.-t. bovine graft
glutathione modification
gluteal
    g. hernia
    g. line
    g. lymph nodes
    region

gluteofemoral
    g. bursa
gluteoinguinal
glutethimide
gluteus
    g. maximus flap
    g. maximus muscle
    g. medius bursae
    g. minimus bursa
glycerinated
    g. extract
    g. gelatin
glycerin method
glycerin-preserved graft
glycerol
    g. chemoneurolysis
    g. rhizotomy
glycogen infiltration
glycopyrrolate
Glynn-Neibauer technique
gnathic index
gnathoplasty
gnathoschisis
goblet incision
Godman fascia
Goebell-Frangenheim-Stoeckel technique
Goebell procedure
Goebell-Stoeckel-Frangenheim procedure
Goethe bone
Goffe colporrhaphy
Gohil-Cavolo method
goiter
Golaski knitted Dacron graft
gold
    g. foil condensation
    g. plate technique
    g. ring
    g. seed implantation technique
    g. weight and wire spring
    operation
Goldberg technique
Goldblatt
    G. kidney
    G. phenomenon
Golden closing wedge osteotomy
Goldman
    G. classification
    G. classification operative risk
    G. vaporizer
Goldmann
    G. coherent radiation
    G. kinetic technique
    G. static technique
Goldmann-Larson
    G.-L. foreign body
    G.-L. foreign body operation
Goldner-Clippinger technique
Goldner-Hayes procedure

Goldner reconstruction
Goldsmith operation
Goldstein spinal fusion technique
Goldthwait-Hauser procedure
golf-hole ureteral orifice
Golgi membrane
Goligher extraperitoneal ileostomy
GoLYTELY solution
Gomco
    G. suction
    G. suction tube
    G. technique
Gomez
    G. fundoplasty
    G. horizontal gastroplasty
    G. horizontal gastroplasty with
      reinforced stoma
Gomez-Marquez lacrimal operation
gomitoli
gomphosis
gonad
    female g.
    male g.
gonadal
    g. complication
    g. cords
    g. endocrine disorder
gonadectomy
gonadoblastoma
gonadopathy
gonadorelin hydrochloride
gonadotrophic
gonaduct
gonangiectomy
gonatocele
gonecyst
gonecystolith
Gonin cautery operation
gonioma
goniophotocoagulation
gonioplasty
gonioscopy
    indentation g.
goniotomy
    g. operation
gonocele
gonococcal infection
gonodoblastoma
Goodall-Power operation
Goode
    G. Trim tube
    G. T-tube ventilating tube

Good 'N Bed wedge
Goodwin
    G. cup-patch principle
    G. technique
Goodwin-Hohenfellner technique
Goodwin-Scott technique
gooseneck deformity
Gordon
    G. approach
    G. body
    G. elementary body
    G. joint injection technique
Gordon-Broström technique
Gordon-Taylor
    G.-T. hindquarter amputation
    G.-T. technique
Gore-Tex
    G.-T. AF fistula
    G.-T. aortofemoral fistula
    G.-T. cardiovascular patch
    G.-T. jump graft
    G.-T. nonabsorbable suture
    G.-T. soft tissue patch
    G.-T. surgical membrane
    G.-T. tube
    G.-T. vascular graft
Gorlin-Chaudhry-Moss syndrome
gossamer silk suture
Gosselin fracture
Gothic arch formation
Gott tube
Gouffon pin fixation
Gould
    G. ES 1000 recorder
    G. Godard pneumotachograph
    G. procedure
    G. suture
    G. suture technique
Gould-Brush 481 eight-channel recorder
Goulding procedure
Gowers
    G. solution
    G. tract
grabbing technique
gracilis
    g. flap technique
    g. muscle flap
    g. procedure
graciloplasty
    dynamic g.
gradation
    Levine g. 1–6 of cardiac murmurs

G

NOTES

grade

    fusion g.

    g. I, II oscillation

    g.'s of mobilization

    g. 1–5 mobilization

graded

    g. exposure

    g. spinal anesthesia

gradient

    alveolocapillary partial pressure g.

    aortic pressure g.

    aortic valve g.

    biliary-duodenal pressure g.

    Doppler pressure g.

    duodenobiliary pressure g.

    gastrosphincteric pressure g.

    hepatic venous pressure g.

    intracavitary pressure g.

    g. method

    mitral valve g.

    peak systolic g. (PSG)

    peak transaortic valve g.

    pressure g.

    pullback pressure g.

    pulmonary valve g.

    temperature g.

    transaortic valve g.

    transcapillary hydrostatic pressure g.

    transmural hydrostatic pressure g.

gradient-echo

    2DFT g.-e. imaging

    3DFT g.-e. MR imaging

    g.-e. method

    g.-e. MR image

    g.-e. MR imaging

gradient-recalled

    g.-r. echo image

    multiple planar g.-r. (MPGR)

gradient-reversal fat suppression method

grading of manipulation

Gradle keratoplasty operation

graduated

    g. compression stocking

    g. tenotomy

Graefenberg ring

Graefe operation

Grafco Martin laryngectomy tube

graft

    AAA bone g.

    accordion g.

    acetabular augmentation g.

    acrylic g.

    adipodermal g.

    adipose g.

    advancement flap g.

    Albee bone g.

    albumin-coated vascular g.

    albuminized woven Dacron tube g.

    aldehyde-tanned bovine carotid artery g.

    AlloDerm universal dermal tissue g.

    allogeneic fetal g.

    allogenic bone g.

    allogenous bone g.

    alloplastic g.

    alveolar cleft g.

    Amsler corneal g.

    anastomosed g.

    g. anastomosis

    animal g.

    annular corneal g.

    antebrachial fascial g.

    anterior sliding tibial g.

    anterosuperior iliac spine g.

    aorticorenal g.

    aortic tube g.

    aortocoronary bypass g.

    aortocoronary snake g.

    aortoenteric g.

    aortofemoral bypass g.

    aortohepatic arterial g.

    aortoiliac bypass g.

    araldehyde-tanned bovine carotid artery g.

    arterial bypass g.

    augmentation g.

    auricular cartilage g.

    autoclaved g.

    autodermic g.

    autogeneic g.

    autogenous bone g.

    autogenous dermis fat g.

    autogenous fibular g.

    autogenous tunica vaginalis g.

    autogenous vein bypass g.

    autologous fat g.

    autologous iliac crest bone g.

    autologous rib bone g.

    autologous vein g.

    autoplastic g.

    AV Gore-Tex g.

    axillobifemoral bypass g.

    Banks bone g.

    Bard PTFE g.

    basilic vein g.

    batten g.

    B-B g.

    g. bed

    Berens g.

    bicondylar g.

    bifemoral g.

    bifid g.

    bifurcated vascular g.

    bilateral myocutaneous g.

    Biocoral g.

Biograft g.
Bionit vascular g.
BioPolyMeric femoropopliteal
 bypass g.
BioPolyMeric vascular g.
Björk-Shiley g.
Blair-Brown skin g.
bone autogenous g.
bone marrow g.
bone peg g.
bone-tendon-bone g.
bone-to-bone g.
Bonfiglio bone g.
Boplant g.
bovine g.
Boyd dual onlay bone g.
branched vascular g.
Braun-Wangensteen g.
brephoplastic g.
Brescia-Cimino g.
Brett bone g.
bridge g.
buccal mucosal patch g.
bulk g.
B-W g.
bypass g.
C g.
cable g.
cadaver g.
Calcitite bone g.
Campbell onlay bone g.
cancellous chip bone g.
cancellous and cortical bone g.
cancellous insert g.
cantilevered bone g.
carbon fiber g.
Carbo-Seal cardiovascular
 composite g.
carotid-vertebral vein bypass g.
cartilage g.
cephalic vein g.
chessboard g.'s
chip g.
Clancy patellar tendon g.
clip g.
clothespin spinal fusion g.
Codivilla bone g.
collagen-impregnated knitted Dacron
 velour g.
compilation autogenous vein g.
composite rib g.
composite skin g.

compressed Ivalon patch g.
conjunctival patch g.
connective tissue g.
Cooley woven Dacron g.
corneal g.
coronary artery bypass g. (CABG)
cortical bone g.
cortical strut g.
corticocancellous bone g.
costal cartilage g.
Cotton cartilage g.
Cragg endoluminal g.
Creech aortoiliac g.
Crescent corneal g.
cross-facial nerve g.
Cryolife valve g.
cutis g.
Dacron aortic bifurcation g.
Dacron aortobifemoral g.
Dacron interposition g.
Dacron knitted g.
Dacron preclotted g.
Dacron Sauvage g.
Dacron tightly-woven g.
Dacron tube g.
Dacron velour g.
Dacron Weave Knit g.
Daniel iliac bone g.
Dardik umbilical g.
Davis muscle-pedicle g.
DeBakey g.
delayed g.
demineralized bone g.
Dermagraft g.
dermal g.
dermal-fat g.
dermis patch g.
devitalized bone g.
diamond inlay bone g.
Diastat vascular access g.
discrete blood supply to a bone g.
donor iliac Y g.
dorsal vein patch g.
double-looped gracilis g.
double papilla pedicle g.
double velour knitted g.
Douglas g.
dowel bone g.
Dragstedt g.
dual onlay cortical bone g.
Edwards-Tapp arterial g.

NOTES

G

287

graft *(continued)*

Edwards woven Teflon aortic
bifurcation g.
endovascular g.
epidermic g.
EPTFE g.
Esser g.
expanded polytetrafluoroethylene
vascular g.
g. expulsion
EXS femoropopliteal bypass g.
extra-articular g.
g. failure
fascial g.
fascia lata freeze-thawed g.
fascicular g.
fat g.
fat-patch g.
Favaloro saphenous vein bypass g.
femoropopliteal bypass g.
femur g.
FEP-ringed Gore-Tex vascular g.
fiberglass g.
fibular strut g.
filler g.
filleted g.
fillet local flap g.
g. fixation
Flanagan-Burem apposing
hemicylindric g.
flap g.
flat bone g.
flexor tendon g.
Forbes onlay bone g.
g. fragmentation
free fat g.
free gingival g.
free jejunal g.
free muscle g.
free peritoneal g.
free skin g.
freeze-dried g.
freeze-thawed g.
full-thickness corneal g.
full-thickness periodontal g.
full-thickness skin g.
funicular g.
GEA g.
Gillies bone g.
Gill massive sliding g.
gingival onlay g.
glutaraldehyde-tanned bovine g.
glycerin-preserved g.
Golaski knitted Dacron g.
Gore-Tex jump g.
Gore-Tex vascular g.
H g.
Haldeman bone g.

hamstring g.
Hancock pericardial valve g.
Hancock vascular g.
Harris superior acetabular g.
g. harvest
Hemashield collagen-enhanced g.
hemicondylar g.
hemicylindrical bone g.
Henderson onlay bone g.
Henry bone g.
heterodermic g.
heterogeneous g.
heterogenous g.
heterologous g.
heteroplastic g.
heterospecific g.
heterotopic g.
Hey-Groves-Kirk bone g.
H-graft bone g.
HLA identical kidney g.
Hoaglund bone g.
homogeneous g.
homogenous g.
homologous g.
homoplastic g.
Horton-Devine dermal g.
human dural substitute g.
Huntington bone g.
HUV bypass g.
hydroxyapatite g.
hyperplastic g.
IEA g.
iliac crest bone g.
iliac crest-inlay g.
iliac slot g.
iliac strut bone g.
IMA g.
g. impingement
implantation g.
Impra bypass g.
Impra Flex vascular g.
Impra-Graft microporous PTFE
vascular g.
Impra microporous PTFE
vascular g.
Inclan bone g.
g. infection
infusion g.
inlay bone g.
insert g.
in situ tricortical iliac crest block
bone g.
in situ vein g.
interbody bone g.
intercalary g.
interfascicular Millesi nerve g.
internal mammary g. (IMA)
interposition Dacron g.

interposition vein g.
interspecific g.
g. interstices
intracranial-extracranial nerve g.
intracranial-intratemporal nerve g.
intramedullary g.
Ionescu-Shiley pericardial valve g.
Ionescu-Shiley vascular g.
island g.
isogeneic g.
isogenic g.
isologous g.
isoplastic g.
ITA g.
Ivalon compressed patch g.
Jeb g.
Judet g.
jump g.
Kebab g.
Keystone g.
Kiel g.
Kimura cartilage g.
knitted g.
Koenig g.
Krause-Wolfe g.
Kutler V-Y flap g.
lamellar corneal g.
Langenskiöld bone g.
lateral pedicle g.
latex sponge g.
Lee anterosuperior iliac spine g.
Lee bone g.
ligament g.
load-bearing g.
loop forearm g.
Lo-Por vascular g.
lower extremity bypass g.
lyophilized bone g.
mammary artery g.
mandrel g.
Mangoldt epithelial g.
Marlex mesh g.
Marqez-Gomez conjunctival g.
Massie sliding g.
massive sliding g.
matchstick g.
material g.
g. material alternative
Matti-Russe bone g.
McFarland bone g.
McFarland tibial g.
McMaster bone g.

Meadox Microvel double-velour
  Dacron g.
Meadox vascular g.
Mediform dural g.
medullary bone g.
meniscus g.
Mersilene g.
mesenteric bypass g.
mesh g.
methyl methacrylate g.
Meyerding bone g.
Meyers quadratus muscle-pedicle
  bone g.
Microknit patch g.
Microknit vascular g.
Microvel double velour g.
g. migration
Millesi interfascicular g.
Millesi nerve g.
Milliknit g.
Moberg dowel g.
mucoperiosteal periodontal g.
mucosal periodontal g.
mucous membrane g.
Mueller patellar tendon g.
Mules g.
multiple cancellous chip g.
murine g.
muscle pedicle bone g.
muscular g.
mushroom corneal g.
Mustardé g.
nail bed g.
nerve g.
neuromuscular pedicle g.
neurovascular island g.
Nicoll cancellous bone g.
Nicoll cancellous insert g.
nonisometric g.
nontubed closed distant flap g.
nontubed open distant flap g.
Ollier thick split free g.
Ollier-Thiersch g.
omental pedicle flap g.
onlay bone g.
onlay cancellous iliac g.
orthotopic g.
osteoarticular g.
osteochondral g.
osteoperiosteal bone g.
Ostrup vascularized rib g.
Overton dowel g.

G

NOTES

graft *(continued)*
Padgett mesh skin g.
Paladon g.
papilla g.
papillary pedicle g.
Papineau bone g.
paraffin g.
partial-thickness periodontal g.
partial-thickness skin g.
particulate cancellous bone g.
patch g.
patellar tendon g.
pattern-cut corneal g.
pedicle bone g.
pedicle fat g.
peg bone g.
penetrating full-thickness corneal g.
Peri-Guard vascular g.
periosteal g.
Perma-Flow coronary g.
petrous carotid-to-intradural carotid saphenous vein g.
Phemister onlay bone g.
pie-crusting skin g.
pigskin g.
pinch skin g.
g. placement
plantaris tendon g.
plasma TFE vascular g.
Plexiglas g.
Plystan g.
polyethylene g.
Poly-Plus Dacron vascular g.
polytetrafluoroethylene g.
polyurethane g.
polyvinyl g.
porcine skin g.
porous polyethylene g.
portacaval H g.
postage stamp skin g.
posterior bone g.
posterior cruciate ligament g.
posterolateral bone g.
preclotted g.
g. preparation
g. preservation solution
primary skin g.
prophylactic bone g.
Proplast g.
prosthetic arterial g.
PTFE Gore-Tex g.
punch g.'s
Rastelli g.
reanastomosis of blood supply to bone g.
reduced-size g.
g. rejection
renal artery bypass g.

revascularization of g.
Reverdin epidermal free g.
reversed saphenous vein g.
reversed vein g.
rib g.
roof-patch g.
Ruese bone g.
Russe bone g.
Ryerson bone g.
sandwiched iliac bone g.
saphenous vein bypass g.
saphenous vein patch g.
Sauvage Bionit g.
Sauvage Dacron g.
Sauvage filamentous velour g.
SCA-EX 7F g.
scapular g.
scleral patch g.
scotty-dog g.
seamless g.
Seddon nerve g.
segmental liver g.
segmental tendon g.
semitendinosus-gracilis g.
seromuscular intestinal patch g.
serum chemistry g.
Sheen tip g.
Shiley Tetraflex vascular g.
sieve g.
Silastic g.
Silovi saphenous vein g.
Siloxane g.
single-condylar g.
single onlay cortical bone g.
single-stage tendon g.
g. site
skin bone free g.
skip g.
sleeve g.
sliding inlay bone g.
sliding tibial bone g.
snake g.
Solvang g.
Soto-Hall bone g.
soybean lectin T-lymphocyte-depleted marrow g.
Sparks mandrel g.
g. spatulation
Speed osteotomy g.
split calvarial g.
split skin g.
split-thickness periodontal g.
split-thickness skin g.
split thin g.
sponge g.
spongiosa bone g.
spreader g.
Stark g.

Stent g.
St. Jude composite valve g.
g. strength
g. structure
strut g.
subclavian artery bypass g.
subclavius tendon g.
subcutaneous arterial bypass g.
subepithelial connective tissue g.
g. suction tube
suprailiac aortic mesenteric g.
Supramid g.
sural nerve bridge g.
sural nerve cable g.
g. survival
syngeneic g.
synthetic bone g.
synthetic vascular bypass g.
Taylor-Townsend-Corlett iliac crest bone g.
Teflon tube g.
tendon g.
tension-free Millesi nerve g.
Thiersch-Duplay tube g.
Thiersch medium split free g.
Thiersch thin split free g.
Thomas extrapolated bar g.
tibial bone g.
tricortical iliac crest bone g.
tubed free skin g.
tube flap g.
Tudor-Thomas g.
tunnel g.
Varivas R denatured homologous vein g.
vascular bypass g.
vascularized bone g.
vascularized fibular g.
vascularized rib g.
vascular patch g.
g. vasculopathy
Vascutek gelseal vascular g.
Vascutek knitted vascular g.
Vascutek woven vascular g.
vein g.
Velex woven Dacron vascular g.
velour collar g.
venous interposition g.
g. versus host
vertebral artery bypass g.
Vitagraft vascular g.

Weavenit patch g.
wedge g.
Weiland iliac crest bone g.
Wesolowski bypass g.
Wesolowski Teflon g.
white g.
Whitecloud-LaRocca fibular strut g.
Wilson-Jacobs patellar g.
Windson-Insall-Vince bone g.
Wolfe-Kawamoto bone g.
Wolfe-Krause g.
Wolf full-thickness free g.
woven Dacron tube g.
wraparound flap bone g.
xenogeneic g.
Y g.
zooplastic g.
Z-plasty local flap g.

graft-enteric fistula
graft-host interface
grafting
g. anastomosis
coronary artery bypass g. (CABG)
endarterectomy and coronary artery bypass g.
port-access coronary artery bypass g.
surgical patch g.
graft-versus-host
g.-v.-h. disease
g.-v.-h. disease reaction
Graham
G. closure with omental pouch
G. plication
Gram
G. iodine
grammatic method
Gram-negative, gram-negative
G.-n. micro-organism
G.-n. pneumonia
G.-n. sepsis
Gram-positive, gram-positive
G.-p. micro-organism
G.-p. sepsis
Gram-stain morphology
Granger
G. line
G. method
G. projection
granisetron HCl
granny knot

NOTES

G

Grantham
    G. classification of femoral fracture
    G. femur fracture classification
Grant-Small-Lehman supracondylar
  extension osteotomy
Grant-Ward operation
granular
    g. kidney
    g. pits
    g. respiration
granulation
    arachnoid g.
    extradural g.
    pacchionian g.
    g. phase
    red g.
    g. stenosis
    g. tissue
    toxic g.
granule
    extracellular g.
    membrane-coating g.
    ProOsteon Implant 500 g.
    rod g.
    seminal g.
granuloma
granulomatous
    g. bacterial infection
    g. fungal infection
    g. inflammation
    g. tissue
gras
    tulle g.
Graseby
    G. anesthesia pump
    G. 3300 pump
grasping
    g. suture
    g. technique
grasp reflex
grass-line ligature
Grass pressure-recording device
Gratiolet radiation
grattage
Gräupner method
Graves technique
graviditas examnialis
gravimetric technique
gravitation abscess
gravitational
    g. line
    g. particle collection
gravity
    line of g.
    g. line
    g. method of Stimson
gray
    g. hepatization
    g. induration
    g. infiltration
    g. line
    g. patch
    g. rami communicantes
    g. scale examination
grayline incision
gray-white corneal scar
great
    g. anastomotic artery
    g. auricular nerve
    g. cardiac vein
    g. cerebral vein
    g. foramen
    G. Ormond Street pediatric
      tracheostomy tube
    G. Ormond Street tracheostomy
    G. Ormond Street tracheostomy
      tube
    g. pancreatic artery
    g. radicular artery
    g. saphenous vein
    g. superior pancreatic artery
    g. toe
    g. vein of Galen
greater
    g. cul-de-sac
    g. curvature banded gastroplasty
    g. curvature of stomach
    g. curve position
    g. horn of hyoid bone
    g. multangular bone
    g. occipital nerve
    g. omentectomy
    g. omentectomy with splenectomy
    g. omentum
    g. palatine artery
    g. pelvis
    g. peritoneal cavity
    g. peritoneal sac
    g. petrosal nerve
    g. posterior rectus muscle of head
    g. psoas muscle
    g. rhomboid muscle
    g. ring
    g. saphenous phlebectomy
    g. splanchnic nerve
    g. superficial petrosal nerve
    g. supraclavicular fossa
    g. trochanter
    g. trochanteric femoral fracture
    g. tubercle of humerus
    g. tuberosity fracture
    g. vestibular gland
    g. wing of sphenoid bone
    g. zygomatic muscle
Greaves operation

green
- g. braided suture
- g. monofilament polyglyconate suture
- G. procedure

Green-Banks technique

Greenfield
- G. IVC filter
- G. osteotomy
- G. spinocerebellar ataxia classification
- G. titanium inferior vena cava filter

Green-Reverdin osteotomy

greenstick
- g. dorsal proximal metatarsal osteotomy
- g. fixation
- g. fracture

Greenwald and Lewman method

Green-Watermann osteotomy

Greer EZ Access drainage pouch

Gregoir-Lich procedure

Greiling gastroduodenal tube

grenz ray therapy

Greulich-Pyle technique

Grice
- G. incision
- G. procedure

Grice-Green technique

grid
- external g.

gridiron incision

Griffith incision

Grimelius
- G. argyrophil method
- G. technique

Grimsdale operation

griseotomy
- circular g.

Gristina-Webb total shoulder arthroplasty

gristle

Gritti-Stokes
- G.-S. amputation
- G.-S. knee amputation technique

gritty tumor

Grocott-Gomori methenamine-silver method

groin
- g. dissection
- g. exploration
- g. flap
- g. hernia
- g. incision
- g. laparoscopy
- g. mass

grommet
- g. drain tube
- g. ventilating tube

Grondahl esophagoplasty

Grondahl-Finney
- G.-F. esophagogastroplasty
- G.-F. operation

groove
- alar g.
- alveololabial g.
- anterior auricular g.
- arterial g.'s
- auriculoventricular g.
- bicipital g.
- carotid g.
- cavernous g.
- chiasmatic g.
- corneal lamellar g.
- costal g. for subclavian artery
- g. of crus of the helix
- digastric g.
- ethmoidal g.
- g. extension
- gingivolabial g.
- g. of greater petrosal nerve
- inferior petrosal g.
- g. for inferior petrosal sinus
- g. for inferior venae cava
- infraorbital g.
- interosseous g. of calcaneus
- interosseous g. of talus
- intertubercular g.
- lateral bicipital g.
- g. of lesser petrosal nerve
- Lucas g.
- g. of lung for subclavian artery
- medial bicipital g.
- median g. of tongue
- middle meningeal artery g.
- g. for middle temporal artery
- musculospiral g.
- mylohyoid g.
- nail g.
- nasolabial g.
- nasopharyngeal g.
- obturator g.
- occipital g.

NOTES

G

groove *(continued)*
>   palatovaginal g.
>   paraglenoid g.
>   peroneal g.
>   pharyngotympanic g.
>   popliteal g.
>   posterior auricular g.
>   preauricular g.
>   g. of pterygoid hamulus
>   pterygopalatine g.
>   g. for radial nerve
>   Sibson g.
>   skin g.'s
>   g. for spinal nerve
>   spiral g.
>   subclavian g.
>   g. for subclavian vein
>   subcostal g.
>   g. for superior petrosal sinus
>   g. for superior vena cava
>   supra-acetabular g.
>   g. suture
>   transverse anthelicine g.
>   g. for ulnar nerve
>   urethral g.
>   venous g.'s
>   vertebral g.
>   g. for vertebral artery
>   vomerovaginal g.

grooved incision

gross
>   g. deformity
>   g. lesion
>   g. manipulation
>   G. tracheoesophageal fistula

Grosse-Kempf tibial technique

Grossmann operation

ground
>   lateral g. (LG)

ground-glass
>   g.-g. body of Hadziyannis
>   g.-g. lesion

group
>   g. A beta-hemolytic streptococcal
>   infection
>   g. A streptococcus infection
>   g. fascicular repair
>   g. pressure

grouping
>   tumor stage g.

Groves-Goldner technique

growing
>   g. fracture
>   g. point

growth
>   g. acceleration
>   g. arrest line
>   exophytic g.

>   g. plate complex
>   g. retardation
>   tumor g.

Gruber cul-de-sac

Gruber-Landzert fossa

Gruca stabilization

grunt
>   expiratory g.

grunting
>   g. maneuver
>   g. respiration

Grüntzig
>   G. balloon dilation
>   G. technique

Grynfeltt triangle

G syndrome

GU
>   genitourinary

guard
>   hypoxic g.

guarding
>   abdominal g.
>   involuntary g.
>   voluntary g.

gubernacular canal

gubernaculum
>   Hunter g.
>   g. testis

Gubler line

Gudas
>   G. scarf Z-plasty
>   G. scarf Z-plasty osteotomy

Guéneau de Mussy point

Guérin
>   G. fold
>   G. fracture
>   G. glands
>   G. sinus
>   valve of G.

Guhl technique

Guibor
>   G. duct tube
>   G. Silastic tube
>   G. tube

guidance-cooperation model

guide
>   image g. (IG)

guided
>   g. fine-needle aspiration
>   g. transcutaneous biopsy

guided-needle aspiration cytology

guide plane

guidewire
>   g. exchange technique
>   g. manipulation
>   g. and mini-snare technique
>   g. perforation
>   g. reflection

guiding plane
Guilford-Wright suction tube
guillotine
    g. amputation
    g. needle biopsy
guinea worm infection
Guisez tube
Guleke-Stookey approach
Guller resection
gullet
gullwing incision
gum
    g. line
    g. resection
Gunderson conjunctival flap
Gunderson-Sosin modification
gunpowder lesion
gunshot
    g. fracture
    g. wound
Gunston arthroplasty
Gurd
    G. procedure
    G. resection
Gussenbauer suture
gustation
gustatory anesthesia
Gustilo
    G. classification of puncture wound
    G. puncture wound classification
Gustilo-Anderson
    G.-A. open clavicular fracture
    G.-A. open fracture classification
gut
    blind g.

congenital malrotation of the g.
    g. suture
gut-associated lymphoid tissue (GALT)
Guthrie muscle
gutta-percha point
gutter
    abdominal g.
    g. fracture
    paracolic g.'s
    paravertebral g.
    g. wound
guttered T tube
guttering
    corneal g.
Guttmann technique
Gutzeit dacryostomy operation
Guyon
    G. ankle amputation technique
    G. canal
guy steading suture
Guyton-Noyes fixation
Guyton ptosis operation
Gwathmey suction tube
gynandroblastoma
gynecoid pelvis
gynecologic
    g. anesthesia
    g. laparoscopy
gynecological carcinoma
gynoplasty
gyration
gyrectomy
    frontal g.
gyrose
gyrus, pl. gyri

NOTES

H
  H graft
  H space
H-600 normothermic irrigation
habena
habenula
habenulointerpeduncular tract
Haber-Kraft osteotomy
habitual
  h. dislocation
  h. temporomandibular joint luxation
habitus
  body h.
Hackethal
  H. intramedullary bouquet fixation
  H. stacked nailing technique
Haddad metatarsal osteotomy
Hadju-Cheney acro-osteolysis syndrome
Hadziyannis
  ground-glass body of H.
haemodynamic (*var. of* hemodynamic)
Haering tube
Hagan surface suction tube
Hagedorn and Jansen method
Haggitt classification
Haglund deformity
Hahnenkratt root canal post
Hahn-Steinthal
  H.-S. fracture
  H.-S. fracture of capitellum
HAI
  hepatic arterial infusion
hair bulb incubation test
hairline fracture
Hajek incision
Håkanson technique
Hakim valve and pump
Halban
  H. culdoplasty
  H. procedure
Haldane-Priestley tube
Haldeman bone graft
half-and-half
  h.-a.-h. exposure
  h.-a.-h. nail
half-axial projection
half-body irradiation
half-hitch knot
half-mouth technique
half-pin fixation
half ring
half-time method
Halifax clamp posterior cervical fixation
Hall
  H. facet fusion

  H. method
  H. technique
Halle point
Haller
  H. annulus
  H. ansa
  H. insula
  H. membrane
  H. plexus
  H. rete
  H. tripod
Hallermann-Streiff-François syndrome
Hallermann-Streiff syndrome
hallex
Hallpike maneuver
hallucal
hallucis
  extensor h.
  h. longus laceration
hallus
hallux
  h. extensus
  h. valgus deformity
  h. valgus procedure
  h. varus correction
halo
  h. fracture frame
  h. head frame
  h. ring
halogenated volatile anesthetic
halothane
  h. analyzer
  h. anesthesia
  h. anesthetic
  h. hepatitis
  1-MAC h.
halothane-ether azeotrope
halothane/narcotic/nitrous oxide anesthesia
Halpin operation
Halsted
  H. inguinal herniorrhaphy
  H. maneuver
  H. mastectomy
  H. operation
  H. suture
  H. suture technique
Halsted-Bassini
  H.-B. hernia repair
  H.-B. herniorrhaphy
HAM
  human T cell lymphotropic virus type 1-associated myelopathy
hamartoblastoma
hamartoma

H

hamartomatous lesion
Hamas technique
hamate
    h. bone
    h. tail fracture
hamatum
Hamazaki-Wesenberg body
Hambly procedure
Hamilton method
Hammerschlag method
hammertoe deformity
Hammon procedure
Hamou technique
Hampton
    H. line
    H. maneuver
    H. operation
hamstring
    h. graft
    h. ligament augmentation
    h. muscles
    h. tendon
hamular
    h. procedure
hamulus
    pterygoid h.
    h. pterygoideus
Hancock
    H. pericardial valve graft
    H. procedure
    H. vascular graft
hand
    h. amputation
    h. anomaly
    h. deformity
    h. infection
    h. ratio
    h. reconstruction
    h. ventilation
hand-sewn
    h.-s. anastomosis
    h.-s. ileoanal anastomosis with
       mucosectomy
hand-sutured ileoanal anastomosis
hanger
    yoke h.
hanging
    h. chain method
    h. hip operation
    h. toe operation
hangman fracture
hangnail
Hanhart syndrome
Hankin reduction
Hanks
    H. balanced salt solution
    H. buffer solution
Hanley-McNeil method

Hanley rectal bladder procedure
Hannover
    H. canal
    H. classification
Hansen classification of fracture
Hantavirus infection
Hapsburg jaw
Hara
    H. classification of gallbladder
      inflammation
    H. infiltration block
Harada-Ito procedure
hard
    h. adhesion
    h. calculus
    h. callus stage
    h. cataract
    h. chancre
    h. corn
    h. exudate
    h. metal disease
    h. pad disease
    h. palate
    h. palate cancer
    h. palate dissection
    h. percussion
    h. socket
    h. and soft tissue
    h. solder
    h. sore
    h. stool
    h. tubercle
Hardcastle classification of
    tarsometatarsal joint injury
hard-copy image
hardening solution
Hardinge
    H. lateral approach
    H. technique
hardness
    indentation h.
hard-soft palate junction
Hardy suction tube
Har-el pharyngeal tube
Harewood suspension procedure
Hark
    H. procedure
    H. technique
Harman operation
Harmon
    H. cervical approach
    H. hip reconstruction
    H. incision
    H. modified posterolateral approach
    H. procedure
    H. shoulder approach
    H. transfer technique
harmonic suture

Harms-Dannheim trabeculotomy
  operation
Harper-Warren incision
harpoon extraction
Harriluque
  H. sublaminar wiring modification
  H. technique
Harrington
  H. esophageal diverticulectomy
  H. hernia repair
  H. rod fixation
  H. rod instrumentation failure
  H. rod instrumentation force
  application
  H. total hip arthroplasty
Harrington-Allison repair
Harris
  H. anterolateral approach
  H. femoral component removal
  H. four-wire trochanter reattachment
  H. growth arrest line
  H. lateral approach
  H. superior acetabular graft
  H. suture technique
  H. tube
Harris-Beath projection
Harrison method
Harris-Smith cervical fusion
harsh respiration
Hartel technique
Harting body
Hartman dental solution
Hartmann
  H. colostomy
  H. operation
  H. point
  H. pouch
  H. procedure
  H. reconstruction technique
  H. solution
Harvard criteria of irreversible coma
harvest
  graft h.
  organ h.
harvesting
Hasner
  H. fold
  H. operation
  valve of H.
Hassall body
Hassmann-Brunn-Neer elbow technique
Hasson blunt port

Hass procedure
Hastings
  H. bipolar hemiarthroplasty
  H. open reduction
Hatafuku fundus onlay patch
  esophageal repair
hatchet-head deformity
Hatle method
Haultain operation
Hauri technique
Hauser
  H. bunionectomy
  H. patellar realignment technique
  H. patellar tendon procedure
haustra (*pl. of* haustrum)
haustral
  h. indentation
  h. pouch
haustration
  h.'s of colon
haustrum, pl. haustra
  haustra coli
  haustra of colon
Havers glands
haversian canal
Hawkins
  H. classification of talar fracture
  H. inside-out nephrostomy
  technique
  H. line
  H. method
  H. procedure
  H. single-stick technique
  H. talar fracture classification
Hayem solution
Hay lateral approach
hazardous concentration
HBOC-201
HCl
  esmolol HCl
  granisetron HCl
  Marcaine HCl
  midazolam HCl
  ondansetron HCl
  proparacaine HCl
HDR intracavitary radiation therapy
head
  Austin-Moore h.
  avascular necrosis of the
  femoral h.
  breech h.
  bulldog h.

NOTES

H

299

head *(continued)*
h. of caudate nucleus
h. circumference/abdominal
circumference ratio
h. compression
h. compression test
condyle h.
countersink screw h.
coupling h.
crown of h.
deep h. of flexor pollicis brevis
DePuy hip prosthesis with
Scuderi h.
h. distraction test
dolichocephalic h.
engaged h.
h. of epididymis
femoral h.
h. of femur
fetal h.
h. of fibula
fibular h.
Giliberty bipolar femoral h.
H. hip arthroplasty
hourglass h.
humeral h.
h. of humerus
h. injury
ischemic necrosis of femoral h.
lateral h.
H. line
little h. of humerus
long h.
h. of malleus
h. of mandible
mandibular h.
Matroc femoral h.
medial h.
Medusa h.
h. of metacarpal bone
metatarsal h.
h. of metatarsal bone
molding of h.
Morse h.
h. movement
h. and neck cancer
oblique h.
Omniflex h.
optic nerve h.
h. of pancreas
pancreatic h.
H. paradoxical reflex
h. of phalanx
h. posture
radial h.
h. of radius
h. rest
h. of rib

h. ring
rotatable coupling h.
screw h.
series-II humeral h.
short h.
short h. of biceps brachii muscle
short h. of biceps femoris muscle
h. of stapes
sternocostal h. of pectoralis major
muscle
superficial h. of flexor pollicis
brevis muscle
h. and tail fold
h. of talus
terminal h.
h. tetanus
h. of thigh bone
h. titubation
transillumination of h.
transverse h.
h. trauma
h. turn technique
h. of ulna
ulnar h.
Vitox femoral h.
h. weaving
Ziramic femoral h.
Zirconia orthopaedic prosthetic h.
H. zone
Zyranox femoral h.
headache
brain tumor h.
postdural puncture h. (PDPH)
spinal h.
traction h.
head-bobbing doll syndrome
head:body ratio
head-down tilt test
head-dropping test
head-splitting humeral fracture
head-tilt
h.-t. method
h.-t. test
head-turning reflex
head-up
h.-u. tilt
h.-u. tilt position
h.-u. tilt-table test
h.-u. tilt test
heal
healed fracture
healing
h. by first intention
h. fracture
fracture h.
h. retardation
h. by second intention

soft tissue h.
h. by third intention
Healon solution
Heaney
H. operation
H. technique
hearing aid evaluation
heart
h. anomaly
decortication of h.
dilation of h.
electrical alternation of h.
explanted h.
extracorporeal h.
fatty degeneration of h.
h. laser revascularization
mechanical alternation of h.
myocytolysis of h.
h. position
h. rate (HR)
h. rate variability (HRV)
h. sac
septation of h.
h. synchronized ventilation
h. transplantation
transverse section of h.
h. valve leaflet
h. valve replacement
heart-lung
h.-l. preparation
h.-l. resuscitation
heart-shaped pelvis
heat
h. application
h. balance
h. exposure
h. of formation
h. and moisture exchanger (HME)
h. production temperature
h. of solution
h. of sublimation
h. of vaporization
heater probe coagulation
heat-seal pouch
heavy
h. condensation
Marcaine spinal h.
h. metal injection
h. monofilament suture
h. retention suture
h. silk retention suture
h. wire suture

heavy-gauge suture
heavy-ion irradiation
heaxafluoroisopropranolol
Hedley procedure
hedrocele
heel
h. bone
h. fat pad
h. pad thickening
h. tendon
heel-to-ear maneuver
Heerman incision
Heifetz procedure
height
anterior facial h. (AFH)
facial h.
first twitch h. (T1)
nasal h.
orbital h.
twitch h.
height-length index
Heimlich
H. maneuver
H. tube
Heimlich-Gavrilu gastric tube
Heinecke method
Heineke-Mikulicz
H.-M. gastroenterostomy
H.-M. incision
H.-M. pyloroplasty
Heine operation
Heinz body
Heinz-Ehrlich body
Heisrath operation
Heister
valve of H.
Helal flap arthroplasty
helcoma
helcoplasty
Held
H. bundle
H. decussation
helical suture
helicine arteries of the penis
helicis
h. major muscle
h. minor muscle
helicoid ginglymus
helicotrema
helium
h. dilution method

NOTES

H

helium *(continued)*
    h. equilibration time
    h. insufflation
helix-loop-helix
    h.-l.-h. structure
Heller
    H. cardiomyotomy
    H. esophagomyotomy
    H. myotomy
    H. myotomy with Dor
      fundoplication
    H. myotomy with Dor
      fundoplication method
    II. myotomy with Dor
      fundoplication procedure
    H. myotomy with Dor
      fundoplication technique
    H. operation
    H. plexus
Heller-Belsey operation
Heller-Dor operation
Heller-Nissen operation
Helmholtz line
helminthic infection
helminth infection
helminthoma
heloma
helotomy
Helsper tracheostomy vent tube
Helweg bundle
Hemagard collection tube
hemal
    h. arches
    h. spine
hemangiectasia
    Klippel-Trenaunay
      osteohypertrophic h.
hemangiectasis
hemangiectatic hypertrophy
hemangioameloblastoma
hemangioblastoma
hemangioendothelioblastoma
hemangioendothelioma
hemangioendotheliosarcoma
hemangioepithelioma
hemangiofibroma
    juvenile h.
hemangiolipoma
hemangiolymphangioma
hemangioma
    port-wine h.
hemangioma-thrombocytopenia syndrome
hemangiomatous tissue
hemangiopericytoma
hemangiosarcoma
Hemashield collagen-enhanced graft
hematencephalon
hemathorax

hematobilia
    h. evacuation
hematocele
    pelvic h.
    pudendal h.
    scrotal h.
hematocystis
hematogenic metastasis
hematogenous
    h. metastasis
    h. micrometastasis
    h. spread of infection
hematologic complication
hematolymphangioma
hematolysis
hematoma
    acute subdural h.
    aneurysmal h.
    aortic intramural h.
    axillary h.
    basal ganglia h.
    bladder flap h.
    bowel wall h.
    cerebellar h.
    chronic subdural h.
    communicating h.
    corpus luteum h.
    dissecting intramural h.
    h. drainage
    duodenal h.
    epidural h.
    esophageal intramural h.
    h. evacuation
    expanding retroperitoneal h.
    extradural h.
    facial h.
    follicular h.
    iliopsoas muscle h.
    interhemispheric subdural h.
    interstitial loculated h.
    intracerebral h.
    intracranial h.
    intrahepatic h.
    intramural h.
    intraparenchymal h.
    intrauterine h.
    isodense subdural h.
    mesenteric h.
    nasopharyngeal h.
    orbital h.
    organized h.
    para-aortic h.
    parenchymal h.
    perianal h.
    periaortic mediastinal h.
    pericardial h.
    peridiaphragmatic h.
    perigraft h.

perinephric h.
perirenal h.
puerperal h.
pulsatile h.
rectal sheath h.
rectus sheath h.
renal h.
retroperitoneal h.
retropharyngeal h.
retroplacental h.
sciatic nerve palsy h.
septal h.
subcapsular renal h.
subchorionic h.
subdural interhemispheric h.
subfascial h.
subgaleal h.
subgluteal h.
sublingual h.
submembranous placental h.
submental h.
subperiosteal h.
subungual h.
sylvian h.
traumatic intracranial h.
umbilical cord h.
uterine h.
vaginal h.
vulvar h.
warfarin-associated subcapsular h.
hematomphalocele
hematomyelia
hematomyelopore
hematopoietic
    h. gland
    h. metastasis
    h. tissue
hematorrhachis
    h. externa
    extradural h.
    h. interna
    subdural h.
hematospermatocele
hematospermia
hematoxylin body
hemendothelioma
hemiacidrin irrigation
hemiacrosomia
hemiarthroplasty
    Bateman h.
    Hastings bipolar h.
    I-beam hip h.

    large-humeral-head h.
    McKeever and MacIntosh h.
    Neer h.
    prosthetic h.
    Smith-Petersen h.
hemiazygos vein
hemibody irradiation
hemic calculus
hemicentrum
hemicolectomy
    Duecollement h.
    laparoscopic-assisted h.
hemicondylar
    h. fracture
    h. graft
hemicorporectomy
hemicorticectomy
    cerebral h.
hemicraniectomy
hemicraniosis
hemicraniotomy
hemicylindrical bone graft
hemidiaphragm rupture
hemi-double stapling method
hemifacial
hemi-Fontan
    h.-F. operation
    h.-F. procedure
hemifundoplication
    Toupet h.
hemigastrectomy
hemiglossal
hemiglossectomy
hemihepatectomy
hemihydranencephaly
hemi-Kock procedure
hemilaminectomy
    complete lateral h.
    lumbar h.
    partial h.
    unilateral h.
hemilaryngectomy
hemilingual
hemimandible reconstruction
hemimandibulectomy
hemimaxillectomy
hemimyelocele
hemimyelomeningocele
heminephroureterectomy
hemi-orchiectomy
hemipancreatectomy
hemipancreaticosplenectomy

NOTES

H

hemipelvectomy
    complete internal h.
    external h.
    formal h.
    internal h.
    partial internal h.
hemipelvis
hemipulp flap
hemiresection
    h. interposition arthroplasty
hemiscrotectomy
hemisection
    tooth h.
    triple h.
hemisectomy
hemisphere
    h. of bulb of penis
    cerebellar h.
    cerebral h.
hemispherectomy
hemispheric disconnection syndrome
hemispherium
    h. bulbi urethrae
    h. cerebelli
    h. cerebri
hemistrumectomy
hemithoracic duct
hemithorax
hemithyroidectomy
hemitongue flap
hemivertebral excision
hemivulvectomy
hemobilia
hemocholecyst
hemocholecystitis
hemocryoscopy
hemocytoblastoma
hemocytolysis
hemocytometer
    Coulter MD 16 h.
hemodilution
    acute normovolemic h. (ANH)
hemodynamic, haemodynamic
    h. maneuver
    h. monitoring
    h. pertubation
    h. response
hemofiltration
    arteriovenous h.
    continuous arteriovenous h.
    continuous venovenous h.
    h. therapy
hemoglobin-oxygen dissociation curve
hemolith
hemolymphangioma
hemolytic uremic syndrome
hemomediastinum
hemonephrosis

hemoperfusion
    hepatic venous isolation by
      direct h. (HVI-DHP)
hemopericardium
hemoperitoneum
HEMOPHAN membrane
hemoplasty
hemopneumopericardium
hemopyelectasis
hemorrhage
    abdominal h.
    accidental h.
    acute nonvariceal upper
      gastrointestinal h.
    adrenal h.
    alveolar h.
    aneurysmal h.
    antepartum h.
    arachnoid h.
    arterial h.
    artery of cerebral h.
    bladder h.
    blot h.
    brainstem h.
    catheter-induced pulmonary
      artery h.
    cerebellar h.
    cerebral h.
    choroidal h.
    colonic diverticular h.
    colorectal h.
    concealed h.
    conjunctival h.
    h. control
    diffuse pulmonary alveolar h.
    disk drusen h.
    diverticular h.
    dot h.
    dot-and-blot h.
    Duret h.
    eight-ball h.
    endoscopic stigmata of h.
    epidural h.
    expulsive h.
    exsanguinating h.
    external h.
    extradural h.
    extraluminal h.
    fetal h.
    fetal-maternal h.
    fetomaternal h.
    flame h.
    flame-shaped h.
    gastric h.
    gastrointestinal tract h.
    germinal matrix h.
    gingival h.
    hepatic h.

Icelandic form of intracranial h.
intermediate h.
internal h.
intestinal h.
intra-abdominal arterial h.
intra-alveolar h.
intracapsular h.
intracerebral h.
intracranial h. (ICH)
intraluminal h.
intramural intestinal h.
intraocular h.
intraparenchymal h.
intrapartum h.
intraperitoneal h.
intraventricular h.
laryngeal h.
lobar h.
lower gastrointestinal h.
mediastinal h.
mesencephalic h.
nasal h.
neonatal intracranial h.
neonatal intraventricular h.
nonaneurysmal perimesencephalic
  subarachnoid h.
nonvariceal upper GI h.
ochre h.
pancreatitis-related h.
parenchymatous intracerebral h.
perianeurysmal h.
perinephric space h.
periventricular-intraventricular h.
h. per rhexis
petechial h.
placental h.
pontine h.
postextraction h.
postgastrectomy h.
postpartum h.
postpolypectomy h.
posttraumatic h.
preplacental h.
preretinal h.
primary h.
pulmonary alveolar h.
pulmonary artery h.
punctate h.
refractory variceal h.
renal cyst h.
reperfusion-induced h.
retinal h.

retinopathy h.
retrobulbar h.
retroperitoneal h.
retropharyngeal h.
round h.
salmon-patch h.
scleral h.
secondary h.
signal h.
slit h.
small bowel h.
splinter h.
spontaneous renal h.
sternocleidomastoid h.
stigmata of recent h.
stress ulcer h.
subarachnoid h.
subcapsular h.
subchorial h.
subchorionic h.
subconjunctival h.
subcortical h.
subdural h.
subependymal h.
subepithelial h.
subgaleal h.
subhyaloid h.
subintimal h.
subjunctival h.
submucosal gastric h.
subperiosteal h.
subretinal h.
suprachoroidal h.
syringomyelic h.
thalamic-subthalamic h.
torrential h.
transplacental h.
unavoidable h.
upper GI h.
variceal h.
venous h.
vitreal h.
vitreous break-through h.
white-centered h.
yellow-ochre h.

hemorrhagic
  h. ascites
  h. endovasculitis
  h. infarction
  h. inflammation
  h. lesion
  h. metastasis

NOTES

H

hemorrhagic *(continued)*
    h. radiation injury
    h. shock
hemorrhoid
    cutaneous h.
    dilation of h.
    external h.
    internal h.
    ligation of h.
    Lord dilation of h.
    rubber band ligation of h.
    thrombosed internal and external h.
hemorrhoidal
    h. nerve
    h. plexus
    h. veins
    h. zone
hemorrhoidectomy
    ambulatory h.
    closed h.
    diathermy h.
    laser h.
    Lord h.
    modified Whitehead h.
    open h.
    radical h.
    semiopen h.
hemospermia
hemostasia
hemostasis
    chemical h.
    endoscopic h.
    immaculate h.
    proactive h.
hemostatic
    h. collodion
    h. plug formation
    h. staple line
    h. suture
hemostat technique
hemostyptic
hemothorax
Hemovac suction tube
Henderson
    H. classification
    H. fracture
    H. onlay bone graft
    H. posterolateral approach
    H. posteromedial approach
    H. skin incision
Hendler unitunnel technique
Henke space
Henle
    H. body
    H. elastic membrane
    H. fenestrated membrane
    H. loop
    H. tubules

Henning inside-to-outside technique
Henry
    H. acromioclavicular technique
    H. anterior strap approach
    H. anterolateral approach
    H. bone graft
    H. extensile approach
    H. incision
    H. knot
    H. posterior interosseous nerve approach
    H. posterior interosseous nerve exposure
    H. radial approach
    H. resection
Henry-Geist spinal fusion
Hensen
    H. body
    H. canal
    H. duct
    H. plane
Hensing ligament
hepar
    h. lobatum
heparin
    h. injection
    h. irrigation
    h. neutralization
heparinase correction
heparin-bonded Bott-type tube
heparin-induced lipolysis
heparinization
    h. procedure
heparinized Ringer lactate solution
heparin-protamine titration
HepatAmine amino acid solution
hepatectomize
hepatectomy
    donor h.
    partial h.
    recipient h.
    triple lobe h.
hepatic
    h. adenoma
    h. arterial infusion (HAI)
    h. arterial therapy
    h. arteries
    h. artery ligation
    h. artery-portal vein fistula
    h. branches of vagus nerve
    h. candidal infection
    h. capsule
    h. circulation
    h. coma
    h. complication
    h. dearterialization
    h. duct
    h. flexure

h. fungal infection
h. hemorrhage
h. laminae
h. lobectomy
h. lobule
h. lymph nodes
h. mass lesion
h. metastasis
h. outflow tract
h. plexus
h. portal vein
h. resection
h. rupture
h. segments
h. subsegmentectomy
h. triad
h. tumor
h. vascular exclusion (HVE)
h. vascular exclusion and in situ perfusion procedure
h. vein catheterization
h. vein wedge pressure
h. venous isolation by direct hemoperfusion (HVI-DHP)
h. venous pressure
h. venous pressure gradient
h. venous segments
h. venous web disease
h. web
h. web dilation
h. wedge pressure
hepaticocutaneous jejunostomy
hepaticocystojejunostomy
hepaticodochotomy
hepaticoduodenostomy
hepaticoenterostomy
hepaticogastrostomy
hepaticojejunostomy
Roux-en-Y h.
hepaticolithotomy
hepaticolithotripsy
hepaticopulmonary
hepaticostomy
hepaticotomy
hepatitis
h. A-E infection
anesthetic h.
fulminant h.
halothane h.
long incubation h.
peliosis h.

radiation h.
short incubation h.
hepatization
gray h.
red h.
yellow h.
hepatobiliary manifestation
hepatoblastoma
hepatocarcinoma
hepatocele
hepatocholangioenterostomy
hepatocholangiojejunostomy
hepatocholangiostomy
hepatocolic ligament
hepatocystic
h. duct
hepatocyte transplantation
hepatoduodenal
h. ligament
h. reflection
hepatoduodenal-peritoneal reflection
hepatoduodenostomy
hepatoenteric
hepatoesophageal ligament
hepatofugal
h. flow
hepatogastric
h. ligament
hepatojejunal anastomosis
hepatolith
hepatolithectomy
hepatolithiasis
hepatoma
hepatomphalocele
hepatomphalos
hepatonephric
hepatonephromegaly
hepatopancreatic
h. ampulla
h. sphincter
hepatopathy
radiation h.
hepatoperitonitis
hepatopetal
h. flow
hepatopexy
hepatopleural fistula
hepatopneumonic
hepatoportal
h. biliary fistula
hepatoportoenterostomy
Kasai-type h.

NOTES

hepatoptosis
hepatopulmonary
hepatorenal
    h. ligament
    h. pouch
    h. recess
    h. syndrome
hepatorrhagia
hepatorrhaphy
hepatorrhexis
hepatoscopy
hepatostomy
hepatotomy
hepatotoxemia
hepatotoxicity
    anesthetic h.
HEPES
    4-(2-hydroxyethyl)-1-
    piperazineethanesulfonic acid
    HEPES solution
Hep-Lock injection
herald patch
Herbert
    H. operation
    H. screw fixation
Herculon suture
hereditary
    h. flat adenoma syndrome
    h. multiple exostoses
Hering
    canal of H.
Hering-Breuer reflex
heritable connective tissue disease
Herman-Gartland osteotomy
Hermodsson
    H. fracture
    H. internal rotation technique
    H. tangential projection
hernia
    abdominal wall h.
    antevesical h.
    axial hiatal h.
    Barth h.
    Béclard h.
    bilocular femoral h.
    bladder h.
    Bochdalek h.
    broad ligament h.
    cecal h.
    cerebral h.
    Cheatle-Henry h.
    Cloquet h.
    combined hiatal h.
    complete h.
    concealed h.
    concentric h.
    congenital diaphragmatic h.
    Cooper h.

    crural h.
    diaphragmatic h.
    direct inguinal h.
    double loop h.
    dry h.
    duodenal h.
    duodenojejunal h.
    easily reducible h.
    h. en bissac
    epigastric h.
    esophageal h.
    extrasaccular h.
    fascial h.
    fatty h.
    femoral h.
    funicular inguinal h.
    gastric h.
    gastroesophageal h.
    Gironcoli h.
    gluteal h.
    groin h.
    Hesselbach h.
    Hey h.
    hiatal h.
    hiatus h.
    Holthouse h.
    iliacosubfascial h.
    incarcerated h.
    h. incarceration
    incisional h.
    incomplete h.
    indirect inguinal h.
    infantile h.
    inguinal h.
    inguinocrural h.
    inguinofemoral h.
    inguinolabial h.
    inguinoscrotal h.
    inguinosuperficial h.
    internal h.
    intersigmoid h.
    interstitial h.
    intraepiploic h.
    intrailiac h.
    intrapelvic h.
    irreducible h.
    ischiatic h.
    Krönlein h.
    labial h.
    Larrey h.
    lateral ventral h.
    Laugier h.
    Lesgaft h.
    lesser sac h.
    levator h.
    Littré h.
    lumbar h.
    Madden repair of incisional h.

Malgaigne h.
Maydl h.
meningeal h.
mesenteric h.
mesocolic h.
h. metastasis
Morgagni h.
multiorgan h.
muscle h.
obturator h.
orbital h.
pannicular h.
pantaloon h.
paraduodenal h.
paraesophageal diaphragmatic h.
paraesophageal hiatal h.
parahiatal h.
paraileostomal h.
h. paralysis
paraperitoneal h.
parapubic h.
parasaccular h.
parastomal h.
parietal h.
perineal h.
peritoneal h.
peritoneopericardial diaphragmatic h.
Petit h.
pleuroperitoneal h.
posterior vaginal h.
h. pouch
properitoneal inguinal h.
pudendal h.
reducible h.
h. repair
retrocecal h.
retrocolic h.
retrograde h.
retroperitoneal h.
retropubic h.
retrosternal h.
Richter h.
Rieux h.
Rokitansky h.
rolling hiatal h.
h. rupture
h. sac
sciatic h.
scrotal h.
Serafini h.
short esophagus type hiatal h.
sliding abdominal h.

sliding esophageal hiatal h.
slipped h.
spigelian h.
Spigelius h.
strangulated h.
transient hiatal h.
transmesenteric h.
traumatic diaphragmatic h.
Treitz h.
umbilical h.
h. uteri inguinale
Velpeau h.
ventral h.
vesicle h.
vitreous h.
voluminous hiatus h.
W h.

hernial
    h. aneurysm
    h. repair
    h. sac
herniated
    h. disk
    h. preperitoneal fat
    h. presacral fat pad
herniation
    brain h.
    cardiac h.
    caudal transtentorial h.
    central h.
    cerebral h.
    cervical midline disk h.
    cingulate h.
    cisternal h.
    disk h.
    fat h.
    foraminal h.
    free fragment h.
    intercervical disk h.
    intervertebral disk h.
    intraspongy nuclear disk h.
    lumbar disk h.
    midline disk h.
    nucleus pulposus h.
    h. pit
    posterolateral h.
    rostral transtentorial h.
    sphenoidal h.
    subfalcial h.
    synovial h.
    tentorial h.
    thoracic disk h.

NOTES

H

herniation *(continued)*
  tonsillar h.
  transtentorial h.
  traumatic cervical disk h.
  uncal h.
  ureteroneocystostomy h.
  visceral h.
  vitreous h.
hernioenterotomy
hernioid
herniolaparotomy
hernioplasty
  massive incisional h.
  mesh plug h.
herniopuncture
herniorrhaphy
  Bassini inguinal h.
  extraperitoneal laparoscopic h.
  Halsted-Bassini h.
  Halsted inguinal h.
  Hill-type hiatus h.
  inguinal h.
  laparoscopic inguinal h.
  Lichtenstein h.
  Macewen h.
  Madden incisional h.
  McVay h.
  open h.
  pants-over-vest h.
  Ponka h.
  Shouldice inguinal h.
  umbilical h.
  ventral h.
  vest-over-pants h.
herniotomy
  Petit h.
herpes
  h. epithelial tropic ulceration
  h. simplex virus infection
  h. zoster infection
  h. zoster pain
herpetic infection
herpetoid lesion
herpkinetic circulation
Herring
  H. lateral pillar classification
  H. tube
hersage
HES
  hydroxyethyl starch
  hydroxyethyl starch solution
hesitation phenomenon
Hespan
Hess
  H. eyelid operation
  H. ptosis operation
Hesselbach
  H. fascia

  H. hernia
  H. ligament
  H. triangle
hetastarch
heterocheiral
heterodermic
  h. graft
heterogeneous
  h. attenuation
  h. graft
heterogenous
  h. graft
  h. keratoplasty
heterograft
heterokeratoplasty
heterolateral
heterologous
  h. graft
  h. insemination
heterolysis
hetero-osteoplasty
heterophoric position
heteroplastic
  h. graft
heteroplastid
heteroplasty
heteroscopy
heterospecific
  h. graft
heterotopic
  h. bone formation
  h. graft
  h. ossification prevention
  h. transplantation
heterotransplantation
Hetzel forward triangle method
heuristic method
Heuser membrane
Hewlett Packard monitor 78341 A
hexafluorenium
  h. bromide
hexafluoroisopropranolol (HFIP)
hexametazime
hexamethylpropyleneamine oxime
  (HMPAO)
hexastarch
Hex-Fix external fixation
hexokinase method
hex procedure
hexylcaine
Hey-Groves
  H.-G. fascia lata technique
  H.-G. ligament reconstruction
    technique
Hey-Groves-Kirk
  H.-G.-K. bone graft
  H.-G.-K. technique
Hey hernia

Heyman-Herndon clubfoot procedure
Heyman-Herndon-Strong technique
Heyman procedure
HFIP
> hexafluoroisopropranolol
HFJ
> high-frequency jet
> HFJ ventilation
H-flap incision
HFO
> high-frequency oscillation
> HFO ventilation
HFPP
> high-frequency positive pressure
> HFPP ventilation
H-graft
> H-g. bone graft
> H-g. fusion
HHCA
> hypothermic hypokalemic cardioplegic arrest
hiatal hernia
hiatotomy
hiatus
> adductor h.
> h. adductorius
> aortic h.
> h. aorticus
> Breschet h.
> h. of canal for greater petrosal nerve
> h. canalis facialis
> h. canalis nervi petrosi majoris
> h. canalis nervi petrosi minoris
> h. of canal of lesser petrosal nerve
> esophageal h.
> h. esophageus
> h. ethmoidalis
> h. of facial canal
> fallopian h.
> h. hernia
> h. maxillaris
> maxillary h.
> pleuroperitoneal h.
> sacral h.
> h. sacralis
> saphenous h.
> h. saphenus
> scalene h.
> Scarpa h.
> semilunar h.

> h. semilunaris
> h. subarcuatus
> h. tendineus
Hibbs-Jones spinal fusion
Hibbs procedure
hibernal epidemic viral infection
hibernation
> myocardial h.
hibernoma
Hibiclens solution
Hibond N+ nylon membrane
Hickman line
hickory-stick fracture
hidden
> h. nail skin
> h. part
hidradenitis
hidradenoma
> clear cell h.
> cystic h.
> nodular h.
> papillary h.
> poroid h.
> solid h.
hidrocystoma
hiemalis
> erythrokeratolysis h.
Hiff operation
Higgins
> H. incision
> H. technique
high
> h. blood pressure
> h. endothelial venule
> H. Flex D 700 S bubble oxygenator
> h. intraluminal pressure
> h. intrauterine insemination
> h. level disinfection
> h. ligation
> h. ligation of hernia sac
> h. lip line
> h. lithotomy
> h. neurological lesion
> H. Oxygen PRM resuscitator
> h. pressure zone (HPZ)
> h. smile line
> h. spinal anesthesia
> h. subtotal gastrectomy
> h. thoracic level epidural anesthesia
> h. tibial osteotomy

NOTES

high-altitude
    h.-a. endoscopy
    h.-a. simulation test
high-amplitude sucking technique
high-attenuation
high-capacity fluid warmer
high-dose therapy
high-energy fracture
highest
    h. intercostal artery
    h. intercostal vein
    h. nuchal line
    h. thoracic artery
high-flow regulator
high-flux dialysis membrane
high-frequency
    h.-f. jet (HFJ)
    h.-f. jet ventilation
    h.-f. oscillation (HFO)
    h.-f. oscillation ventilation
    h.-f. oscillatory ventilation
    h.-f. percussive ventilation
    h.-f. positive pressure (HFPP)
    h.-f. positive pressure ventilation
high-grade squamous intraepithelial
    lesion
high-heat casting technique
high-intensity lesion
high-kV technique
high-loop cutaneous ureterostomy
highly selective vagotomy
high-magnification
    h.-m. colonoscopy
    h.-m. endoscopy
    h.-m. gastroscopy
Highmore body
high-pressure
    h.-p. relief valve
high-risk angioplasty
high-speed rotational atherectomy
high-tension suturing technique
high-voltage
    h.-v. pulsed galvanic stimulation
    h.-v. therapy
hila (*pl. of* hilum)
hilar
    h. biopsy
    h. carcinoma
    h. lymph nodes
    h. mass
    h. region
    h. structure scar tissue
Hilgenreiner horizontal Y line
Hilgenreiner-Perkins line
Hill
    H. antireflux operation
    H. hiatus hernia repair
    H. median arcuate repair

    H. posterior gastropexy
    H. procedure
Hillis-Müller maneuver
Hill-Nahai-Vasconez-Mathes technique
hillock
    seminal h.
Hill-Sachs
    H.-S. deformity
    H.-S. fracture
    H.-S. shoulder dislocation
    H.-S. shoulder lesion
Hill-type hiatus herniorrhaphy
Hi-Lo Jet tracheal tube
Hilton
    H. method
    H. sac
    H. white line
hilum, pl. hila
    h. of kidney
    h. lienis
    h. of lung
    h. of lymph node
    h. nodi lymphatici
    h. pulmonis
    h. renalis
    h. of spleen
    h. splenicum
    h. stimulation
Hinchey classification
hindbrain deformity
hindfoot
    h. amputation
    h. deformity
hindgut
hindquarter amputation
hinge
    h. joint
    h. osteotomy
    h. position
    soft tissue h.
hinge-axis point
hinged
    h. flap
    h. fragment
Hinman
    H. procedure
    H. syndrome
Hinsberg operation
hip
    h. arthroplasty
    h. bone
    congenital dislocation of h.
    h. deformity
    h. disarticulation
    h. dislocation
    h. extension
    h. extension range of motion
    h. fracture

Leinbach head and neck total h.
h. pinning
Precision Osteolock h.
h. reduction
h. rotation
transient osteoporosis of h.
Hippel operation
hippocampectomy
Hippocrates manipulation
Hippocratic maneuver
Hirano body
Hirayma osteotomy
Hirschberg method
Hirschfeld
H. canal
H. method
Hirst operation
hirudin
hirudinization
His
bundle of H.
H. bundle
H. bundle ablation
H. bundle heart block
H. canal
H. line
H. perivascular space
H. plane
His-Haas procedure
His-Purkinje tissue
Histaject injection
histangic
histiocyte
histiocytic tissue
histiocytoma
histiocytosis
histioma
histoacryl glue patch
histoangic
histochemical method
histocompatibility
histologic
h. lesion
h. tooth repair
histology
histolysis
histonectomy
Histoplasma **infection**
histotoxic anoxia
Hitchcock tendon technique
HIV-1, -2 infection

HIV classification
HLA
human leukocyte antigen
HLA identical kidney graft
HME
heat and moisture exchanger
HMPAO
hexamethylpropyleneamine oxime
Hoaglund bone graft
Hoaglund-States classification
hobnail liver
Hoche
H. bundle
H. tract
hockey-stick
h.-s. deformity
h.-s. fracture
h.-s. incision
Hodge
H. maneuver
H. plane
Hodgson
H. technique
H. technique of modified Lich
procedure
Hodor-Dobbs procedure
Hoechst dye method
Hoffa
H. fat pad
H. fracture
Hoffman jejunoplasty
Hoffmann
H. approach
H. duct
H. panmetatarsal head resection
Hoffmann-Clayton procedure
Hoffmann-Vidal-Adrey frame
Hofmeister
H. anastomosis
H. gastrectomy
H. gastroenterostomy
H. operation
H. procedure
H. technique
Hofmeister-Pólya anastomosis
Hogan operation
Hoguet
H. maneuver
H. pantaloon hernia repair
**Hohl-Luck tibial plateau fracture
classification**

NOTES

H

Hohl-Moore
    H.-M. classification
    H.-M. technique
Hohl tibial condylar fracture classification
Hohmann procedure
Hoke-Kite technique
Hoke-Miller procedure
Hoke procedure
Holdaway line
Holden line
hold-relax
    h.-r. method
    h.-r. technique
Holdsworth spinal fracture classification
hole
    lag screw thread h.
    h. preparation method
hole-in-one technique
Hollander test
Hollande solution
Hollister
    H. First Choice pouch
    H. Holligard pouch
    H. Karaya 5 ostomy pouch
    H. Karaya Seal pouch
    H. Premium pouch
Holl ligament
hollow
    h. bone
    Sebileau h.
    h. visceral tonometer
Holmes method
Holmgren method
holoacrania
holocord
hologastroschisis
holoprosencephaly
holorachischisis
Holstein fracture of humerus
Holstein-Lewis fracture
Holter tube
Holth
    H. iridencleisis
    H. operation
    H. sclerectomy
Holthouse hernia
Holzer method
Holzknecht space
homatropine dilatation
home
    H. lobe
    h. program
homocladic
homogeneity
    tissue h.

homogeneous
    h. ablation
    h. graft
homogenous
    h. graft
    h. keratoplasty
    h. radiation
    h. tooth transplantation
homograft
    h. aortic valve replacement
    cryopreserved aortic h.
    h. reaction
    h. rejection
homokeratoplasty
homolateral
homologous
    h. artificial insemination
    h. graft
homolysis
homomorphic
homonomous
homonomy
homonymous
homoplastic graft
homoplasty
homotopic
    h. transplantation
homotransplantation
homotype
homotypic
homozygous achondroplasia
honeycomb lesion
hood
    laminar flow h.
    H. procedure
    H. technique
hook
    h. fixation
    h. of the hamate fracture
hooked
    h. bone
    h. bundle of Russell
    h. intramedullary nail
    h. wire localization
hook-nail deformity
hook-plate fixation
hook-to-screw L4-S1 compression construct
hoop stress fracture
Hope
    H. resuscitation bag
    H. resuscitator
Hoppenfeld-Deboer
    H.-D. approach
    H.-D. technique
Horay operation

hordeolum
>external h.
>h. externum

Hori technique

horizontal
>h. angulation
>h. canal
>h. external rotation
>h. fissure of right lung
>h. flap
>h. gastroplasty
>h. incision
>h. mattress suture
>h. maxillary fracture
>h. osteotomy
>h. part of duodenum
>h. part of facial canal
>h. plane
>h. plate of palatine bone
>h. position
>h. projection
>h. section
>h. tube

hormonal evaluation

horn
>coccygeal h.
>dorsal h.
>greater h. of hyoid bone
>h.'s of hyoid bone
>inferior h. of thyroid cartilage
>lesser h. of hyoid bone
>nail h.
>sacral h.'s
>h.'s of saphenous opening
>superior h. of thyroid cartilage
>h.'s of thyroid cartilage
>tip of posterior h.

Horner muscle
hornification
horripilation
horseshoe
>h. fistula
>h. incision

horseshoe-shaped flap
Horsley
>H. anastomosis
>H. gastrectomy
>H. suture

Horton-Devine dermal graft
Horvath operation
Horwitz-Adams ankle fusion
Hoskins razor blade fragment

hospital-acquired infection
Hossli suction tube
host
>graft versus h.
>reservoir h.

hot
>h. abscess
>h. biopsy
>h. biopsy technique
>h. dog technique
>h. lesion
>h. line
>h. wire respirometer

Hotchkiss-McManus PAS technique
hot-knife conization
HOTLINE
>H. blood and fluid warmer
>H. fluid-warming device

hot-wire
>h.-w. anemometer
>h.-w. pneumotachometer

Hotz-Anagnostakis operation
Hotz entropion operation
Hough-Cadogan suction tube
Houghton-Akroyd
>H.-A. fracture technique
>H.-A. open reduction

Hounsfield unit (HU)
hourglass
>h. deformity
>h. head
>h. membrane
>h. stomach

24-hour urine collection
House
>H. advancement anoplasty
>H. endolymphatic shunt tube
>H. flap anoplasty
>H. reconstruction
>H. stapedectomy
>H. suction tube
>H. technique

House-Baron suction tube
House-Brackmann classification
House-Radpour suction tube
House-Stevenson suction tube
House-Urban tube
Houston
>H. folds
>H. muscle
>valve of H.

NOTES

H

315

Hovanian
    H. procedure
    H. transfer technique
Hovius
    H. canal
    H. membrane
Howard
    H. method
    H. technique
    H. test
Howe silver precipitation method
Howland lock
Howorth
    H. approach
    H. procedure
Howorth-Keillor procedure
Ho:YAG laser angioplasty
Hoyer
    H. anastomoses
    ′ H. canals
HPV
    hypoxic pulmonary vasoconstriction
H.P. Wright method
HPZ
    high pressure zone
    anal HPZ
HR
    heart rate
    PC Polygraf HR
HRV
    heart rate variability
HSE
    hypertonic saline-epinephrine
HSE solution
H-shaped
    H-s. capsular incision
    H-s. ileal pouch-anal anastomosis
H-type tracheoesophageal fistula
HU
    Hounsfield unit
Hubbard airplane vent tube
hub contamination
Huber adductor digiti quinti opponensplasty
Hubscher maneuver
Hucker-Conn crystal violet solution
Hudson
    H. Lifesaver resuscitator
    H. line
    H. type oxygen mask
Hudson-Stähli line
hue
    salmon patch h.
Hueck ligament
Hueter
    H. incision
    H. line
    H. maneuver

Hugenholtz method
Huggins operation
Hughes
    H. modification of Burch technique
    H. operation
    H. tarsoconjunctival flap
Hughston
    H. classification
    H. external rotation recurvatum test
    H. procedure
Hughston-Degenhardt reconstruction
Hughston-Hauser procedure
Hughston-Jacobson
    H.-J. lateral compartment reconstruction
    H.-J. technique
Huguier
    H. canal
    canal of H.
    H. circle
    H. sinus
Hui-Linscheid procedure
human
    h. AML cell line
    h. bite infection
    h. dural substitute graft
    h. fibrin foam
    h. leukocyte antigen (HLA)
    h. lyophilized dura cystoplasty
    h. ovum fertilization test
    h. papillomavirus infection
    h. T cell lymphotropic virus type 1-associated myelopathy (HAM)
    h. thrombin
    h. umbilical vein (HUV)
humeral
    h. artery
    h. articulation
    h. canal
    h. epiphysis
    h. fracture malunion
    h. head
    h. head-splitting fracture
    h. line
    h. physeal fracture
    h. shaft fracture
    h. supracondylar fracture
humeroperoneal neuromuscular disease
humeroradial
    h. articulation
humeroscapular
humeroulnar
    h. articulation
humerus
    condyle of h.
    Holstein fracture of h.
HumidFilter heat and moisture exchanger

Humid-Vent Port 1 elbow connector
Hummelsheim
    H. operation
    H. procedure
humpback deformity
Humphrey coronary sinus-sucker suction
    tube
hump removal
Hungerford-Krackow-Kenna knee
    arthroplasty
Hungerford technique
Hunt-Early technique
Hunter
    H. canal
    H. gubernaculum
    H. line
    H. operation
hunterian ligation
Hunter-Schreger line
Huntington
    H. bone graft
    H. rod insertion
    H. tibial technique
Hunt and Kosnik classification
Hunt-Lawrence pouch
Hunt-Transley operation
Hustead epidural needle
Hutchinson
    H. fracture
    H. patch
Hutchison syndrome
Hutch ureteral reflux operation
HUV
    human umbilical vein
    HUV bypass graft
HVE
    hepatic vascular exclusion
HVI-DHP
    hepatic venous isolation by direct
    hemoperfusion
hyaline
    h. basement membrane
    h. body
    h. mass
    h. membrane disease
    h. membrane syndrome
hyalitis anterior membrane
hyalocapsular ligament
hyaloid
    h. body
    h. canal
    h. posterior membrane

hyaloidotomy
Hyam conization
hybridization-subtraction technique
hybridoma
    h. technique
hydatid cyst intrahepatic rupture
hydatidocele
hydatidoma
hydatidostomy
Hydeltrasol injection
Hydeltra-TBA injection
hydradenoma
hydralazine
hydranencephaly
hydration
    adequate h.
    intravenous h.
    h. layer water
    maternal h.
    vigorous h.
hydraulic dissection
hydrencephalocele
hydrencephalomeningocele
hydrencephalus
hydroappendix
hydrocalycosis
hydrocele
    h. sac
hydrocelectomy
hydrocephalic
hydrocephalocele
hydrocephaloid
hydrocephalus
hydrocephaly
hydrochloride
    alfentanil h.
    amylocaine h.
    bupivacaine h.
    buprenorphine h.
    butethamine h.
    chloroprocaine h.
    cocaine h.
    dibucaine h.
    dihydromorphinone h.
    doxapram h.
    dyclonine h.
    ethoxazene h.
    etidocaine h.
    euprocin h.
    flavoxate h.
    flurazepam h.
    gonadorelin h.

NOTES

H

hydrochloride (*continued*)
   hydromorphone h.
   ketamine h.
   lidocaine h.
   lucanthone h.
   meperidine h.
   mepivacaine h.
   methotrimeprazine h.
   methoxamine h.
   midazolam h.
   nalbuphine h.
   nalmefene h.
   naloxone h.
   oxophenarsine h.
   oxymorphone h.
   phenacaine h.
   phenazopyridine h.
   piperocaine h.
   pramoxine h.
   prilocaine h.
   procaine h.
   α-prodine h.
   promethazine h.
   proparacaine h.
   propiomazine h.
   propitocaine h.
   propoxyphene h.
   proxymetacaine h.
   spectinomycin h.
   tetracaine h.
   thenyldiamine h.
hydrocholecystis
hydrocirsocele
hydrocodone
hydrocolpocele
hydrocortisone
   lidocaine and h.
hydrocystoma
hydrodelamination
hydrodelineation
hydrodissection
hydroencephalocele
hydroflotation
hydroflow technique
hydrogen
   h. inhalation technique
   h. peroxide solution
   h. washout method
hydrogenation
hydrogenolysis
hydrolysis
   ATP h.
   intragastric h.
   h. of solution
   h. of surfactant
   urea h.
hydrolysis-resistant
hydroma

hydromeningocele
hydromeningoencephalocele
hydromorphone hydrochloride
hydromyelia
hydromyelocele
hydromyelomeningocele
hydromyoma
hydronephrosis
hydronephrotic
hydroperitoneum
hydropertubation
hydrophilic drug
hydropneumoperitoneum
hydrops
hydropyonephrosis
hydrorchis
hydrosarca
hydrosarcocele
hydrostatic
   h. balloon dilation
   h. pressure
hydrosyringomyelia
hydrotubation
hydroureter
hydroxyapatite graft
hydroxyethyl
   h. methacrylate polymerizing solution
   h. starch (HES)
   h. starch solution (HES)
hyfrecation
Hy-Gestrone injection
hygroma
hygroscopic
   h. expansion
   h. heat and moisture exchanger
   h. technique
hyla
hyloma
Hylutin injection
hymenal
   h. caruncula
   h. membrane
   h. ring
hymenectomy
hymenoplasty
hymenorrhaphy
hymenotomy
Hymlek portable chest tube
Hynes pharyngoplasty
hyoepiglottic
   h. ligament
hyoepiglottidean
hyoglossal
   h. membrane
   h. muscle
hyoglossus
   h. muscle

hyoid
  h. apparatus
  h. bone
  h. bone fracture
  h. bone resection
hyopharyngeus
hyothyroid
Hypaque enema
hyparterial
  h. bronchi
hypaxial
hypencephalon
hyperacute
  h. graft-vs-host disease
  h. rejection
hyperaeration
hyperalgesia
  barbiturate-related h.
hyperbaric
  h. bupivacaine
  h. lidocaine spinal solution
  h. local anesthetic
  h. oxygen
  h. oxygenation
  h. oxygen therapy
  h. pressure
  h. spinal anesthesia
  h. tetracaine
hypercapnia
  permissive h.
hypercapnic
  h. drive
  h. ventilatory response
hypercarbia
hypercoagulation
**hypercontractile external sphincter
  response**
hyperdense brain lesion
hyperdeviation
hyperdynamic
  h. circulation
  h. shock
hyperemia
hyperemic
hypereuryprosopic
hyperexplexia
hyperextension deformity
hyperextension-hyperflexion injury
hyperfibrinolysis
hyperfiltration
  capillary h.
  glomerular h.

  h. injury
  renal h.
Hyperflex tracheostomy tube
hyperfractionated total body irradiation
hyperhydration
hyperhydropexy
hyperinfection
hyperinflation
hyperintense brain lesion
hyperkeratotic lesion
hyperlactation
hypernephroma
hypernephronia
hyperorchidism
hyperosmolar
  h. diabetic coma
  h. hyperglycemic nonketotic coma
hyperostosis
  generalized cortical h.
hyperparathyroidism
  brown tumor of h.
hyperpigmented lesion
hyperplasia
hyperplastic
  h. graft
  h. inflammation
  h. polyp
  h. tissue
hyperpronation
hyperpyrexia
  fulminant h.
  malignant h.
hyperreflexic bladder
hypersalivation
hypersensitive xiphoid syndrome
hypersensitivity
  denervation h.
hypersensitization
hypertelorism
hypertension
  extrahepatic portal venous h.
  lithotripsy-induced h.
  malignant h.
  primary pulmonary h. (PPH)
  pulmonary artery h. (PAH)
  renal h.
  renovascular h.
hyperthermia
  malignant h. (MH)
  h. therapy
  whole-body h.
hyperthymization

NOTES

H

hypertonic
    h. bladder
    h. saline
    h. saline-epinephrine (HSE)
    h. saline-epinephrine solution
hypertonic/hyperoncotic
    h. fluid resuscitation
    h. solution
hypertrophic granulation tissue
hypertrophy
    benign prostatic h.
    eccentric h.
    hemangiectatic h.
hypervalvular phonation
hypervascular fragment
hypervascularity
hyperventilation
    alveolar h.
    isocapnic h.
    h. maneuver
    h. syndrome
    h. test
    h. tetany
hyphema
hypnoplasty
hypnosis
hypnotic
    h. dissociation
    h. effect
    intravenous h.
    h. response
hypoaeration
hypobaria
hypobaric
    h. spinal anesthesia
hypocalcemia
hypocapnia
hypocarbia
hypochondriac region
hypochondrium
hypochordal
hypocystotomy
hypodense brain lesion
hypoderm
hypodermic
    h. implantation
hypoeccrisis
hypoechoic lesion
hypogastric
    h. artery
    h. artery ligation
    h. flap
    h. ganglia
    h. nerve
    h. plexus block anesthetic
      technique
    h. vein
hypogastrium

hypogastrocele
hypogastroschisis
hypogenitalism
hypoglossal
    h. canal
    h. facial nerve anastomosis
    h. facial transfer procedure
hypoglossis
hypoglossus
hypoglottis
hypognathous
hypogonadism
hypohyloma
hypoinflation of the lung
hypolepidoma
hypolobulation
hypo-oncotic plasma substitute
hypoperfusion
hypopharynx
hypophyseal
    h. portal circulation
hypophysectomize
hypophysectomy
    partial central h.
    total h.
    transsphenoidal h.
    unilateral h.
hypophysial
    h. duct
    h. fossa
hypophysis, pl. hypophyses
    alpha cell of h.
    anterior lobe of h.
    beta cell of h.
    h. cerebri
    distal part of anterior lobe of h.
    infundibular part of anterior lobe
      of h.
    pharyngeal h.
    posterior lobe of h.
    h. staining procedure
    tentorium of h.
hypopigmentation
    postinflammatory h.
hypoplasia
hyposalivation
hyposcheotomy
hypospadiac
hypospadias
hypostasis
    postmortem h.
    pulmonary h.
hypostatic abscess
hypostomia
HypoTears PF solution
hypotension
    induced h.

hypotensive
    h. anesthesia
    h. surgery
hypothalamic-hypophyseal-ovarian-
    endometrial axis
hypothalamic-hypophyseal portal
    circulation
hypothalamohypophysial tract
hypothenar
    h. eminence
    h. prominence
hypothermia
    accidental h.
    h. anesthetic technique
    core h.
    extracorporeal exchange h.
    intraoperative core h.
    moderate h.
    pediatric h.
    profound h.
    redistribution h.
    regional h.
    total body h.
hypothermic
    h. anesthesia
    h. circulatory arrest
    h. effect
    h. hypokalemic cardioplegic arrest
      (HHCA)
    h. perfusion
hypotonic solution
hypotympanum
hypouresis
hypoventilation
    alveolar h.
    benzodiazepine-induced h.
    sedation-induced h.
hypovolemia
hypovolemic shock
hypoxia
    diffusion h.
    hypoxic h.
    ischemic h.
    stagnant h.
    tumor h.
hypoxia-induced rhabdomyolysis
hypoxic
    h. guard
    h. hypoxia
    h. pulmonary vasoconstriction
      (HPV)

    h. ventilatory decrease
    h. ventilatory response
Hyprogest injection
hypsibrachycephalic
hypsiconchous
hypsiloid
    h. angle
    h. cartilage
hypsistaphylia
hypsistenocephalic
Hyrtl
    H. anastomosis
    H. foramen
    H. loop
    H. sphincter
hysterectomy
    abdominal h.
    abdominovaginal h.
    Bell-Buettner h.
    Bonney abdominal h.
    cesarean h.
    classic abdominal Semm h.
    Dellepiane h.
    Döderlein method of vaginal h.
    Doyen vaginal h.
    Eden-Lawson h.
    extrafascial h.
    Gelpi-Lowry h.
    laparoscopic-assisted vaginal h.
    laparoscopic Döderlein h.
    laparoscopic radical h.
    Latzko radical abdominal h.
    Mayo h.
    Meigs-Werthein h.
    modified radical h.
    obstetrical h.
    paravaginal h.
    pelviscopic intrafascial h.
    Porro h.
    radical abdominal h.
    radical vaginal h.
    Reis-Wertheim vaginal h.
    supracervical h.
    total abdominal h.
    vaginal h.
    Ward-Mayo vaginal h.
hysterical anesthesia
hysterocele
hysterocleisis
hysterocystopexy
hysterolysis
hysteromyoma

NOTES

H

hysteromyomectomy
hysteromyotomy
hystero-oophorectomy
hysteropexy
    abdominal h.
    Alexander-Adams h.
hysteroplasty
hysterorrhaphy
hysterosacropexy
    Ivalon sponge h.
    polyvinyl alcohol sponge h.
hysterosalpingectomy
    laparoscopic h.

hysterosalpingo-oophorectomy
hysterosalpingostomy
hysteroscopic surgery
hysteroscopy
    laparoscopic-assisted vaginal h.
hysterotomy
    abdominal h.
    vaginal h.
hysterotrachelectomy
hysterotracheloplasty
hysterotrachelorrhaphy
hysterotrachelotomy

IA
inferior apical
IA segment
IAP
intra-abdominal pressure
IAR
immediate asthmatic reaction
IAS
internal anal sphincter
iatrogenic
i. arteriovenous fistula
i. injury
i. tension pneumothorax
i. transmission
iatrotechnique
IB
inferior basal
IB segment
I-beam
I.-b. hip hemiarthroplasty
I.-b. hip operation
ICDA
International Classification of Diseases,
Adapted for Use in the United States
ice
i. application
i. point
i. skater fracture
iced lactated Ringer solution
**Icelandic form of intracranial
hemorrhage**
ICH
intracranial hemorrhage
icing liver
ICLH
Imperial College London Hospital
ICLH double cup arthroplasty
ICP
intracranial pressure
ICS
intracellular-like, calcium-bearing
crystalloid solution
ICS cardioplegic solution
ICU
intensive care unit
ICU sedation
ideal
i. body weight
i. flap
i. solution
Ideberg glenoid fracture classification
identical point
identification
colonic lesion i.
film i.

lesion i.
nasal mucosal i.
i. phenomenon
identifying canal
identity formation
IdI
point I.
idiographic approach
idiopathic
i. bone cavity
i. brown induration
i. dilation
i. eczematous disease
i. paroxysmal rhabdomyolysis
i. preretinal membrane
i. pulmonary fibrosis (IPF)
i. ventricular fibrillation
IdS
point I.
IEA
inferior epigastric artery
IEA graft
IG
image guide
IG bundle
IGF-1
exogenous I.
ignition point
IINB
ilioinguinal/iliohypogastric nerve block
IKI catgut suture
IL-282 co-oximeter
ileac
ileal
i. arteries
i. biopsy
i. bladder
i. conduit
i. conduit urinary diversion
i. inflow tract
i. J-pouch
i. loop
i. neobladder urinary pouch
i. outflow tract
i. patch ureteroplasty
i. perforation
i. pouch-anal anastomosis
i. pouch-distal rectal anastomosis
i. pouch surgery
i. resection
i. reservoir construction
i. sphincter
i. S-pouch
i. veins
i. W-pouch

ileectomy
ileitis
> pouch i.

ileoanal
> i. anastomosis
> i. endorectal pull-through
> i. pouch
> i. pouch procedure
> i. pull-through procedure

ileoascending colostomy
ileocecal
> i. cystoplasty
> i. eminence
> i. fat pad
> i. fold
> i. junction
> i. opening
> i. orifice
> i. pouch
> i. ureterosigmoidostomy

ileocecocolic sphincter
ileocecocystoplasty
> i. bladder augmentation

ileocecostomy
ileocecum
ileocolectomy
ileocolic
> i. artery
> i. conduit
> i. lymph nodes
> i. resection
> i. vein

ileocolonic
> i. pouch
> i. pouch urinary diversion
> i. resection

ileocolonoscopy
ileocolostomy
> end-loop i.
> LeDuc-Camey i.

ileocystoplasty
> Camey i.
> clam i.
> LeDuc-Camey i.

ileocystostomy
> cutaneous i.

ileoduodenal fistula
ileoentectropy
ileofemoral wing fracture
ileogastrostomy
ileoileostomy
ileopexy
ileoproctostomy
ileorectal anastomosis
ileorectostomy
ileorrhaphy
ileoscopy

ileosigmoid
> i. colostomy
> i. fistula
> i. knot

ileosigmoidostomy
ileostomy
> blow-hole i.
> Brooke i.
> i. closure
> continent i.
> Dennis-Brooke i.
> diversionary i.
> diverting loop i.
> double-barrel i.
> end i.
> end-loop i.
> Goligher extraperitoneal i.
> incontinent i.
> J-loop i.
> Kock continent i.
> Kock reservoir i.
> loop i.
> permanent loop i.
> pouched i.
> split i.
> i. stoma
> temporary loop i.
> terminal i.
> Turnbull end-loop i.

ileotomy
ileotransverse
> i. colon anastomosis
> i. colostomy

ileotransversostomy
ileovesical
> i. anastomosis
> i. fistula

ileovesicostomy
> incontinent i.

ileum
ileus
> adhesive i.

iliac
> i. apophysis
> i. arterial tree
> i. arteries
> i. bone
> i. branch of iliolumbar artery
> i. bursa
> i. buttressing procedure
> i. colon
> i. compression test
> i. crest
> i. crest bone graft
> i. crest bone graft stabilization
> i. crest free flap
> i. crest-inlay graft
> i. crest osseous flap

i. crest osteocutaneous flap
i. crest osteomuscular flap
i. crest resection
i. epiphysis
i. fascia
i. fixation
i. fossa
i. muscle
i. osteotomy
i. plexus
i. region
i. roll
i. slot graft
i. spine
i. steal
i. strut bone graft
i. tubercle
i. wing resection

iliacosubfascial
    i. fossa
    i. hernia

iliacus
    i. minor muscle

Iliff
    I. approach
    I. exenteration
    I. operation

Iliff-Haus operation

Iliff-House sclerectomy

iliococcygeal
    i. muscle

iliococcygeus muscle

iliocolotomy

iliocostal
    i. muscle

iliocostalis
    i. cervicis muscle
    i. lumborum muscle
    i. muscle
    i. thoracis muscle

iliofemoral
    i. approach
    i. flap artery
    i. pedicle flap

iliohypogastric
    i. nerve
    i. nerve block

ilioinguinal
    i. acetabular approach
    i. incision
    i. nerve

i. nerve block
i. ring

ilioinguinal/iliohypogastric nerve block (IINB)

iliolumbar
    i. artery
    i. ligament

ilioneoureterocystotomy

iliopectinate line

iliopectineal
    i. arch
    i. bursa
    i. eminence
    i. fascia
    i. fossa
    i. line

iliopelvic
    i. sphincter

iliopsoas
    i. muscle
    i. muscle hematoma
    i. ring

iliopubic
    i. eminence
    i. tract

iliosacral
    i. and iliac fixation construct

iliosciatic

iliospinal

iliotibial
    i. band
    i. band graft augmentation
    i. tract

iliotrochanteric

ilium
    external i.
    in-ex i.
    internal-external i.

Ilizarov
    I. external fixation
    I. limb-lengthening technique
    I. method
    I. procedure
    I. ring

ill-defined mass

illuminating stylet

illumination
    axial i.
    background i.
    central i.
    coaxial i.
    contact i.

NOTES

illumination *(continued)*
    critical i.
    dark-field i.
    dark-ground i.
    diffuse i.
    direct i.
    erect i.
    focal i.
    Köhler i.
    lateral i.
    narrow-slit i.
    oblique i.
    slit i.
    vertical i.
ILP
    isolated limb perfusion
IM
    intramuscular
IMA
    internal mammary graft
      IMA graft
image
    i. analysis
    AP-T i.
    axial spin-echo i.
    body i.
    2C-L i.
    i. compression
    4C-T i.
    5C-T i.
    degradation of i.
    DG-L i.
    DG-T i.
    ejection-fraction i.
    ejection shell i.
    field-echo i.
    flow-on gradient-echo i.
    i. formation
    i. formation principle
    gradient-echo MR i.
    gradient-recalled echo i.
    i. guide (IG)
    i. guide bundle
    hard-copy i.
    i. intensification
    left ventricular cross section i.
    long pulse repetition time/echo
      time i.
    MP-L i.
    MP-T i.
    MV-T i.
    i. point
    point-counting i.
    real-time echo-planar i.
    sagittal spin-echo i.
    second-echo i.
    short pulse repetition time/echo
      time i.

    single-slice gradient-echo i.
    spin-echo i.
    surface-projection rendering i.
    thin-section axial i.
    T1-weighted spin-echo i.
    T2-weighted spin-echo i.
image-guided stereotactic brain biopsy
image-integrated surgery treatment
  planning
image-selected in vivo spectroscopy
image-space
    i.-s. focus
imaginal exposure
imaging
    2DFT gradient-echo i.
    3DFT gradient-echo MR i.
    direct Fourier transformation i.
    Dixon method opposed i.
    Doppler color flow i.
    Doppler tissue i.
    echo i.
    echoplanar magnetic resonance i.
    endocrine i.
    endometrial chemical shift i.
    endorectal coil magnetic
      resonance i.
    endoscopic ultrasonographic i.
    endovaginal i.
    exercise i.
    field-echo i.
    gradient-echo MR i.
    intravenous digital subtraction i.
    krypton-8lm ventilation i.
    LaparoScan laparoscopic
      ultrasonic i.
    low flip angle gradient-echo i.
    magnetic source i. (MSI)
    multiple-echo i.
    multiple line scan i.
    multiple plane i.
    multiple spin-echo i.
    oblique sagittal gradient-echo
      MR i.
    paramagnetic enhancement
      accentuation by chemical shift i.
    phase-sensitive gradient-echo MR i.
    point i.
    projection-reconstruction i.
    projection tract i.
    rapid acquisition radiofrequency-
      echo-steady state i.
    rotating frame i.
    sagittal-plane i.
    selective excitation projection
      reconstruction i.
    sensitive plane projection
      reconstruction i.
    sequential line i.

sequential plane i.
sequential point i.
short inversion recovery i. (STIR)
single-echo diffusion i.
spin-echo magnetic resonance i.
spoiled gradient-echo i.
steady-state gradient-echo i.
stress-redistribution-reinjection
  thallium-201 i.
three-dimensional Fourier transform
  gradient-echo i.
three-dimensional projection
  reconstruction i.
tissue Doppler i.
transverse section i.
tumor i.
two-dimensional Fourier
  transformation i.
two-dimensional Fourier transform
  gradient-echo i.
ventilation/perfusion i.
xenon lung ventilation i.

imbricate
imbrication
  capsular i.
  i. lines of Ebner
  i. lines of Pickerill
  i. lines of von Ebner
  MacNab line for facet i.
  medial i.
  medial capsular i.
  medialis obliquus i.
  retinal i.
IMED infusion pump
Imitrex injection
IML
  internal mammary lymphoscintigraphy
Imlach ring
immaculate hemostasis
immediate
  i. amputation
  i. asthmatic reaction (IAR)
  i. extension technique
  i. flap
  i. transfusion
Immergut suction tube
immersion
  i. method
  i. technique
imminens
immobilization
  cast i.

i. method
postoperative i.
Rowe-Zarins shoulder i.
sling i.
sternal-occipital-mandibular i.
tooth i.
Treponema pallidum i.
Webril i.
immotile cilia syndrome
immovable joint
ImmTher therapy
immune
  i. electron microscopy
  i. inflammation
  i. modulation
  i. system anatomy
immune-mediated coagulation disorder
immunocompetent tissue therapy
immunocytoma
immunodepression
immunodiagnostic method
immunofluorescence
  i. method
  i. microscopy
immunofluorescent examination
immunohistochemical method
immunoincompetent
immunologic
  i. classification
  i. complication
  i. method of purging
immunometric sandwich method
immunomodulating infection
immunoperoxidase method
immunoproliferative lesion
immunostimulation
immunosympathectomy
impact
impacted
  i. fracture
impaction
  endoscope i.
  fecal i.
  i. lesion
  i. point
  stool i.
impaired regeneration syndrome
impatent
impedance
  electrode i.
  i. method
  pacemaker i.

NOTES

impedance *(continued)*
    i. plethysmography
    i. pneumography
imperfecta
    lethal osteogenesis i.
    osteogenesis i.
    severe deforming osteogenesis i.
    Sillence type II-IV osteogenesis i.
imperforation
Imperial College London Hospital
  (ICLH)
impetiginization
impingement
    graft i.
implant
    i. abutment
    i. alloy aluminum
    i. arthroplasty
    i. biocompatibility
    i. cervix
    i. entry
    i. erosion
    i. extrusion
    i. failure
    i. fatigue
    i. fixture
    i. fracture
    i. framework
    i. gingival sulcus
    i. infrastructure
    i. mesostructure
    i. migration
    i. model
    i. neck
    i. placement
    i. post
    i. reaction
    i. removal
    i. restoration
    i. stage
    i. structure
    i. substructure interspace
    i. superstructure frame
    i. superstructure neck
    i. survival rate
implantable
    i. cardioverter-defibrillator/atrial
    tachycardia pacing
    i. infusion port
    i. neural stimulator
implantation
    i. bleeding
    circumferential i.
    collared Press-Fit femoral stem i.
    cortical i.
    displacement i.
    i. failure
    fusion i.

    gastric balloon i.
    i. graft
    hypodermic i.
    interstitial i.
    in-the-bag i.
    intracavitary i.
    intraocular lens i.
    intrusive i.
    i. metastasis
    metastatic i.
    nerve i.
    noncollared Press-Fit femoral
      stem i.
    periosteal i.
    i. phase
    placental i.
    Press-Fit collared femoral stem i.
    Press-Fit noncollared femoral
      stem i.
    radioactive seed i.
    radon seed i.
    real-time 3-D biplanar transperineal
      prostate i.
    i. response
    screw i.
    i. site
    stent i.
    subcutaneous i.
    subdural grid i.
    submuscular i.
    subpectoral i.
    superficial i.
    Surgicel i.
    i. test
    tubouterine i.
    ureter i.
implant-bearing surface
implant-cement interface
implanted suture
implicit memory
implosive therapy
impotence
Impra
    I. bypass graft
    I. Flex vascular graft
    I. microporous PTFE vascular graft
Impra-Graft microporous PTFE
  vascular graft
impregnation
impressio, pl. impressiones
    i. cardiaca hepatis
    i. cardiaca pulmonis
    i. colica
    impressiones digitatae
    i. duodenalis
    i. esophagea
    i. gastrica
    i. renalis

i. suprarenalis
i. trigeminalis
impression
cardiac i. of liver
cardiac i. of lung
i. for cerebral gyri
colic i.
digitate i.'s
duodenal i.
esophageal i.
i.'s of esophagus
extrinsic esophageal i.
i. fracture
gastric i.
i. preparation
prepared cavity i.
renal i.
suprarenal i.
surgical bone i.
i. technique
trigeminal i.
imprint
tissue i.
impulse
ectopic i.
i. formation
mobilization with i.
point of maximum i.
Imre
I. keratoplasty
I. lateral canthoplasty
I. lateral canthoplasty operation
I. sliding flap
imus
IMV
intermittent mandatory ventilation
IMZ type restoration
in
i. situ
i. situ bypass
i. situ carcinoma of vagina
i. situ dissection
i. situ photocoagulation
i. situ procedure
i. situ spinal fusion
i. situ tricortical iliac crest block
bone graft
i. situ uterine repair
i. situ vein graft
i. utero exposure
i. utero repair
i. vitro contracture test

i. vitro fertilization
i. vitro fertilization-embryo transfer
i. vivo fertilization
i. vivo optical spectroscopy
inadequate
i. dilation
i. surgery
inadvertent enterotomy
in-and-out catheterization
inapparent infection
Inapsine
incarcerated
i. hernia
incarceration
colon i.
colonoscopy-related i.
hernia i.
iris i.
penile i.
retrograde i.
string method for treatment of
penile i.
incarial bone
incarnant
incarnative
incidence
plane of i.
incident
i. exposure
i. point
incidental
i. appendectomy
i. splenectomy
incidentaloma
incineration
incisal
i. canal
i. cavity
i. mandibular plane angle
i. point
i. preparation
incise
incised wound
incision
abdominal i.
abdominoinguinal i.
ab externo i.
ab interno i.
Agnew-Verhoeff i.
Alexander i.
Amussat i.
angular i.

NOTES

incision *(continued)*
- anterolateral thoracotomy i.
- apron skin i.
- Auvray i.
- Banks-Laufman i.
- Battle i.
- battledore i.
- Bergmann i.
- Bergmann-Israel i.
- Bevan abdominal i.
- bikini skin i.
- bilateral subcostal i.
- bilateral transabdominal i.
- bisubcostal i.
- Blair i.
- boutonnière i.
- Brackin i.
- Brockman i.
- Bruser skin i.
- bucket handle i.
- Burns-Haney i.
- buttonhole i.
- Caldwell-Luc i.
- capsular i.
- celiotomy i.
- cervical i.
- Chang-Miltner i.
- Charnley i.
- Cherney i.
- Chernez i.
- chevron i.
- Chiene i.
- choledochotomy i.
- chord i.
- Cincinnati i.
- circum-umbilical i.
- classical transverse i.
- i. closure
- Codman i.
- Coffey i.
- collar i.
- Colonna-Ralston i.
- colpotomy i.
- conjunctival i.
- Conley i.
- Connell i.
- corneal i.
- corneoscleral i.
- corridor i.
- Courvoisier i.
- Couvelaire i.
- Crawford i.
- crosshatch i.
- crucial i.
- cruciate i.
- Cubbins i.
- Curtin i.
- curvilinear i.
- cutdown i.
- darting i.
- Deaver i.
- deltoid-splitting i.
- dorsal linear i.
- dorsal longitudinal i.
- dorsal lumbotomy i.
- dorsal transverse i.
- dorsomedial i.
- double i.
- i. and drainage
- Dührssen i.
- dural i.
- DuVries i.
- Dwyer i.
- Edebohls i.
- eleventh rib flank i.
- eleventh rib transperitoneal i.
- elliptical uterine i.
- endaural i.
- endaural mastoid i.
- endoscopic i.
- endourological cold-knife i.
- epigastric i.
- extended left subcostal i.
- external bevel i.
- fascia-splitting i.
- Fergusson i.
- fiber-splitting i.
- fish-mouth i.
- flank i.
- Fowler-Philip i.
- Frazier i.
- Gaenslen split-heel i.
- Gatellier-Chastang i.
- Gibson i.
- Gibson-type i.
- goblet i.
- grayline i.
- Grice i.
- gridiron i.
- Griffith i.
- groin i.
- grooved i.
- gullwing i.
- Hajek i.
- Harmon i.
- Harper-Warren i.
- Heerman i.
- Heineke-Mikulicz i.
- Henderson skin i.
- Henry i.
- H-flap i.
- Higgins i.
- hockey-stick i.
- horizontal i.
- horseshoe i.
- H-shaped capsular i.

I

Hueter i.
ilioinguinal i.
i. inferius
inframammary i.
infraumbilical i.
inguinal i.
inner bevel i.
internal bevel i.
i. into eyelid
intraoral i.
inverse bevel i.
inverted bevel i.
inverted-U abdominal i.
inverted-Y i.
Jergesen i.
J-shaped skin i.
Kammerer-Battle i.
Kehr i.
Killian i.
Kocher i.
Koenig-Schaefer i.
Küstner i.
Lanz i.
laparotomy i.
LaRoque herniorrhaphy i.
lateral utility i.
lazy-C i.
lazy-S i.
L-curved i.
Lempert i.
Lilienthal i.
limbal i.
i. line
lip-splitting i.
Loeffler-Ballard i.
longitudinal i.
lower abdominal midline i.
lower abdominal transverse i.
lower lip-splitting i.
low-segment transverse i.
low transverse i.
L-shaped capsular i.
Ludloff i.
Lynch i.
MacFee i.
Mackenrodt i.
Mallard i.
marginal i.
Martin i.
Mayfield i.
Maylard i.
McBurney i.

McLaughlin-Ryder i.
medial parapatellar i.
median sternotomy i.
Meyer i.
midabdominal transverse i.
midaxillary line i.
midline lower abdominal i.
midline oblique i.
midline upper abdominal i.
modified Gibson i.
Morison i.
multiple-port i.'s
muscle-splitting i.
Nicola i.
non-rib-spreading thoracotomy i.
Ober i.
oblique i.
Ollier i.
omega-shaped i.
paramedial i.
paramedian i.
parapatellar i.
pararectus i.
Parker i.
perineal i.
periumbilical i.
Perthes i.
Pfannenstiel i.
Picot i.
plantar longitudinal i.
plaque i.
port i.
postauricular i.
posterior transthoracic i.
posterolateral costotransversectomy i.
preauricular i.
precut i.
Pridie i.
racquet i.
racquet-shaped i.
relaxing i.
relief i.
relieving i.
reverse bevel i.
reverse-Y i.
right-sided submandibular
  transverse i.
Risdon i.
Rockey-Davis i.
Rollet i.
saber-cut i.
Sanger i.

NOTES

incision *(continued)*
    scalp i.
    Schobinger i.
    Schuchardt relaxing i.
    scived i.
    Sellheim i.
    serpentine i.
    S-flap i.
    single midline extraperitoneal i.
    skin i.
    smiling i.
    split i.
    split-heel i.
    S-shaped i.
    stab i.
    standard retroperitoneal flank i.
    steri-stripped i.
    sternal-splitting i.
    stocking-seam i.
    subcostal flank i.
    subcostal transperitoneal i.
    sublabial i.
    i. superius
    supraumbilical i.
    surgical i.
    Sutherland-Rowe i.
    Swan i.
    T i.
    i. terminus
    thoracoabdominal i.
    thoracotomy i.
    transmeatal tympanoplasty i.
    transpubic i.
    transverse abdominal i.
    transverse semilunar skin i.
    trap i.
    trapezoid i.
    trapezoidal i.
    T-shaped i.
    unilateral subcostal i.
    upright-Y i.
    U-shaped i.
    uterine i.
    vertical midline i.
    volar midline oblique i.
    volar zig-zag finger i.
    von Noorden i.
    V-shaped i.
    Wagner skin i.
    Watson-Jones i.
    Weir i.
    Westin-Hall i.
    Wilde i.
    W-shaped i.
    xiphoid-to-pubis midline
      abdominal i.
    xiphoid-to-umbilicus i.
    Y i.

    Y-shaped i.
    Y-V-plasty i.
    zig-zag finger i.
    Z-plasty i.
incisional
    i. biopsy
    i. corporoplasty
    i. hernia
incisive
    i. canal
    i. duct
    i. suture
incisor
    i. point
    point i.
incisura, pl. **incisurae**
    i. acetabuli
    i. angularis
    i. clavicularis
    i. costalis
    i. ethmoidalis
    i. frontalis
    i. ischiadica major
    i. ischiadica minor
    i. jugularis ossis occipitalis
    i. jugularis ossis temporalis
    i. jugularis sternalis
    i. lacrimalis
    i. ligamenti teretis hepatis
    i. mandibulae
    i. mastoidea
    i. nasalis
    i. pancreatis
    i. parietalis
    i. pterygoidea
    i. radialis
    i. scapulae
    i. sphenopalatina
    i. supraorbitalis
    i. tentorii
    i. thyroidea inferior
    i. thyroidea superior
    i. umbilicalis
    i. vertebralis
incisural
    i. dissection
    i. epidermoidoma
    i. space
Inclan bone graft
Inclan-Ober procedure
inclinatio
    i. pelvis
inclination
    angle of thoracic i.
    axial i.
    condylar guidance i.
    condylar guide i.
    crown i.

enamel rod i.
lateral condylar i.
lingual i.
pelvic i.
i. of pelvis
inclusion body disease
incompetent sphincter
incomplete
i. amputation
i. atrioventricular dissociation
i. A-V dissociation
i. compound fracture
i. dislocation
i. duplication
i. fistula
i. hernia
i. polypectomy
i. reduction
i. regeneration
i. relaxation
i. resection
i. right bundle-branch block
Inconel tube
incontinence
exercise-induced i.
fecal i.
neurogenic i.
overflow i.
paradoxical i.
passive i.
postprostatectomy i.
reflex i.
stress urinary i.
urge i.
urinary exertional i.
incontinent
i. ileostomy
i. ileovesicostomy
incorporation
bone graft i.
increased
i. lateral joint space
i. pressure
i. systemic vascular resistance
incremental
i. line of Retzius
i. therapy
incrustation
stent i.
incudal fold

incudomalleolar
i. articulation
i. joint
indenization
indentation
i. gonioscopy
i. hardness
haustral i.
i. operation
prominent i.
i. tonometer
i. tonometry
independent exercise program
index, pl. **indices**
alveolar i.
American Rheumatism
Association i.
American Urological Association
symptom i.
anesthetic i.
articulation i.
atherectomy i.
atrial stasis i.
auricular i.
basilar i.
biliary saturation i.
body mass i. (BMI)
cephalic i.
cephalo-orbital i.
cephalorrhachidian i.
cerebral i.
cerebrospinal i.
chest i.
cholesterol saturation i.
compliance, rate, oxygenation, and
pressure i.
cranial i.
dental i.
diastolic pressure-time i.
eccentricity i.
ejection phase i.
exercise i.
facial i.
Flower dental i.
frequency-duration i.
gnathic i.
height-length i.
irritation i.
juxtaglomerular granulation i.
length-breadth i.
length-height i.
limb salvage i.

NOTES

index *(continued)*
  maturation i.
  mean shunt i.
  i. metacarpophalangeal joint reconstruction
  mitral valve closure i.
  nasal i.
  orbital i.
  orbitonasal i.
  oxygenation i. (OI)
  oxygen saturation indices
  palatal i.
  palatomaxillary i.
  penile-brachial pressure i.
  phosphate excretion i.
  portal shunt i.
  pressure-volume i.
  pulmonary vascular resistance i. (PVRI)
  i. ray amputation
  relaxation time i.
  Röhrer i.
  sacral i.
  saturation i.
  sedimentation i.
  segmental pressure i.
  Singh osteoporosis i.
  systolic pressure time i.
  thoracic i.
  transversovertical i.
  ventilation i. (VI)
  vertical i.
  zygomaticoauricular i.
Indian
  I. flap
  I. method
  I. operation
  I. rhinoplasty
Indiana
  I. continent reservoir urinary diversion
  I. urinary pouch
India rubber suture
indicator
  Crystaline i.
  i. dilution technique
  finger i.
  i. fractionation
  redox i.
  thyration i.
  i. tube
  xylol pulse i.
indicator-dilution curve
indices (*pl. of* index)
indicis
  extensor i.
indifferent genitalia
indigotin disulfonate sodium

indirect
  i. fracture
  i. hernial sac
  i. inguinal hernia
  i. laryngoscopy
  i. manipulation
  i. memory
  i. method for making inlays
  i. obturator nerve block
  i. ophthalmoscopy
  i. pulpal therapy
  i. reduction
  i. restorative method
  i. technique
  i. transfusion
  i. triangulation
indiscriminate lesion
Indocin
  I. I.V. injection
  I. ophthalmic solution
indocyanine
  i. green indicator dilution technique
  i. green method
Indoklon therapy
indomethacin
indophenol method
induced
  i. apnea
  i. hypotension
  i. hypotension anesthetic technique
inducer
  ANNE anesthesia i.
induction
  i. of anesthesia
  i. anesthetic technique
  Carlens endotracheal i.
  dorsal i.
  electric i.
  enzyme i.
  Faraday law of i.
  gene i.
  labor augmentation i.
  lysogenic i.
  magnetic i.
  menstrual cycle i.
  negative control enzyme i.
  neuromuscular system electric i.
  ovulation i.
  pain i.
  Pitocin i.
  positive control enzyme i.
  rapid sequence i. (RSI)
  remission i.
  Spemann i.
  sputum i.
  superovulation i.
induration
  brawny i.

cyanotic i.
Froriep i.
gray i.
idiopathic brown i.
plastic i.
red i.
industrial exposure
indwelling line
inequality
ventilation/perfusion i.
in-ex ilium
In-Exsufflator respiratory device
infant Ambu resuscitator
infantile
i. articulation
i. choriocarcinoma syndrome
i. hernia
i. perseveration
infarct
i. expansion
i. extension
infarction
hemorrhagic i.
Thrombolysis in Myocardial I.
(TIMI)
infarctive lesion
infected tract
infection
abortive i.
Absidia i.
active systemic bacterial i.
adenoviral type 40/41 i.
adenovirus i.
adnexal i.
aerobic i.
airborne i.
amebic i.
anaerobic ocular i.
antifungal esophageal i.
antifungal-resistant opportunistic i.
apical i.
aspergillosis i.
Aspergillus i.
asymptomatic i.
atypical mycobacterial i.
bacterial i.
benign papillomavirus i.
beta hemolytic streptococci i.
blood-borne i.
blood stream i.
brain i.
buccal space i.

i. calculus
Candida i.
candidal i.
catheter-related i.
catheter tunnel i.
cervical i.
cervicovaginal i.
chlamydial i.
Chlamydia trachomatis i.
chorioamnionic i.
chronic Epstein-Barr virus i.
closed-space i.
clostridial i.
CMV i.
Coccidioides i.
coliform urinary i.
colonization i.
community-acquired i.
congenital i.
congenital HIV i.
cross i.
cryptococcal i.
Cryptococcus i.
cryptogenic i.
cryptosporidial i.
cutaneous bacterial i.
cutaneous viral i.
cysticercal i.
cytomegalovirus i.
deep delayed i.
deep-seated fungal i.
deep wound i.
dengue hemorrhagic fever i.
dental i.
dermatophyte fungal i.
disk space i.
disseminated CMV i.
disseminated gonococcal i.
dragon worm i.
droplet i.
EBV i.
echovirus i.
ectothrix i.
endemic fungal i.
endogenous i.
endothrix i.
enteric i.
enteroviral i.
environmental mycobacterial i.
epidural space i.
Epstein-Barr viral i.
esophageal i.

NOTES

infection *(continued)*
  esophageal fungal i.
  exit site i.
  exogenous i.
  extrapulmonary *Pneumocystis carinii* i.
  eyelid molluscum contagiosum i.
  fascial space i.
  felon i.
  fetal i.
  fever caused by i.
  focal i.
  fungal i.
  fungous i.
  gas-forming pyogenic liver i.
  gas-producing streptococcal i.
  gastrointestinal i.
  gay bowel i.
  genital i.
  genitourinary i.
  gonococcal i.
  graft i.
  granulomatous bacterial i.
  granulomatous fungal i.
  group A beta-hemolytic streptococcal i.
  group A streptococcus i.
  guinea worm i.
  hand i.
  Hantavirus i.
  helminth i.
  helminthic i.
  hematogenous spread of i.
  hepatic candidal i.
  hepatic fungal i.
  hepatitis A-E i.
  herpes simplex virus i.
  herpes zoster i.
  herpetic i.
  hibernal epidemic viral i.
  Histoplasma i.
  HIV-1, -2 i.
  hospital-acquired i.
  human bite i.
  human papillomavirus i.
  immunomodulating i.
  inapparent i.
  intestinal i.
  intra-abdominal i.
  intra-amniotic i.
  intrauterine i.
  IUD-related i.
  kala-azar i.
  laryngeal i.
  latent herpes simplex virus i.
  liver cyst i.
  lower genital tract i.
  lower respiratory tract i.

MAC i.
MAI i.
mass i.
masticator space i.
maternal i.
Medina i.
Mcleney i.
metasynchronous bacterial urinary tract i.
middle ear i.
mixed nail i.
monilial i.
mucor i.
multiple hepatitis virus i.
musculoskeletal i.
mycobacterial i.
mycobacterial nodal i.
Mycobacterium avium complex i.
Mycobacterium avium-intracellulare i.
Mycoplasma i.
mycotic i.
natural focus of i.
necrotizing i.
neisserial i.
nematode i.
neonatal i.
neutropenia-related bacterial i.
nondermatophyte fungal i.
nonopportunistic i.
nontuberculous mycobacterial i.
nosocomial fungal i.
odontogenic i.
opportunistic systemic fungal i.
oral i.
orbital i.
overwhelming postsplenectomy i.
papillomavirus i.
parainfluenza virus i.
parasitic i.
paravaccinia virus i.
paronychial i.
pelvic i.
percutaneous bone marrow i.
perianal i.
periapical i.
perinatal i.
perineal i.
periorbital i.
peristomal i.
peritoneal fungal i.
persistent tolerant i.
pharyngeal gonococcal i.
pin tract i.
pneumococcal i.
polymicrobial i.
postoperative i.
postpartum i.

postsplenectomy i.
i. prevention
primary herpes simplex i.
protozoal i.
Pseudomonas i.
puerperal i.
pulmonary bacterial i.
pulmonary fungal i.
pulmonary parenchymal i.
pyodermatous i.
pyogenic spinal i.
recurrent i.
recurrent upper respiratory tract i.
renal cyst i.
renal fungal i.
repeated respiratory i.
reservoir of i.
respiratory syncytial virus i.
respiratory tract i.
retroperitoneal i.
retrovirus i.
rhinocerebral i.
Rhizopus i.
rickettsial i.
rotavirus i.
salivary gland i.
scalp i.
secondary i.
serpent i.
Shigella i.
shunt i.
spinal i.
spirochetal i.
spirochete i.
staphylococcal i.
streptococcal i.
Streptococcus i.
subcutaneous fungal i.
subcutaneous necrotizing i.
subperiosteal i.
superficial i.
surgical i.
sycosiform fungous i.
symptomatic i.
synchronous urinary tract i.
systemic fungal i.
tarsal joint i.
temporal space i.
torulopsis i.
trematode i.
Trichomonas i.
tunnel i.

unusual opportunistic i.
upper genital tract i.
upper respiratory tract i.
urinary tract i.
uterine i.
vaccinia i.
vaginal i.
varicella i.
varicella-zoster virus i.
vertically-acquired i.
vesicular viral i.
Vibrio fetus i.
Vincent i.
viral respiratory i.
vulvar i.
vulvovaginal premenarchal i.
web space i.
Western blot i.
whipworm i.
wound i.
yeast i.
zoonotic i.
infectious complication
InFed injection
inferior
   i. aberrant ductule
   i. accessory fissure
   i. alveolar nerve
   i. anastomotic vein
   i. angle of scapula
   i. apical (IA)
   i. apical aspect of the myocardium
   i. arcuate bundle
   i. articular facet of atlas
   i. articular pit of atlas
   i. basal (IB)
   i. basal vein
   i. belly of omohyoid muscle
   i. border of liver
   i. border of lung
   i. border of pancreas
   i. branches of transverse cervical
     nerve
   i. branch of pubic bone
   i. branch of superior gluteal artery
   i. bursa of biceps femoris
   i. cardiac vein
   i. carotid triangle
   i. cerebral veins
   i. cervical cardiac branches of
     vagus nerve
   i. cervical ganglion

I

NOTES

inferior *(continued)*
  i. complete closed dislocation
  i. complete compound dislocation
  i. constrictor muscle of pharynx
  i. costal facet
  i. costal pit
  i. dental foramen
  i. duodenal fold
  i. duodenal fossa
  i. duodenal recess
  i. epigastric artery (IEA)
  i. epigastric lymph nodes
  i. epigastric vein
  i. esophageal sphincter
  i. extradural approach
  i. fascia of pelvic diaphragm
  i. fascia of urogenital diaphragm
  i. flexure of duodenum
  i. fornix reformation
  i. ganglion of vagus nerve
  i. gluteal artery
  i. hemorrhoidal artery
  i. hemorrhoidal nerve
  i. hemorrhoidal plexuses
  i. hemorrhoidal veins
  i. horn of thyroid cartilage
  i. hypogastric plexus
  i. hypophysial artery
  i. ileocecal recess
  i. internal parietal artery
  i. labial artery
  i. labial branches of mental nerve
  i. labial vein
  i. laryngeal artery
  i. laryngeal cavity
  i. laryngeal vein
  i. laryngotomy
  i. lateral genicular artery
  i. ligament of epididymis
  i. lingular segment
  i. longitudinal muscle of tongue
  i. longitudinal sinus
  i. meatal antrostomy
  i. meatus antrostomy
  i. medial genicular artery
  i. mediastinum
  i. mesenteric artery
  i. mesenteric ganglion
  i. mesenteric lymph nodes
  i. mesenteric plexus
  i. mesenteric vein
  i. nuchal line
  i. oblique extraocular muscle
  i. oblique muscle of head
  i. occipital triangle
  i. omental recess
  i. orbital fissure
  i. pancreatic artery

  i. pancreaticoduodenal artery
  i. part of duodenum
  i. pelvic aperture
  i. petrosal groove
  i. petrosal sinus
  i. petrosal sulcus
  i. phrenic artery
  i. phrenic lymph nodes
  i. phrenic vein
  i. pole
  i. pole of kidney
  i. pole of testis
  i. posterior serratus muscle
  i. pubic ligament
  i. rectal artery
  i. rectal nerve
  i. rectal plexuses
  i. rectal veins
  i. rectus extraocular muscle
  i. root of cervical loop
  i. sagittal sinus
  i. segment
  i. segmental artery of kidney
  i. suprarenal artery
  i. surface of petrous part of temporal bone
  i. surface of tongue
  i. tarsus
  i. temporal line
  i. temporal venule of retina
  i. thoracic aperture
  i. thyroid artery
  i. thyroid notch
  i. thyroid plexus
  i. thyroid tubercle
  i. thyroid vein
  i. tracheobronchial lymph nodes
  i. transvermian approach
  i. transverse scapular ligament
  i. trunk of brachial plexus
  i. ulnar collateral artery
  i. vena cava (IVC)
  i. vena cava pressure (IVCP)
  i. vesical artery
  i. vesical nerve
  i. vesical plexus
inferior-lateral endonasal transsphenoidal approach
inferius
  incision i.
InFerno moist heat therapy
inferolateral surface of prostate
inferomedial aspect
infertility evaluation
infiltrate
infiltrating duct adenocarcinoma
infiltration
  adipose i.

i. anesthesia
i. anesthetic technique
bacterial mucosal i.
i. block
bone marrow i.
brachial plexus i.
calcareous i.
cellular i.
choroidal i.
colonic i.
diffuse fatty i.
epituberculous i.
fatty i.
focal fatty i.
gastric epithelial cell i.
gelatinous i.
glomerular macrophage i.
glomerular neutrophil i.
glycogen i.
gray i.
leukemic i.
leukocyte i.
leukocytic i.
lipomatous i.
local i.
local tissue i.
lymphocytic i.
lymphoid i.
massive malignant i.
mononuclear cell i.
neutrophilic i.
panmucosal inflammatory cell i.
paraneural i.
patchy i.
peribronchiolar lymphocyte i.
pericapsular fat i.
perineural i.
plasma cell portal i.
root i.
sanguineous i.
tuberculous i.
tumor i.

inflamed synovial pouch
inflammation
active chronic i.
acute and chronic i.
acute hemorrhagic i.
adhesive i.
allergic i.
alterative i.
atrophic i.
blenorrhagic i.

bronchial i.
bullous granulomatous i.
calcified granulomatous i.
cartilage i.
caseating granulomatous i.
caseous i.
catarrhal i.
cavitating i.
central zone i.
cervical i.
chronic jejunal i.
circumscribed i.
confluent i.
i. of connective tissue
croupous i.
cystic acute i.
cystic chronic i.
cystic granulomatous i.
degenerative i.
diffuse acute i.
diffuse chronic i.
disseminated i.
ear cartilage i.
erosive i.
esophageal i.
exanthematous i.
exudative granulomatous i.
i. of eyelid
fibrinoid necrotizing i.
fibrinopurulent i.
fibrinous i.
fibrocaseous i.
fibroid i.
focal granulomatous i.
follicular i.
gangrenous granulomatous i.
gelatinous acute i.
gingival i.
granulomatous i.
hemorrhagic i.
hyperplastic i.
immune i.
interstitial i.
intralobular i.
ischemic ocular i.
localized i.
membranous acute i.
microbiliary i.
miliary granulomatous i.
mucosal i.
multifocal i.
myocardial i.

NOTES

inflammation *(continued)*
    necrotic i.
    necrotizing granulomatous i.
    neutrophilic i.
    nonnecrotizing granulomatous i.
    obliterative i.
    ocular i.
    organizing i.
    ossifying i.
    pelvic i.
    periodontal i.
    perirectal i.
    portal eosinophilic i.
    portal tract i.
    prepatellar bursa i.
    productive i.
    proliferative i.
    pseudomembranous acute i.
    purulent i.
    pustular i.
    i. reaction
    recurrent i.
    retrodiskal temporomandibular joint
      pad i.
    sanguineous i.
    sclerosing i.
    serofibrinous i.
    serous acute i.
    spinal i.
    subacute i.
    suppurative acute i.
    suppurative chronic i.
    suppurative granulomatous i.
    transudative i.
    traumatic i.
    ulcerative i.
    urate-associated i.
    uremic i.
    vaginal i.
    vesicular acute i.
    vesicular granulomatous i.
inflammatory
    i. bowel disease
    i. cavity
    i. exudate
    i. fistula
    i. fracture
    i. lesion
    i. membrane
    i. pain
    i. perforation
    i. renal mass
    i. rupture
    i. sinus tract
inflatable tracheal tube cuff
inflation
    balloon i.
    i. reflex

inflection, inflexion
    point of i.
inflow tract
infold
informal method
informed consent
infra-auricular
    i.-a. deep parotid lymph nodes
    i.-a. mass
    i.-a. subfascial parotid lymph nodes
infraclavicular
    i. fossa
    i. part of brachial plexus
    i. triangle
infraclinoid aneurysm
infracostal line
infracotyloid
infraction fracture
infradentale
infradiaphragmatic
infraduodenal fossa
infragastric pancreoscopy
infraglenoid
    i. tubercle
infraglottic
    i. space
infrahepatic
    i. cavotomy
    i. inferior vena cava
infrahyoid
    i. branch of superior thyroid artery
    i. bursa
    i. muscles
infralabyrinthine approach
inframammary
    i. crease
    i. incision
    i. region
inframandibular
inframarginal
inframaxillary
inframesocolic space
infraorbital
    i. anesthesia
    i. artery
    i. canal
    i. groove
    i. injection
    i. nerve
    i. region
    i. space
    i. space abscess
    i. suture
infrapatellar
    i. branch of saphenous nerve
    i. fat body
    i. fat pad
    i. tendon rupture

infrapopliteal transluminal angioplasty
infrared
    i. coagulation
    i. laser-Doppler flowmeter
    i. photocoagulation
    i. spectroscopy
    i. therapy
    i. transillumination gastroscopy
infrarenal
    i. aortic cross-clamping
    i. template procedure
infrascapular
    i. artery
    i. region
infraspinatus
    i. bursa
    i. insertion erosion
infraspinous
    i. fossa
infrasplenic
infrasternal
    i. angle
infrastructure
    implant i.
infratemporal
    i. crest
    i. fossa
    i. fossa approach
    i. space
    i. surface of maxilla
infratentorial
    i. arteriovenous malformation
    i. supracerebellar approach
infrathoracic
infratrochlear nerve
infraumbilical
    i. incision
    i. omphalocele
infraversion
infundibular
    i. part of anterior lobe of hypophysis
    i. wedge resection
infundibulectomy
    Brock i.
infundibuliform
    i. fascia
    i. sheath
infundibuloma
infundibulo-ovarian ligament
infundibulopelvic
    i. ligament

infundibulotomy
infundibulum
    caliceal i.
    ethmoid i.
    ethmoidal i.
    i. ethmoidale
Infuse-A-Port
    I.-A.-P. port
    I.-A.-P. pump
infuser
    ANNE anesthesia i.
infusion
    chronic subcutaneous i.
    dexmedetomidine i.
    epidural i.
    epidural opioid i.
    i. graft
    hepatic arterial i. (HAI)
    intravariceal i.
    i. port
    target-controlled i. (TCI)
    i. tube
Infu-Surg pressure infuser bag
Ingelman-Sundberg gracilis muscle procedure
ingested foreign body
Inglis-Cooper technique
Inglis-Ranawat-Straub
    I.-R.-S. elbow synovectomy
    I.-R.-S. technique
Inglis triaxial total elbow arthroplasty
Ingram-Bachynski classification of hip fracture
Ingram bony bridge resection
Ingram-Canle-Beaty epiphyseal-metaphyseal osteotomy
Ingram-Withers-Speltz motor test
Ingrassia wing
ingrown nail
ingrowth
    i. fixation
    local i.
inguen
inguinal
    i. aponeurotic fold
    i. approach
    i. branches of external pudendal arteries
    i. canal
    i. canal dissection
    i. crest
    i. fossa

NOTES

inguinal *(continued)*
    i. glands
    i. hernia
    i. herniorrhaphy
    i. incision
    i. ligament of the kidney
    i. lymphadenectomy
    i. lymph node metastasis
    i. plexus
    i. region
    i. triangle
    i. trigone
inguinal-femoral node dissection
inguinocrural
    i. hernia
inguinofemoral hernia
inguinolabial
    i. hernia
inguinoperitoneal
inguinoscrotal
    i. hernia
inguinosuperficial hernia
inhalant anesthesia
inhalation
    i. aerosol
    i. agent
    i. analgesia
    i. anesthesia
    i. anesthetic
    i. anesthetic technique
    i. method
    i. pneumonia
    i. therapy
    i. tuberculosis
inhalational
    i. anesthesia
    i. anesthetic
inhaled anesthetic
inhaler
    Cyprane i.
    Oxford miniature vaporizer i.
inhibitor
inhibitory-excitatory mechanism
inhibitory nerve
initial
    i. consonant position
    i. preparation
    i. syphilitic lesion
initialization
injected
injection
    Abbokinase i.
    Activase i.
    Adenocard i.
    Adlone i.
    adrenaline i.
    Adrucil i.
    air i.

alcohol i.
Alfenta i.
A-methaPred i.
Amidate i.
Amikin i.
amphotericin B lipid complex i.
Anectine Chloride i.
Apresoline i.
AquaMEPHYTON i.
Arfonad i.
Articulose-50 i.
Astramorph PF i.
Baci-IM i.
Bactocill i.
Bena-D i.
Benadryl i.
Benahist i.
Benoject i.
Bicillin C-R 900/300 i.
Bicillin L-A i.
bismuth i.
Black peroneal tendon sheath i.
block i.
blood patch i.
bolus i.
Brethine i.
Brevibloc i.
Bricanyl i.
Bronkephrine i.
Calciferol i.
Carbocaine i.
Caverject i.
Ceredase i.
cervical nerve root i.
Chlor-Pro i.
Chlor-Trimeton i.
ciliary i.
Cipro i.
circumcorneal i.
collagen i.
Compazine i.
conjunctival i.
continuous subcutaneous insulin i.
contrast i.
Cophene-B i.
Cortone Acetate i.
Cortrosyn i.
Corvert i.
Crysticillin A.S. i.
cyanocobalamin i.
Cyklokapron i.
Cytoxan i.
DDAVP i.
Dehist i.
Demadex i.
Demerol i.
depMedalone i.
Depoject i.

Depo-Medrol i.
Depopred i.
Depo-Provera i.
depot i.
D.H.E. 45 i.
diazepam emulsified i.
Diflucan i.
Diprivan i.
Dizac i.
D-Med i.
Dobutrex i.
Dopram i.
Doxychel i.
Duralone i.
Duralutin i.
Duramorph i.
Duranest i.
dye i.
Edecrin Sodium i.
endoscopic India ink i.
Enlon i.
epidural steroid i.
Ethamolin i.
ethanol i.
etomidate i.
extra-arachnoid i.
facet joint i.
Flolan i.
Floxin i.
Foscavir i.
Garamycin i.
Gesterol i.
heavy metal i.
heparin i.
Hep-Lock i.
Histaject i.
Hydeltrasol i.
Hydeltra-TBA i.
Hy-Gestrone i.
Hylutin i.
Hyprogest i.
Imitrex i.
Indocin I.V. i.
InFed i.
infraorbital i.
i. injury
intra-articular i.
intracavernosal i.
intracavernous i.
intracytoplasmic sperm i.
intralesional i.
intralesional steroid i.

intramuscular i.
intraosseous i.
intraperiapical i.
intrapulpal i.
intratendinous i.
intrathecal i.
intratumoral i.
intravariceal i.
intravascular i.
intraventricular i.
intravitreal i.
Intropin i.
iopromide i.
ipsilateral i.
Isocaine HCl i.
Jenamicin i.
Kantrex i.
Keflin i.
Kefurox i.
Kenalog i.
Ketalar i.
Key-Pred i.
Key-Pred-SP i.
Konakion i.
Largon i.
Lasix i.
Levo-Dromoran i.
Levophed i.
Lincocin i.
Lincorex i.
lipiodol i.
Liquaemin i.
i. of local anesthetic
local depot i.
local methotrexate i.
Lovenox i.
lumbar facet i.
lumbar nerve root i.
Lyphocin i.
i. mass
Medralone i.
mental block i.
i. method
Metro I.V. i.
Minocin I.V. i.
i. molding
moxisylyte i.
M-Prednisol i.
Nafcil i.
Nallpen i.
Narcan i.
Nasahist B i.

NOTES

343

injection *(continued)*
    nasopalatine i.
    ND-Stat i.
    Nebcin i.
    Neosar i.
    nerve root i.
    Netromycin i.
    Neupogen i.
    Neut i.
    Neutrexin i.
    Nitro-Bid I.V. i.
    Nordryl i.
    Normodyne i.
    Novocain i.
    Numorphan i.
    Nuromax i.
    Nydrazid i.
    Octocaine i.
    Oncovin i.
    Oraminic II i.
    Ornidyl i.
    Osmitrol i.
    papaverine i.
    paracervical i.
    paramagnetic contrast i.
    paravariceal i.
    Pentacarinat i.
    Pentam-300 i.
    percutaneous alcohol i.
    percutaneous ethanol i. (PEI)
    peribulbar i.
    periocular i.
    Permapen i.
    peroneal tendon sheath i.
    Pfizerpen i.
    Pfizerpen-AS i.
    PGE1 i.
    Phenazine i.
    Phenergan i.
    Pitressin i.
    polidocanol i.
    Polocaine i.
    polytetrafluoroethylene paste i.
    Pontocaine i.
    Predaject i.
    Predalone i.
    Predcor i.
    Predicort-50 i.
    Prednisol TBA i.
    Priscoline i.
    Pro-Depo i.
    Prodrox i.
    Prometh i.
    Prorex i.
    Prostaphlin i.
    Prostin VR Pediatric i.
    Prothazine i.
    Quelicin i.

    retrobulbar i.
    Retrovir i.
    Reversol i.
    Rifadin i.
    root i.
    saline i.
    Sandimmune i.
    i. sclerotherapy
    Seconal i.
    selective i.
    sensitizing i.
    sham i.
    silicone i.
    i. site
    sodium morrhuate i.
    sodium tetradecyl i.
    Solu-Medrol i.
    somatropin i.
    Sotradecol i.
    Spectam i.
    steroid i.
    i. study
    subarachnoid i.
    subconjunctival i.
    subcutaneous i.
    Sublimaze i.
    submucosal Teflon i.
    Sucostrin i.
    Sufenta i.
    tangential colonic submucosal i.
    i. technique
    Teflon periurethral i.
    Tensilon i.
    Terramycin I.M. i.
    test i.
    i. therapy
    Toposar i.
    Toradol i.
    Trandate i.
    Tridil i.
    trigger point i.
    Trobicin i.
    ultrasonographically-guided i.
    Ultravist i.
    Unipen i.
    Ureaphil i.
    Valium i.
    Vancocin i.
    Vancoled i.
    Van Lint i.
    VePesid i.
    V-Gan i.
    Vibramycin i.
    Vincasar PFS i.
    vocal cord i.
    Vumon i.
    Wellcovorin i.
    Wyamine Sulfate i.

Wycillin i.
Zantac i.
Zetran i.
Zinacef i.
Zovirax i.
injection-molded method
injury
acceleration i.
acceleration/deceleration i.
axial compression i.
blast i.
brachial plexus traction i.
Callahan extension of cervical i.
closed head i.
closed soft tissue i.
compression i.
contrecoup i. of brain
coup i. of brain
crush i.
current of i.
decompensation i.
endothelial i.
epiphyseal plate i.
explosion i.
extension i.
extension-type cervical spine i.
extensor tendon i.
extravasation i.
first degree radiation i.
flexion-extension i.
fourth degree radiation i.
head i.
hemorrhagic radiation i.
hyperextension-hyperflexion i.
hyperfiltration i.
iatrogenic i.
injection i.
innominate vascular i.
i. of intervertebral disk
intestinal radiation i.
irradiation i.
kneecapping i.
lateral compression i.
levator i.
liver transplantation preservation i.
medication-induced i.
microwave radiation i.
missile i.
needlestick i.
nonsevered i.
obstetrical traction i.
obturator nerve i.

open head i.
osteochondral i.
percutaneous i. (PI)
perigenicular vascular i.
peroneal nerve i.
pronation i.
pronation-abduction i.
pronation-eversion i.
pronation-eversion-external
rotation i.
radiation i.
second degree radiation i.
I. Severity Score
soft tissue i.
stretch i.
suction i.
supination i.
supination-eversion i.
supination-external rotation i.
supination-inversion rotation i.
supination-plantar flexion i.
third degree radiation i.
transfusion-related lung i. (TRALI)
translation i.
trifurcation i.
trocar-related i.
valgus-external rotation i.
whiplash i.
inlay
i. bone graft
corneal i.'s
direct method for making i.'s
epithelial i.
indirect method for making i.'s
i. restoration
inlet
i. patch mucosa
pelvic plane of i.
i. port
in-line
inner
i. bevel incision
i. cell mass
i. ear tack procedure
i. heel wedge
i. limiting membrane
i. table of skull
innermost intercostal muscle
innervation
striated muscle i.
innominatal

NOTES

innominate
    i. artery compression syndrome
    i. bone
    i. bone resection
    i. cardiac veins
    i. line
    i. osteotomy
    i. vascular injury
    i. vessel
Innovar
innovative therapy
inoperable
    i. canal
inoscopy
inotropic state
inotropism
inotropy
    negative i.
Inoue balloon mitral valvotomy
Insall
    I. anterior cruciate ligament
      reconstruction
    I. ligament reconstruction technique
    I. patella alta method
    I. patellar injury classification
    I. procedure
Insall-Burstein-Freeman knee
  arthroplasty
inscriptio
    i. tendinea
inscription
    tendinous i.
insemination
    artificial intravaginal i.
    cervical i.
    cup i.
    direct intraperitoneal i.
    heterologous i.
    high intrauterine i.
    homologous artificial i.
    intrafollicular i.
    intratubal i.
    intrauterine i.
    Makler i.
    subzonal i.
    i. swim-up technique
    therapeutic i.
    washed intrauterine i.
insert
    Dischler rectoscopic suction i.
    Endostat calibration pod i.
    i. graft
    United Surgical Convex i.
insertion
    anatomic i.
    anomalous i.
    biliary endoprosthesis i.
    Bosworth bone peg i.

    catheter i.
    caval i.
    C-D rod i.
    CLS stem i.
    depth of i. (DOI)
    endovascular graft i.
    i. equipment
    flatus tube i.
    Huntington rod i.
    jejunal tube i.
    J-tube i.
    lag screw i.
    i. loss
    marginal i.
    oblique screw i.
    path of i.
    pedicle screw i.
    PEG i.
    percutaneous catheter i.
    percutaneous pin i.
    Pierrot-Murphy advancement i.
    rerouting i.
    retrograde catheter i.
    route of i.
    screw i.
    Sengstaken-Blakemore tube i.
    subclavian central venous
      catheter i.
    tendinous i.
    tensor i.
    i. tube
    velamentous i.
    wire i.
insertional excursion
inside-out technique
inside-to-outside technique
insight-oriented
    exploratory i.-o.
insolation
inspiration
    crowing i.
    degree of i.
    duration of i.
    shallow i.
    suspended i.
    i. time
inspiratory
    i. bulbospinal neuron
    i. intercostal activity
    i. occlusion pressure
    i. positive airway pressure
    i. pressure support
    i. rib cage depression
    i. time (Ti)
    i. vapor concentration
inspiratory/expiratory
inspiratory-to-expiratory ratio

inspired
  i. gas
  i. ventilation (VI)
inspissate
inspissation
instability
  catheter i.
  detrusor i.
  extension i.
  ligamentous repair of the knee for
    rotatory i.
  membrane i.
  one-plane i.
  repair of the knee for rotatory i.
  sagittal plane i.
  spinal i.
installation procedure
install method
instantaneous axis of rotation
instillation
  i. of anesthetic
  contrast material i.
  lavage i.
  i. therapy
instrument
  automated analysis i.
  i. migration
  i. recirculation
instrumentarium
instrumentation
  i. failure
  segmental spinal i. (SSI)
instrument-tract seeding
insufficiency
  aortic valve i.
  atrioventricular valve i.
  exocrine i.
  exocrine pancreatic i.
  i. fracture
  mitral valve i.
  pulmonary valve i.
  transverse plane motion i.
  venous i.
insufflate
insufflation
  air i.
  i. anesthesia
  i. anesthetic technique
  constant flow i.
  cranial i.
  endotracheal i.
  extraperitoneal carbon dioxide i.

extraperitoneal CO_2 i.
gas i.
gastric i.
helium i.
intraperitoneal carbon dioxide i.
intraperitoneal CO_2 i.
perirenal i.
peritoneal i.
presacral i.
i. pressure
retroperitoneal gas i.
Rubin tubal i.
i. of stomach
talc i.
i. test set
thoracoscopic talc i.
tubal i.
insula, pl. insulae
  Haller i.
insular arteries
insulin
  i. coma therapy
  i. coma treatment
  i. preparation
  i. shock therapy
insult
intact membrane
Intal Nebulizer solution
integration
  binaural i.
  body side i.
  competing messages i.
  large-scale i.
  medium-scale i.
  very large scale i.
integrity
  anatomic i.
  soft tissue i.
integument
integumentary
  i. barrier
integumentum commune
intensification
  image i.
intensive care unit (ICU)
intent
  curative i.
  palliative i.
intention
  secondary i.
intentional
  i. rebreathing

NOTES

intentional *(continued)*
    i. replantation
    i. rotation
    i. tooth reimplantation
interaction
    additive i.
    synergistic i.
interalveolar space
interarticular
    i. fibrocartilage
    i. joints
interarytenoid notch
interatrial septum
interaural attenuation
interbody
    i. bone graft
    i. graft tamp
    i. spinal fusion
intercalary
    i. allograft procedure
    i. graft
    i. resection
intercalated disk
intercapillary
intercapitular veins
intercarotic
intercarpal articulation
intercartilaginous
intercavernous
    i. sinuses
intercellular
    i. fenestration
    i. space
intercentral
intercervical disk herniation
interchondral
    i. articulations
interclavicular
    i. ligament
    i. notch
interclinoid ligament
intercoccygeal
intercolonoscopy
intercolumnar
    i. fasciae
    i. fibers
intercondylar
    i. eminence
    i. femoral fracture
    i. fossa
    i. humeral fracture
    i. line of femur
    i. space
    i. tibial fracture
intercondyloid
    i. fossa
    i. notch
intercoronary anastomosis

intercostal
    i. anesthesia
    i. arteries
    i. flap
    i. lymph nodes
    i. membranes
    i. nerve
    i. nerve block
    i. nerve block anesthetic technique
    i. neuralgia
    i. space
    i. veins
intercostalis externus muscle
intercostohumeral
    i. nerve
intercostohumeralis
intercricothyrotomy
intercristal space
intercrural
    i. fibers
intercuspal position
intercuspation
intercutaneomucous
interdeferential
interdental
    i. canal
    i. denudation
    i. excision
    i. ligation
    i. resection
    i. space
    i. tissue
interdigit
interdigital
interdigitation
interendognathic suture
interesophageal variceal pressure
interface
    bone-cement i.
    bone-implant i.
    cement i.
    cement-bone i.
    cup-cement i.
    electrode-skin i.
    graft-host i.
    implant-cement i.
    long-term bone-instrumentation i.
    pin-bone i.
    prosthesis i.
    prosthesis-cement i.
    soft tissue i.
interfacet wiring and fusion
interfacial canal
interfascial
    i. approach
    i. space
interfascicular
    i. epineurectomy

i. epineurotomy
i. fibrous tissue
i. Millesi nerve graft
interfemoral
interference
i. dissociation
i. fit fixation
i. modification
i. screw technique
interforniceal approach
interfoveolar ligament
interfragmentary compression
interfrontal
interganglionic rami
interglobular space of Owen
intergluteal
intergonial
interhemispheric
i. approach
i. propagation time
i. subdural hematoma
interiliac lymph nodes
interilioabdominal amputation
interincisoral distance
interincisor gap
interinnominoabdominal amputation
interischiadic
interlamellar
i. space
interlesional therapy
interlobar
i. arteries of kidney
i. surfaces of lung
i. veins of kidney
interlobular
i. arteries
i. arteries of kidney
i. arteries of liver
i. ductules
i. veins of kidney
i. veins of liver
intermaxilla
intermaxillary
i. fixation
i. relation
i. suture
intermediary nerve
intermediate
i. amputation
i. basilic vein
i. bronchus
i. bundle

i. cephalic vein
i. cuneiform bone
i. dorsal cutaneous nerve
i. ganglia
i. great muscle
i. hemorrhage
i. lacunar lymph node
i. laryngeal cavity
i. line of iliac crest
i. lumbar lymph nodes
i. mesoderm
i. phalangectomy
i. restoration
i. sacral crests
i. supraclavicular nerve
i. temporal artery
i. vastus muscle
intermediate-acting insulin preparation
intermediolateral
intermedius
intermedullary rod fixation
intermesenteric
i. arterial anastomosis
i. plexus
intermetacarpal articulation
intermetameric
intermittent
i. catheterization
i. demand ventilation
i. flow machine
i. mandatory ventilation (IMV)
i. mechanical ventilation
i. pneumatic compression
i. positive pressure
i. positive pressure breathing (IPPB)
i. positive pressure ventilation (IPPV)
i. self-obturation
i. sterilization
i. subclavian vein obstruction
intermodulation
intermuscular
i. gluteal bursa
i. membrane
i. septum
internal
i. abdominal ring
i. anal sphincter (IAS)
i. auditory canal
i. auditory foramen
i. base of skull

NOTES

internal *(continued)*
   i. bevel incision
   i. branch of accessory nerve
   i. branch of superior laryngeal
     nerve
   i. canthus
   i. carotid (nervous) plexus
   i. carotid venous plexus
   i. decompression
   i. drainage
   i. elastic membrane
   i. ethmoidectomy
   i. female genital organs
   i. fixation, closed reduction
   i. fixation fracture
   i. hemipelvectomy
   i. hemorrhage
   i. hemorrhoid
   i. hernia
   i. iliac artery
   i. iliac lymph nodes
   i. inguinal ring
   i. intercostal membrane
   i. intercostal muscle
   i. jugular vein
   i. jugular vein cannulation
     anesthetic technique
   i. jugular vein catheterization
     anesthetic technique
   i. jugular vein puncture anesthetic
     technique
   i. lacrimal fistula
   i. limiting membrane
   i. male genital organs
   i. mammary artery
   i. mammary graft (IMA)
   i. mammary lymphoscintigraphy
     (IML)
   i. mammary plexus
   i. maxillary plexus
   i. neurolysis
   i. oblique line
   i. oblique muscle
   i. oblique osteomuscular flap
   i. occipital crest
   i. occipital protuberance
   i. pterygoid muscle
   i. pudendal artery
   i. pudendal vein
   i. radiation therapy
   i. ramus of accessory nerve
   i. respiration
   i. rotation
   i. rotation deformity
   i. rotation in extension
   i. rotator
   i. spermatic artery
   i. spermatic fascia

   i. sphincter muscle of anus
   i. sphincterotomy
   i. spinal fixation
   i. spiral sulcus
   i. surface
   i. surface of frontal bone
   i. surface of parietal bone
   i. thoracic artery (ITA)
   i. thoracic lymphatic plexus
   i. thoracic plexus
   i. thoracic vein
   i. urethral opening
   i. urethral orifice
   i. urethral sphincter
   i. urethrotomy
internal-external
   i.-e. ilium
   i.-e. rotation
internarial
internasal
   i. suture
International
   I. classification of cancer of cervix
   I. Classification of Diseases,
     Adapted for Use in the United
     States (ICDA)
   I. Federation of Gynecology and
     Obstetrics (FIGO)
   I. Federation of Gynecology and
     Obstetrics classification
   I. Union Against Cancer (UICC)
interne
   fixator i.
internervous plane
internodal tract of Bachmann
internus
   obturator i.
interocclusal rest space
interorbital
interosseal
interosseous
   i. border
   i. border of fibula
   i. border of radius
   i. border of tibia
   i. border of ulna
   i. cartilage
   i. crest
   i. groove of calcaneus
   i. groove of talus
   i. margin
   i. membrane of forearm
   i. membrane of leg
   i. muscles
   i. sacroiliac ligaments
   i. wire fixation
interosseus, pl. interossei
interpalpebral

interparietal
    i. bone
    i. suture
interpectoral lymph nodes
interpediculate
interpeduncular
    i. cistern
    i. fossa lesion
interpeduncularis
    cisterna i.
interpelviabdominal amputation
interperiosteal fracture
interphalangeal
    i. amputation
    i. articulation
    distal i. (DIP)
    i. joint dislocation
interpleural
    i. administration
    i. analgesia
    i. anesthesia
    i. anesthetic technique
    i. application
interpolated flap
interpolation flap
Interpore IMZ restoration
interposition
    i. Dacron graft
    i. membrane
    soft tissue i.
    tissue i.
    i. vein graft
interpositional
    i. elbow arthroplasty
    i. shoulder arthroplasty
interpretation
    intraoperative i.
    mirror-image i.
    i. variability
interprismatic space
interproximal
    i. reduction
    i. space
interproximate space
interpubic
    i. disk
interpulmonary septum
interradicular
    i. alveoloplasty
    i. lesion
    i. septa
    i. space

interrenal
interrogation
    deep Doppler velocity i.
    Doppler i.
    stereoscopic i.
interrupted
    i. pledgeted suture
    i. respiration
interscalene
    i. approach
    i. blockade
    i. block anesthetic technique
    i. brachial plexus block
    i. triangle
interscapulum
intersection syndrome
intersegmental rotation
intersheath spaces of optic nerve
intersigmoid
    i. hernia
    i. recess
interspace
    implant substructure i.
interspecific graft
intersphincteric
    i. anal fistula
    i. anorectal space
interspinal
    i. line
    i. muscles
    i. plane
interspinales muscles
interspinalis
interspinous
    i. ligament
    i. segmental spinal instrumentation technique
interstice, pl. interstices
    graft interstices
interstimulus interval (ISI)
interstitial
    i. brachytherapy
    i. cell tumor of testis
    i. hernia
    i. implantation
    i. inflammation
    i. irradiation
    i. loculated hematoma
    i. neovascularization
    i. photodynamic therapy
    i. pulmonary fibrosis (IPF)
    i. radiation therapy

NOTES

interstitial *(continued)*
    i. rejection
    i. space
    i. tissue
intersymphyseal stitch
Intertech
    I. anesthesia breathing circuit
    I. Perkin-Elmer gas sampling line
intertransversalis
intertransversarii muscles
intertransverse
    i. fusion
    i. ligament
    i. muscles
intertrigo with ulceration
intertrochanteric
    i. crest
    i. femoral fracture
    i. four-part fracture
    i. line
    i. varus osteotomy
intertubercular
    i. groove
    i. line
    i. plane
    i. sheath
    i. sulcus
interureteral
interureteric
    i. fold
intervaginal
    i. space of optic nerve
interval
    i. appendectomy
    interstimulus i. (ISI)
    i. operation
    pacemaker escape i.
    rupture-delivery i.
interval-strength relation
intervascular
intervening connective tissue
intervention
    surgical i.
interventional
    i. cardiac catheterization
    i. procedure
interventricular
    i. septal rupture
    i. septum
intervertebral
    i. cartilage
    i. disk
    i. disk herniation
    i. foramen
    i. ganglion
    i. notch
    i. symphysis
    i. vein

intervolar plate ligament
intestina (*pl. of* intestinum)
intestinal
    i. anastomosis
    i. arterial arcades
    i. arteries
    i. biopsy
    i. bypass procedure
    i. calculus
    i. conduit
    i. endoscopy
    i. fistula
    i. fixation
    i. glands
    i. hemorrhage
    i. infection
    i. loop
    i. malrotation
    i. perforation
    i. radiation injury
    i. rotation
    i. surface of uterus
    i. surgery
    i. tract
    i. trunks
    i. tube
    i. ulceration
    i. villi
    i. web
intestine
    large i.
    malrotation of i.
    nonrotation of i.
    papillary adenoma of large i.
    small i.
intestinum, pl. intestina
    i. cecum
    i. crassum
    i. ileum
    i. jejunum
    i. rectum
    i. tenue
    i. tenue mesenteriale
in-the-bag implantation
intima
intimal
    i. flap
intonation contour
intortor
intoxification amaurosis
intra-abdominal
    i.-a. abscess
    i.-a. adhesion
    i.-a. arterial hemorrhage
    i.-a. infection
    i.-a. mass
    i.-a. pressure (IAP)
    i.-a. surgery

intra-adenoidal
intra-alveolar hemorrhage
intra-amniotic infection
intra-anal pressure
intra-anesthetic event
intra-aortic balloon counterpulsation
intra-arterial
    i.-a. counterpulsation
    i.-a. therapy
intra-articular
    i.-a. anesthetic technique
    i.-a. cartilage
    i.-a. injection
    i.-a. knee fusion
    i.-a. ligament of costal head
    i.-a. loose body
    i.-a. osteotomy
    i.-a. procedure
    i.-a. proximal tibial fracture
    i.-a. reconstruction
    i.-a. sternocostal ligament
intrabuccal
intrabulbar fossa
intracameral suture
intracanalicular irradiation
intracapsular
    i. cataract extraction
    i. cataract extraction operation
    i. dissection
    i. extraction of cataract
    i. fracture
    i. hemorrhage
    i. ligaments
    i. metastasis
    i. osteotomy
    i. temporomandibular joint arthroplasty
intracardiac
    i. mass
    i. pressure
    i. pressure curve
    i. suction tube
    i. sump tube
intracatheter
intracavernosal
    i. injection
    i. injection treatment
intracavernous
    i. injection
    i. injection therapy
    i. plexus

intracavitary
    i. anesthesia
    i. implantation
    i. pressure-electrogram dissociation
    i. pressure gradient
    i. radiation boost therapy
intracellular-like, calcium-bearing crystalloid solution (ICS)
intracerebral
    i. arteriovenous malformation
    i. ganglioma
    i. hematoma
    i. hemorrhage
    i. leukostasis
    i. vascular malformation
intracerebroventricular
intracholedochal pressure
intracisternal
intracolic
intraconal lesion
intracorneal
intracoronal-extracoronal retention
intracoronary thrombolysis balloon valvuloplasty
intracorporeal
    i. injection therapy
    i. knotting technique
    i. laser lithotripsy
    i. shock wave lithotripsy
    i. suturing
intracostal
intracranial
    i. anatomy
    i. aneurysm
    i. arteriovenous fistula
    i. arteriovenous malformation
    i. cavity
    i. circulation
    i. dural vascular anomaly
    i. ganglion
    i. hematoma
    i. hemorrhage (ICH)
    i. mass
    i. mass lesion
    i. part of vertebral artery
    i. pressure (ICP)
    i. pressure monitoring
    i. pressure monitoring device
    i. rhizotomy
    i. stimulation
    i. vascular malformation
intracranial-extracranial nerve graft

NOTES

intracranial-intratemporal nerve graft
intracristal space
intractable
    i. nausea and vomiting
    i. pain
intracuticular
    i. stitch
    i. suture
intracystic
intracytoplasmic sperm injection
intradermal
    i. anesthetic
    i. suture
    i. tattooing technique
intradiscal pressure
intraductal
    i. cholangioscopy
    i. pressure
intradural
    i. approach
    i. dissection
    i. dorsal spinal root rhizotomy
    i. epidermoidoma
    i. extramedullary lesion
    i. extramedullary mass
    i. tumor surgery
intraepiphyseal osteotomy
intraepiploic hernia
intraepithelial
    i. excementosis
    i. lesion
intraesophageal peristaltic pressure
intrafaradization
intrafollicular insemination
intragalvanization
intragastric
    i. hydrolysis
    i. pressure
    i. provocation under endoscopy
intraglandular deep parotid lymph
  nodes
intraglomerular pressure
intrahaustral contraction ring
intrahepatic
    i. arterial-portal fistula
    i. AV fistula
    i. biliary cystic dilation
    i. ductal dilation
    i. hematoma
    i. lesion
    i. spontaneous arterioportal fistula
intrahyoid
intrailiac hernia
intrajugular process
intralabyrinthine fistula
intralesional
    i. excision
    i. injection

    i. steroid injection
    i. therapy
intraligamentary anesthesia
intralobular
    i. connective tissue
    i. inflammation
intraluminal
    i. esophageal pressure
    i. foreign body
    i. hemorrhage
    i. intubation
    i. pH-pressure relationship
    i. pouch
    i. urethral pressure
intramedullary
    i. anesthesia
    i. arteriovenous malformation
    i. canal
    i. demyelination
    i. graft
    i. lesion
    i. nailing
    i. rod fixation
    i. tractotomy
    i. tumor biopsy
intramembranous
    i. formation
    i. space
intramucosal metastasis
intramural
    i. air dissection
    i. esophageal rupture
    i. extramucosal lesion
    i. fistulous tract
    i. hematoma
    i. intestinal hemorrhage
    i. pH
intramuscular (IM)
    i. anesthetic
    i. injection
    i. preanesthetic medication
    anesthetic technique
    i. venous malformation
intramyocardial
    i. air
    i. pressure
intranasal
    i. analgesic
    i. anesthesia
    i. ethmoidectomy
    i. polypectomy
intraneural pressure
in-transit metastasis
intraocular
    i. administration
    i. cataract extraction
    i. fistula
    i. foreign body

i. hemorrhage
i. lens dislocation
i. lens implantation
i. lesion
i. part of optic nerve
i. pressure

intraoperative
i. biliary endoscopy
i. cavernous nerve stimulation
i. cholangiogram (IOC)
i. complication
i. core body temperature
i. core hypothermia
i. enteroscopy
i. fentanyl (IOF)
i. fracture
i. interpretation
i. neurophysiologic monitoring (IOM)
i. normothermia
i. penile erection
i. radiation
i. rupture
i. stress relaxation
i. transcranial Doppler monitoring

intraoperatively donated autologous blood

intraoral
i. anesthesia
i. antrostomy
i. cone irradiation
i. flap
i. incision
i. pressure
i. trauma

intraorbital
i. anesthesia
i. foreign body
i. lesion
i. surgery

intraosseous
i. anesthesia
i. bone lesion
i. fixation
i. injection
i. membrane

intraparavariceal procedure

intraparenchymal
i. hematoma
i. hemorrhage

intraparotid plexus of facial nerve

intrapartum
i. asphyxiation
i. hemorrhage

intrapelvic
i. hernia

intraperiapical
i. injection
i. pressure

intrapericardial pressure

intraperitoneal
i. abscess
i. adhesion
i. air
i. anesthesia
i. anesthetic
i. blood transfusion
i. carbon dioxide insufflation
i. cavity
i. CO_2 insufflation
i. drug administration
i. endometrial metastatic disease
i. fetal transfusion
i. hemorrhage
i. hyperthermic perfusion
i. method
i. onlay mesh (IPOM)
i. perforation
i. procedure
i. radiation therapy
i. technique
i. viscus
i. viscus rupture
i. volume

intrapial

intrapleural
i. block
i. pressure
i. rupture

intraprostatic

intrapulmonary
i. shunt ratio

intrapulpal
i. anesthesia
i. injection
i. pressure

intrapyretic amputation

intrarenal
i. chemolysis

intrarrhachidian

intrascrotal

intrasellar
i. extension

NOTES

intrasellar *(continued)*
    i. lesion
    i. mass
intraseptal alveoloplasty
intrasheath tenotomy
intraspinal
    i. administration
    i. anesthesia
intrasplenic
intraspongy nuclear disk herniation
intrasynovial
intratendinous injection
intratentorial supracerebellar approach
intrathecal
    i. administration
    i. analgesic
    i. anesthesia
    i. anesthetic
    i. antinociception
    i. cannulation anesthetic technique
    i. injection
    i. morphine anesthetic technique
    i. opioid labor analgesia
    i. therapy
intrathoracic
    i. esophagogastroscopy
    i. esophagogastrostomy
    i. Nissen fundoplication
    i. pressure
intrathyroid cartilage
intratracheal
    i. anesthesia
    i. intubation
    i. tube
intratubal insemination
intratumoral injection
intraurethral pressure
intrauterine
    i. amputation
    i. foreign body
    i. fracture
    i. growth retardation
    i. hematoma
    i. infection
    i. insemination
    i. intraperitoneal fetal transfusion
    i. pressure measurement
    i. respiration
    i. resuscitation
intravaginal
    i. electrical stimulation
    i. pouch
    i. torsion
intravariceal
    i. infusion
    i. injection
    i. pressure
    i. sclerotherapy

intravasation
    venous i.
intravascular
    i. coagulation screen
    i. endothelial proliferative lesion
    i. fluid therapy
    i. foreign body
    i. foreign body retrieval
    i. injection
    i. ligature
    i. lipolysis
    i. mass
    i. oxygenator
    i. pressure
    i. volume expansion
intravenous
    i. administration
    i. alimentation
    i. analgesic
    i. anesthetic
    i. block anesthesia
    i. cannulation
    i. cannulation anesthetic technique
    i. digital subtraction imaging
    i. drip
    i. hydration
    i. hypnotic
    i. line
    i. medication
    i. oxygen-15 water bolus technique
    i. ozone therapy
    i. regional anesthesia (IVRA)
    i. sedation
intraventricular
    i. aberration
    i. endoscopy
    i. hemorrhage
    i. injection
    i. mass
    i. therapy
intravesical
    i. alum irrigation
    i. anastomosis
    i. migration
    i. pressure
    i. ureterolysis
intravital microscopy
intravitreal injection
intrinsic
    i. brainstem lesion
    i. compression
    i. end-expiratory pressure
    i. minus deformity
    i. minus position
    i. muscles
    i. plus deformity
    i. positive end-expiratory pressure (PEEPi)

i. restoration
i. sphincter
introducer
Eschmann endotracheal tube i.
introduction
introgastric
introitus
i. canalis
i. of facial canal
introjection
intromittent organ
Intropin injection
introspective method
introvert
intrusive implantation
intubate
intubated ureterotomy
intubation
altercursive i.
i. anesthetic technique
aqueductal i.
blind nasal i.
blind nasotracheal i.
bronchoscope-guided i.
catheter-guided endoscopic i.
emergency tracheal i.
emergent i.
endobronchial i.
endotracheal i.
esophageal i.
esophagogastric i.
failed i.
i. failure
fiberoptic i.
intraluminal i.
intratracheal i.
lighted stylet-guided oral i.
mainstem i.
nasal i.
nasogastric i.
nasotracheal i. (NTI)
O'Dwyer i.
oral endotracheal i.
oral lighted-stylet i.
orotracheal i.
pyloric i.
RSI orotracheal i.
Silastic i.
silicone i.
terminal ileum i.
total time to i. (TTI)

tracheal i.
translaryngeal tracheal i.
intumescence
intumescent
intumescentia
i. ganglioformis
i. lumbalis
i. tympanica
intussusception
inulin solution
inundation fever
invaded furcation
invaginate
invaginated membrane
invagination
i. of the ampulla
basilar i.
endplate i.
epithelial i.
stomal i.
stump i.
i. technique
invasion
perineural i.
invasive
i. pressure measurement
i. therapy
i. tumor
inverse
i. bevel incision
i. ratio ventilation
inverse-ratio ventilation
Inversine
inversion
i. appendectomy
inversion-eversion rotation
inverted
i. bevel incision
i. L-form osteotomy
i. pelvis
i. skin flap
inverted-U
i.-U. abdominal incision
i.-U. pouch
inverted-V peritoneotomy
inverted-Y
i.-Y. fracture
i.-Y. incision
inverting
i. knot technique
i. suture
invertor

NOTES

investing
  i. cartilage
  i. fascia
  i. layer of deep cervical fascia
investment expansion
involuntary
  i. guarding
  i. sterilization
involved-field radiation
involvement
  bifurcation i.
  extramedullary i.
  extraocular muscle i.
  nervous system i.
  trifurcation i.
inward-going rectification
inward rotation
IOC
  intraoperative cholangiogram
Iocare balanced salt solution
Iodide
  Metubine I.
iodide-containing medication
iodine
  butanol-extractable i.
  i. catgut suture
  Gram i.
  i. solution
  tamed i.
iodine-131 whole-body scan
iodized
  i. oil
  i. surgical gut suture
iodochromic catgut suture
iodophor
  i. solution
IOF
  intraoperative fentanyl
iohexol 300
IOM
  intraoperative neurophysiologic monitoring
iomeprol
Ionalyzer analyzer
Ionescu-Shiley
  I.-S. pericardial patch
  I.-S. pericardial valve graft
  I.-S. vascular graft
ionization
  i. chamber pocket
  root canal i.
  specific i.
ionizing irradiation
Ion Phosphate Fluoride Topical solution
iopamidol 300
iopromide injection
I-Paracaine

IPF
  idiopathic pulmonary fibrosis
  interstitial pulmonary fibrosis
I-Phrine Ophthalmic solution
IPOM
  intraperitoneal onlay mesh
IPPB
  intermittent positive pressure breathing
IPPV
  intermittent positive pressure ventilation
ipsilateral
  i. adrenalectomy
  i. femoral neck fracture
  i. femoral shaft fracture
  i. injection
  i. nerve root lesion
Iradicav acidulated phosphate fluoride solution
iridectomy
  argon laser i.
  basal i.
  Bethke i.
  buttonhole i.
  Castroviejo i.
  central i.
  Chandler i.
  complete i.
  Elschnig central i.
  laser i.
  i. operation
  optic i.
  optical i.
  patent i.
  peripheral i.
  preliminary i.
  preparatory i.
  pupil-to-root i.
  i. scar
  sector i.
  stenopeic i.
  superior sector i.
  therapeutic i.
iridencleisis
  Holth i.
  i. operation
iridization
iridocapsulotomy
iridocele
iridocoloboma
iridocorneal
  i. angle
  i. endothelial syndrome
  i. epithelial syndrome
iridocorneosclerectomy
iridocyclectomy
iridocyclochoroidectomy
  Peyman i.
iridocystectomy

iridodialysis operation
iridodiastasis
iridogoniocyclectomy
iridolysis
iridoplasty
iridosclerotomy
iridotasis operation
iridotomy
    Abraham i.
    Castroviejo i.
    Castroviejo radial i.
    laser i.
    i. operation
    radial i.
iris
    i. diastasis
    i. ectasia
    i. incarceration
    i. neovascularization
    i. ring
    i. suture
iritoectomy
iritomy
iron
    i. Fleischer ring
    i. line
    i. lung
iron-ferry line
iron-Hudson-Stähli line
iron-stocker line
irotomy
irradiation
    abdominal i.
    abdominopelvic i.
    adjuvant i.
    cardiac i.
    i. cataract
    cataract i.
    cesium i.
    charged-particle i.
    convergent beam i.
    cranial i.
    craniospinal i.
    i. damage
    external beam i.
    external orthovoltage i.
    extracorporeal i.
    i. failure
    fractionated external beam i.
    gamma i.
    half-body i.
    heavy-ion i.

    hemibody i.
    hyperfractionated total body i.
    i. injury
    interstitial i.
    intracanalicular i.
    intraoral cone i.
    ionizing i.
    local i.
    low LET external beam i.
    mantle i.
    mediastinal i.
    Nd:YAG laser i.
    para-aortic node i.
    pelvic i.
    prophylactic i.
    selective i.
    single-fraction total body i.
    surface i.
    therapeutic i.
    total axial node i.
    total body i.
    total lymphoid i.
    total nodal i.
    ultraviolet blood i.
    UV i.
    whole-abdomen i.
    whole abdominopelvic i.
    whole-body i.
    whole-pelvis i.
irreducible
    i. fracture
    i. hernia
irregular bone
irrespirable
irresuscitable
irreversible
    i. coma
    i. shock
irrigate
irrigating solution
irrigation
    acetohydroxamic acid i.
    antral i.
    i. and aspiration
    bacitracin i.
    i. bulb
    i. burn
    caloric i.
    canal i.
    closed i.
    Colon-A-Sun colonic i.
    i. of colostomy

NOTES

irrigation *(continued)*
    continuous bladder i.
    copious i.
    endodontic i.
    hemiacidrin i.
    heparin i.
    H-600 normothermic i.
    intravesical alum i.
    oral i.
    pulsed i.
    rectal pulsed i.
    rectum i.
    Renacidin i.
    sinus i.
    i. solution
    i. tube
    whole-gut i.
    wound i.
irrigation-aspiration
irrigation-suction
    postoperative i.-s.
irritability
    soft tissue i.
irritable lesion
irritant
    i. patch-test reaction
    i. patch-test response
irritation
    i. callus
    i. index
irritative lesion
irruption
irruptive
Irvine operation
Irving tubal ligation
Irwin osteotomy
ischemia, ischaemia
    exercise i.
    exercise-induced silent myocardial i.
    extremity i.
    limb i.
    normothermic i.
    radiation-induced i.
    tourniquet i.
ischemia-guided medical therapy
ischemic
    i. compression
    i. hypoxia
    i. necrosis of femoral head
    i. ocular inflammation
    i. preconditioning
ischemic-tourniquet technique
ischiadic
    i. plexus
    i. spine
ischial
    i. bone
    i. bursa

    i. ramus
    i. spine
    i. weightbearing ring
ischiatic hernia
ischioanal
    i. fossa
ischiobulbar
ischiocavernous muscle
ischiocele
ischiococcygeal
ischiococcygeus
ischioperineal
ischiopubic
    i. ramus
ischiopubiotomy
    Farabeuf i.
    Galbiati bilateral fetal i.
ischiorectal
    i. abscess
    i. anorectal space
    i. fat pad
    i. fossa
    i. fossa plane
ischiovertebral
ischuretic
I-shaped scalp flap
Isherwood projection
ISI
    interstimulus interval
island
    endometrial i.
    i. flap procedure
    i. graft
    i. pedicle scalp flap
    i. skin flap
islet
    i. cell cancer
    i.'s of Langerhans
isobaric spinal anesthesia
isobologram analysis
isobolographic analysis
isobolography
Isocaine
    I. HCl injection
isocapnia
isocapnic hyperventilation
isodense subdural hematoma
isodose line
isoelectric
    i. line
    i. point
isoflurane
    i. anesthesia
    1-MAC i.
isoflurane-induced vasoconstriction
isoflurane/narcotic/nitrous oxide
    anesthesia
isoflurane/nitrous oxide anesthesia

isogeneic graft
isogenic graft
isograft
isokinetic collection
Isola
    I. spinal implant system application
    I. spinal implant system iliac post
isolated
    i. dislocation
    i. limb perfusion (ILP)
isolation
    i. face mask
    i. perfusion therapy
    total vascular i. (TVI)
isologous graft
isolysis
isomethadone
isometric
    i. cervical extension strength
    i. force dynamometry
    i. point
    i. technique
    i. tubular vacuolization
    i. venous tension
isoperistaltic anastomosis
isoplastic graft
isoproterenol
Isopto
    I. Frin ophthalmic solution
    I. Plain solution
    I. Tears solution
isoquinoline
isorhythmic dissociation
isosbestic point
Iso-Thermex 16-channel electronic
    thermometer
isotonic sodium chloride solution
isotope dilution-mass spectrometry
isotransplantation
isotropic tissue
isovolumetric relaxation
isovolumic
    i. relaxation
    i. relaxation time
Israel
    I. method
    I. suction tube
israpidine
iSTAT hand-held blood analyzer
isthmectomy
isthmointerstitial anastomosis
isthmorrhaphy

isthmus
    i. of fauces
    i. faucium
    i. glandulae thyroideae
    i. prostatae
    i. of prostate
    i. of thyroid
ITA
    internal thoracic artery
    ITA graft
Italian
    I. flap
    I. method
    I. operation
    I. rhinoplasty
itchy soft palate
iteration
iterative reconstruction
Itinerol B_6 suppository
Itis
    bundle of I.
Ito
    I. method
    I. procedure
itraconazole
IUD-related infection
I.V.
    Cardene I.V.
    I.V. fluid therapy
IVAC 831 drip controller
Ivalon
    I. compressed patch graft
    I. sponge hysterosacropexy
    I. sponge rectopexy
    I. sponge wrap operation
    I. suture
IVC
    inferior vena cava
IVCP
    inferior vena cava pressure
Ivor
    I. Lewis esophagogastrectomy
    I. Lewis two-stage subtotal
        esophagectomy
ivory membrane
I.V.-PCA
    Pain Management Provider I.-P.
IVRA
    intravenous regional anesthesia
Ivy
    I. loop wiring
    I. method of bleeding time

NOTES

J

J loop technique
J point
J versus S versus W pelvic ileal
pouch

Jaboulay

J. amputation
J. gastroduodenostomy
J. pyloroplasty

Jaboulay-Doyen-Winkleman

J.-D.-W. operation
J.-D.-W. technique

jackknife position

Jackson

J. cane-shaped tracheal tube
J. cone-shaped tracheal tube
J. laryngectomy tube
J. membrane
J. open-end aspirating tube
J. and Parker classification of
Hodgkin disease
J. silver tracheostomy tube
J. tracheal tube
J. veil
J. velvet-eye aspirating tube

Jackson-Pratt suction tube

Jackson-Rees

J.-R. apparatus
J.-R. circuit
J.-R. endotracheal tube

Jacobaeus procedure

Jacob membrane

Jacobs

J. locking-hook spinal rod
instrumentation modification
J. locking-hook spinal rod
technique

Jacobson cartilage

Jacoby

border tissue of J.

Jacquart facial angle

Jacquemet recess

Jacques

J. gastric tube
J. plexus

Jaeger-Hamby procedure

Jaesche-Arlt operation

Jaesche operation

Jaffe procedure

Jahss

J. maneuver
J. ninety-ninety method
J. procedure

Jaime lacrimal operation

Jako

J. laryngeal suction tube
J. suction tube

James

J. bundle
J. position

Jameson operation

Janecki-Nelson shoulder girdle resection

Janeway lesion

**Jannetta microvascular decompression
procedure**

Jansey

J. procedure
J. technique

Jansky classification

Japanese

J. cancer classification
J. standard operation

Japas

J. osteotomy
J. V-osteotomy

jar

bubble j.

Jarit-Poole abdominal suction tube

Jarit-Yankauer suction tube

Jarjavay ligament

Jatene arterial switch procedure

jaundice

obstructive j.
regurgitation j.

Javid bypass tube

jaw

j. bone
Hapsburg j.
j. joint
lower j.
j. relation
j. relation record
j. thrust maneuver
upper j.

Jaworski body

jaw-to-jaw

j.-t.-j. position
j.-t.-j. relation

Jeb graft

Jefferson

J. fracture
J. fracture of atlas

Jeffery

J. classification of radial fracture
J. technique

jejunal

j. arteries
j. feeding tube
j. free flap

J

jejunal *(continued)*
    j. and ileal veins
    j. interposition of Henle loop
    j. loop
    j. pouch
    j. tube insertion
jejunectomy
jejunization
jejunocolic fistula
jejunocolostomy
jejunoileal
    j. anastomosis
    j. bypass (JIB)
    j. bypass reversal method
    j. bypass reversal procedure
    j. bypass reversal technique
    j. bypass surgery
jejunoileostomy
    Roux-en-Y distal j.
jejunojejunal anastomosis
jejunojejunostomy
jejunoplasty
    Hoffman j.
jejunostomy
    j. elemental diet feeding
    endoscopic j.
    hepaticocutaneous j.
    loop j.
    needle-catheter j.
    percutaneous endoscopic j. (PEJ)
    j. tract choledochoscopy
    j. tube
    j. tube feeding
    Witzel j.
jejunotomy
jejunum
    Roux-en-Y loop of j.
Jena method
Jenamicin injection
Jenckel cholecystoduodenostomy
Jendrassik-Grof method
Jendrassik maneuver
jennerization
Jensen
    J. classification
    J. operation
    J. transposition procedure
Jergesen
    J. incision
    J. tube
jerky respiration
Jerne
    J. technique
    J. theory of antibody formation
jet
    high-frequency j. (HFJ)
    j. lesion
    j. stylet

    transtracheal j.
    j. ventilation
    j. ventilation anesthetic technique
Jeune syndrome
Jewett
    J. and Strong staging
    J. and Whitmore classification
JIB
    jejunoileal bypass
    JIB reversal
Jiffy tube
J-loop
    J-l. ileostomy
J-needle
    Unimar J-n.
job capacity evaluation
Jobe-Glousman capsular shift procedure
Jobert
    J. de Lamballe fossa
    J. de Lamballe suture
Jobst extremity pump
Johner-Wruhs tibial fracture classification
Johnson
    J. chevron osteotomy
    J. esophagogastroscopy
    J. esophagogastrostomy
    J. intestinal tube
    J. method of ventilation
    J. operation
    J. pelvic fracture technique
    J. procedure
    J. pronator advancement
    J. root canal filling method
    J. staple technique
Johnson-Spiegl
    J.-S. hallux varus correction
    J.-S. procedure
Johnston
    J. buttonhole procedure
    J. method
    J. pursestring suture technique
joint
    anterior intraoccipital j.
    arthrodial j.
    j. aspiration
    atlantoaxial j.
    atlanto-occipital j.
    axial rotation j.
    ball-and-socket j.
    biaxial j.
    bicondylar j.
    bilocular j.
    j. branches
    capitular j.
    j. capsule
    j. cavity
    coccygeal j.

composite j.
compound j.
costochondral j.
costotransverse j.
costovertebral j.'s
cotyloid j.
cricothyroid j.
j. deformity
deltoid insertion over j.
dentoalveolar j.
j. depression fracture
diarthrodial j.
j. disarticulation
j.'s of ear bones
ellipsoidal j.
enarthrodial j.
extra-articular subtalar j.
facet j.'s
fibrous j.
j. fusion
ginglymoid j.
gliding j.
j. of head of rib
hinge j.
immovable j.
incudomalleolar j.
interarticular j.'s
jaw j.
lateral atlantoaxial j.
j. line
j. line pain
lumbosacral j.
Luschka j.'s
mandibular j.
j. manipulation
manubriosternal j.
median atlantoaxial j.
j. mobilization
j. mouse
movable j.
multiaxial j.
neurocentral j.
j. oil
peg-and-socket j.
j.'s of pelvic girdle
petro-occipital j.
pivot j.
plane j.
polyaxial j.
posterior intraoccipital j.
j. protection training
j. reconstruction

rotary j.
rotation j.
sacrococcygeal j.
screw j.
SI j.
simple j.
socket j.
j. space
j. space narrowing
spheno-occipital j.
spheroid j.
spiral j.
sternal j.'s
sternoclavicular j.
sternocostal j.'s
suture j.
synarthrodial j.
synchondrodial j.
syndesmodial j.
synovial j.
temporomandibular j.
tenotomy of metatarsophalangeal j.
thigh j.
trochoid j.
uncovertebral j.'s
uniaxial j.
unilocular j.
wedge-and-groove j.
xiphisternal j.
zygapophyseal j.'s
Jonas modification of Norwood procedure
Jones
    J. and Boadi-Boatang method
    J. first-toe repair
    J. fracture
    J. and Jones wedge technique
    J. operation
    J. position
    J. Pyrex tube
    J. resection arthroplasty
    J. tear duct tube
    J. tube procedure
Jones-Barnes-Lloyd-Roberts classification
Jones-Brackett technique
Jones-Politano technique
Jonnesco fossa
Jonnson maneuver
Joplin bunionectomy
Jorgensen technique
Joseph rhinoplasty
Jostra arterial blood filter

NOTES

J-pexy
    omental J-p.
J-pouch
    colonic J-p.
    ileal J-p.
J. R. Moore procedure
J-sella deformity
J-shaped
    J-s. ileal pouch
    J-s. ileal pouch-anal anastomosis
    J-s. skin incision
    J-s. tube
J-sign
J-tube insertion
J-type maneuver
Judd pyloroplasty technique
Judet
    J. graft
    J. quadricepsplasty
Judkins-Sones
    J.-S. technique
    J.-S. technique of cardiac catheterization
Judkins technique
juga (*pl. of* jugum)
jugal
    j. bone
    j. point
jugomaxillary
    j. point
jugular
    j. bulb
    j. bulb anomaly
    j. bulb catheter placement assessment
    j. bulb venous oxygen saturation
    j. compression maneuver
    j. duct
    j. foramen
    j. foramen syndrome
    j. fossa
    j. ganglion
    j. lymphatic trunk
    j. nerve
    j. notch of occipital bone
    j. notch of temporal bone
    j. plexus
    j. process
    j. sinus
    j. technique
    j. tubercle
    j. vein dissection
    j. veins
    j. venous arch
    j. venous bulb
    j. venous oxygen saturation (SjVO$_2$)
    j. venous pressure
    j. wall of middle ear
jugulodigastric
    j. lymph node
    j. node
jugulo-omohyoid
    j.-o. lymph node
    j.-o. node
jugulum
jugum, pl. **juga**
    j. alveolare
    j. sphenoidale
juice
    cancer j.
jumbo biopsy
jump
    j. flap
    j. graft
jumper-knee position
junction
    anorectal j.
    choledochoduodenal j.
    costochondral j.
    duodenojejunal j.
    esophagogastric j.
    hard-soft palate j.
    ileocecal j.
    j. of lips
    manubriosternal j.
    neuroeffector j.
    pancreaticobiliary j.
    rectosigmoid j.
    sacrococcygeal j.
    sclerocorneal j.
    scotoma j.
    sternomanubrial j.
    ureteropelvic j. (UPJ)
junctional
    j. dilatation
    j. dilation
    j. ectopic tachycardia
junctura, pl. **juncturae**
    juncturae cinguli membri superioris
    j. fibrosa
    juncturae ossium
    j. synovialis
    juncturae tendinum
    juncturae zygapophyseales
Jung muscle
Junod procedure
Jurkat T-cell line
justo
    j. major
    j. minor
Just Tears solution
Jutte tube
Juvara procedure

juvenile
- j. hemangiofibroma
- j. nevoxanthoendothelioma
- j. pelvis
- j. polyp

juxta-anal colostomy
juxta-articulation
juxtacardiac pleural pressure
juxtacortical fracture
juxtacrine stimulation

juxtacubital reconstruction
juxtaepiphysial
juxtaesophageal pulmonary lymph nodes
juxtaglomerular
- j. body
- j. complex
- j. granulation index

juxtaintestinal lymph nodes
juxtaposition
juxtarestiform body

J

NOTES

K

K Sol preservation solution

K-141

Dianeal K-141

K-37 pediatric arterial blood filter
K562 erythroid line
KACT

kaolin-activated clotting time

Kader gastrostomy
Kader-Senn gastrotomy technique
Kaes

line of K.

Kajava classification
kala-azar infection
Kalamchi classification
Kal-Dermic suture
Kaliscinski ureteral procedure
Kalish osteotomy
Kammerer-Battle incision
kangaroo

K. gastrostomy feeding tube
k. pouch
K. silicone gastrostomy feeding
tube
k. tendon suture

Kantrex injection
kaolin-activated clotting time (KACT)
Kapandji technique
Kapel elbow dislocation technique
Kaplan

K. oblique line
K. open reduction
K. osteotomy
K. technique

Kaplan-Meier method
Kapp Surgical Instrument prosthetic
knee
Karakousis-Vezeridis

K.-V. procedure
K.-V. resection

Karapandzic flap
Karhunen-Loeve procedure
Karlsson procedure
Karnofsky scale
Karr method
Kasai

K. operation
K. portoenterostomy
K. procedure

Kasai-type hepatoportoenterostomy
Kashiwagi

K. resection
K. technique

Kaslow

K. gastrointestinal tube
K. intestinal tube

Kasser-Kennedy method
Kasugai classification
Katena ring
Kates arthroplasty
Kates-Kessel-Kay technique
Kato thick smear technique
Katzin operation
Kaufer tendon technique
Kauffman-White classification
Kaufmann technique
Kavanaugh-Brower-Mann fixation
Kawaii-Yamamoto procedure
Kawamura

K. dome osteotomy
K. pelvic osteotomy

Kay-Cross suction tip suction tube
Kayser-Fleischer cornea ring
Kazanjian operation
Keasbey lesion
Keating-Hart method
Kebab graft
Keen

K. operation
K. point

Keflin injection
Kefurox injection
Kehr

K. incision
K. technique

Keil tumor cell classification
Keith bundle
Keith-Wagener-Barker (KWB)

K.-W.-B. classification

Keith-Wagener classification
Kelami classification
Kelikian-Clayton-Loseff

K.-C.-L. surgical syndactyly
K.-C.-L. technique

Kelikian-McFarland procedure
Kelikian procedure
Kelikian-Riashi-Gleason

K.-R.-G. patellar tendon repair
K.-R.-G. technique

Kellam-Waddel classification
Keller

K. bunionectomy
K. procedure
K. resection arthroplasty

Keller-Madlener operation
Kelling-Madlener procedure

K

Kellogg-Speed
K.-S. fusion technique
K.-S. lumbar spinal fusion
Kelly
K. operation
K. plication
K. plication procedure
K. suture technique
K. tube
Kelly-Keck osteotomy
Kelly-Kennedy modification
Kelman operation
keloid formation
keloplasty
Kelsey unloading exercise therapy
Kelvin body
Kempf-Grosse-Abalo Z-step osteotomy
Kenalog injection
Kendall
K. endotracheal tube cuff
K. rank correlation
Kendrick
K. method
K. method below-knee amputation
K. procedure
K. technique
**Kendrick-Sharma-Hassler-Herndon
technique**
Kennedy
K. area-length method
K. classification
K. ligament technique
K. procedure
Kennedy-Pacey operation
Kent
K. bundle
K. bundle ablation
bundle of Stanley K.
Kent-His bundle
Keofeed feeding tube
keratectomy
Castroviejo k.
excimer laser photorefractive k.
k. operation
photorefractive k.
phototherapeutic k.
superficial k.
keratin
keratinized tissue
keratitis
k. lesion
keratitis-deafness cornification disorder
keratoacanthoma
keratoangioma
keratocele
keratocentesis operation
keratoconjunctivitis
keratocricoid

keratodermatocele
keratoepithelioplasty
keratoglossus
keratohyal
keratoleukoma
keratolysis
pitted k.
keratoma
keratometry
surgical k.
keratomileusis operation
keratomy
prospective evaluation of radial k.
keratopathy
exposure k.
keratophakic keratoplasty
keratoplasty
allopathic k.
Arroyo k.
Arruga k.
autogenous k.
Durr nonpenetrating k.
Elschnig k.
epikeratophakic k.
Filatov k.
heterogenous k.
homogenous k.
Imre k.
keratophakic k.
lamellar refractive k.
layered k.
Morax k.
nonpenetrating k.
k. operation
optic k.
optical k.
partial k.
Paufique k.
penetrating k.
perforating k.
photorefractive k.
punctate epithelial k.
refractive k.
Sourdille k.
superficial lamellar k.
tectonic k.
thermal k.
total k.
keratoscopy
keratostomy
keratotomy
arcuate transverse k.
astigmatic k.
delimiting k.
laser k.
k. operation
radial k.
refractive k.

Ruiz trapezoidal k.
trapezoidal k.
Kerckring folds
kerectomy
kerion formation
Kerley A, B, C, lines
Kernohan
K. notch
K. system of glioma classification
Kern technique
Kerr cesarean section
Kessel-Bonney
K.-B. extension osteotomy
K.-B. procedure
Kessler
K. grasping suture
K. repair
K. suture technique
Kessler-Klcinert suture
Kessler-Tajima suture
Kestenbaum procedure
Ketalar injection
ketamine
k. hydrochloride
ketanserin
ketone body formation
ketoprofen analgesic therapy
ketorolac
k. tromethamine
Kety-Schmidt
K.-S. inert gas saturation technique
K.-S. method
Kevorkian punch biopsy
Key
K. operation
Key-Conwell classification of pelvic fracture
keyed filling device
Keyes punch biopsy
keyhole
k. approach
k. deformity
k. method
k. surgery
k. tenodesis technique
keyhole-shaped craniectomy
key-in-lock maneuver
KeyMed esophageal tube
Key-Pred injection
Key-Pred-SP injection

Keystone
K. graft
K. technique
keyway
OEC lag screw component with k.
Khafagy modified ileocecal cystoplasty urinary diversion
Khodadoust line
Kidde cannula technique
Kidner
K. foot procedure
K. lesion
K. procedure for accessory navicular
kidney
k. adenocarcinoma
k. adenoma
amyloid k.
k. anomaly
arteriolosclerotic k.
arteriosclerotic k.
artificial k.
Ask-Upmark k.
atrophic k.
k. biopsy
k. carbuncle
clear cell carcinoma of k.
contracted k.
cystic k.
decapsulation of k.
ectopic k.
embryoma of the k.
floating k.
Goldblatt k.
granular k.
k. internal splint/stent (KISS)
maximal tubular excretory capacity of k.'s
medullary sponge k.
mortar k.
movable k.
nonrotation of k.
pelvic k.
putty k.
pyelonephritic k.
sclerotic k.
sigmoid k.
simultaneous pancreas and k. (SPK)
thoracic k.
k. transplantation
unicaliceal k.

K

NOTES

kidney *(continued)*
    wandering k.
    waxy k.
kidney-sparing operation
Kiehn-Earle-DesPrez procedure
Kiel
    K. classification
    K. graft
    K. Pediatric Tumor Registry
Kienböck dislocation
Kiernan space
Kikuchi-MacNap-Moreau approach
Kilfoyle classification of humeral medial condylar fracture
Kilian line
killer
    flow artifact k. (FLAK)
Killian
    K. bundle
    K. frontal sinusotomy
    K. frontoethmoidectomy procedure
    K. incision
    K. suction tube
Killip classification of heart disease
Killip-Kimball heart failure classification
kilogram per meter squared
kilovolt (kV)
Kilsyn-Evans principle of frontal plane correction
Kimerle anomaly
Kimmelstiel-Wilson lesion
Kim-Ray
    K.-R. Greenfield antiembolus filter
    K.-R. Greenfield vena cava filter
Kimura cartilage graft
Kinast indirect reduction
kinesthetic method
King
    K. ASD umbrella closure
    K. biopsy method
    K. intra-articular hip fusion
    K. open reduction
    K. operation
    K. technique
    K. type IV curve posterior correction
King-Richards dislocation technique
King-Steelquist
    K.-S. hindquarter amputation
    K.-S. technique
kinking
    catheter k.
Kinsey
    K. atherectomy
    K. rotation atherectomy extrusion angioplasty
Kinzie method
Kirby-Bauer disk diffusion method

Kirby operation
Kirk thigh amputation technique
Kirner deformity
Kirschner
    K. pin fixation
    K. wire fixation
    K. wire placement
Kirstein method
KISS
    kidney internal splint/stent
kissing
    k. balloon angioplasty
    k. balloon technique
Kistner plastic tracheostomy tube
Kitano knot
Kitaoka-Leventen medial displacement metatarsal osteotomy
Kitzinger method of childbirth
Kjeldahl method
Kjolbe technique
kleeblatschädel deformity
Klein
    K. muscle
    K. technique
    K. ventilation tube
Kleinert
    K. modification
    K. repair
Klein-Tolentino ring
Klippel-Feil
    K.-F. anomaly
    K.-F. deformity
Klippel-Trenaunay osteohypertrophic hemangiectasia
Klippel-Trenaunay-Weber syndrome
Klisic-Jankovic technique
Kluge method
Knapp
    K. operation
    K. procedure
Knapp-Imre operation
Knapp-Wheeler-Reese operation
knee
    k. anatomy
    k. arthroplasty
    articular vascular network of k.
    k. dislocation
    k. extension
    k. extensor
    k. fracture
    k. fusion
    Kapp Surgical Instrument prosthetic k.
    Mazet disarticulation of k.
    k. replacement surgery
    k. rotation
kneecap
kneecapping injury

knee-chest position
knee-elbow position
kneeling position
knife-edged finishing line
knitted
  k. graft
  k. sewing ring
knitting
knob
  aortic k.
  lateral deflection control k.
Knobby-Clark procedure
Knoche tube
knock-knee deformity
Knoll
  K. glands
  K. refraction technique
Knoop hardness indenter point
knot
  Aberdeen k.
  Ahern k.
  bow-tie k.
  clinch k.
  curved-needle surgeon k.
  Dangel slip k.
  enamel k.
  externally releasable k.
  false k.
  friction k.
  granny k.
  half-hitch k.
  Henry k.
  ileosigmoid k.
  Kitano k.
  laparoscopic k.
  one-handed k.
  partial-throw surgeon k.
  primitive k.
  Roeder loop k.
  self-tightening slip k.
  surgeon's k.
  syncytial k.
  Tim k.
  Topel k.
  Tripier operation throw square k.
  true k.
  vital k.
  wire k.
knotting
  catheter k.
Knott technique
Knowles pinning

knuckle
  k. of tube
Ko-Airan bleeding control procedure
Kocher
  K. anastomosis
  K. classification
  K. curved L approach
  K. fracture
  K. incision
  K. lateral J approach
  K. maneuver
  K. method
  K. point
  K. pylorectomy
  K. ureterosigmoidostomy procedure
Kocher-Gibson posterolateral approach
Kocher-Langenbeck
  K.-L. approach
  K.-L. exposure
Kocher-Lorenz fracture of capitellum
Kocher-McFarland hip arthroplasty
Kock
  K. continent ileostomy
  K. pouch cutaneous urinary diversion
  K. reservoir ileostomy
  K. technique
  K. urinary pouch
Kocks operation
Koenig graft
Koenig-Schaefer
  K.-S. incision
  K.-S. medial approach
Koerner flap
Koerte-Ballance operation
Koffler operation
KOH
  KOH examination
  KOH preparation
Köhler
  K. illumination
  K. line
Kohlrausch muscle
Kolmogorov-Smirnov procedure
Kolobow membrane lung
Konakion injection
Kondoleon operation
Kondoleon-Sistrunk elephantiasis procedure
Konno
  K. biopsy method
  K. operation

K

NOTES

Konno *(continued)*
  K. procedure
  K. repair
koronion
koroscopy
Korotkoff test
Kortzeborn procedure
Kotz-Salzer rotationplasty
Koutsogiannis
  K. calcaneal displacement
    osteotomy
  K. procedure
Koutsogiannis-Fowler-Anderson
  osteotomy
Kovalevsky canal
Kozlowski tube
Krackow
  K. maneuver
  K. point
Kramer-Craig-Noel basilar femoral neck
  osteotomy
Kraske
  K. operation
  K. parasacral approach
  K. position
Kraupa operation
Krause
  K. bone
  K. denervation
  K. ligament
  K. method
  K. muscle
  K. respiratory bundle
  transverse suture of K.
Krause-Wolfe graft
Krawkow-Cohn technique
Krawkow-Thomas-Jones technique
Krebs-Henseleit solution
Krebs-Ringer solution
Krebs solution
Kreiker operation
Kreiselman resuscitation unit
Krempen-Craig-Sotelo tibial nonunion
  technique
Krempen-Silver-Sotelo nonunion
  operation
Kreuscher bunionectomy
Krimsky method
Kristeller
  K. maneuver
  K. method
Kristiansen-Kofoed external fixation
Kritter irrigation tube
Kroner tubal ligation
Krönig technique
Krönlein
  K. hernia
  K. operation

  K. orbitotomy
  K. procedure
Krönlein-Berke operation
Kronner external fixation
Kropp
  K. cystourethroplasty
  K. operation
  K. procedure
Krukenberg
  K. corneal spindle
  K. hand reconstruction
  K. procedure
Krupin valve with disk
Kruskal-Wallis
  K.-W. nonparametric analysis
  K.-W. test
krypton-81m ventilation imaging
k space
  k. s. segmentation
Kugel anastomosis
Kugelberg reconstruction
Kuhn endotracheal tube
Kuhnt
  K. dacryostomy
  K. eyelid operation
  K. tarsectomy
Kuhnt-Helmbold operation
Kuhnt-Junius repair
Kuhnt-Szymanowski
  K.-S. operation
  K.-S. procedure
Kuhnt-Thorpe operation
Kumar
  K. application
  K. spica cast technique
Kumar-Cowell-Ramsey technique
Küntscher technique
Kurze suction tube
Kussmaul
  K. coma
  K. respiration
Kussmaul-Kien respiration
Küstner
  K. incision
  K. uterine inversion correction
Kutes arthroplasty
Kutler
  K. double lateral advancement flap
  K. finger amputation technique
  K. V-Y flap
  K. V-Y flap graft
kV
  kilovolt
kV fluoroscopy
KWB
  Keith-Wagener-Barker
  KWB classification
K-wire placement

Kwitko operation
Kyle-Gustilo classification
Kyle-Gustilo-Premer classification
Kyle internal fixation
kyphectomy
    Sharrard-type k.
kyphos
    k. resection
kyphosis
    k. correction

    k. creation
    Luque rod fixation for k.
    postlaminectomy k.
    postradiation k.
kyphotic
    k. angulation
    k. deformity
    k. deformity pathomechanics
Kytril

NOTES

K

LA
  lateral apical
    LA segment
Labbé
    L. gastrotomy technique
    L. triangle
    L. vein
labeling
    MPF l.
labia (*pl. of* labium)
labial
    l. cavity
    l. fusion
    l. glands
    l. hernia
    l. line
    l. pad
    l. tubercle
    l. ulceration
    l. veins
    l. vestibule
labialization
labile blood pressure
labioglossolaryngeal
labioglossomandibular approach
labioglossopharyngeal
labioincisal line angle
labiolingual
    l. plane
    l. technique
labiomandibular
    l. approach
    l. glossotomy
labiomental
labionasal
labiopalatine
labioperineal pouch
labioplasty
labioscrotal folds
labium, pl. **labia**
    l. inferius oris
    labia oris
    l. superius oris
    l. vocale
labor
    l. augmentation induction
    l. pain
LaBorde method
labored respiration
labral lesion
labyrinth
    bony l.
    ethmoidal l.
    Ludwig l.
    osseous l.

renal l.
    Santorini l.
    vestibular l.
labyrinthectomy
labyrinthine
    l. fistula
    l. fistula test
    l. veins
labyrinthotomy
labyrinthus
    l. ethmoidalis
    l. osseus
    l. vestibularis
lacerable
lacerated
    l. foramen
laceration
    aortic l.
    birth canal l.
    bladder l.
    brain l.
    burst-type l.
    canalicular l.
    central stellate l.
    cervical l.
    chevron l.
    concurrent hepatic l.
    conjunctival l.
    corneal l.
    corneoscleral l.
    eyebrow l.
    falx l.
    flexor tendon l.
    hallucis longus l.
    lid margin l.
    longitudinal l.
    lower pole l.
    parenchymal l.
    perineal l.
    rectal l.
    scalp l.
    stellate l.
    tarsal l.
    tentorial l.
    through-and-through l.
    vaginal l.
    vascular l.
lacertus
    l. of lateral rectus muscle
    l. musculi recti lateralis
Lachman maneuver
lachrymal
lacidem suture
lacmoid staining solution
Lacor tube

L

Lacril ophthalmic solution
lacrimal
>l. angle duct anomaly
>l. apparatus
>l. canal
>l. fascia
>l. fistula
>l. fold
>l. gland repair
>l. gland tumor
>l. irrigation test
>l. margin of maxilla
>l. mass
>l. nerve
>l. notch
>l. papilla
>l. point
>l. sac
>l. sac fossa
>l. surgery

lacrimation
>excessive l.
>l. reflex

lacrimoconchal suture
lacrimomaxillary suture
lacrimotomy
Lacroix
>fibro-osseous ring of L.
>osseous ring of L.
>L. osseous ring

lactated Ringer solution
lactate extraction
lactation letdown response
lacteal
>l. fistula
>l. vessel

lactiferous
>l. ducts
>l. gland
>l. sinus

lactobacilli preparation
lactoperoxidase radioiodination
lacuna, pl. lacunae
>lateral venous lacunae
>l. magna
>Morgagni l.
>osteocytic l.
>urethral l.
>l. urethralis

lacunar
>l. abscess
>l. ligament

Ladd
>L. band
>L. operation
>L. procedure

Laerdal
>L. infant resuscitator
>L. silicone resuscitator

Lafora body disease
lag
>dilation l.
>l. dilation
>l. screw fixation
>l. screw insertion
>l. screw thread hole

Lagleyze operation
Lagleyze-Trantas operation
Lagrange
>L. classification of humeral supracondylar fracture
>L. operation

Lahey Y-tube tube
Laird-McMahon anorectoplasty
laissez-faire lid operation
lake
>lateral l.'s

Lallemand bodies
Lallemand-Trousseau body
Lallouette pyramid
LAMA
>laser-assisted microanastomosis

Lamaze
>L. method
>L. technique

lambda suture line
lambdoid
>l. border of occipital bone
>l. margin of occipital bone
>l. suture

lambdoidal suture
Lambert canal
Lambl excrescences
Lamb-Marks-Bayne technique
Lambrinudi
>L. osteotomy
>L. technique

lamella, pl. lamellae
>corneal l.
>elastic l.

lamellar
>l. corneal graft
>l. corneal transplant
>l. exfoliation
>l. refractive keratoplasty

lamellation
lamina, pl. laminae
>l. anterior vaginae musculi recti abdominis
>l. arcus vertebrae
>basal l. of ciliary body
>basal l. of semicircular duct
>basilar l.
>l. cartilaginis cricoideae

l. cartilaginis lateralis tubae auditivae
l. cartilaginis medialis tubae auditivae
l. cartilaginis thyroideae
l. choriocapillaris
l. choroidocapillaris
l. cribrosa ossis ethmoidalis
l. cribrosa sclerae
cribrous l.
deep l.
l. densa
elastic laminae of arteries
l. externa cranii
external elastic l.
l. fibrocartilaginea interpubica
hepatic laminae
l. interna cranii
l. interna ossium cranii
l. lateralis processus pterygoidei
l. medialis processus pterygoidei
l. modioli
orbital l. of ethmoid bone
l. orbitalis ossis ethmoidalis
osseous spiral l.
l. papyracea
l. parietalis
l. parietalis pericardii
l. parietalis tunicae vaginalis testis
l. perpendicularis
l. perpendicularis ossis ethmoidalis
l. perpendicularis ossis palatini
l. posterior vaginae musculi recti abdominis
l. pretrachealis
l. prevertebralis
l. profunda fasciae temporalis
l. propria of semicircular duct
pterygoid laminae
l. superficialis fasciae cervicalis
l. superficialis fasciae temporalis
l. of thyroid cartilage
l. of vertebral arch
l. visceralis tunicae vaginalis testis
laminaplasty
expansive l.
Tsuji l.
laminar
l. cortex posterior aspect
l. flow hood
l. fracture
laminated acellular mass

lamination
laminectomy
cervical spine l.
decompression l.
decompressive l.
Gill l.
Girdlestone l.
multilevel l.
4-place l.
radial l.
laminoforaminotomy
laminoplasty
laminotomy
l. and diskectomy
Lam procedure
Lancaster operation
lance
Lancefield classification
lanceolate deformity
lancet suture
Lanchner operation
landmark
bony l.
cephalometric l.
developmental l.
pedicle l.
surface l.
Winnie l.'s
Landolt
L. body
L. broken ring
L. operation
Landzert fossa
Lane
L. band
L. operation
L. procedure
Lange
L. procedure
L. solution
L. tendon lengthening and repair
Langenbeck
L. operation
L. triangle
Langendorff
L. heart preparation
L. method
L. perfusion
Langenskiöld
L. bone graft
L. bony bridge resection

L

NOTES

Langenskiöld *(continued)*
    L. fusion
    L. procedure
Langer
    L. arch
    L. line
Langevin updating procedure
Langhans line
Lannelongue ligaments
Lanz
    L. incision
    L. line
    L. low-pressure cuff endotracheal
    tube
    L. point
    L. pressure regulating valve
LAO
    left anterior oblique
    left anterior occipital
        LAO position
Lap
    L. Sac
laparectomy
laparocele
laparogastroscopy
laparohysterectomy
laparohystero-oophorectomy
laparohysteropexy
laparohysterosalpingo-oophorectomy
laparohysterotomy
laparomyomectomy
laparomyositis
laparorrhaphy
laparosalpingectomy
laparosalpingo-oophorectomy
laparosalpingotomy
LaparoScan laparoscopic ultrasonic
    imaging
laparoscopic
    l. adrenalectomy
    l. biopsy
    l. cholecystectomy (LC)
    l. cholecystotomy
    l. clip application
    l. colectomy
    l. colposuspension technique
    l. dismembered pyeloplasty
    l. Döderlein hysterectomy
    l. fenestration
    l. hysterosalpingectomy
    l. inguinal herniorrhaphy
    l. knot
    l. lymph node dissection method
    l. lymph node dissection procedure
    l. lymph node dissection technique
    l. lymphocelectomy
    l. management
    l. multiple-punch resection

l. needle colposuspension
l. nephrectomy
l. Nissen fundoplication
l. Nissen fundoplication method
l. Nissen fundoplication procedure
l. Nissen fundoplication technique
l. orchiopexy
l. para-aortic lymph node sampling
l. para-aortic lymph node sampling
    method
l. para-aortic lymph node sampling
    procedure
l. para-aortic lymph node sampling
    technique
l. pelvic lymphadenectomy
l. pelvic lymph node dissection
l. photography
l. pneumodissection
l. PROST
l. radical hysterectomy
l. retropubic colposuspension
l. seromyotomy
l. surgery
l. total occlusion (LTO)
l. transcystic common bile duct
    exploration (LTCBDE)
l. trocar wound
l. tubal banding procedure
l. ureteral reanastomosis
l. ureterolithotomy
l. uterolysis
l. vagotomy
l. varicocelectomy
l. varicocele repair
l. varix ligation
laparoscopically
    l. assisted surgery
    l. guided cryoablation
    l. guided transcystic exploration
laparoscopic-assisted
    l.-a. hemicolectomy
    l.-a. vaginal hysterectomy
    l.-a. vaginal hysteroscopy
laparoscopist
laparoscopy
    ambulatory gynecologic l.
    Cavitron ultrasonic surgical
        aspirator for l.
    closed l.
    double-puncture l.
    flexible l.
    gaseous l.
    gasless l.
    groin l.
    gynecologic l.
    laser l.
    open l.
    operative l.

pelvic l.
second-look l.
single-puncture l.
therapeutic l.
laparoscopy-guided subhepatic cholecystostomy
Laparostat with fiber diversion
laparotomy
emergency l.
exploratory l.
l. incision
negative l.
second-look l.
l. sponge ring
staging l.
laparotrachelotomy
laparouterotomy
Lapides-Ball urethropexy
Lapides technique
Lapidus
L. bunionectomy
L. hammertoe technique
lappet formation
Lapra-Ty suture
lap seatbelt fracture
LAR
low anterior resection
Lar-A-Jext laryngectomy tube
lardaceous liver
large
l. bowel carcinoma
l. canal
l. intestine
l. loop excision
l. loop excision of transformation zone
l. muscle of helix
l. pelvis
l. restoration
l. saphenous vein
large-bore gastric lavage tube
large-core
l.-c. needle biopsy
l.-c. technique
large-humeral-head hemiarthroplasty
large-particle biopsy
large-scale integration
Largon injection
Larmon
L. forefoot arthroplasty
L. forefoot procedure
LaRocca nasolacrimal tube

LaRoque herniorrhaphy incision
Laroyenne operation
Larrey
L. cleft
L. hernia
Larsen syndrome
Larson
L. ligament reconstruction
L. technique
laryngeal
l. anesthesia
l. anomaly
l. aperture
l. bursa
l. carcinoma
l. cartilage fracture
l. framework surgery
l. glands
l. hemorrhage
l. infection
l. keel operation
l. mask
l. mask airway (LMA)
l. mask insertion anesthetic technique
l. oscillation
l. part of pharynx
l. pharynx
l. pouch
l. prominence
l. respiration
l. sinus
l. suction tube
l. veins
l. ventricle
l. web
laryngectomy
anterior partial l.
frontolateral l.
narrow-field l.
near-total l.
subtotal supraglottic l.
supraglottic l.
total l.
l. tube
vertical partial l.
wide-field total l.
larynges (*pl. of* larynx)
laryngocele
Laryngoflex reinforced endotracheal tube

NOTES

L

laryngopharyngectomy
    partial l.
    total l.
laryngopharynx
laryngoplasty
    sternothyroid muscle flap l.
laryngopyocele
laryngoscopy
    l. anesthetic technique
    direct l.
    indirect l.
    laser l.
    mirror-image l.
    suspension l.
laryngospasm
    postextubation l.
laryngotomy
    inferior l.
laryngotracheoplasty (LTP)
larynx, pl. **larynges**
    external auditory l.
    extrinsic muscles of the l.
    folding l.
lase
laser
    l. arthroscopy
    l. biliary lithotripsy
    l. cavity
    l. cervical conization
    l. coagulation
    l. diode
    l. hemorrhoidectomy
    l. hemorrhoid excision
    l. iridectomy
    l. iridotomy
    l. keratotomy
    l. laparoscopic vagotomy
    l. laparoscopy
    l. laryngeal suction tube
    l. laryngoscopy
    l. manipulation
    l. method
    l. partial nephrectomy
    l. photoablation
    l. photocoagulation
    l. photovaporization
    l. plume
    l. recanalization
    l. surgery
    l. therapy
    l. tissue weld
    l. tissue welding
    l. tissue welding solder
    l. trabeculoplasty
    l. uterosacral nerve ablation
    l. vaporization
    l. welding technique

laser-assisted
    l.-a. balloon angioplasty
    l.-a. microanastomosis (LAMA)
    l.-a. spinal endoscopy
    l.-a. uvulopalatoplasty
laser-Doppler flowmetry
laser-filtering surgery
laser-induced
    l.-i. fragmentation
    l.-i. intracorporeal shock wave lithotripsy
lasering
Laser-Trach endotracheal tube
lasertripsy
Lash
    L. operation
    L. procedure
Lasix injection
Latarget nerve
Latarjet procedure
late graft dysfunction
latency
    postdrug l.
latent herpes simplex virus infection
latera (*pl. of* latus)
lateral
    l. aberration
    l. adenoidectomy
    l. angle of eye
    l. angle of scapula
    l. angle of uterus
    l. antebrachial cutaneous nerve
    l. antebrachial cutaneous nerve block
    l. anterior thoracic nerve
    l. apical (LA)
    l. arcuate ligament
    l. aspiration
    l. atlantoaxial joint
    l. band mobilization
    l. basal (LB)
    l. basal branch
    l. basal segment
    l. bending technique
    l. bicipital groove
    l. border of forearm
    l. border of humerus
    l. border of kidney
    l. border of scapula
    l. calcaneal branches of sural nerve
    l. canal
    l. canal entrapment
    l. canthotomy
    l. canthus
    l. central palmar space
    l. circumflex artery of thigh
    l. circumflex femoral artery

l. closing wedge osteotomy
l. column
l. compartment reconstruction
l. compression
l. compression injury
l. condensation
l. condensation root canal filling method
l. condylar humeral fracture
l. condylar inclination
l. condyle
l. condyle of femur
l. condyle of tibia
l. cord of brachial plexus
l. corticospinal tract
l. costal branch of internal thoracic artery
l. costotransverse ligament
l. crus of facial canal
l. crus of the superficial inguinal ring
l. cuneiform bone
l. cutaneous branch
l. cutaneous branches of intercostal nerves
l. cutaneous nerve of calf
l. cutaneous nerve of forearm
l. cutaneous nerve of thigh
l. decubitus position
l. deep cervical lymph nodes
l. deflection control knob
l. deltoid splitting approach
l. deviation angle
l. displacement osteotomy
l. dissection
l. dorsal cutaneous nerve
l. electrical surface stimulation
l. epicondylar crest
l. epicondylar ridge
l. epicondyle of femur
l. epicondyle of humerus
l. excursion
l. extensor expansion
l. extensor release
l. extracavitary approach
l. femoral circumflex artery
l. femoral cutaneous nerve
l. frontobasal artery
l. fusion
l. Gatellier-Chastung approach
l. geniculate body
l. ginglymus

l. glossoepiglottic fold
l. great muscle
l. ground (LG)
l. ground bundle
l. group of axillary lymph nodes
l. head
l. head of gastrocnemius
l. hip arthroscopy
l. humeral condyle fracture
l. illumination
l. inferior genicular artery
l. inguinal fossa
l. intradural approach
l. J approach
l. jaw projection
l. joint line
l. joint space
l. jugular lymph nodes
l. Kocher approach
l. lacunar lymph node
l. lakes
l. lemniscus tract
l. ligaments of the bladder
l. ligament of temporomandibular articulation
l. listhesis
l. lithotomy
l. lumbar intertransversarii muscles
l. lumbar intertransverse muscles
l. lumbocostal arch
l. malleolar fracture
l. malleolar network
l. malleolar subcutaneous bursa
l. malleolus bursa
l. mammary branches
l. mass
l. mass fracture
l. meniscectomy
l. midpalmar space
l. midpapillary
l. nail fold
l. nasal branches of anterior ethmoidal nerve
l. oblique projection of mandible
l. occipital artery
l. occlusal position
l. occlusion relation
l. Ollier approach
l. opening wedge osteotomy
l. orbitofrontal branch
l. palpebral ligament
l. pancreaticojejunostomy

L

NOTES

lateral *(continued)*
l. parapatellar approach
l. parotidectomy
l. part of occipital bone
l. part of sacrum
l. part of vaginal fornix
l. patellar compression syndrome
l. patellar retinaculum
l. pectoral nerve
l. pedicle graft
l. perforation
l. pericardiac lymph nodes
l. pharyngeal space
l. plantar artery
l. plantar nerve
l. pole
l. popliteal nerve
l. process of calcaneal tuberosity
l. process of talus
l. pterygoid muscle
l. puboprostatic ligament
l. pyramidal tract
l. rectus extraocular muscle
l. rectus muscle of the head
l. rectus recession
l. rectus resection
l. recumbent position
l. reflection of colon
l. region of neck
l. rhachotomy
l. root of median nerve
l. root of optic tract
l. root pressure
l. sac
l. sacral artery
l. sacral crests
l. sacrococcygeal ligament
l. sesamoidectomy
l. sinus
l. sling procedure
l. spinothalamic tract
l. striate arteries
l. superficial cervical lymph nodes
l. superior genicular artery
l. supraclavicular nerve
l. supracondylar crest
l. supracondylar ridge
l. sural cutaneous nerve
l. surface of testis
l. surface of zygomatic bone
l. tarsal artery
l. tarsorrhaphy
l. temporal resection
l. thigh flap
l. thoracic artery
l. thoracic flap
l. thoracic vein
l. thyrohyoid ligament

l. tibial plateau fracture
l. trapezius flap
l. trap suture
l. tubercle of posterior process of talus
l. umbilical fold
l. umbilical ligament
l. upper arm flap
l. utility incision
l. vastus muscle
l. venous lacunae
l. ventral hernia
l. window technique
laterality
lateralization
cortical l.
lateral-lateral pouch
lateriflexion
lateroabdominal
laterodeviation
lateroflexion
laterolisthesis
lateroposition
lateropulsion of body movement
latex sponge graft
lathing procedure
latissimus
l. dorsi muscle
l. dorsi muscle flap
l. dorsi musculocutaneous flap
l. dorsi myocutaneous flap
l. dorsi procedure
latissimus/scapular muscle flap
latissimus/serratus muscle flap
lattice
l. degeneration of retina
l. space
latus, pl. latera
Latzko
L. cesarean section
L. partial colpocleisis
L. radical abdominal hysterectomy
laudable
laudonosine
Lauenstein procedure
Lauge-Hansen
L.-H. classification
L.-H. classification of ankle fracture
laughing gas
Laugier
L. fracture
L. hernia
Laumonier ganglion
Laurell
L. method
L. technique
Lauren gastric carcinoma classification

Lauth
L. canal
L. ligament
lavage
l. bowel preparation
continuous postoperative closed l.
diagnostic peritoneal l.
Exeter bone l.
external biliary l.
l. instillation
peritoneal l.
pulsatile pressure l.
saline l.
l. solution
l. and suction
laveur
Lavine reduction
law
l. of association
l. of denervation
Laws
L. gastroplasty
L. gastroplasty with Silastic collar-reinforced stoma
layer
barrier l.
echographic l.
echo-poor l.
meningeal l. of dura mater
molecular external l.
nerve fiber bundle l.
nuclear external l.
orbital l. of ethmoid bone
parietal l. of leptomeninges
parietal l. of tunica vaginalis
periosteal l. of dura mater
plexiform external l.
posterior l. of rectus abdominis sheath
pretracheal l.
prevertebral l.
serous l. of peritoneum
superficial l. of deep cervical fascia
superficial l. of temporalis fascia
suprachoroid l.
visceral l. of tunica vaginalis of testis
layered
l. closure
l. keratoplasty
laying-open fistulotomy

Lazarus-Nelson technique
Lazepen-Gamidov anteromedial approach
lazy-C incision
lazy-S incision
LB
lateral basal
LB segment
LC
laparoscopic cholecystectomy
L-Caine
L-curved incision
LDR intracavitary radiation therapy
Le
L. Bag ileocolonic pouch
L. Bag urinary pouch
L. Chatelier principle
L. Dentu suture technique
L. Dran suture technique
L. Fort classification
L. Fort fibular fracture
L. Fort I-III fracture
L. Fort mandibular fracture
L. Fort-Neugebauer operation
L. Fort operation
L. Fort osteotomy
L. Fort partial colpocleisis
L. Fort procedure
L. Fort suture technique
L. Fort-Wagstaffe fracture
L. Fort-Wehrbein-Duplay hypospadias repair
Leach-Igou step-cut medial osteotomy
Leach-Schepsis-Paul augmentation
Leach technique
lead
l. incrustation of cornea
l. line
l. suture
64-lead
64-l. epidural electrode array
64-l. subdural electrode array
Leadbetter
L. cystourethroplasty
L. hip manipulation
L. maneuver
L. modification technique
L. procedure
L. tunneling technique
Leadbetter-Politano
L.-P. procedure
L.-P. reimplantation

L

NOTES

lead-pipe
 l.-p. colon
 l.-p. fracture
lead-shot tie suture
leaflet
 aortic valve l.
 bowing of mitral valve l.
 heart valve l.
 mitral valve l.
 posterior mitral valve l.
 valve l.
Leahey operation
leak
 glue patch l.
 mask l.
 l. point pressure
leakage
 anastomotic l.
 chylous l.
 corneal l.
 silicone implant l.
 tube l.
lean
 l. body mass
 l. body weight
leapfrog position
least-squares method
leather-bottle stomach
Leboyer
 L. method
 L. technique
Lecompte maneuver
ledge
 eccentric l.
LeDuc-Carney
 L.-C. ileocolostomy
 L.-C. ileocystoplasty
LeDuc technique
Lee
 L. anterosuperior iliac spine graft
 L. bone graft
 L. ganglion
 L. procedure
 L. reconstruction
 L. technique
leech
 mechanical l.
LEEP
 loop electrocautery excision procedure
 LEEP conization
leeway space
Lee-White clotting time method
Lefèvre gastrectomy technique
left
 l. anterior oblique (LAO)
 l. anterior oblique position
 l. anterior oblique projection
 l. anterior occipital (LAO)

l. atrial isolation procedure
l. atrial pressure
l. bundle-branch block
l. colic artery
l. colic flexure
l. colic lymph nodes
l. colic vein
l. coronary artery
l. coronary vein
l. crus of diaphragm
l. decubitus position
l. dominant coronary circulation
l. duct of caudate lobe
l. erector spinae musculature
l. fibrous trigone
l. frontoanterior position
l. frontoposterior position
l. frontotransverse position
l. gastric artery
l. gastric lymph nodes
l. gastric vein
l. gastroepiploic artery
l. gastroepiploic lymph nodes
l. gastroepiploic vein
l. gastro-omental artery
l. gastro-omental nodes
l. gastroomental vein
l. heart catheterization
l. hepatic artery
l. hepatic duct
l. hepatic veins
l. inferior pulmonary vein
l. lateral decubitus position
l. lateral projection
l. lateral Sims position
l. lobe of liver
l. lower extremity
l. lumbar lymph nodes
l. main bronchus
l. mentoanterior position
l. mentoposterior position
l. mentotransverse position
l. occipitoanterior position
l. occipitoposterior position
l. occipitotransverse position
l. ovarian vein
l. rotation
l. sacroanterior position
l. sacroposterior position
l. sacrotransverse position
l. sagittal fissure
l. scapuloanterior position
l. scapuloposterior position
l. superior intercostal vein
l. superior pulmonary vein
l. suprarenal vein
l. testicular vein
l. triangular ligament

l. umbilical vein
l. upper extremity
l. upper quadrant peritonectomy
l. ventricle
l. ventricle-aorta conduit surgery
l. ventricular cross section image
l. ventricular diastolic relaxation
l. ventricular ejection time
l. ventricular end-diastolic area
(LVEDa)
l. ventricular end-diastolic pressure
l. ventricular end-systolic area
(LVESa)
l. ventricular filling pressure
l. ventricular inflow tract
obstruction
l. ventricular mass
l. ventricular outflow tract (LVOT)
l. ventricular outflow tract
obstruction
l. ventricular pressure-volume curve
l. ventricular puncture
l. ventricular-right atrial
communication murmur
l. ventricular systolic pressure
left-sided
l.-s. nail
l.-s. thoracotomy
left-side-down position
left-to-right subtotal pancreatectomy
leg
l. of antihelix
Legat point
leg-compression stocking
Lehman technique
Leibolt technique
Leinbach head and neck total hip
leiomyoblastoma
leiomyofibroma
lciomyoma
l. enucleation
l. of uveal tract
leiomyomectomy
leiomyosarcoma
Leishman classification
Leiter tube
Leksell technique
Lelièvre osteotomy
Lell tracheal tube
Lembert inverting seromuscular suture

Lempert
L. fenestration
L. incision
Lenart-Kullman technique
length
pedicle screw chord l.
pedicle screw path l.
peripheral capillary filtration slit l.
restriction fragment l.
l. of stay (LOS)
length-breadth index
lengthening
distal catheter l.
extensor l.
surgical crown l.
length-height index
length-resting tension relation
length-tension relation
Lennarson tube
Lennert
L. classification
L. lesion
lens
l. aberration
accommodation of crystalline l.
aspiration of l.
C-loop intraocular l.
coloboma of l.
corneal l.
decentration of contact l.
dislocation of l.
l. dislocation
l. equator
l. exchange
exfoliation of l.
luxation of l.
l. plane
l. removal
subluxation of l.
suture of l.
l. sutures
lensectomy
Charles l.
coal-mining l.
lentectomy
lenticular
l. fossa of vitreous body
l. loop
l. papillae
l. process of incus
l. ring
lenticulostriate arteries

L

NOTES

lentiform bone
Lepird procedure
L'Episcopo hip reconstruction
L'Episcopo-Zachary procedure
Lepley-Ernst tracheal tube
leprosy
    anesthetic l.
leptomeningeal
    l. anastomosis
    l. metastasis
    l. space
leptomyelolipoma
Leriche
    L. operation
    L. sympathectomy
Leri-Weill disease
LES
    lower esophageal sphincter
    LES pressure
Lesgaft
    L. hernia
    L. space
lesion
    acetowhite l.
    acneform l.
    acute gastric mucosal l.
    acute traumatic l.
    admixture l.
    aggressive l.
    ALPSA l.
    anal squamous intraepithelial l.
    angiocentric immunoproliferative l.
    angiocentric lymphoproliferative l.
    angiodysplastic l.
    angioinvasive l.
    angioproliferative l.
    annular constricting l.
    anterior labrum periosteum shoulder arthroscopic l.
    aortic valve l.
    aorto-ostial l.
    aphthous-type l.
    apple-core l.
    l. arrangement
    articular cartilage l.
    atherosclerotic l.
    atlantoaxial l.
    axillary skin l.
    Baehr-Lohlein l.
    Bankart shoulder l.
    barrel-shaped l.
    basal ganglionic l.
    benign bone l.
    benign lymphoepithelial l.
    benign lymphoproliferative l.
    benign vascular l.
    Bennett l.
    biceps interval l.

    bifurcation l.
    bilobed polypoid l.
    bird's nest l.
    blanchable red l.
    blastic l.
    bleeding l.
    blue-gray l.
    Blumenthal l.
    bone l.
    bone marrow l.
    bony l.
    boomerang-shaped l.
    Bracht-Wachter l.
    braid-like l.
    brain l.
    branch l.
    breast l.
    bridge-like l.
    brown-black l.
    bubbly bone l.
    bullous skin l.
    bull's-eye macular l.
    Bywaters l.
    calcified l.
    carpet l.
    cauda equina l.
    cavitary lung l.
    cavitary small bowel l.
    cemental l.
    central l.
    centrilobular l.
    cervical l.
    chiasmal l.
    choroidal l.
    cleavage l.
    cochlear l.
    coin l.
    cold l.
    colonic vascular l.
    complete common peroneal nerve l.
    concentric l.
    conjunctival melanotic l.
    constricting l.
    cornea guttate l.
    corneal punctate l.
    coronary artery l.
    Councilman l.
    culprit l.
    cutaneous l.
    cylindromatous l.
    cystic bone l.
    cystic lymphoepithelial AIDS-related l.
    demyelinating l.
    dendritic l.
    de novo l.
    dermal l.
    desmoid l.

destructive bone l.
Dieulafoy l.
Dieulafoy-like l.
diffuse ulcerative l.
dilatable l.
discoid skin l.
discrete coronary l.
disk l.
l. distribution
division I–IV l.
dorsal root entry zone l.
Dreulofoy l.
DREZ l.
ductal-dependent l.
duodenal l.
Duret l.
dye sham intrarenal l.
dysarthric l.
dysplasia-associated l.
ectatic vascular l.
eczematous l.
elementary l.
enhancing brain l.
entry zone l.
eosinophilic fibrohistiocytic l.
epididymis l.
epidural extramedullary l.
erysipelas-like skin l.
erythrodermatous l.
l. evolution
expansile unilocular well-demarcated
  bone l.
extracranial mass l.
extrahepatic l.
extramural l.
extratesticular l.
fibrocalcific l.
fibrohistiocytic l.
fibromusculoelastic l.
fibro-osseous l.
fibrous bone l.
fibrous polypoid l.
fingertip l.
firm l.
flat depressed l.
flat elevated l.
floor-of-mouth l.
florid duct l.
focal parenchymal brain l.
focal splenic l.
Forest I, II l.
gastric l.

gastrointestinal l.
genetic l.
genital papulosquamous l.
genitourinary l.
Ghon primary l.
giant cell l.
Gill l.
glomerular tip l.
gross l.
ground-glass l.
gunpowder l.
hamartomatous l.
hemorrhagic l.
hepatic mass l.
herpetoid l.
high-grade squamous
  intraepithelial l.
high-intensity l.
high neurological l.
Hill-Sachs shoulder l.
histologic l.
honeycomb l.
hot l.
hyperdense brain l.
hyperintense brain l.
hyperkeratotic l.
hyperpigmented l.
hypodense brain l.
hypocchoic l.
l. identification
immunoproliferative l.
impaction l.
indiscriminate l.
infarctive l.
inflammatory l.
initial syphilitic l.
interpeduncular fossa l.
interradicular l.
intraconal l.
intracranial mass l.
intradural extramedullary l.
intraepithelial l.
intrahepatic l.
intramedullary l.
intramural extramucosal l.
intraocular l.
intraorbital l.
intraosseous bone l.
intrasellar l.
intravascular endothelial
  proliferative l.
intrinsic brainstem l.

L

NOTES

lesion *(continued)*

ipsilateral nerve root l.
irritable l.
irritative l.
Janeway l.
jet l.
Keasbey l.
keratitis l.
Kidner l.
Kimmelstiel-Wilson l.
labral l.
Lennert l.
Libman-Sacks l.
lichenified l.
linear l.
lipocytic l.
localized l.
Löhlein-Baehr l.
long l.
low-attenuation l.
lower motor neuron l.
low-grade squamous
  intraepithelial l.
lucent lung l.
lumbar spinal cord l.
lumbar spine l.
lumbosacral plexus l.
lumbosacral root l.
lung l.
lymphoepithelial l.
lymphoproliferative l.
lytic bone l.
macroscopic l.
macrovascular coronary l.
malignant pituitary l.
Mallory-Weiss l.
l. margination
mass l.
medium l.
melanocytic conjunctival l.
melanotic l.
mesencephalic low density l.
mesenchymal l.
mesenteric vascular l.
metastatic l.
minute polypoid l.
mixed fat-water density l.
mixed sclerotic and lytic bone l.
molecular l.
monotypic l.
Monteggia equivalent l.
Morel-Lavele l.
morphea-like l.
l. morphology
mucocutaneous l.
mucosal l.
mucous membrane l.
mulberry l.

multifocal enhancing l.
multilocular cystic l.
nail l.
napkin-ring annular l.
neoplastic l.
nerve root l.
neural l.
neurovascular l.
nickel-and-dime l.
nodular l.
nodule-in-nodule l.
nonbacterial thrombotic
  endocardial l.
nonblanchable, abnormally
  colored l.
nonerosive gastric mucosal l.
nonmeningiomatous malignant l.
nonneoplastic tumor-like l.
nonperforative l.
nucleus ambiguus l.
nummular l.
occipital lobe l.
occult talar l.
ocular adnexal l.
oil drop l.
onion scale l.
optic nerve l.
optic tract l.
l. of orbit
orbital l.
organic l.
Osgood-Schlatter l.
osseous l.
osteoblastic l.
osteochondral l.
osteolytic bone l.
osteopathic l.
osteosclerotic l.
ostial l.
pancreatic l.
papillary l.
papulopustular l.
papulosquamous l.
papulovesicular l.
paraorbital l.
parasagittal l.
patch l.
penile l.
perforative l.
perianal l.
periodontal l.
peripheral l.
perisellar vascular l.
periventricular hyperintense l.
periventricular white matter l.
Perthes l.
photon-deficient bone l.
pigmented l.

pigment epithelial l.
plaque-like l.
plexiform l.
plexus l.
polypoid l.
polypoidal l.
postfracture l.
precancerous l.
prechiasmal optic nerve l.
precursor l.
premalignant l.
preoperative l.
presacral cystic l.
primary glomerular l.
proliferative l.
pruritic l.
pseudocancerous l.
pseudomedial longitudinal
  fasciculus l.
pulmonary l.
pulpoperiapical l.
punched-out l.
purpuric l.
pustular l.
pyodermatous skin l.
radial sclerosing l.
radiodense l.
radiofrequency l.
radiolucent l.
radiopaque l.
reactive lymphoid l.
regurgitant l.
rcstenosis l.
reticular l.
retroacetabular l.
retrochiasmal l.
retrogeniculate l.
reverse Hill-Sachs l.
right-sided l.
rim-enhancing l.
ring l.
ring-wall l.
rolled shoulder l.
rotationally induced shear-strain l.
rotator cuff l.
ruptured peliotic l.
saddle l.
satellite l.
scaling skin-colored l.
scirrhous l.
sclerosing l.
sclerotic l.

secondary l.
semipedunculated l.
sessile l.
short-segment l.
SIL/ASCUS l.
Sinding-Larsen-Johansson l.
sinonasal l.
sinusoidal l.
l. size
skeletal l.
skin l.
skin-colored l.
skip l.
SLAP l.
slope-shouldered l.
smooth skin-colored l.
soft l.
soft tissue l.
space-occupying brain l.
special l.
spiculated l.
spinal l.
spleen l.
splenic l.
spontaneous l.
squamous intraepithelial l.
square-shouldered l.
stellate border breast l.
Stener l.
stenotic l.
stress l.
structural l.
subglottic l.
submucosal upper gastrointestinal
  tract l.
subtentorial l.
superior labrum anterior and
  posterior l.
supranuclear l.
suprasellar low-density l.
supratentorial l.
synchronous l.
systemic l.
tandem l.
target l.
trabeculated bone l.
transient l.
traumatic l.
trophic l.
tuberculous l.
tubulovillar l.
ulcer l.

L

NOTES

lesion (*continued*)
    uncommitted metaphyseal l.
    unifocal optic nerve l.
    unilocular cystic l.
    upper motor neuron l.
    uremic gastrointestinal l.
    varicelliform l.
    vascular l.
    vasculitic l.
    vegetative l.
    venular l.
    verrucous l.
    vesicobullous l.
    violaceous l.
    visceral l.
    vulvar pigmented l.
    vulvovaginal l.
    Waldeyer ring l.
    weeping l.
    well-circumscribed l.
    white l.
    white-spot l.
    wire-loop l.
    wraparound periapical l.
    Wrisberg l.
    yellow l.
Leslie-Ryan anterior axillary approach
lesser
    l. cul-de-sac
    l. curvature of stomach
    l. horn of hyoid bone
    l. internal cutaneous nerve
    l. multangular bone
    l. occipital nerve
    l. omentectomy
    l. omentectomy with cholecystectomy
    l. omentum
    l. palatine artery
    l. pancreas
    l. pelvis
    l. peritoneal cavity
    l. peritoneal sac
    l. resection
    l. rhomboid muscle
    l. ring
    l. sac
    l. sac hernia
    l. splanchnic nerve
    l. supraclavicular fossa
    L. triangle
    l. trochanter
    l. trochanter fracture
    l. vestibular glands
    l. wing of sphenoid bone
    l. zygomatic muscle
Lesshaft triangle
Lester-Jones operation

Lester Martin modification of Duhamel operation
LET
    liposome-encapsulated tetracaine
lethal
    l. concentration
    l. osteogenesis imperfecta
Letournel-Judet
    L.-J. acetabular fracture classification
    L.-J. approach
letterbox technique
leucotomy
leukemia
leukemic infiltration
leukochloroma
leukocyte infiltration
leukocytic
    l. infiltration
    l. margination
leukocytoma
leukoencephalopathy
    radiation-induced l.
leukolymphosarcoma
leukolysis
leukoma
    l. adherens
    adherent l.
leukosarcoma
leukostasis
    intracerebral l.
leukotomy
    prefrontal l.
    transorbital l.
Leung thumb loss classification
Levaditi method
levator
    l. anguli oris muscle
    l. ani
    l. ani muscle
    l. ani syndrome
    l. aponeurosis repair
    l. costae muscle
    l. glandulae thyroidea muscle
    l. hernia
    l. injury
    l. labii superioris alaeque nasi muscle
    l. muscle of angle of mouth
    l. muscle of thyroid gland
    l. muscle of upper eyelid
    l. palati muscle
    l. palpebrae
    l. palpebrae superioris
    l. palpebrae superioris muscle
    l. palpebrae superiosus
    l. prostatae muscle
    l. resection

l. scapulae
l. scapulae muscle
l. scapulae syndrome
l. span
l. swelling
l. trochlear muscle
l. veli palatini
l. veli palatini muscle
levatores costarum muscles
Lev classification
level
l. of analgesia
l. of aspiration
attenuation l.
Clark l.
endothelin plasma l.
l. foundation
multiple shunt l.'s
L. One normothermic IV fluid set
L. One pressure infusion system
  250 fluid warmer
overall sound l.
pentane excretion l.
saturation sound pressure l.
sensation l.
sound pressure l.
uterine lysosome l.
level-dependent
blood oxygenation l.-d.
lever
leverage
Levin-Davol tube
Levin duodenal tube
Levine
L. dislocation operation
L. gradation 1–6 of cardiac
  murmurs
Levine-Harvey classification
levitation
levobunolol
levodopa dopaminergic medication
Levo-Dromoran
L.-D. injection
L.-D. Oral
levonordefrin
mepivacaine with l.
Levophed injection
Levoprome
levorphanol tartrate
levosmendan
levo-transposed position
Levret maneuver

Levy, Rowntree, and Marriott method
Lewis
L. and Benedict method
L. intercalary resection
L. laryngectomy tube
L. operation
L. thoracotomy
Lewis-Chekofsky resection
Lewis-Leigh valve
Lewissohn method
Lewis-Tanner procedure
Lewit stretch technique
Lexer operation
Lezius suction tube
LG
lateral ground
LG bundle
Liang and Pardee method
Libman-Sacks lesion
Libritabs
Librium
Lich
L. extravesical technique
L. procedure
lichenification
lichenified lesion
lichenization
lichenoid graft-versus-host disease
Lich-Gregoire
L.-G. anastomosis
L.-G. repair
L.-G. technique
L.-G. ureterolysis
Lichtblau osteotomy
Lichtenstein
L. hernial repair
L. herniorrhaphy
Lichtman technique
lid
l. closure reaction
lower l.
l. margin laceration
upper l.
lid-loading technique
lidocaine
bacitracin, neomycin, polymyxin B,
  and l.
l. hydrochloride
l. and hydrocortisone
l. and prilocaine
l. test
l. topical anesthetic

L

NOTES

lidocaine *(continued)*
    viscous l.
    l. with epinephrine
lidocaine-prilocaine cream
LidoPen
Lieberkühn
    L. crypts
    L. glands
Liebolt radioulnar technique
lien
    l. accessorius
    l. mobilis
    l. succenturiatus
lienal
    l. artery
lienculus
lienectomy
lienopancreatic
lienophrenic ligament
lienorenal
    l. ligament
lienunculus
Lieutaud
    L. body
    L. triangle
    L. trigone
    L. uvula
life
    l. expectancy
    l. space
    l. table method
Lifemask infant resuscitator
Lifesaver disposable resuscitator bag
life-saving tube
lift-and-cut biopsy
lifting
    abdominal wall l.
ligament
    accessory plantar l.'s
    accessory volar l.'s
    acromioclavicular l.
    alar l.'s
    anococcygeal l.
    anterior costotransverse l.
    anterior cruciate l. (ACL)
    anterior sacrococcygeal l.
    anterior sacroiliac l.'s
    anterior sacrosciatic l.
    anterior sternoclavicular l.
    apical l. of dens
    Arantius l.
    arcuate pubic l.
    auricular l.'s
    Berry l.'s
    Camper l.
    capsular l.
    Carcassone perineal l.
    cardinal l.

caroticoclinoid l.
caudal l.
ceratocricoid l.
cervical l. of uterus
check l.'s of eyeball, medial and lateral
check l.'s of odontoid
chondroxiphoid l.
ciliary l.
Civinini l.
Clado l.
collateral l.
Colles l.
Cooper l.'s
coracoacromial l.
coracoclavicular l.
coracohumeral l.
coronary l. of knee
coronary l. of liver
costoclavicular l.
costocolic l.
costotransverse l.
costoxiphoid l.
cotyloid l.
Cowper l.
cricothyroid l.
cricotracheal l.
cruciate l. of the atlas
cruciform l. of atlas
cystoduodenal l.
deep dorsal sacrococcygeal l.
deep posterior sacrococcygeal l.
Denonvilliers l.
denticulate l.
duodenorenal l.
l. of epididymis
epihyal l.
external l.
extra-articular knee l.
extracapsular l.'s
falciform l. of liver
fallopian l.
Ferrein l.
fibulocalcaneal l.
fundiform l. of penis
gastrocolic l.
gastrodiaphragmatic l.
gastrolienal l.
gastrophrenic l.
gastrosplenic l.
genitoinguinal l.
Gimbernat l.
l. graft
Hensing l.
hepatocolic l.
hepatoduodenal l.
hepatoesophageal l.
hepatogastric l.

hepatorenal l.
Hesselbach l.
Holl l.
Hueck l.
hyalocapsular l.
hyoepiglottic l.
iliolumbar l.
inferior l. of epididymis
inferior pubic l.
inferior transverse scapular l.
infundibulo-ovarian l.
infundibulopelvic l.
inguinal l. of the kidney
interclavicular l.
interclinoid l.
interfoveolar l.
interosseous sacroiliac l.'s
interspinous l.
intertransverse l.
intervolar plate l.
intra-articular l. of costal head
intra-articular sternocostal l.
intracapsular l.'s
Jarjavay l.
Krause l.
lacunar l.
Lannelongue l.'s
lateral arcuate l.
lateral l.'s of the bladder
lateral costotransverse l.
lateral palpebral l.
lateral puboprostatic l.
lateral sacrococcygeal l.
lateral thyrohyoid l.
lateral umbilical l.
Lauth l.
l. of left superior vena cava
left triangular l.
l. of left vena cava
lienophrenic l.
lienorenal l.
Lockwood l.
longitudinal l.
lumbocostal l.
Luschka l.'s
Mackenrodt l.
Mauchart l.'s
Meckel l.
medial arcuate l.
medial palpebral l.
medial puboprostatic l.
medial umbilical l.

median arcuate l.
median thyrohyoid l.
median umbilical l.
middle costotransverse l.
middle umbilical l.
nuchal l.
ossification of the posterior
  longitudinal l.
pectineal l.
peridental l.
periodontal l.
Petit l.
phrenicocolic l.
phrenicolienal l.
phrenicosplenic l.
phrenogastric l.
phrenosplenic l.
posterior costotransverse l.
posterior longitudinal l.
posterior occipitoaxial l.
posterior sacroiliac l.'s
posterior sacrosciatic l.
posterior sternoclavicular l.
Poupart l.
pterygomandibular l.
pterygospinal l.
pterygospinous l.
puboprostatic l.
pulmonary l.
radiate l. of head of rib
radiate sternocostal l.'s
l. reconstruction
reflected inguinal l.
reflex l.
rhomboid l.
right triangular l.
round l. of liver
round l. of uterus
sacrodural l.
sacrospinous l.
sacrotuberous l.
serous l.
sphenomandibular l.
splenorenal l.
stellate l.
sternoclavicular l.
sternopericardial l.
stylohyoid l.
stylomandibular l.
stylomaxillary l.
superficial dorsal sacrococcygeal l.

L

NOTES

ligament *(continued)*
    superficial posterior sacrococcygeal l.
    superior costotransverse l.
    superior l. of epididymis
    superior pubic l.
    superior transverse scapular l.
    suprascapular l.
    supraspinous l.
    suspensory l. of axilla
    suspensory l.'s of breast
    suspensory l. of clitoris
    suspensory l.'s of Cooper
    suspensory l. of penis
    suspensory l. of testis
    suspensory l. of thyroid gland
    sutural l.
    synovial l.
    temporomandibular l.
    Teutleben l.
    Thompson l.
    thyroepiglottic l.
    transverse atlantal l.
    transverse l. of the atlas
    transverse l. of pelvis
    transverse perineal l.
    transverse l. of perineum
    Treitz l.
    triangular l.'s of liver
    urachal l.
    uterosacral l.
    uterovesical l.
    venous l.
    ventral sacrococcygeal l.
    ventricular l.
    vertebropelvic l.'s
    vesicoumbilical l.
    vesicouterine l.
    vestibular l.
    vocal l.
    yellow l.
    Zaglas l.
    Zinn l.
ligamenta *(pl. of* ligamentum)
ligamental anesthesia
ligamentopexy
ligamentoplasty
ligamentous
    l. repair of the knee for rotatory instability
    l. support tissue
ligamentum, pl. **ligamenta**
    l. acromioclaviculare
    ligamenta alaria
    l. anococcygeum
    l. apicis dentis
    l. arcuatum laterale
    l. arcuatum mediale

l. arcuatum medianum
l. arcuatum pubis
ligamenta auricularia
l. capitis costae intra-articulare
l. capitis costae radiatum
l. capsulare
l. caudale
l. ceratocricoideum
l. collaterale
l. colli costae
l. coracoacromiale
l. coracoclaviculare
l. coracohumerale
l. coronarium hepatis
l. costoclaviculare
l. costotransversarium
l. costotransversarium anterius
l. costotransversarium laterale
l. costotransversarium posterius
l. costotransversarium superius
l. costoxiphoideum
l. cotyloideum
l. cricothyroideum
l. cricotracheale
l. cruciatum atlantis
l. denticulatum
l. ductus venosi
l. duodenorenale
l. epididymidis
l. epididymidis inferius
l. epididymidis superius
l. falciforme
l. falciforme hepatis
l. flavum
l. fundiforme penis
l. gastrocolicum
l. gastrolienale
l. gastrophrenicum
l. gastrosplenicum
l. genitoinguinale
l. hepatocolicum
l. hepatoduodenale
l. hepatoesophageum
l. hepatogastricum
l. hepatorenale
l. hyaloideo-capsulario
l. hyoepiglotticum
l. hyothyroideum laterale
l. hyothyroideum medium
l. iliolumbale
l. inguinale
l. interclaviculare
l. interfoveolare
l. interspinale
l. intertransversarium
ligamenta intracapsularia
l. lacunare
l. latum pulmonis

l. latum uteri
l. lienorenale
l. longitudinale
l. longitudinale anterius
l. longitudinale posterius
l. lumbocostale
l. medialis
l. menisci lateralis
ligamenta meniscofemorale
l. meniscofemorale anterius
l. meniscofemorale posterius
l. natatorium
l. orbiculare radii
ligamenta ossiculorum auditus
l. ovarii proprium
ligamenta palmaria
l. palpebrale externum
l. palpebrale laterale
l. palpebrale mediale
l. patellae
l. pectinatum
l. pectinatum anguli iridocornealis
l. pectinatum iridis
l. pectineale
l. phrenicocolicum
l. phrenicolienale
l. phrenicosplenicum
l. pisohamatum
l. pisometacarpeum
l. plantare longum
ligamenta plantaria
l. popliteum arcuatum
l. popliteum obliquum
l. pterygospinale
l. pubicum superius
l. pubocapsulare
l. pubofemorale
l. puboprostaticum
l. puboprostaticum laterale
l. puboprostaticum mediale
l. pubovesicale
l. pulmonale
l. quadratum
l. radiatum
l. reflexum
l. sacrococcygeum anterius
l. sacrococcygeum laterale
l. sacrococcygeum posterius
  profundum
l. sacrococcygeum posterius
  superficiale
l. sacrodurale

ligamenta sacroiliaca anteriora
ligamenta sacroiliaca interossea
ligamenta sacroiliaca posteriora
l. sacroiliacum posterius
l. sacrospinale
l. sacrospinosum
l. sacrotuberale
l. sacrotuberosum
l. serosum
l. sphenomandibulare
l. spirale cochleae
l. splenorenale
l. sternoclaviculare
l. sternoclaviculare anterius
l. sternoclaviculare posterius
l. sternocostale intra-articulare
ligamenta sternocostalia radiata
ligamenta sternopericardiaca
l. stylohyoideum
l. stylomandibulare
l. supraspinale
ligamenta suspensoria mammae
l. suspensorium clitoridis
l. suspensorium ovarii
l. suspensorium penis
l. talocalcaneare
l. talocalcaneare interosseum
l. talocalcaneare laterale
l. talocalcaneare mediale
l. talofibulare anterius
l. talofibulare posterius
l. talonaviculare
l. talotibiale anterius
l. talotibiale posterius
l. tarsale externum
l. tarsale internum
ligamenta tarsi
l. temporomandibulare
l. teres cardiopexy
l. teres hepatis
l. teres uteri
l. thyroepiglotticum
l. thyrohyoideum laterale
l. thyrohyoideum medianum
l. tibionaviculare
ligamenta trachealia
l. transversale colli
l. transversum acetabuli
l. transversum atlantis
l. transversum cruris
l. transversum genus
l. transversum pelvis

L

NOTES

ligamentum *(continued)*
l. transversum perinei
l. transversum scapulae inferius
l. transversum scapulae superius
l. trapezoideum
l. triangulare
l. triangulare dextrum
l. triangulare sinistrum
l. tuberculi costae
l. umbilicale laterale
l. umbilicale mediale
l. umbilicale medianum
l. venae cavae sinistrae
l. ventriculare
l. vestibulare
l. vocale
ligand
tissue l.
Ligapak suture
ligate
ligated
doubly l.
suture l.
ligate-divide-staple
ligation
band l.
Bardenheurer l.
Barron l.
bidirectional l.
bile duct l.
Blalock-Taussig shunt l.
bleeding site l.
elastic band l.
endoscopic band l.
endoscopic esophagogastric
variceal l.
esophageal band l.
l. of hemorrhoid
hepatic artery l.
high l.
hunterian l.
hypogastric artery l.
interdental l.
Irving tubal l.
Kroner tubal l.
laparoscopic varix l.
modified Irving-type tubal l.
open retroperitoneal high l.
parotid duct l.
pole l.
Pomeroy tubal l.
postureteral l.
rubber band l.
sigmoid sinus l.
sling l.
spermatic vein l.
stump l.
surgical l.

teeth l.
transesophageal varix l.
transgastric l.
tubal l.
variceal band l.
varicose vein stripping and l.
varix l.
vessel l.
ligature
chromic gut pelviscopic loop l.
elastic l.
grass-line l.
intravascular l.
nonabsorbable l.
occluding l.
provisional l.
simple proximal l.
soluble l.
suboccluding l.
Surgiwip suture l.
suture l.
light
l. coagulation
l. exposure
l. guide bundle
l. microscopy
l. projection
l. wire torque
light-around-wire technique
lighted
l. stylet
l. stylet-guided oral intubation
light-reflecting wedge
lignocaine
M l.
Lilienthal incision
Liliequist
membrane of L.
Lillie allochrome method
Lilliput neonatal oxygenator
limb
anterior l. of stapes
l. deformity
l. of helix
l. ischemia
l. ischemia pain
l. length angulation
pelvic l.
phantom l.
posterior l. of stapes
l. reduction
l. reduction abnormality
l. reduction anomaly
l. replantation
l. salvage
l. salvage index
thoracic l.

limbal
  l. approach
  l. compression
  corneal inferior l.
  l. incision
  l. parallel orientation
limbal-based flap
limb-body wall complex
Limberg
  L. flap
  L. technique
limbi (*pl. of* limbus)
limb-lengthening procedure
limb-salvage
  l.-s. procedure
  l.-s. surgery
limb-saving
  l.-s. method
  l.-s. procedure
  l.-s. technique
limb-sparing
  l.-s. operation
  l.-s. procedure
  l.-s. surgery
limbus, pl. limbi
  l. acetabuli
  l. alveolaris
  corneal l.
  l. mass
  limbi palpebrales
  l. palpebrales anteriores
  l. parallel orientation straddling
    tattoo mark
  Vieussens l.
limen
  l. nasi
limitation
  l. of exposure
  l. of joint motion
  l. of movement
limited
  l. examination
  l. fasciectomy
  l. obturator node dissection
  l. resection
limit of flocculation
limiting
  l. membrane
  l. plate erosion
limoge current
lincocin injection
lincoff operation

Lincorex injection
Lindell classification
Lindeman procedure
Lindeman-Silverstein
  L.-S. Arrow tube
  L.-S. ventilation tube
Lindesmith operation
Linde Walker Oxygen Program
Lindholm
  L. technique
  L. tendo calcaneus repair
  L. tracheal tube
Lindner
  L. operation
  L. sclerotomy
Lindsay operation
Lindseth osteotomy
Lindsjö method
line
  accretion l.
  AC-PC l.
  action l.
  air-fluid l.
  alveolar point-basion l.
  alveolar point-nasal point l.
  alveolar point-nasion l.
  alveolobasilar l.
  alveolonasal l.
  Amberg lateral sinus l.
  aneuploid cell l.
  l. angle
  angular l.
  anocutaneous l.
  anterior axillary l., ant ax l.
  anterior commissure-posterior
    commissure l.
  anterior humeral l.
  anterior junction l.
  anterior median l.
  antitension l.
  arcuate l. of ilium
  arcuate l. of rectus sheath
  Arlt l.
  arterial l., art l.
  arterial mean l.
  atopic l.
  axillary l.
  azygoesophageal l.
  basal l.
  base l.
  basinasal l.
  B cell l.

L

NOTES

line *(continued)*

Beau l.
l. of Bechterew
BeWo choriocarcinoma cell l.
bimastoid l.
bisector l.
bismuth l.
black l.
Blaschko l.
blue l.
Blumensaat l.
Bolton-nasion l.
Brödel bloodless l.
Burton l.
calcification l.
calciotraumatic l.
Camper l.
canthomeatal l.
Cantlie l.
CaSki cell l.
cell l.
cement l.
cemental l.
cementing l.
CEM/HIV-1 cell l.
central venous pressure l.
cervical l.
Chamberlain palato-occipital l.
Chaussier l.
Clapton l.
cleavage l.
clinoparietal l.
clivus canal l.
clivus torcula l.
Codman ICP monitoring l.
colonic mucosal l.
Conradi l.
contour l.
corneal iron l.
coronoid l.
Correra l.
costoclavicular l.
costophrenic septal l.'s
Crampton l.
craze l.
cross-arch fulcrum l.
curved radiolucent l.
CVP l.
cyma l.
D l.
Daubenton l.
delay l.
l. of demarcation
demarcation l.
Dennie l.
Dennie-Morgan l.
dentate l.
developmental l.

diagastric l.
l. of direction
Donders l.
Douglas l.
Dul45 cell l.
Ebner l.
Egger l.
Ehrlich-Türck l.
cmission l.
epiphysial l.
equipotential l.
established cell l.
external oblique l.
facc l.
Farre white l.
fat l.
fat-density l.
feather-edged proximal finishing l.
Feiss l.
femoral head l.
Ferry l.
fingerprint l.
finish l.
Fishgold l.
l. of fixation
Fleischner l.
l. focus principle
foramen magnum l.
fracture l.
Fränkel white l.
Frankfort horizontal light l.
Fraunhofer l.
fulcrum l.
Futcher l.
gallbladder-vena cava l.
Garrett orientation l.
gas density l.
gaussian l.
l. of Gennari
George l.
germ l.
gingival finishing l.
gluteal l.
Granger l.
gravitational l.
l. of gravity
gravity l.
gray l.
growth arrest l.
Gubler l.
gum l.
Hampton l.
Harris growth arrest l.
Hawkins l.
Head l.
Helmholtz l.
hemostatic staple l.
Hickman l.

highest nuchal l.
high lip l.
high smile l.
Hilgenreiner horizontal Y l.
Hilgenreiner-Perkins l.
Hilton white l.
His l.
Holdaway l.
Holden l.
hot l.
Hudson l.
Hudson-Stähli l.
Hueter l.
human AML cell l.
humeral l.
Hunter l.
Hunter-Schreger l.
iliopectinate l.
iliopectineal l.
incision l.
indwelling l.
inferior nuchal l.
inferior temporal l.
infracostal l.
innominate l.
intercondylar l. of femur
intermediate l. of iliac crest
internal oblique l.
interspinal l.
Intertech Perkin-Elmer gas
  sampling l.
intertrochanteric l.
intertubercular l.
intravenous l.
iron l.
iron-ferry l.
iron-Hudson-Stähli l.
iron-stocker l.
isodose l.
isoelectric l.
joint l.
Jurkat T-cell l.
l. of Kaes
Kaplan oblique l.
Kerley A, B, C, l.'s
K562 erythroid l.
Khodadoust l.
Kilian l.
knife-edged finishing l.
Köhler l.
labial l.
lambda suture l.

Langer l.
Langhans l.
Lanz l.
lateral joint l.
lead l.
Linton l.
lip l.
load l.
long l.
lorentzian l.
lower anterior axillary l.
lower midclavicular l.
low lip l.
lumbar gravitational l.
lymphoblastoid cell l.
M l.
Mach l.
MacNab l.
mamillary l.
mammary l.
mare's tail l.
McGregor basal l.
McKee l.
McRae foramen magnum l.
medial joint l.
median l.
Mees l.
mercurial l.
Meyer l.
Meyerding spondylolisthesis
  classification l.
midaxillary l.
midclavicular l.
middle axillary l.
middle cranial fossa l.
midheel l.
midhumeral l.
midmalleolar l.
midpoint to meatal l.
midsternal l.
Moloney l.
Monro l.
Monro-Richter l.
Morgan l.
mucogingival l.
mucosal l.
Muehrcke l.
Muerhrcke l.
murine mesangial cell l.
myelomonocytic cell l.
mylohyoid l.
Nafion dryer l.

NOTES

L

line *(continued)*

nasion-alveolar point l.
nasobasilar l.
nasolabial l.
Nélaton l.
neonatal l.
neuronal cell l.
nipple l.
Obersteiner-Redlich l.
oblique l. of mandible
oblique metacarpal l.
oblique l. of thyroid cartilage
obturator l.
l. of occlusion
odontoid perpendicular l.
Ohngren l.
orbital l.
orbitomeatal l.
l. of Owen
Owen l.
oxygen supply l.
palato-occipital l.
pararectal l.
paraspinal l.
parasternal l.
paravertebral l.
Pastia l.
pectinate l.
pectineal l. of pubis
percutaneous l.
peripheral arterial l.
Perkins vertical l.
physeal l.
PICC l.
Pickerill imbrication l.
pigmentary demarcation l.
pleural l.'s
pleuroesophageal l.
plumb l.
Poirier l.
postaxillary l.
posterior axillary l.
posterior canal l.
posterior cervical l.
posterior junction l.
posterior median l.
Poupart l.
preaxillary l.
principal l.
properitoneal fat l.
protrusive l.
psoas l.
pubic hair l.
pubococcygeal l.
pupillary l.
radial arterial l.
radiocapitellar l.
radiolucent l.

radiolucent crescent l.
radio signal l.
recessional l.
Reid base l.
rejection l.
resonance l.
resting l.
retentive fulcrum l.
l. of Retzius
reversal l.
Rex-Cantli-Serege l.
Richter-Monro l.
Rolandic l.
Roser-Nélaton l.
sacral arcuate l.
sacral horizontal plane l.
sagittal suture l.
Salter incremental l.
Sampoelesi l.
S-BP l.
scapular l.
Schreger l.
Schwalbe l.
sclerotic l.
scurvy l.
semicircular l. of Douglas
semilunar l.
septal l.'s
Seraflo blood l.
Sergent white l.
Shenton l.
simian l.
sinus l.
S-N l.
Snellen l.
soleal l.
spectral l.
Spigelius l.
spinolamellar l.
spinolaminar l.
spinous interlaminar l.
spiral l.
stabilizing fulcrum l.
Stähli pigment l.
sternal l.
Stocker l.
stromal l.
subclavian l.
subcostal l.
superficial corneal l.
superior nuchal l.
superior temporal l.
supracrestal l.
survey l.
suture l.
Sydney l.
sylvian l.
T-cell l.

teardrop l.
temporal l.
tender l.
terminal l.
l. test
Thompson l.
tibiofibular l.
l. of Toldt
tram l.'s
transverse l.'s of sacrum
transverse umbilical l.
trapezoid l.
triradiate l.
trough l.
Turk l.
Twining l.
Tycos pressure infusion l.
Ullmann l.
umbilical artery l.
upper midclavicular l.
venous l.
Vesling l.
vibrating l.
visual l.
Voigt l.
von Ebner l.
Wackenheim clivus canal l.
water density l.
Wegner l.
white l. of anal canal
white l. of Toldt
l. width
Winberger l.
Z. l.
Zahn l.'s
l.'s of Zahn
zero l.
Zöllner l.
linea, pl. lineae
  l. alba
  l. anocutanea
  l. arcuata ossis ilii
  l. arcuata vaginae musculi recti
   abdominis
  l. axillaris anterior
  l. axillaris media
  l. axillaris posterior
  l. epiphysialis
  l. glutea
  l. glutea anterior
  l. glutea inferior
  l. glutea posterior

l. intercondylaris femoris
l. intermedia cristae iliacae
l. interspinalis
l. intertrochanterica
l. intertubercularis
l. mamillaris
l. mediana anterior
l. mediana posterior
l. medio-axillaris
l. medioclavicularis
l. musculi solei
l. mylohyoidea
l. nuchae inferior
l. nuchae mediana
l. nuchae superior
l. nuchae suprema
l. obliqua
l. obliqua cartilaginis thyroidea
l. obliqua mandibulae
l. parasternalis
l. paravertebralis
l. pectinea
l. postaxillaris
l. preaxillaris
l. scapularis
l. semicircularis
l. semilunaris
l. spiralis
l. sternalis
l. subcostalis
l. supracristalis
l. temporalis inferior
l. temporalis superior
l. terminalis
lineae transversa ossi sacri
l. trapezoidea
linear
  l. craniectomy
  l. lesion
  l. osteotomy
  l. salpingostomy
  l. skull fracture
  l. thermal expansion
lined flap
Linell-Ljungberg classification
linen suture
lingual
  l. approach
  l. artery
  l. bone
  l. branches
  l. branch of facial nerve

L

NOTES

lingual *(continued)*
    l. cavity
    l. frenulum
    l. inclination
    l. lymph nodes
    l. mucosa
    l. plexus
    l. split-bone technique
    l. tongue flap
    l. vein
lingualplasty
lingula
    l. sphenoidalis
lingular branch
linguofacial trunk
linguoincisal line angle
linguo-occlusal line angle
lining
    cavity l.
linitis
    l. plastica
linkage
    rod l.
linnaean system of nomenclature
lint
Linton
    L. esophageal tube
    L. flap
    L. line
    L. procedure
Linton-Nachlas tube
lip
    acetabular l.
    anterior l. of uterine os
    cleft l.
    junction of l.'s
    l. line
    lower l.
    l.'s of mouth
    mucous membrane of l.
    posterior l. of uterine os
    l. switch flap
    upper l.
lipectomy
    abdominal l.
lipid peroxidation product
lipiodol
    l. injection
    l. transarterial embolization treatment
lipoatrophy
    postinfection l.
lipoblastoma
lipocele
lipocytic lesion
lipofibroadenoma
lipofibroma
lipogranuloma

lipoleiomyoma
lipolysis
    heparin-induced l.
    intravascular l.
    LPL-mediated l.
lipoma
    l. of cord
    l. sarcomatosum
lipoma-like tissue
lipomatous
    l. infiltration
    l. tissue
lipomeningocele
lipomyelocele
lipomyelocystocele
lipomyelomeningocele
lipomyxoma
lipophilic
    l. drug
    l. opioid
liposarcoma
liposomal preparation
liposome-encapsulated tetracaine (LET)
liposuction
liposuctioning
Liposyn II fat emulsion solution
Lipscomb
    L. procedure
    L. technique
Lipscomb-Anderson procedure
lip-splitting incision
Liquaemin injection
liquid
    l. extraction
    l. scintillation spectrometer
Liquifilm
    L. Forte solution
    L. Tears solution
liquor
    l. entericus
    Scarpa l.
Lisfranc
    L. amputation
    L. articulation
    L. disarticulation
    L. dislocation
    L. fracture
    L. fracture-dislocation
    L. tubercle
Lison-Dunn method
Lissauer
    L. bundle
    L. tract
lissosphincter
Lister
    L. method
    L. technique
    L. tubercle

listerism
listhesis
    lateral l.
Listing plane
lithagogue
lithectomy
lithiasis
    biliary l.
    pancreatic l.
lithium
    fractional excretion of l.
lithocystotomy
litholapaxy
    Bigelow l.
litholysis
    chemical l.
litholyte
litholytic
lithomyl
lithotomist
lithotomy
    bilateral l.
    dorsal l.
    high l.
    lateral l.
    marian l.
    median l.
    perineal l.
    l. position
    prerectal l.
    suprapubic l.
    vaginal l.
    vesical l.
lithotresis
    ultrasonic l.
lithotripsy
    biliary l.
    blind l.
    candela l.
    coumarin green tunable dye laser l.
    cystoscopic electrohydraulic l.
    Dornier extracorporeal shock wave l.
    Dornier MPL 9000 gallstone l.
    electrohydraulic shock wave l. (ESWL)
    endoscopic-controlled l.
    endoscopic electrohydraulic l.
    endoscopic pulsed dye laser l.
    external shock wave l.

    extracorporeal piezoelectric shock wave l.
    intracorporeal laser l.
    intracorporeal shock wave l.
    laser biliary l.
    laser-induced intracorporeal shock wave l.
    mechanical l.
    Medstone extracorporeal shock wave l.
    piezoelectric l.
    pressure regulated electrohydraulic l.
    l. retreatment
    rotational contact l.
    shock wave l.
    tunable dye laser l.
    ultrasonic l.
lithotripsy-induced hypertension
lithotriptic
lithotriptoscopy
lithotrity
lithuresis
litigation reaction
little
    l. head of humerus
    L. technique
Littler
    L. technique
    wing excision of L.
Littler-Cooley technique
Littré
    L. glands
    L. hernia
Littre suture technique
Livadatis circular myotomy
live donor nephrectomy
liver
    l. biopsy
    l. cyst infection
    echogenic l.
    fatty infiltration of l.
    l. flap
    focal fatty infiltration of l.
    focal nonfatty infiltration of l.
    frosted l.
    hobnail l.
    icing l.
    lardaceous l.
    l. mass
    l. metastasis
    nodular transformation of l.

L

NOTES

liver *(continued)*
    nutmeg l.
    polycystic l.
    l. resection
    split l.
    stasis l.
    sugar-icing l.
    l. transplantation
    l. transplantation preservation injury
    l. tumor
    undifferentiated embryonal sarcoma of l.
    wandering l.
    waxy l.
living-related donor transplantation (LRLT)
Livingstone therapy
Livingston peribulbar wedge
LKB Optiphase 2 scintillation fluid
Lloyd-Roberts
    L.-R. fracture technique
    L.-R. open reduction of Monteggia fracture
Lloyd-Roberts-Catteral-Salamon classification
LMA
    laryngeal mask airway
    LMA cuff
LMW
    low molecular weight
load-bearing graft
load-deflection
    l.-d. curve
    l.-d. rate
load-deformation curve
load-displacement
    l.-d. curve
    l.-d. plot
load line
lobar
    l. bronchi
    l. hemorrhage
    l. nephronia
lobate
lobe
    ear l.
    Home l.
    left l. of liver
    l.'s of mammary gland
    middle l. of prostate
    l. of prostate
    pyramidal l. of thyroid gland
    renal l.
    Riedel l.
    right l. of liver
    spigelian l.
    Spigelius l.
    l.'s of thyroid gland

lobectomy
    anterior temporal l.
    anteromesial temporal l.
    Falconer l.
    hepatic l.
    sleeve l.
    temporal l.
    thyroid l.
lobi *(pl. of lobus)*
lobose
lobotomy
    frontal l.
    prefrontal l.
    radical prefrontal l.
    transorbital l.
Lobstein ganglion
lobster-claw deformity
lobular
lobulate
lobulated mass
lobule
    cortical l.'s of kidney
    l.'s of epididymis
    hepatic l.
    l.'s of mammary gland
    renal cortical l.
    secondary pulmonary l.
    l.'s of testis
    l.'s of thymus
    l.'s of thyroid gland
lobulet
lobulus, pl. lobuli
    l. auriculae
    coloboma lobuli
    l. corticalis renalis
    lobuli epididymidis
    lobuli glandulae mammariae
    lobuli glandulae thyroideae
    l. hepatis
    lobuli testis
    lobuli thymi
lobus, pl. lobi
    l. appendicularis
    lobi glandulae mammariae
    lobi glandulae thyroideae
    l. hepatis dexter
    l. hepatis sinister
    l. inferior pulmonis
    l. medius prostatae
    l. medius pulmonis dextri
    l. prostatae
    l. pyramidalis glandulae thyroideae
    l. renalis
    l. sinister
local
    l. anesthesia
    l. anesthetic
    l. anesthetic reaction

l. bloodletting
l. depot injection
l. epineurotomy
l. excision
l. excitatory state
l. exhaust ventilation
l. infiltration
l. ingrowth
l. irradiation
l. methotrexate injection
l. muscle flap
l. radical resection
l. recurrence
l. skin flap
l. standby anesthesia technique
l. surgery
l. tissue infiltration
l. tumor extension

Localio-Francis-Rossano resection
Localio procedure
localization
anatomic l.
bleeding site l.
estrogen receptor l.
eye tumor l.
hooked wire l.
methylene blue dye l.
needle l.
needle l. of breast lesion
pancreatic tumor l.
pedicle l.
percutaneous l.
placental l.
l. technique
localized
l. inflammation
l. lesion
l. leukocyte mobilization
l. plaque formation
locating canal
lock
Howland l.
l. suture
Locke-Ringer solution
Locke solution
locking
l. horizontal mattress suture
l. nail
lock-stitch suture
Lockwood ligament

loculation
l. of fluid
l. syndrome
Loeffler-Ballard incision
Loesche classification
Loewenthal
L. bundle
L. tract
lofentanil
Löffler suture technique
logadectomy
Logan traction bow with teeth
logical
l. method
l. operation
log relative exposure
log-rolling maneuver
Löhlein-Baehr lesion
Löhlein operation
loin
lollipop
fentanyl l.
Londermann operation
lone atrial fibrillation
long
l. abductor muscle of thumb
l. adductor muscle
l. anterior flap
l. axis
l. axis of body
l. bone
l. bone fracture
l. buccal nerve
l. cone technique
l. deltopectoral approach
l. extensor
l. external rotator
l. head
l. head of biceps
l. head biceps tendon
l. incubation hepatitis
l. intestinal tube
l. lesion
l. levatores costarum muscles
l. line
l. muscle of head
l. muscle of neck
l. oblique fracture
l. palmar muscle
l. posterior flap
l. posterior flap technique

L

NOTES

long (*continued*)
    l. pulse repetition time/echo time image
    l. saphenous vein
    l. segment spinal fusion
    l. and short lever rotational manipulation
    l. subscapular nerve
    l. thoracic artery
    l. thoracic nerve
    l. thoracic vein
    l. vinculum

long-acting insulin preparation
longer-segment obstruction
longissimus
    l. capitis muscle
    l. cervicis muscle
    l. thoracis muscle

longitudinal
    l. aberration
    l. arc of skull
    l. bands of cruciform ligament
    l. canals of modiolus
    l. choledochotomy
    deep-gastric l. (DG-L)
    l. dissociation
    l. duct of epoöphoron
    l. enterotomy
    l. fold of duodenum
    l. fracture
    l. incision
    l. laceration
    l. layer of muscular coat
    l. ligament
    l. ligament rupture
    l. method
    midpapillary l. (MP-L)
    l. myotomy
    l. nephrotomy of Boyce
    l. oval pelvis
    l. pancreaticojejunostomy
    l. relaxation
    l. ridge of hard palate
    l. section
    l. suture of palate
    two-chamber l. (2C-L)
    l. vertebral venous sinus

Longmire
    L. operation
    L. valvotomy

long-term
    l.-t. bone-instrumentation interface
    l.-t. central venous access catheter placement
    l.-t. epidural catheterization
    l.-t. oxygen therapy

longus
    l. capitis muscle
    l. colli muscle
    extensor carpi radialis l. (ECRL)
    extensor digitorum l.
    extensor hallucis l.
    extensor pollicis l.

Lonnecken tube
Look suture
loop
    air-filled l.
    Biebl l.
    bowel l.
    l. of bowel
    central chemoreflex l.
    cerebral-sacral l.
    cervical l.
    l. choledochojejunostomy
    colonic l.
    contiguous l.
    l. diathermy cervical conization
    l. distribution
    duodenal l.
    efferent l.
    l. electrocautery excision procedure (LEEP)
    l. electrosurgical excision procedure
    l. esophagojejunostomy
    expressor l.
    l. fixation
    l. forearm graft
    foreign body l.
    l. gastric bypass
    l. gastric bypass method
    l. gastric bypass procedure
    l. gastric bypass technique
    l. gastrojejunostomy
    Henle l.
    Hyrtl l.
    ileal l.
    l. ileostomy
    inferior root of cervical l.
    intestinal l.
    jejunal l.
    jejunal interposition of Henle l.
    l. jejunostomy
    lenticular l.
    nephronic l.
    N-shaped sigmoid l.
    open l.
    ostomy l.
    l. ostomy bridge
    peduncular l.
    peripheral chemoreflex l.
    puborectalis l.
    Roux-en-Y l.
    l. stoma
    subclavian l.
    superior root of cervical l.
    l. suture

3-l. technique
l. transverse colostomy
vascular l.
venous l.

loose
l. body
l. fracture
l. fragment
l. intra-articular body
l. knee procedure

loosening
screw l.

Loosett maneuver
lop-ear
Lopez-Enriquez operation
Lo-Por
L.-P. tracheal tube
L.-P. vascular graft

lorazepam
Lord
L. dilation of hemorrhoid
L. hemorrhoidectomy

Lord-Blakemore tube
lordosis
l. creation
l. preservation

Lore-Lawrence
L.-L. trachea tube
L.-L. tracheotomy tube

lorentzian line
Lorenz procedure
Lore suction tube
lorry-driver fracture
Lortat-Jacob approach
LOS
length of stay

Losee
L. modification
L. modification of MacIntosh
technique
L. sling and reef technique

loss
l. of contact point
cutaneous heat l.
discrimination l.
excessive blood l.
excessive weight l.
extreme hearing l.
insertion l.
memory l.
percutaneous anesthetic l.

l. of resistance
surgical weight l.
loss-of-resistance technique
lost wax pattern technique
Lotheissen hernia repair
Lothrop frontoethmoidectomy procedure
Lotrimin AF solution
lotus position
Lougheed-White coccygectomy
Louis angle
loupe magnification
Lovenox injection
Lovset maneuver
low
l. anterior resection (LAR)
l. cervical approach
l. cervical cesarean section
l. current monopolar coagulation
l. flip angle gradient-echo imaging
l. intermittent suction
l. LET external beam irradiation
l. lip line
l. lumbar spine fracture
l. molecular weight (LMW)
l. pressure bladder substitute
l. rectal resection
l. spinal anesthesia
l. thoracic level epidural anesthesia
l. transverse cesarean section
l. transverse incision

low-attenuation
l.-a. lesion
l.-a. mass

low-density mass
low-dose anesthetic
LowDye taping technique
Lowell reduction
Löwenberg canal
low-energy fracture
Löwenstein operation
lower
l. abdominal midline incision
l. abdominal transverse incision
l. anterior axillary line
l. body negative pressure
l. cervical spine fusion
l. cervical spine posterior
stabilization
l. cervical spine procedure
l. esophageal B ring
l. esophageal mucosal ring
l. esophageal sphincter (LES)

NOTES

lower *(continued)*
    l. esophageal sphincter pressure
    l. extremity
    l. extremity bypass graft
    l. extremity nerve block
    l. extremity noninvasive
    l. extremity revascularization
    l. extremity surgery
    l. eyelid
    l. gastrointestinal hemorrhage
    l. genital tract infection
    l. GI tract foreign body
    l. incisor angulation
    l. jaw
    l. lid
    l. lid sling procedure
    l. lip
    l. lip-splitting incision
    l. midclavicular line
    l. motor neuron lesion
    l. nephron syndrome
    l. panendoscopy
    l. pole laceration
    l. posterior lumbar spine and sacrum surgery
    l. respiratory tract infection
    L. ring
    l. trapezius flap
    l. uterine segment (LUS)
    l. uterine segment transverse (LUST)
    l. uterine segment transverse cesarean section
    l. uterine segment transverse C-section
Lowery method
lowest
    l. lumbar arteries
    l. splanchnic nerve
    l. thyroid artery
low-flow
    l.-f. anesthetic technique
    l.-f. circuit
    l.-f. regulator
    l.-f. sevoflurane anesthesia
low-flux
    l.-f. cellulose-based membrane
    l.-f. cuprophane membrane
    l.-f. dialysis membrane
low-frequency jet ventilation
low-grade
    l.-g. squamous intraepithelial lesion
    l.-g. suction unit
low-loop cutaneous ureterostomy
Lowman procedure
Lown
    L. classification

    L. technique
    L. and Woolf method
low-pressure
    l.-p. tamponade
low-segment transverse incision
Lowsley
    L. lobar anatomy
    L. ribbon gut method
low-speed rotational angioplasty
lozenge
    Oralet l.
LPL-mediated lipolysis
LRLT
    living-related donor transplantation
L-shaped capsular incision
LTCBDE
    laparoscopic transcystic common bile duct exploration
L.T. Jones tear duct tube
LTO
    laparoscopic total occlusion
LTP
    laryngotracheoplasty
lubrication
    skin l.
LubriTears solution
lucanthone hydrochloride
Lucas groove
lucent lung lesion
lückenschädel
Luc operation
Ludloff
    L. bunionectomy
    L. incision
    L. medial approach
    L. osteotomy
    L. technique
Ludwig
    L. angle
    L. ganglion
    L. labyrinth
    L. plane
Luer
    L. connection
    L. connector
    L. speaking tube
    L. tracheal tube
Luer-Lok
    L.-L. jet ventilator connector
    L.-L. port
Lugol
    L. dye esophagoscopy
    L. iodine solution
Lukens catgut suture
Luke procedure
Lukes and Butler classification of Hodgkin disease
Lukes-Collins classification

lumbar
l. accessory movement technique
l. anesthetic technique
l. approach
l. artery
l. branch of iliolumbar artery
l. canal
l. cistern
l. diskectomy
l. disk herniation
l. epidural anesthesia
l. epidural endoscopy
l. extension
l. extension test
l. facet injection
l. flexure
l. ganglia
l. gravitational line
l. hemilaminectomy
l. hernia
l. iliocostal muscle
l. interspinales muscles
l. interspinal muscle
l. lordosis preservation
l. lymph nodes
l. nephrectomy
l. nerve root injection
l. part of diaphragm
l. part of spinal cord
l. pedicle fixation
l. plexus
l. plexus block
l. port
l. puncture
l. quadrate muscle
l. region
l. rib
l. rotation
l. rotation test
l. rotator muscles
l. segments of spinal cord
l. spinal cord lesion
l. spinal fusion
l. spine biopsy
l. spine burst fracture
l. spine fusion
l. spine kyphotic deformity
l. spine lesion
l. spine segmental fixation
l. spine stabilization
l. spine transpedicular fixation
l. spine vertebral osteosynthesis

l. splanchnic nerve
l. sympathectomy
l. sympathetic block
l. triangle
l. trunks
l. tumor
l. veins
l. vertebrae
l. vertebral interbody fusion
lumbarization
lumbar-peritoneal
l.-p. shunting
lumbi (*pl. of* lumbus)
lumboabdominal
lumbocolostomy
lumbocolotomy
lumbocostal
l. ligament
lumbocostoabdominal triangle
lumbodorsal fascia
lumboinguinal
l. nerve
lumbo-ovarian
lumbosacral
l. angle
l. canal
l. dislocation
l. fusion
l. joint
l. junction fracture
l. plexus
l. plexus lesion
l. root lesion
l. trunk
lumbrical
l. muscle of foot
l. muscle of hand
lumbus, pl. lumbi
lumen, pl. lumina
luminal
lumpectomy
endoscopic aspiration l.
lunate
l. bone
l. dislocation
lung
acinic cell tumor of l.
aeration of l.
l. biopsy
brown induration of l.
l. carcinoma
l. cavity

NOTES

411

lung *(continued)*
    coin lesion of l.
    consolidation of l.
    decortication of l.
    endstage l.
    eosinophilic granuloma of l.
    essential brown induration of l.
    giant cell tumor of l.
    hypoinflation of the l.
    iron l.
    Kolobow membrane l.
    l. lesion
    membrane artificial l.
    nonventilated l.
    pigment induration of l.
    pump l.
    respirator l.
    Sci-Med-Kolobow membrane l.
    Sci-Med Life Systems, Inc.,
      membrane artificial l.
    shock l.
    shunt to the l.
    l. tumor
    l. volume reduction (LVR)
    l. volume reduction surgery
    l. water
    wet l.
lung-imaging fluorescent endoscopy
lunotriquetral
    l. dissociation
    l. fusion
lunula
Luomanen oral airway
lupus-associated valve disease
lupus erythematosus preparation
Luque
    L. instrumentation concave
      technique
    L. instrumentation convex technique
    L. loop fixation
    L. ring
    L. rod fixation
    L. rod fixation for kyphosis
    L. rod migration
    L. sublaminar wiring technique
Luque-Galveston fixation
Luria-Delbruck fluctuation test
Luride topica solution
LUS
    lower uterine segment
Luschka
    L. cartilage
    L. gland
    L. joints
    L. ligaments
    L. sinus

LUST
    lower uterine segment transverse
      LUST C-section
luster
    corneal l.
lustrous central yellow point
luteal
luteectomy
luteinization
luteinized thecoma
luteinoma
luteolysis
luteoma
    pregnancy l.
luteus
luxatio erecta shoulder dislocation
luxation
    l. of eyeball
    habitual temporomandibular joint l.
    l. of lens
    rotatory l.
    temporomandibular l.
luxurians
    ectropion l.
Luys
    L. body
    L. body syndrome
LVEDa
    left ventricular end-diastolic area
LVESa
    left ventricular end-systolic area
LVOT
    left ventricular outflow tract
LVR
    lung volume reduction
      LVR procedure
Lyden-Lehman technique
Lyden technique
lymph
    l. gland
    l. node biopsy
    l. node dissection
    l. node metastasis
    l. node sampling
    l. space
    tissue l.
    l. vessels
lymphadenectomy
    bilateral l.
    endocavitary pelvic l. (ECPL)
    extended pelvic l.
    inguinal l.
    laparoscopic pelvic l.
    mediastinal l.
    Meigs pelvic l.
    para-aortic l.
    pelvic l.
    prophylactic l.

retroperitoneal l.
thoracoabdominal retroperitoneal l.
lymphadenoma
lymphadenopathy
lymphangiectasis
lymphangiectomy
lymphangioendothelioma
lymphangiohemangioma
lymphangioma
lymphangioplasty
lymphangiosarcoma
lymphangiotomy
Lymphapress compression therapy
lymphatic
l. canal
l. duct
l. malformation
l. metastasis
l. permeation
l. plexus
l. ring of cardiac part of stomach
l. valvule
l. vessels
lymphaticostomy
lymphaticovenous anastomosis
lymphatolysis
lymphedema
lymph node
l. n.'s of abdominal organs
accessory nerve l. n.'s
anorectal l. n.'s
anterior deep cervical l. n.'s
anterior group of axillary l. n.'s
anterior jugular l. n.'s
anterior mediastinal l. n.'s
anterior superficial cervical l. n.'s
anterior tibial l. n.
apical group of axillary l. n.'s
appendicular l. n.'s
axillary l. n.'s
l. n. of azygos arch
bifurcation l. n.'s
brachial l. n.'s
bronchopulmonary l. n.'s
buccal l. n.
carinal l. n.'s
celiac l. n.'s
central group of axillary l. n.'s
central mesenteric l. n.'s
colic l. n.'s
common iliac l. n.'s

companion l. n.'s of accessory nerve
cubital l. n.'s
cystic l. n.
deep inguinal l. n.'s
deep parotid l. n.'s
l. n.'s of elbow
external iliac l. n.'s
facial l. n.'s
fibular l. n.
gastroduodenal l. n.'s
gluteal l. n.'s
hepatic l. n.'s
hilar l. n.'s
ileocolic l. n.'s
inferior epigastric l. n.'s
inferior mesenteric l. n.'s
inferior phrenic l. n.'s
inferior tracheobronchial l. n.'s
infra-auricular deep parotid l. n.'s
infra-auricular subfascial parotid l. n.'s
intercostal l. n.'s
interiliac l. n.'s
intermediate lacunar l. n.
intermediate lumbar l. n.'s
internal iliac l. n.'s
interpectoral l. n.'s
intraglandular deep parotid l. n.'s
jugulodigastric l. n.
jugulo-omohyoid l. n.
juxtaesophageal pulmonary l. n.'s
juxtaintestinal l. n.'s
lateral deep cervical l. n.'s
lateral group of axillary l. n.'s
lateral jugular l. n.'s
lateral lacunar l. n.
lateral pericardiac l. n.'s
lateral superficial cervical l. n.'s
left colic l. n.'s
left gastric l. n.'s
left gastroepiploic l. n.'s
left lumbar l. n.'s
l. n. of ligamentum arteriosum
lingual l. n.'s
lumbar l. n.'s
malar l. n.
mandibular l. n.
mastoid l. n.'s
medial lacunar l. n.
mesenteric l. n.'s
mesocolic l. n.'s

NOTES

lymph node (*continued*)
 middle colic l. n.'s
 middle group of mesenteric l. n.'s
 middle rectal l. n.
 nasolabial l. n.
 obturator l. n.'s
 occipital l. n.'s
 pancreatic l. n.'s
 pancreaticoduodenal l. n.'s
 pancreaticosplenic l. n.'s
 paramammary l. n.'s
 pararectal l. n.'s
 parasternal l. n.'s
 paratracheal l. n.
 parauterine l. n.'s
 paravaginal l. n.'s
 paravesical l. n.'s
 parietal l. n.'s
 pectoral group of axillary l. n.'s
 popliteal l. n.'s
 posterior group of axillary l. n.'s
 posterior mediastinal l. n.'s
 posterior tibial l. n.
 preauricular deep parotid l. n.'s
 prececal l. n.'s
 prelaryngeal l. n.'s
 prepericardiac l. n.'s
 pretracheal l. n.'s
 prevertebral l. n.'s
 promontory common iliac l. n.'s
 pulmonary l. n.'s
 pyloric l. n.'s
 retroauricular l. n.'s
 retrocecal l. n.'s
 retropharyngeal l. n.'s
 retropyloric l. n.'s
 right colic l. n.'s
 right gastric l. n.'s
 right gastroepiploic l. n.'s
 right gastro-omental l. n.'s
 right lumbar l. n.'s
 sacral l. n.'s
 sigmoid l. n.'s
 splenic l. n.'s
 subaortic l. n.'s
 submandibular l. n.'s
 submental l. n.'s
 subpyloric l. n.'s
 subscapular group of axillary l. n.'s
 superficial inguinal l. n.'s
 superficial parotid l. n.'s
 superior gastric l. n.'s
 superior mesenteric l. n.'s
 superior phrenic l. n.'s
 superior rectal l. n.'s
 superior tracheobronchial l. n.'s
 supraclavicular l. n.'s

 suprapyloric l. n.
 thyroid l. n.'s
 tracheal l. n.'s
 visceral l. n.'s
lymphoadenoma
lymphoblastoid cell line
lymphocelectomy
 laparoscopic l.
 pelvic l.
lymphocele drainage
lymphocyte migration
lymphocytic infiltration
lymphocytoma
lymphoepithelial lesion
lymphoepithelioma
lymphogenous metastasis
lymphogranuloma
lymphoid
 l. infiltration
 l. ring
 l. tissue
lymphoidectomy
lymphoma
lymphomyeloma
lymphoplasty
lymphoproliferation
lymphoproliferative lesion
lymphosarcoma
lymphoscintigraphy
 internal mammary l. (IML)
Lynch
 L. frontoethmoidectomy procedure
 L. incision
Lynn
 L. technique
 L. tendo calcaneous repair
Lyon
 L. ring
 L. ring-constrictive band
 L. tube
Lyon-Horgan procedure
lyophilization of bone
lyophilized
 l. bone graft
 l. dural patch
 l. extract
Lyphocin injection
lyse
lysed
Lysholm
 L. Knee Scale
 L. score
lysing
lysis
 adhesion l.
 l. of adhesions
 endothelial l.

lysogenic
l. induction
l. strain
lysosomal
l. enzyme disorder
l. membrane
l. storage disease
l. swelling

lyssa bodies
lytic
l. blockade
l. bone lesion
Lytren electrolyte solution

NOTES

L

M

M lignocaine
M line

M1156A monitoring system

MABP

mean arterial blood pressure

MAC

minimal anesthetic concentration
minimum alveolar anesthetic
concentration
minimum alveolar concentration
monitored anesthesia care
MAC anesthesia
MAC infection
MAC multiples
MAC ratio

1-MAC

1-minimum alveolar concentration
1-MAC halothane
1-MAC isoflurane

MacAusland procedure
MAC-Awake ratio
MacCallan classification
MacCallum patch
MacCarthy procedure
maceration
Macewen

M. classification
M. hernia operation
M. herniorrhaphy
M. triangle

Macewen-Shands osteotomy
MacFee incision
Machek-Blaskovics operation
Machek-Brunswick operation
Machek-Gifford operation
Machek ptosis operation
machination
machine

demand flow m.
intermittent flow m.

Mach line
MAC-hour
MacIntosh

M. blade anesthesia
M. extra-articular tenodesis
M. laryngoscope blade
M. over-the-top ACL reconstruction
M. over-the-top repair
M. technique

MAC-intubation ratio
Mack-Brunswick operation
Mackenrodt

M. incision
M. ligament

MacKenty laryngectomy tube
Mackenzie point
Mackler intraluminal tube
Mackray short-cuffed endobronchial tube
MAC-minute
MacNab

M. line
M. line for facet imbrication
M. operation
M. shoulder repair

MacNichol-Voutsinas classification
macroadenoma
macrocalcification
macrocirculation
macrocolon
macroelectrode technique
macro-Kjeldahl method
macroorchidism
macropenis
macroperforation
macrophallus
macroprolactinoma
macroprosopia
macroscopic

m. lesion
m. sphincter

macrosigmoid
macrovascular coronary lesion
MAC-Skin incision ratio
MAC-Surgical incision ratio
macula, pl. **maculae**

m. densa
vitelliform degeneration of m.

macular

m. ectopia
m. photocoagulation

maculopapillary bundle
maculopapular bundle
maculopathy
Madajet XL local anesthesia
Madden

M. incisional herniorrhaphy
M. repair
M. repair of incisional hernia
M. technique

Maddox

M. rod test
M. wing test

Madelung deformity
Madlener operation
Madoff suction tube
maduromycetoma
Magendie spaces
magenstrasse

M

Magerl
  M. posterior cervical screw fixation
  M. translaminar facet screw
    fixation technique
maggot
  surgical m.
Magilligan measuring technique
**Magill Safety Clear Plus endotracheal
  tube**
Magitot keratoplasty operation
magna, pl. **magnae**
  cisterna m.
  cisterna venae magnae
magnetic
  m. extraction
  m. induction
  m. operation
  m. radiation exposure
  m. resonance imaging scan
  m. resonance spectroscopy
  m. source imaging (MSI)
  m. stimulation
magnetite in tumor targeting
magnetization precession angle
**magnetization prepared-rapid gradient
  echo (MP-RAGE)**
magnetoelectric stimulation
magnet operation
magnification
  area of interest m.
  electronic m.
  loupe m.
  relative spectacle m.
  spot m.
**magnitude preparation-rapid acquisition
  gradient echo (MP-RAGE)**
Magnuson-Stack
  M.-S. operation
  M.-S. procedure
  M.-S. shoulder arthrotomy
Magnuson technique
Magnus operation
Magpi
  M. hypospadius repair
  M. operation
Ma-Griffith
  M.-G. technique
  M.-G. tendo calcaneus repair
Mahaim bundle
Mahan procedure
MAI
  Mycobacterium avium-intracellulare
  MAI infection
maim
main
  m. bundle
  m. pancreatic duct (MPD)
mainstem intubation

maintainer cast space
maintenance of anesthesia
Mainz
  M. pouch augmentation
  M. pouch cutaneous urinary
    diversion
  M. pouch operation
  M. urinary pouch
Maisonneuve fibular fracture
Maissiat band
Maitland technique
Majestro-Ruda-Frost tendon technique
Majewsky operation
major
  m. amputation
  m. calices
  m. duodenal papilla
  m. fissure
  justo m.
  m. liver resection (MLR)
  m. operation
  m. surgery
Makler insemination
mala
Malacarne space
malacotomy
Maladie de Graeffe operation
malangulation
malar
  m. fat pad
  m. fold
  m. foramen
  m. fracture
  m. lymph node
  m. node
Malawer
  M. excision technique
  M. resection
Malbec operation
Malbran operation
male
  m. breast
  m. castration
  m. gonad
  m. urethra
maleate
  thiethylperazine m.
Malecot
  M. gastrostomy tube
  M. nephrostomy tube
malformation
  angiographically occult intracranial
    vascular m. (AOIVM)
  anorectal m.
  Arnold-Chiari m.
  arteriovenous m.
  atrioventricular m.
  AV m.

Bing-Siebenmann m.
bronchopulmonary foregut m.
capillary m.
cardiac valvular m.
cardiovascular m.
cavernous m.
central nervous system m.
cerebral arteriovenous m.
cerebral vascular m.
cerebrovascular m.
Chiari I–III m.
cloacal m.
clomiphene fetal m.
congenital brain m.
congenital cystic adenomatoid m.
congenital heart m.
congenital vascular m.
craniofacial m.
cutaneous m.
cystic adenomatoid m.
Dandy-Walker m.
DeMyer system of cerebral m.
Dieulafoy vascular m.
dural arteriovenous m.
dysraphic m.
Ebstein m.
extremity m.
faciotelencephalic m.
fetal cystic adenomatoid m.
flocculonodular arteriovenous m.
foregut m.
frontal arteriovenous m.
frontoparietal arteriovenous m.
galenic venous m.
gastric arteriovenous m.
glomus arteriovenous m.
infratentorial arteriovenous m.
intracerebral arteriovenous m.
intracerebral vascular m.
intracranial arteriovenous m.
intracranial vascular m.
intramedullary arteriovenous m.
intramuscular venous m.
lymphatic m.
medial hemispheric
  arteriovenous m.
mermaid m.
Michel m.
mixed venous-lymphatic m.
Mondini-Alexander m.
Mondini pulmonary
  arteriovenous m.

neural axis vascular m.
neural crest m.
occipital m.
occult cerebrovascular m.
occult vascular m.
orbital arteriovenous m.
pulmonary arterial m.
pulmonary arteriovenous m.
radiculomeningeal spinal
  vascular m.
retinal arteriovenous m.
Scheibe m.
sink-trap m.
spinal vascular m.
split-cord m.
supratentorial arteriovenous m.
telencephalic m.
teratogen-induced m.
thalamocaudate arteriovenous m.
Uhl m.
vascular m.
vein of Galen m.
venous m.
malfunction
  cuff m.
  pacemaker m.
Malgaigne
  M. fossa
  M. hernia
  M. pelvic fracture
  M. triangle
malignancy
malignant
  m. adenoma
  m. external otitis syndrome
  m. fasciculation
  m. giant cell tumor of bone
  m. hyperpyrexia
  m. hypertension
  m. hyperthermia (MH)
  m. pituitary lesion
  m. renal mass
  m. synovioma
  m. tumor of cervix
malinterdigitation
Malis-Frazier suction tube
maljunction
Mallampati
  M. oropharyngeal classification
  M. pharyngeal visibility
    classification
Mallard incision

M

NOTES

malleable multipore suction tube
malleoincudal
malleolar
  m. fracture
  m. osteotomy
malleolus, pl. malleoli
  tip of medial m.
mallet
  m. finger deformity
  m. fracture
  m. toe deformity
Mallinckrodt
  M. endotracheal tube
  M. Laser-Flex tube
  M. sensory system
Mallory technique
Mallory-Weiss
  M.-W. lesion
  M.-W. mucosal rupture
  M.-W. syndrome
  M.-W. tear
malocclusion
maloccurrence
malpighian
  m. body
  m. pyramid
  m. stigmas
malposition
  catheter m.
  extension m.
malpresentation
  fetal m.
malprojection
malrelation
malrotation
  intestinal m.
  m. of intestine
  midgut volvulus with m.
  renal m.
malunion
  humeral fracture m.
malunited
  m. calcaneus fracture
  m. forearm fracture
  m. radial fracture
malutinization
mamillary
  m. body
  m. ducts
  m. line
  m. process
  m. tubercle
mamillothalamic tract
mamma, pl. mammae
  m. masculina
  m. virilis
mammalian cell membrane

mammaplasty, mammoplasty
  Aries-Pitanguy m.
  augmentation m.
  postreduction m.
  reconstructive m.
  reduction m.
mammary
  m. artery graft
  m. branches
  m. duct ectasia
  m. ducts
  m. fistula
  m. gland
  m. line
  m. plexus
  m. region
  m. tissue
mammectomy
mammillaplasty
mammoplasty (var. of mammaplasty)
mammotomy
management
  m. of anesthesia
  emergency airway m.
  endoscopic m.
  expectant m.
  foreign body m.
  laparoscopic m.
  mechanical endoscopic m.
  operative m.
  pain m.
  surgical m.
  ventilator m.
Manchester
  M. operation
  M. system for radium therapy
Manchester-Fothergill operation
Mancini technique
Mandelbaum-Nartolozzi-Carney patellar
  tendon repair
mandible
  lateral oblique projection of m.
  osteotomy of m.
  space of body of m.
  vertical osteotomy of ramus of m.
mandibula, pl. mandibulae
mandibular
  m. articulation
  m. body fracture
  m. canal
  m. centric relation
  m. condylectomy
  m. condyle fracture
  m. disk
  m. dislocation
  m. equilibration
  m. excess
  m. fixation

m. foramen
m. fossa
m. head
m. hinge position
m. joint
m. lymph node
m. nodes
m. osteotomy advancement
m. plane
m. ramus fracture
m. ramus osteotomy
m. reconstruction
m. rest position
m. space
m. surgery
m. swing operation
m. swing technique
m. symphysis
m. symphysis fracture
m. tongue
mandibulectomy
segmental m.
mandibulofacial
m. dysotosis syndrome
mandibulomaxillary fixation
mandibulo-oculofacial
m.-o. syndrome
mandibulopharyngeal
mandibulotomy
mandibulum
mandrel graft
maneuver
Addison m.
Adson m.
Allen m.
Allis m.
alpha-loop m.
Apley m.
avoidance m.
Barlow m.
Bielschowsky m.
Bigelow m.
Bill m.
Bracht m.
Brandt-Andrews m.
bunching m.
Buzzard m.
Cairns m.
Carlo Traverso m.
circumduction m.
closed manipulative m.
cold pressor testing m.

corkscrew m.
costoclavicular m.
Credé m.
Cushieri m.
Dandy m.
DeLee m.
Dix-Hallpike m.
doll's eye m.
doll's head m.
Duecollement m.
Ejrup m.
Finkelstein m.
flexion-extension m.
forceps m.
Fowler m.
Fowler-Stephens m.
Frenzel m.
grunting m.
Hallpike m.
Halsted m.
Hampton m.
heel-to-ear m.
Heimlich m
hemodynamic m.
Hillis-Müller m.
Hippocratic m.
Hodge m.
Hoguet m.
Hubscher m.
Hueter m.
hyperventilation m.
Jahss m.
jaw thrust m.
Jendrassik m.
Jonnson m.
J-type m.
jugular compression m.
key-in-lock m.
Kocher m.
Krackow m.
Kristeller m.
Lachman m.
Leadbetter m.
Lecompte m.
Levret m.
log-rolling m.
Loosett m.
Lovset m.
Massini m.
Mattox m.
Mauriceau m.
Mauriceau-Levret m.

NOTES

maneuver *(continued)*
 Mauriceau-Smellie-Veit m.
 McDonald m.
 McKenzie extension m.
 McMurray circumduction m.
 McRoberts m.
 midforceps m.
 modified Ritgen m.
 Mueller m.
 Müller m.
 Müller-Hillis m.
 Munro-Kerr m.
 notch-and-roll m.
 Nylen-Barany m.
 oculocephalic m.
 Ortolani m.
 osteoclasis m.
 Pajot m.
 peroral m.
 Phalen m.
 Pinard m.
 postural fixation back m.
 Prague m.
 Prentiss m.
 Pringle m.
 Proetz m.
 pull m.
 push m.
 recruitment m.
 reexpansion m.
 relative response attributable to
  the m.
 reverse Bigelow m.
 Ritgen m.
 rotation-compression m.
 Rubin m.
 Saxtorph m.
 scalene m.
 Scanzoni m.
 Scanzoni-Smellie m.
 scarf m.
 Schatz m.
 Schreiber m.
 Sellick m.
 Slocum m.
 Spurling m.
 Steel m.
 Stimson m.
 straightening m.
 Thorn m.
 U-turn m.
 Valsalva m.
 Van Hoorn m.
 wall push m.
 Wigand m.
 Woods screw m.
 Wright m.
 Zavanelli m.

mangled
 M. Extremity Severity Score
 m. extremity syndrome
Mangoldt epithelial graft
ManHood absorbent pouch
manifestation
 allergic m.
 cardiopulmonary m.
 clinical m.
 cutaneous m.
 hepatobiliary m.
 mucocutaneous m.
 neuro-ophthalmic m.
 ocular m.
 oral m.
 otolaryngologic m.
 presenting clinical m.
 renal m.
manipulation
 bile duct m.
 catheter m.
 cervical m.
 contact m.
 cranial nerve m.
 digital m.
 direct m.
 fine m.
 gamete m.
 general thrust m.
 grading of m.
 gross m.
 guidewire m.
 Hippocrates m.
 indirect m.
 joint m.
 laser m.
 Leadbetter hip m.
 long and short lever rotational m.
 myofascial m.
 noncontact m.
 opening wedge m.
 pancreatic duct m.
 passive joint m.
 pharmacologic m.
 physical m.
 postureteroscopic m.
 specific thrust m.
 spinal m.
 thrust m.
manipulative therapy
Mankin
 M. resection
 M. technique
Manktelow transfer procedure
Mann-Bollman fistula
Mann-Coughlin-DuVries cheilectomy
Mann-Coughlin procedure
Mann-DuVries arthroplasty

Mannis suture
mannitol
    m. fermentation
Mann procedure
Mann-Whitney test
Mann-Williamson operation
manometric evaluation
Mansfield Valvuloplasty Registry
Manske-McCarroll opponensplasty
Manske-McCarroll-Swanson
   centralization
Manske technique
Mansson
    M. operation
    M. urinary pouch
mantle irradiation
Mantou method
manual
    m. method
    m. pressure
    m. push-pull technique
    m. resuscitation bag
    m. rotation
    m. technique
    m. ventilation
    m. ventilation device
manubriosternal
    m. joint
    m. junction
    m. symphysis
manubrium
    m. mallei
    m. of malleus
    m. sterni
    m. of sternum
MAP
   mean arterial pressure
Mapleson D type of T-piece circuit
maplike skull
mapping
    activation-sequence m.
    atrial activation m.
    body surface Laplacian m.
    catheter m.
    dermatome m.
    endocardial m.
    retrograde atrial activation m.
Maquet
    M. anteromedial osteoplasty
    M. dome osteotomy
    M. procedure
    M. technique

Maragiliano body
Marbach-Weil technique
marbleization
Marcacci muscle
Marcaine
    M. HCl
    M. spinal heavy
March
    M. fracture
    M. technique
Marchand adrenals
Marchi tract
Marcille triangle
Marckwald operation
Marcove-Lewis-Huvos shoulder girdle
   resection
Marcus-Balourdas-Heiple ankle fusion
   technique
mare's tail line
Marfan syndrome
margin
    carious restoration m.
    cavity m.
    dissection m.
    m.'s of eyelids
    free m. of eyelids
    frontal m.
    interosseous m.
    lacrimal m. of maxilla
    lambdoid m. of occipital bone
    mastoid m. of occipital bone
    mesovarian m. of ovary
    occipital m.
    parietal m.
    psoas m.
    pupillary m. of iris
    squamous m.
    supraorbital m.
    surgical m.
    m. of the tongue
    tumor-free m.
marginal
    m. artery of colon
    m. degeneration of cornea
    m. excess
    m. excision
    m. incision
    m. insertion
    m. insertion of umbilical cord
    m. mandibular branch of facial
    nerve
    m. myotomy

M

NOTES

marginal *(continued)*
   m. resection
   m. ridge fracture
   m. ring ulcer of cornea
   m. sinuses of placenta
   m. sinus rupture
   m. sphincter
   m. tentorial branch of internal
    carotid artery
   m. tubercle
   m. tubercle of zygomatic bone
   m. ulceration
margination
   lesion m.
   leukocytic m.
marginoplasty
margo, pl. **margines**
   m. anterior fibulae
   m. anterior pancreatis
   m. anterior pulmonis
   m. anterior radii
   m. anterior testis
   m. anterior tibiae
   m. anterior ulnae
   m. frontalis
   m. frontalis ossis parietalis
   m. frontalis ossis sphenoidalis
   m. inferior hepatis
   m. inferior pancreatis
   m. inferior pulmonis
   m. inferior splenis
   m. interosseus
   m. interosseus fibulae
   m. interosseus radii
   m. interosseus tibiae
   m. interosseus ulnae
   m. lacrimalis maxillae
   m. lambdoideus squamae occipitalis
   m. lateralis antebrachii
   m. lateralis humerii
   m. lateralis pedis
   m. lateralis renis
   m. lateralis scapulae
   m. liber ovarii
   m. liber unguis
   m. mastoideus squamae occipitalis
   m. medialis antebrachii
   m. medialis glandulae suprarenalis
   m. medialis humerii
   m. medialis pedis
   m. medialis renis
   m. medialis scapulae
   m. medialis tibiae
   m. mesovaricus ovarii
   m. occipitalis
   m. occipitalis ossis parietalis
   m. occipitalis ossis temporalis
   m. palpebrae
   m. parietalis
   m. parietalis ossis frontalis
   m. parietalis ossis sphenoidalis
   m. parietalis ossis temporalis
   m. posterior partis petrosae ossis
    temporalis
   m. posterior radii
   m. posterior testis
   m. posterior ulnae
   m. pupillaris iridis
   m. radialis antebrachii
   m. sagittalis ossis parietalis
   m. sphenoidalis ossis temporalis
   m. squamosus
   m. squamosus ossis parietalis
   m. squamosus ossis sphenoidalis
   m. superior cerebri
   m. superior glandulae suprarenalis
   m. superior pancreatis
   m. superior partis petrosae ossis
    temporalis
   m. superior scapulae
   m. superior splenis
   m. supraorbitalis
   m. tibialis pedis
   m. ulnaris antebrachii
   m. uteri
   m. zygomaticus alae majoris
marian lithotomy
Marion disease
Marion-Moschcowitz culdoplasty
Mariotte bottle
mark
   ecchymotic m.
   limbus parallel orientation
    straddling tattoo m.
   port-wine m.
   tape m.
marked tube
marker stitch
**Marks-Bayne technique for thumb
  duplication**
Marlen
   M. double-faced adhesive disk
   M. Gas Relief drainage pouch
   M. Odor-Ban ileostomy pouch
   M. Solo ileostomy pouch
   M. Zip Klosed pouch
Marlex
   M. hernial repair
   M. mesh abdominal rectopexy
   M. mesh graft
   M. plug technique
   M. suture
Marmo method
Marqez-Gomez conjunctival graft
Marquardt angulation osteotomy
Marquette Case 12

Marquez-Gomez operation
Marriott method
marrow
    m. ablation
    m. cavity
    m. graft rejection
    m. space
    spinal m.
Marseille pancreatitis classification
Marshall
    M. ligament repair technique
    M. method
    M. oblique vein
    M. test
Marshall-Marchetti
    M.-M. procedure
    M.-M. test
Marshall-Marchetti-Krantz (MMK)
    M.-M.-K. operation
    M.-M.-K. procedure
    M.-M.-K. urethropexy
Marshall-McIntosh technique
Marshall-Taylor vacuum extraction
marsupialization
    renal cyst m.
    Spence and Duckett m.
    m. technique
    transurethral m.
marsupium
Martin
    M. anoplasty
    M. incision
    M. laryngectomy tube
    M. osteotomy
    M. patellar wiring technique
    M. reduction technique
    M. tracheostomy tube
Martinez
    M. corneal transplant centering ring
    M. scleral centering ring
Martin-Gruber anastomosis
Martius
    M. bulbocavernosus fat flap
    M. procedure
masculine
    m. pelvis
    m. uterus
masculinization
    ovarian m.
masculinizing genitoplasty
masculinovoblastoma
Masimo SET pulse oximeter

mask
    bridgeless m.
    ecchymotic m.
    face m.
    Hudson type oxygen m.
    isolation face m.
    laryngeal m.
    m. leak
    medium-concentration oxygen m.
    mouth m.
    nonrebreathing m.
    Patil-Syracuse m.
    Rendell-Baker Soucek m.
    reservoir face m.
    m. seal
    SealEasy resuscitation m.
    surgical m.
    Swiss Therapy eye m.
    ventilation m.
    ventilation by m.
masking technique
Mason
    M. operation
    M. radial head fracture
      classification
    M. suction tube
    M. vertical banded gastroplasty
Mason-Allen suture
Mason-Likar limb lead modification
masquerade technique
mass
    abdominal wall m.
    abdominopelvic m.
    adnexal m.
    adrenal cystic m.
    anterior mediastinal m.
    appendiceal m.
    apperceptive m.
    asymptomatic m.
    atomic m.
    benign m.
    bleeder in tumor m.
    body cell m.
    bone m.
    bony m.
    brain m.
    calcified renal m.
    carbon gelatin m.
    cardiac m.
    cardiophrenic angle m.
    cellular periosteal
      osteocartilaginous m.

M

NOTES

mass *(continued)*
    center of m.
    cicatricial m.
    circumscribed m.
    colonic m.
    complex chest m.
    m. concentration
    congenital nasal m.
    congenital renal m.
    conglomerate m.
    cortical m.
    critical m.
    cul-de-sac m.
    cystic adnexal m.
    cystic adrenal m.
    cystic chest m.
    cystic pelvic m.
    m. defect
    dense brain m.
    discrete m.
    dominant m.
    dumbbell m.
    duodenal m.
    dysplasia-associated m.
    echodense m.
    erythrocyte m.
    esophageal m.
    exchangeable m.
    exophytic gut m.
    expansile abdominal m.
    extracardiac m.
    extramucosal m.
    extrarenal m.
    extrauterine pelvic m.
    extravascular m.
    extrinsic m.
    fallopian tube m.
    fat-free m.
    filar m.
    flank m.
    m. flow controller
    fluctuant m.
    fungating m.
    gastric m.
    groin m.
    hilar m.
    hyaline m.
    ill-defined m.
    m. infection
    inflammatory renal m.
    infra-auricular m.
    injection m.
    inner cell m.
    intra-abdominal m.
    intracardiac m.
    intracranial m.
    intradural extramedullary m.
    intrasellar m.

intravascular m.
intraventricular m.
lacrimal m.
laminated acellular m.
lateral m.
lean body m.
left ventricular m.
m. lesion
limbus m.
liver m.
lobulated m.
low-attenuation m.
low-density m.
malignant renal m.
mediastinal high-attenuation m.
m. memory
mesenteric m.
mixed-density m.
molecular m.
mulberry-shaped m.
multiloculated renal m.
mushroom-shaped m.
mycelial m.
myocardial m.
neoplastic renal m.
noncalcified nodular m.
nonopaque intraluminal m.
ochre m.
ovarian m.
ovoid m.
palpable m.
parasellar m.
parovarian m.
pediatric m.
pelvic m.
periampullary m.
perirectal m.
perivascular m.
persistent ovarian m.
phlegmonous m.
plantar-hindfoot-midfoot bony m.
pleural m.
polypoid m.
posterior mediastinal m.
postmenopausal body m.
presacral m.
pulmonary m.
pulsatile m.
rectal m.
red blood cell m.
m. reflex
renal m.
retrobulbar m.
retrocardiac m.
retrosternal m.
salivary m.
sclerotic cemental m.
scrotal m.

soft tissue m.
solitary pulmonary m.
m. spectrometer
m. spectrometry
stellate m.
Stent m.
submucosal m.
suprasellar m.
testicular m.
thymic m.
tooth m.
transformary m.
traumatic renal m.
tubular excretory m.
tumor m.
umbilical m.
uncinate process m.
unit of m.
uterine m.
vaginal m.
vascular renal m.
vertebral bone m.
well-defined m.

massage
connective tissue m.
external cardiac m.
nerve-point m.
prostatic m.
soft tissue m.

masseter
m. muscle flap

masseteric
m. artery
m. fascia
m. nerve
m. space

masseter-mandibulopterygoid space
Massier solution
Massie sliding graft
Massini maneuver
massive
m. autotransfusion
m. bowel resection syndrome
m. incisional hernioplasty
m. malignant infiltration
m. sliding graft
Masson trichrome method
MASS syndrome
mastadenoma
mastectomy
bilateral subcutaneous m.
extended radical m.

Halsted m.
McKissick m.
McWhirter m.
modified radical m.
Patey modified radical m.
radical m.
simple m.
subcutaneous m.
total m.
Willy Meyer m.

master
m. gland
m. IG bundle

mastication
component of m.
m. disorder
force of m.
m. muscle

masticator
m. nerve
m. space
m. space infection

masticatory
m. fat pad
m. space

mastoccipital
mastocytoma
mastoid
m. angle of parietal bone
m. antrum
m. border of occipital bone
m. branches of posterior auricular artery
m. branch of occipital artery
m. cavity
m. fontanel
m. foramen
m. fossa
m. lymph nodes
m. margin of occipital bone
m. obliteration operation
m. part of the temporal bone
m. wall of middle ear

mastoidectomy
modified radical m.
radical m.
simple m.
tympanoplasty m.

masto-occipital
mastopexy
Benelli m.

mastoplasty

NOTES

mastotomy
Mast-Spieghel-Pappas classification
MAST technique
Matas
    M. aneurysmectomy
    M. operation
Matchett-Brown hip arthroplasty
matchstick graft
Mate
    Soft M.
material
    m. failure break point
    m. graft
maternal
    m. abdominal pressure
    m. anesthesia
    m. birthing position
    m. deprivation syndrome
    m. fracture
    m. hydration
    m. infection
    m. mercury exposure
    m. rejection
    m. tissue
    m. venous (MV)
Mathews classification of olecranon
  fracture
Mathieu
    M. island onlay flap
    M. procedure
    M. technique
Mathieu-Horton-Devine flip-flap
matricectomy
matrilineal
matrixectomy
    chemical m.
    partial m.
    phenol m.
    Steindler m.
    Winograd partial m.
    Zadik total m.
Matroc femoral head
Matsen procedure
Matsura preparation
Matta-Saucedo fixation
Matti-Russe
    M.-R. bone graft
    M.-R. technique
Mattox maneuver
mattress
    m. stitch
    m. suture
    m. suture otoplasty
maturation
    m. division
    m. index
    m. phase
maturing the stoma

Mauchart ligaments
Mauck procedure
Maudsley Mentation Test
Mauksch-Maumenee-Goldberg operation
Mauksch operation
Maumenee-Goldberg operation
Maunsell-Weir operation
Mau osteotomy
Mauriceau-Levret maneuver
Mauriceau maneuver
Mauriceau-Smellie-Veit maneuver
Maxam suture
maxillary
    m. antrum
    m. antrum closure
    m. canal
    m. excess
    m. expansion
    m. fracture
    m. hiatus
    m. nerve
    m. osteotomy
    m. restoration
    m. sinus carcinoma
    m. sinuscopy
    m. sinus mucocele
    m. surface of greater wing of
      sphenoid bone
    m. surface of palatine bone
    m. surface of perpendicular plate
      of palatine bone
    m. surgery
maxillectomy
    Cocke m.
    subtotal m.
maxillofacial
    m. anomaly
    m. fracture
    m. surgery
maxillomandibular
    m. fixation
    m. relation
maxillotomy
    extended m.
maximal
    m. drug concentration
    m. expiratory flow rate
    m. expiratory flow volume
    m. tubular excretory capacity of
      kidneys
    m. ventilation rate
    m. voluntary ventilation
Maxima Plus plasma resistant fiber
  oxygenator
maximum
    m. breathing capacity (MBC)
    m. duration of phonation
    m. mouth opening

m. occipital point
m. permissible concentration
m. stimulation test
m. urethral closure pressure
m. voluntary ventilation (MVV)
maximum-intensity projection
Maxon absorbable suture
Maxwell
M. body
M. ring
Maydl
M. hernia
M. procedure
M. ureterosigmoidostomy
Mayer-hematoxylin solution
Mayfield
M. head fixation
M. incision
May-Hegglin body
Maylard incision
Mayo
M. approach
M. carpal instability classification
M. classification of rheumatoid
elbow
M. hysterectomy
M. linen suture
M. modified total elbow
arthroplasty
M. operation
M. perfusing O ring
M. resection arthroplasty
Mayo-Fueth inversion procedure
Mayo-Heuter bunionectomy
Mayo-Robson position
Maze
M. III procedure
Mazet
M. disarticulation of knee
M. technique
mazolysis
mazopexy
MBC
maximum breathing capacity
MBF3 infrared laser-Doppler flowmeter
McAfee approach
McBride
M. bunionectomy
M. procedure
McBurney
M. incision
M. point

McCall
M. culdoplasty
M. stitch
McCall-Schumann procedure
McCarey-Kaufman solution
McCarroll-Baker procedure
McCauley technique
McConnell
M. extensile approach
M. median and ulnar nerve
approach
M. technique
McCormick-Blount procedure
McCraw gracilis myocutaneous flap
McDonald
M. maneuver
M. procedure
McElfresh-Dobyns-O'Brien technique
McElvenny-Caldwell procedure
McElvenny technique
McFarland
M. bone graft
M. tibial graft
McFarland-Osborne
M.-O. lateral approach
M.-O. technique
McFarlane
M. skin flap
M. technique
McGavic operation
Mcginnis balloon system
McGlamry-Downey procedure
McGoon technique
McGowan-Keeley tube
McGregor basal line
McGuire operation
McIndoe
M. operation
M. procedure
M. vaginal creation
McIndoe-Hayes
M.-H. construction
M.-H. procedure
McKay-Simons clubfoot operation
McKee line
McKees solution
McKeever
M. and MacIntosh hemiarthroplasty
M. medullary clavicle fixation
M. open reduction
M. procedure

M

NOTES

McKeever-Buck
  M.-B. elbow technique
  M.-B. fragment excision
McKenzie extension maneuver
McKinney fixation ring
McKissick mastectomy
McLaughlin
  M. acromioplasty
  M. approach
  M. modification of Bunnell pull-
  out suture
  M. operation
  M. procedure
McLaughlin-Hay technique
McLaughlin-Ryder incision
McLean
  M. operation
  M. suture
  M. technique
MCL port
McMaster
  M. bone graft
  M. technique
McMurray circumduction maneuver
McMurtry-Schlesinger shunt tube
McNeer classification
McNeill-Goldmann scleral ring
McRae foramen magnum line
McReynolds
  M. method
  M. open reduction technique
  M. operation
McRoberts maneuver
McShane-Leinberry-Fenlin acromioplasty
McSpadden method
McVay
  M. herniorrhaphy
  M. inguinal hernial repair
  M. method
  M. operation
  M. procedure
  M. technique
McWhirter mastectomy
McWhorter posterior shoulder approach
Meadox
  M. Microvel double-velour Dacron
  graft
  M. vascular graft
mean
  m. airway resistance
  m. arterial blood pressure (MABP)
  m. arterial pressure (MAP)
  m. circulation time
  m. diastolic left ventricular
  pressure
  m. foundation plane
  m. normalized systolic ejection rate
  m. pulmonary artery pressure

  m. pulmonary artery wedge
  pressure
  m. shunt index
  m. systolic left ventricular pressure
  m. UV/MV ratio
Meares-Stamey technique
Mears-Rubash approach
measurement
  acoustic reflection m.
  alveolar diffusion m.
  ankle-brachial pressure m.
  continuous intramucosal PCO_2 m.
  diurnal intraocular pressure m.
  cnd-point m.
  esophageal m.
  facial excursion m.
  Fick cardiac output m.
  intrauterine pressure m.
  invasive pressure m.
  muscle m.
  near-infrared m.
  negative inspiratory pressure m.
  oxygen saturation m.
  pascal unit of pressure m.
  pressure m.
  pulse-echo distance m.
  skin m.
  skin-temperature gradient m.
  tissue pressure m.
  total exchangeable potassium m.
  transcutaneous oxygen pressure m.
  transstenotic pressure gradient m.
  tympanic membrane m.
  urethral pressure m.
  vasodilator-stimulated rCBF single
  photon emission computed
  tomographic m.
  voiding urethral pressure m.
Measuroll suture
meatal
  m. advancement and glansplasty
  m. cartilage
meati (*pl. of* meatus)
meatoplasty
  V-flap m.
meatorrhaphy
meatoscopy
meatotomy
  ureteral m.
meatus, pl. meati
  external auditory m.
  ureteral m.
  m. urinarius
MEC
  minimum effective concentration
mecamylamine
mechanical
  m. alternation of heart

m. endoscopic management
m. extrahepatic obstruction
m. leech
m. lithotripsy
m. perforation
m. pulp exposure
m. stimulation
m. thrombectomy
m. ureteral dilation
m. variceal compression
m. ventilation
m. ventilation anesthetic technique

mechanism
    m.'s of anesthesia
    antireflux flap-valve m.
    association m.
    central extensor m.
    cholinergic m.
    m. of correction
    countercurrent m.
    digital extensor m.
    extensor hood m.
    extrinsic m.
    flap-valve m.
    inhibitory-excitatory m.
    noradrenergic m.
    screw-home m.
    urethral closure m.

mechanoactivation
mechanogram
mechanomyography
mechanoreflex
mèche
Meckel
    M. band
    M. cavity
    M. ganglion
    M. ligament
    M. scan
    M. space
    M. sphenopalatine ganglionectomy
meconium
    m. aspiration
    m. aspiration syndrome
    m. plug syndrome
Medela membrane regulator
Medena tube
media
    adhesive otitis m.
medial
    m. angle of eye
    m. antebrachial cutaneous nerve

m. anterior thoracic nerve
m. arcuate ligament
m. aspect
m. aspiration
m. basal segment
m. bicipital groove
m. border of forearm
m. border of humerus
m. border of kidney
m. border of scapula
m. border of suprarenal gland
m. border of tibia
m. brachial cutaneous nerve
m. calcaneal branches of tibial nerve
m. canthal repair
m. canthus
m. canthus single injection periocular anesthesia
m. capsular imbrication
m. capsulorrhaphy
m. circumflex artery of thigh
m. circumflex femoral artery
m. clear space
m. condyle
m. condyle of femur
m. condyle of tibia
m. cord of brachial plexus
m. cortical overlap technique
m. crus of facial canal
m. crus of the superficial inguinal ring
m. cuneiform bone
m. cutaneous branch
m. cutaneous nerve of arm
m. cutaneous nerve of forearm
m. cutaneous nerve of leg
m. displacement osteotomy
m. dissection
m. dorsal cutaneous nerve
m. epicondylar apophysis
m. epicondylar crest
m. epicondylar ridge
m. epicondylectomy
m. epicondyle of femur
m. epicondyle humeral fracture
m. epicondyle of humerus
m. extensor expansion
m. extradural approach
m. femoral circumflex artery
m. forebrain bundle
m. frontobasal artery

NOTES

M

431

medial *(continued)*
- m. geniculate body
- m. great muscle
- m. head
- m. heel skive technique
- m. heel wedge
- m. hemispheric arteriovenous malformation
- m. imbrication
- m. inferior genicular artery
- m. inguinal fossa
- m. joint line
- m. lacunar lymph node
- m. longitudinal bundle
- m. lumbar intertransversarii muscles
- m. lumbar intertransverse muscles
- m. lumbocostal arch
- m. malleolar network
- m. malleolar subcutaneous bursa
- m. malleolus fixation
- m. malleolus resection
- m. mammary branches
- m. midpalmar space
- m. nasal branches of anterior ethmoidal nerve
- m. neurovascular bundle
- m. occipital artery
- m. opening wedge osteotomy
- m. palpebral ligament
- m. parapatellar approach
- m. parapatellar capsular approach
- m. parapatellar incision
- m. part of longitudinal arch of foot
- m. patellar retinaculum
- m. plantar artery
- m. plantar nerve
- m. pole of ovary
- m. popliteal nerve
- m. process of calcaneal tuberosity
- m. pterygoid muscle
- m. puboprostatic ligament
- m. repair
- m. root of optic tract
- roots of olfactory tract, lateral and m.
- m. rotation procedure
- m. rotator
- m. superior genicular artery
- m. supraclavicular nerve
- m. supracondylar crest
- m. supracondylar ridge
- m. sural cutaneous nerve
- m. surface of ovary
- m. surface of testis
- m. swivel dislocation
- m. tubercle of posterior process of talus

- m. umbilical fold
- m. umbilical ligament
- m. vastus muscle
- m. wall of tympanic cavity

medialis obliquus imbrication
medialization
median
- m. arcuate ligament
- m. atlantoaxial joint
- m. bar formation
- m. bar of Mercier
- m. basilic vein
- m. cephalic vein
- m. corpectomy
- m. detection threshold
- m. episiotomy
- m. groove of tongue
- m. jaw relation
- m. labiomandibular glossotomy
- m. line
- m. lithotomy
- m. longitudinal raphe of tongue
- m. mandibular point
- m. nerve
- m. nerve compression
- m. occlusal position
- m. palatine suture
- m. retruded relation
- m. sacral artery
- m. sacral crest
- m. sacral vein
- m. sagittal plane
- m. section
- m. sternotomy
- m. sternotomy incision
- m. strumectomy
- m. thyrohyoid ligament
- m. umbilical fold
- m. umbilical ligament
- m. vein of neck

mediastinal
- m. arteries
- m. branches
- m. branches of thoracic aorta
- m. CTD
- m. dissection
- m. hemorrhage
- m. high-attenuation mass
- m. irradiation
- m. lymphadenectomy
- m. lymph node biopsy
- m. part of lung
- m. pleura
- m. shed blood (MSB)
- m. space
- m. tube
- m. tumor

m. veins
m. wedge
mediastinoscopic examination
mediastinoscopy
Chamberlain m.
mediastinotomy
mediastinum
anterior m.
m. anterius
inferior m.
m. inferius
m. medium
middle m.
posterior m.
m. posterius
superior m.
m. superius
m. testis
mediate transfusion
medical
m. care evaluation
m. diathermy
m. dilation
m. ophthalmoscopy
m. record
m. vagotomy
medication
aerosolized m.
anticholinergic m.
anti-inflammatory m.
base m.
beta-blocker m.
m. bezoar
bromocriptine dopaminergic m.
carbidopa dopaminergic m.
concomitant m.
dopaminergic m.
intravenous m.
iodide-containing m.
levodopa dopaminergic m.
nonsteroidal anti-inflammatory m.
over-the-counter m.
parenteral m.
pergolide dopaminergic m.
preanesthetic m.
pressor m.
prophylactic m.
prosyncopal m.
psychopharmacologic m.
psychotropic m.
teratogenic m.
vasoactive m.

medication-induced injury
medicinal preparation
medicine
anesthesiology critical care m.
critical care m. (CCM)
medicochirurgical
Mediform dural graft
Medina
M. infection
M. tube
medioccipital
mediocolic sphincter
mediolateral episiotomy
medisect
Mediterranean exanthematous fever
medium-concentration oxygen mask
medium lesion
medium-scale integration
medium-sized artery
medium/solution
Medoc-Celestin pulsion tube
Medrafil wire suture
Medralone injection
Medstone extracorporeal shock wave lithotripsy
medulla, pl. medullae
m. of adrenal gland
m. glandulae suprarenalis
m. of kidney
m. of lymph node
m. nodi lymphatici
m. ossium
m. ossium flava
m. ossium rubra
renal m.
m. renalis
suprarenal m.
medullar
medullary
m. adenocarcinoma
m. bone graft
m. canal
m. cavity
m. nail fixation
m. oxygenation
m. pyramid
m. pyramidotomy
m. ray
m. space
m. spinal arteries
m. sponge kidney

M

NOTES

medullary *(continued)*
  m. substance
  m. tube
medullated
medullation
medullectomy
medullization
medulloblastoma
  desmoplastic m.
  melanotic m.
  m. metastasis
medulloepithelioma
medullomyoblastoma
medullostomy
  tarsal m.
meduloblastoma
Medusa head
Meek operation
Mees line
mefenamic acid
Mefoxin-saline solution
megacalycosis
megacolon
megacystic syndrome
megacystis
megacystis-megaureter association
megacystitis-megaureter syndrome
megacystitis-microcolon-intestinal
  hypoperistalsis syndrome
megadolichovertebrobasilar anomaly
megaloureter
megalourethra
megasigmoid
megaureter
Mehn-Quigley technique
meibomian
  m. gland carcinoma
  m. glands
Meigs-Okabayashi procedure
Meigs pelvic lymphadenectomy
Meigs-Werthein hysterectomy
Meissner plexus
melamine formaldehyde
melanization
melanoacanthoma
melanoameloblastoma
melanoblastoma
melanocarcinoma
  m. of anus
melanocytic conjunctival lesion
melanocytoma
melanoma of eyelid
melanosarcoma
melanotic
  m. lesion
  m. medulloblastoma

Meleney
  M. gangrene
  M. infection
Meller operation
melocervicoplasty
melolabial flap
Melone distal radius fracture
  classification
melonoplasty
melon seed body
meloplasty
meloschisis
Melrose solution
melting point
Meltzer method
membrana, pl. membranae
  m. abdominis
  m. atlanto-occipitalis anterior
  m. atlanto-occipitalis posterior
  m. carnosa
  m. cricothyroidea
  m. fibroelastica laryngis
  m. hyothyroidea
  membranae intercostalia
  m. intercostalis externa
  m. intercostalis interna
  m. interossea antebrachii
  m. interossea cruris
  m. mucosa
  m. perinei
  m. propria of semicircular duct
  m. quadrangularis
  m. suprapleuralis
  m. tectoria
  m. thyrohyoidea
membrane
  acute inflammatory m.
  acute pyogenic m.
  adamantine m.
  alveolar-capillary m.
  alveolocapillary m.
  alveolodental m.
  amniotic m.
  anterior atlanto-occipital m.
  anterior hyaloid m.
  antibasement m.
  antiglomerular basement m.
  antitubular basement m.
  antral m.
  arachnoid m.
  m. artificial lung
  asymmetric unit m.
  atlanto-occipital m.
  Barkan m.
  basal cell m.
  basement m.
  basilar m.
  basolateral m.

Bichat m.
bilaminar m.
Bowman m.
m. bridge
bronchial mucous m.
Bruch m.
brush-border m.
m. catheter technique
cell m.
cellulose-based m.
chorioallantoic m.
choroidal neovascular m.
cloacal m.
collodion m.
congenital pyloric m.
conjunctival m.
connective tissue m.
contraction of cyclitic m.
cricothyroid m.
cricotracheal m.
cricovocal m.
croupous m.
cuprophane m.
m. current
cyclitic m.
cytoplasmic m.
Debove m.
decidual m.
Demours m.
dentinoenamel m.
Descemet m.
dialyzer m.
diphtheritic m.
drum m.
dry mucous m.
Duddell m.
Duralon-UV nylon m.
dysmenorrheal m.
egg m.
elastic silicone m.
enamel m.
endothelial cell basement m.
epipapillary m.
epiretinal m.
epithelial basement m.
erythrocyte m.
exocelomic m.
external intercostal m.
external limiting m.
extraembryonic fetal m.
false m.
fenestrated m.

fetal m.
fibroelastic m. of larynx
fibroproliferative m.
Fielding m.
filtration-slit m.
focal rupture of basement m.
Fresnel m.
germinal m.
glassy m.
gliotic m.
glomerular basement m.
Golgi m.
Gore-Tex surgical m.
Haller m.
HEMOPHAN m.
Henle elastic m.
Henle fenestrated m.
Heuser m.
Hibond N+ nylon m.
high-flux dialysis m.
hourglass m.
Hovius m.
hyaline basement m.
hyalitis anterior m.
hyaloid posterior m.
hymenal m.
hyoglossal m.
idiopathic preretinal m.
inflammatory m.
inner limiting m.
m. instability
intact m.
intercostal m.'s
intermuscular m.
internal elastic m.
internal intercostal m.
internal limiting m.
interosseous m. of forearm
interosseous m. of leg
interposition m.
intraosseous m.
invaginated m.
ivory m.
Jackson m.
Jacob m.
m. of Liliequist
limiting m.
low-flux cellulose-based m.
low-flux cuprophane m.
low-flux dialysis m.
lysosomal m.
mammalian cell m.

M

NOTES

membrane *(continued)*
    microvillous m.
    moist mucous m.
    MSI nylon m.
    mucous m.'s
    NaK-ATPase m.
    Nasmyth m.
    neovascular m.
    neuronal m.
    nictitating m.
    onion skin-like m.
    otolithic m.
    outer limiting m.
    m. oxygenator
    PAN m.
    Payr m.
    m. peeling
    peridental m.
    perineal m.
    periodontal m.
    periorbital m.
    m. permeability
    phrenoesophageal m.
    pial-glial m.
    placental m.
    plasma m.
    polyacrylonitrile m.
    porous filter m.
    posterior atlanto-occipital m.
    posterior hyaloid m.
    postsynaptic m.
    posttransplant antiglomerular
        basement m.
    m. potential
    Preclude pericardial m.
    Preclude peritoneal m.
    preretinal m.
    presynaptic m.
    prophylactic m.
    pseudoserous m.
    pulpodentinal m.
    pupillary m.
    purpurogenous m.
    pyogenic m.
    quadrangular m.
    Reichert m.
    Reissner m.
    retrocorneal m.
    rolling m.
    m. rupture
    Ruysch m.
    ruyschian m.
    salpingopalatine m.
    salpingopharyngeal m.
    sarcolemmal m.
    schneiderian respiratory m.
    secondary m.
    semi-impermeable m.

semipermeable m.
Seprafilm bioresorbable m.
serous m.
Shrapnell m.
Slavianski m.
small intestinal m.
spiral m.
stripping m.
stylomandibular m.
subepithelial m.
subimplant m.
submucous m.
subretinal neovascular m.
suprapleural m.
surface m.
syncytiovascular m.
synovial m.
tarsal m.
m. tectora
tectorial m.
Tenon m.
thickened synovial m.
thin basement m.
thyrohyoid m.
Toldt m.
Tourtual m.
trabecular m.
m. trafficking
tubular basement m.
tympanic m.
undulating m.
unit m.
urea-impermeable m.
urogenital m.
urorectal m.
urothelial basement m.
vernix m.
vestibular m.
virginal m.
vitelline m.
vitreal m.
vitreous m.
Wachendorf m.
wrinkling m.
XM-50 Dialow m.
yolk m.
Zinn m.
membrane-coating granule
membranectomy
membrane-spanning
membranocartilaginous
membranous
    m. acute inflammation
    m. layer of superficial fascia
    m. part of male urethra
    m. septum
    m. urethra
    m. wall of trachea

Memford-Gurd arthroplasty
memory
    explicit m.
    implicit m.
    indirect m.
    m. loss
    mass m.
    m. recall
    scratch-pad m.
Mendelson syndrome
Menghini
    M. biopsy technique
    M. technique for percutaneous liver biopsy
meningeal
    m. branch of internal carotid artery
    m. branch of mandibular nerve
    m. branch of occipital artery
    m. branch of ophthalmic nerve
    m. branch of spinal nerves
    m. branch of vagus nerve
    m. carcinoma
    m. hernia
    m. layer of dura mater
    m. plexus
    m. veins
meningeorrhaphy
meningioma
    m. of posterior fossa
meningioma-en-plaque
meningiomatosis
meningitic respiration
meningocele
meningoencephalitis
meningoencephalocele
meningomyelocele
meningo-osteophlebitis
meningorrhagia
meningosis
meninguria
meniscal
    m. excision
    m. repair
meniscectomy
    arthroscopic m.
    lateral m.
    partial m.
    Patel medial m.
    subtotal lateral m.
    total m.

meniscoplasty
meniscus, pl. menisci
    Dickhaut-DeLee classification of discoid m.
    m. graft
    resection of m.
    Watanabe classification of discoid m.
Mensor-Scheck
    M.-S. hanging hip operation
    M.-S. technique
menstrual
    m. aspiration
    m. cycle induction
    m. extraction
    m. extraction abortion
mental
    m. artery
    m. block injection
    m. branches of mental nerve
    m. canal
    m. foramen
    m. nerve
    m. point
    m. process
    m. projection
    m. region
    m. spine
    m. status evaluation
    m. status examination
    m. symphysis
    m. tubercle
mentalis muscle
mentoanterior position
mentolabial
    m. furrow
    m. sulcus
mentolabialis
mentoplasty
mentoposterior position
mentotransverse position
mentum
    m. anterior position
    m. posterior position
    m. transverse position
Menzies method
MEP
    motor-evoked potential
    myogenic motor-evoked potential
meperidine
    m. conscious sedation

NOTES

meperidine *(continued)*
    m. hydrochloride
    m. with bupivacaine
mephentermine sulfate
mephobarbital
mepivacaine
    m. hydrochloride
    m. with levonordefrin
MER
    motor-evoked response
MERA F breathing system
meralgia paresthetica
Mercator projection
Mercier bar
mercurial line
mercuroscopic expansion
mercury pressure
Merendino technique
meridian
    corneal m.
meridional aberration
Merindino operation
Merkel
    M. filtrum ventriculi
    M. fossa
    M. muscle
mermaid malformation
Mersilene
    M. braided nonabsorbable suture
    M. graft
Mertz keratoscopy ring
Méry gland
mesangial matrix expansion
mesangiolysis
mesangium
    extraglomerular m.
mesareic
mesatipellic pelvis
mesencephalic
    m. cistern
    m. hemorrhage
    m. low density lesion
    m. reticular formation
    m. tractotomy
    m. tract of trigeminal nerve
mesencephalotomy
mesenchymal
    m. lesion
    m. tissue
mesenchymoma
mesenteric
    m. arteriovenous fistula
    m. bypass graft
    m. circulation
    m. glands
    m. hematoma
    m. hernia
    m. lymph node (MLN)

    m. lymph nodes
    m. mass
    m. portion of small intestine
    m. rupture
    m. vascular lesion
    m. veins
    m. venoconstriction
mesentericoparietal
    m. fossa
    m. recess
mesenteriolum
    m. processus vermiformis
mesenteriopexy
mesenteriorrhaphy
mesenteriplication
mesenteritis
mesenterium
    m. dorsale commune
mesentery
    m. of appendix
    m. of cecum
    m. of lung
    m. of sigmoid colon
    m. of transverse colon
mesethmoid bone
mesh
    m. graft
    intraperitoneal onlay m. (IPOM)
    m. myringotomy tube
    m. plug hernioplasty
    m. suture
mesioangular position
mesiobuccal
    m. canal
    m. line angle
mesiobucco-occlusal point angle
mesiodistal
    m. fracture
    m. plane
mesiolabial
    m. bilobed transposition flap
    m. line angle
mesiolabioincisal point angle
mesiolingual line angle
mesiolinguoincisal point angle
mesiolinguo-occlusal point line angle
mesio-occlusal (MO)
mesio-occlusal line angle
mesio-occlusodistal (MOD)
mesoappendix
mesoblastoma
    m. ovarii
mesocaval anastomosis
mesocecal
mesocecum
mesocolic
    m. hernia

m. lymph nodes
m. tenia
mesocolon
mesocolopexy
mesocoloplication
mesoderm
extraembryonic m.
intermediate m.
mesoduodenal
mesoduodenum
mesoenteriolum
mesoepididymis
mesoileum
mesojejunum
mesolepidoma
mesolimbic-mesocortical tract
mesonephric
m. adenocarcinoma
m. duct
m. ridge
m. tubule
mesonephroma
mesonephros
mesoneuritis
mesopexy
mesophryon
mesorchium
mesorectal
m. excision
m. lymph node
mesorectum
residual m.
mesorrhaphy
mesosigmoid
mesosigmoidopexy
mesostenium
mesosternum
mesostructure
implant m.
mesotendineum
mesotendon
mesothelial tissue
mesothelioma
mesovarian
m. border of ovary
m. margin of ovary
Messerklinger technique
Mestinon
meta-analysis
metabolic
m. coma
m. complication

m. evaluation
m. heat production
m. rate
metabolite
metacarpal
m. neck fracture
m. osteotomy
metacarpophalangeal
m. articulation
m. joint arthroplasty
metadiaphysis
metafacial angle
metal
m. band suture
m. sewing ring
metal-ceramic restoration
metallic
m. biliary stent migration
m. cranioplasty
m. foreign body
m. fragment
m. restoration
m. rod fixation
m. suture
metalloscopy
metal-weighted Silastic feeding tube
metamizol
metamorphosing respiration
metanephric
m. cap
m. duct
metaphyseal
m. osteotomy
m. tibial fracture
metaphysis, pl. metaphyses
distal m.
femoral m.
fibular m.
funnelization of m.
rachitic m.
tibial m.
metaplasia
metastasectomy
pulmonary m.
metastasis, pl. metastases
adnexal m.
adrenal m.
aortic node m.
axillary node m.
biochemical m.
biopsy-proven m.
blastic m.

M

NOTES

metastasis *(continued)*
    bone m.
    bony m.
    brain m.
    breast m.
    calcareous m.
    calcified liver m.
    calcifying m.
    cardiac m.
    cavitating m.
    celiac lymph node m.
    cerebral m.
    cervical m.
    chiasmal m.
    choroidal m.
    clivus m.
    colonic m.
    contact m.
    contralateral axillary m.
    cutaneous m.
    cystic m.
    diffuse m.
    distal m.
    distant m.
    drop m.
    duodenal m.
    echopenic liver m.
    extracapsular m.
    extrahepatic m.
    extralymphatic m.
    extrathoracic m.
    fallopian tube m.
    floxuridine in hepatic m.
    gastrointestinal m.
    hematogenic m.
    hematogenous m.
    hematopoietic m.
    hemorrhagic m.
    hepatic m.
    hernia m.
    implantation m.
    inguinal lymph node m.
    intracapsular m.
    intramucosal m.
    in-transit m.
    leptomeningeal m.
    liver m.
    lymphatic m.
    lymph node m.
    lymphogenous m.
    medulloblastoma m.
    necrotic m.
    neoplasm m.
    nodal m.
    ocular m.
    orbital m.
    osseous m.
    osteoblastic m.
    ovarian cancer m.
    paracardiac m.
    parasellar m.
    parenchymal brain m.
    periesophagogastric lymph node m.
    peritoneal m.
    placental m.
    pulmonary m.
    retrobulbar orbital m.
    satellite m.
    skeletal m.
    skip m.
    soft tissue m.
    sphenoid sinus m.
    spinal m.
    stomach cancer m.
    testicular m.
    tumor, node, m. (TNM)
    unresectable m.
    uterine sarcoma m.
    uveal m.
    vascular m.
    Virchow m.
metastatic
    m. abscess
    m. adenocarcinoma
    m. carcinoma
    m. contamination
    m. implantation
    m. lesion
    m. prostatic carcinoma
    m. renal cell carcinoma
    m. tumor removal
metasternum
metasynchronous bacterial urinary tract infection
metatarsal
    m. artery
    m. bone
    m. fracture
    m. head
    m. head resection
    m. neck osteotomy
    m. oblique osteotomy
    m. pad
    m. proximal dome osteotomy
    m. Reverdin osteotomy
    m. V-shaped osteotomy
metatarsocuneiform articulation
metatarsophalangeal
    m. articulations
    m. joint disarticulation
    m. joint dislocation
metathesis
meter
    Narkotest m.
    Potential Acuity M. (PAM)
meter-kilogram-second (mks)

metesthesiologist
metesthesiology
methacholine
    m. bronchoprovocation challenge
methamphetamine exposure
methanol freezing method
methaqualone
methemoglobin
methemoglobinemia
methitural
method
    Abbott m.
    Abell m.
    Abell-Kendall m.
    acid anhydride m.
    acid guanidine thiocyanate-phenol-
      chloroform m.
    acoupedic m.
    acoustic m.
    acridine orange m.
    agar diffusion m.
    Allain m.
    AMeX m.
    analytic m.
    Anderson-Keys m.
    Anel m.
    antegrade m.
    anthrone m.
    antibody linkage m.
    Antyllus m.
    area-length m.
    aristotelian m.
    artificial m.
    Arvidsson dimension-length m.
    Ashby differential agglutination m.
    Astrand 30-beat stopwatch m.
    atrial extrastimulus m.
    Attwood staining m.
    auditory m.
    Autenrieth and Funk m.
    avidin-biotin-peroxidase complex m.
    Ayoub-Shklar m.
    bacterial agar m.
    Baker Sudan black m.
    Barnett-Bourne acetic alcohol-silver
      nitrate m.
    barostat m.
    Barraquer m.
    barrier m.
    Barnett-Seligman
      dihydroxydinaphthyl disulfide m.

Barrnett-Seligman indoxyl
  esterase m.
Barroso-Moguel and Costero
  silver m.
Bass m.
Bassini m.
Batch least-squares m.
Baumgartner m.
Beaver direct smear m.
Beck m.
Belsey fundoplication m.
Benedict-Talbot body surface
  area m.
Bengston m.
Bennett sulfhydryl m.
Bennhold Congo red m.
Bensley aniline-acid fuchsin-methyl
  green m.
benzo sky blue m.
Berg chelate removal m.
B_0-gradient m.
Bielschowsky m.
Bier m.
bilateral inguinal hernia repair m.
Billings m.
Billroth I m.
bimodal m.
Biogenex antigen retrieval m.
bisensory m.
black periodic acid m.
Bland-Altman m.
Bleck m.
Bobath m.
Bodian m.
Bohr isopleth m.
Bonnaire m.
Borchgrevink m.
Borggreve m.
Brasdor m.
breast-conserving m.
breathing m.
Brecher-Cronkite m.
brine flotation m.
Brisbane m.
Brown-Dodge m.
Brown and Wickham pressure
  profile m.
Bruhn m.
Buck m.
Budin-Chandler m.
Buist m.
bulkhead m.

NOTES

M

method (continued)

Burch bladder suspension m.
Burgess m.
Burkhalter-Reyes m. of phalangeal fracture
Burow quantitative m.
bypass m.
Byrd-Drew m.
Cajal gold-sublimate m.
Cajal uranium silver m.
Caldwell-Moloy m.
Callahan root canal filling m.
Camp-Gianturco m.
carbolfuchsin-methylene blue staining m.
Carpue m.
catheter introduction m.
Celermajer m.
cellophane tape m.
Chang aniline-acid fuchsin m.
Charters m.
Chayes m.
chewing m.
Chiffelle and Putt m.
chloranilate m.
chloropercha m.
cholesterol-cholesteroloxidase-phenol 4-aminophenazone m.
chromate m.
chrome alum hematoxylin-phloxine m.
chromogenic m.
chromolytic m.
Ciaccio m.
cinefluoroscopic m.
Clark-Collip m.
Clausen m.
clean-catch collection m.
closed circuit m.
cobaltinitrite m.
Cockroft m.
Colcher-Sussman m.
cold knife m.
collagen staining m.
Collis-Nissen fundoplication m.
combined m.
composite pelvic resection m.
computer-assisted design-controlled alignment m.
confrontation m.
Con-Lish polishing m.
consonant-injection m.
constitutive heterochromatin m.
contact m.
contoured adduction trochanteric-controlled alignment m.
contraceptive m.
conventional m.

cooled-knife m.
Cope m.
copper sulfate m.
Corning m.
correlational m.
Craigie tube m.
Crawford m.
Credé m.
Cribier m.
Crippa lead tetraacetate m.
cross-consonant injection m.
cross-sectional m.
crown-contouring m.
Cryolife Single Step dilution m.
Cuignet m.
cup and cone m.
Cutler-Ederer m.
cyanogen bromide m.
cysteic acid m.
Dale-Laidlaw clotting time m.
Dane m.
Danielson m.
Defares rebreathing m.
definitive m.
depth caliper-meter stick m.
Devereux-Reichek m.
diazo staining m.
Dick m.
Dieffenbach m.
Dieterle m.
diffusion root canal filling m.
digitonin m.
direct m.
disk diffusion m.
disk sensitivity m.
Dixon fat suppression m.
Döderlein m.
Dodge area-length m.
Dor fundoplication m.
double antibody m.
double-stapled ileoanal reservoir m.
Douglas bag collection m.
Dow m.
downstream sampling m.
dye-dilution m.
dyed starch m.
dye scattering m.
dynamic traction m.
edge-detection m.
Eggleston m.
Eicken m.
ellipsoid m.
Elmslie-Trillat patellar realignment m.
encu m.
endorectal ileoanal pull-through m.
endoscopic mucosal resection m.
end-to-end reconstruction m.

ensu m.
enucleation m.
Epstein m.
estimated Fick m.
Eve m.
excisional biopsy m.
experimental m.
extension block splinting m.
extra-anatomic bypass m.
extracorporeal m.
Fahraeus m.
Fallat-Buckholz m.
Ferguson scoliosis measuring m.
fiberoptic intubation m.
fibrinogen m.
fibrin plate m.
Fick oxygen m.
Fick oxygen extraction m.
field m.
Fisk and Subbarow m.
Fite m.
fixed sediment m.
flat substrate m.
floppy Nissen fundoplication m.
flow convergence m.
fluorescence polarization m.
flush m.
Folin and Wu m.
Fones m.
Fontana-Masson staining m.
Foot reticulin m.
formal m.
formaldehyde-induced
  fluorescence m.
formalin-ether sedimentation m.
forward triangle m.
four-port m.
free-hand m.
freeze-cleave m.
freeze-etch m.
freeze-fracture-etch m.
French m.
frozen section m.
Gabastou hydraulic m.
Galanti-Giusti colorimetric m.
Gärtner m.
gas clearance m.
gaseous laparoscopy m.
gasless laparoscopy m.
gastric valve tightening m.
Gerbert-Mellilo m.
German m.

glass-bead retention m.
glucose oxidase m.
glycerin m.
Gohil-Cavolo m.
gradient m.
gradient-echo m.
gradient-reversal fat suppression m.
grammatic m.
Granger m.
Gräupner m.
Greenwald and Lewman m.
Grimelius argyrophil m.
Grocott-Gomori methenamine-
  silver m.
Hagedorn and Jansen m.
half-time m.
Hall m.
Hamilton m.
Hammerschlag m.
hanging chain m.
Hanley-McNeil m.
Harrison m.
Hatle m.
Hawkins m.
head-tilt m.
Heinecke m.
helium dilution m.
Heller myotomy with Dor
  fundoplication m.
hemi-double stapling m.
Hetzel forward triangle m.
heuristic m.
hexokinase m.
Hilton m.
Hirschberg m.
Hirschfeld m.
histochemical m.
Hoechst dye m.
hold-relax m.
hole preparation m.
Holmes m.
Holmgren m.
Holzer m.
Howard m.
Howe silver precipitation m.
H.P. Wright m.
Hugenholtz m.
hydrogen washout m.
Ilizarov m.
immersion m.
immobilization m.
immunodiagnostic m.

NOTES

method *(continued)*
immunofluorescence m.
immunohistochemical m.
immunometric sandwich m.
immunoperoxidase m.
impedance m.
Indian m.
indirect restorative m.
indocyanine green m.
indophenol m.
informal m.
inhalation m.
injection m.
injection-molded m.
Insall patella alta m.
install m.
intraperitoneal m.
introspective m.
Israel m.
Italian m.
Ito m.
Jahss ninety-ninety m.
jejunoileal bypass reversal m.
Jena m.
Jendrassik-Grof m.
Johnson root canal filling m.
Johnston m.
Jones and Boadi-Boatang m.
Kaplan-Meier m.
Karr m.
Kasser-Kennedy m.
Keating-Hart m.
Kendrick m.
Kennedy area-length m.
Kety-Schmidt m.
keyhole m.
kinesthetic m.
King biopsy m.
Kinzie m.
Kirby-Bauer disk diffusion m.
Kirstein m.
Kjeldahl m.
Kluge m.
Kocher m.
Konno biopsy m.
Krause m.
Krimsky m.
Kristeller m.
LaBorde m.
Lamaze m.
Langendorff m.
laparoscopic lymph node
    dissection m.
laparoscopic Nissen
    fundoplication m.
laparoscopic para-aortic lymph node
    sampling m.
laser m.

lateral condensation root canal
    filling m.
Laurell m.
least-squares m.
Leboyer m.
Lee-White clotting time m.
Levaditi m.
Levy, Rowntree, and Marriott m.
Lewis and Benedict m.
Lewissohn m.
Liang and Pardee m.
life table m.
Lillie allochrome m.
limb-saving m.
Lindsjö m.
Lison-Dunn m.
Lister m.
logical m.
longitudinal m.
loop gastric bypass m.
Lowery m.
Lown and Woolf m.
Lowsley ribbon gut m.
macro-Kjeldahl m.
Mantou m.
manual m.
Marmo m.
Marriott m.
Marshall m.
Masson trichrome m.
McReynolds m.
McSpadden m.
McVay m.
Meltzer m.
Menzies m.
methanol freezing m.
Metzer-Boyce m.
Meyerding m.
microinjection m.
micro-Kjeldahl m.
microsurgery m.
microwave-assisted streptavidin-biotin
    peroxidase m.
minimal-access m.
modified band lid m.
modified Belsey fundoplication m.
modified Seldinger m.
modified Toupe m.
Monte Carlo multiway sensitivity
    analysis m.
Moore m.
Morison m.
mother m.
Movat pentachrome m.
Mueller m.
Mueller-Walle m.
multiple cone root canal filling m.
multiple-port incisions m.

Murphy m.
nail length gauge m.
Narula m.
natural m.
Needles split cast m.
needle thoracentesis m.
Neufeld dynamic m.
Nichols m.
Nikiforoff m.
ninety-ninety m.
Nissen fundoplication m.
Nissen-Rosseti fundoplication m.
Nitchie m.
noninvasive m.
nonresectional m.
non-rib-spreading thoracotomy
  incision m.
numerical cipher m.
odd-even m.
Ogata m.
O'Hara two-clamp m.
Okamoto m.
Oliver-Rosalki m.
Ollier m.
one-inclinometer m.
open circuit m.
optical density m.
oral-aural m.
Orsi-Grocco m.
Ouchterlony m.
oxygen step-up m.
Pachon m.
Palmer m.
Papanicolaou m.
Paris m.
Parker-Kerr closed m.
pause-squeeze m.
Pavlov m.
Payr clamp m.
pedicle m.
Penaz volume-clamp m.
Penfield m.
Penn m.
percutaneous sampling m.
Pfeiffer-Comberg m.
Pfiffner and Myers m.
phosphotungstic acid-magnesium
  chloride precipitation m.
Pichlmayer m.
pilocarpine iontophoresis m.
pin and plaster m.
pinprick m.

Pizzolato peroxide-silver m.
plasma thrombin clot m.
plateau m.
plosive-injection m.
polarographic m.
Politzer m.
Pólya m.
polyvinyl alcohol fixative m.
prick-test m.
Pringle vascular control m.
prism m.
Prochownick m.
Puchtler alkaline Congo red m.
Puchtler Sirius red m.
Purmann m.
Puzo m.
PVA fixative m.
pyramid m.
Quick m.
m. of Quinones
m. of Rackley
Rackley m.
Raff-Glantz derivative m.
rag-wheel m.
Ranawat-Dorr-Inglis m.
Ranawat triangle m.
Read rebreathing m.
reconstruction m.
Reddick-Saye m.
reduction m.
Rees-Ecker m.
reference m.
Rehfuss m.
Reichel-Pólya m.
retrofilling m.
retrograde root canal filling m.
Reverdin m.
rhythm m.
Rideal-Walker m.
Risser m.
Riva-Rocci m.
Rochester m.
Rodeck m.
Russe-Gerhardt m.
Sahli m.
Salzman m.
Sandler-Dodge area-length m.
Sargenti m.
Satterthwaite m.
Scarpa m.
Schäfer m.
Schede m.

NOTES

method *(continued)*
    Schick m.
    Schiller m.
    Schober m.
    Schüller m.
    Schwartz m.
    scientific m.
    Scudder m.
    sectional root canal filling m.
    segmentation root canal filling m.
    Seldinger m.
    Sengstaken-Blakemore m.
    shadowing m.
    Shaffer-Hartmann m.
    Shimazaki area-length m.
    Sigma m.
    silver cone m.
    silver point root canal filling m.
    Silvester m.
    simultaneous m.
    single cone root canal filling m.
    single-stick m.
    sliding scale m.
    Smellie m.
    Smellie-Veit m.
    sniff m.
    Somogyi m.
    special reference m.
    sperm washing insemination m.
    sphincter-saving m.
    sphincter-sparing m.
    split cast m.
    Stammer m.
    standard radioenzymatic m.
    Stanford biopsy m.
    stapled reconstruction m.
    Stegemann-Stalder m.
    stereotactic core biopsy m.
    Stillman m.
    Stimson gravity m.
    Stovall-Black m.
    Strauss m.
    Stroganoff m.
    suction m.
    surgical enucleation m.
    swallow m.
    Sweet m.
    symptothermal m.
    synthetic m.
    systematic m.
    Tajima m.
    Tarkowski m.
    tetanic stimulation m.
    Thal fundoplication m.
    Thane m.
    Theden m.
    thermally active m.
    thermodilution m.

Thiersch m.
thiourea-resorcinol m.
Thom flap laryngeal
  reconstruction m.
Thompson-Hatina m.
Thoms m.
three-dimensional-FATS m.
threshold shift m.
Thrombo-Wellcotest m.
Tilden m.
total fundoplication m.
Toupe m.
Towako m.
trapezoid m.
triangulation stapling m.
triphenyltetrazolium staining m.
trocar drainage m.
Tweed m.
twin m.
twirling m.
two-dye m.
two-inclinometer m.
two-microphone acoustic
  reflection m.
ultropaque m.
uncut Collis-Nissen
  fundoplication m.
unilateral inguinal hernia repair m.
u-score m.
Vecchietti m.
verbotonal m.
vertical condensation root canal
  filling m.
vertical-cut m.
Victor Gomel m.
visual m.
Vogel m.
volumetric m.
von Claus chronometric m.
von Kossa m.
V-slope m.
Wardill four-flap m.
Wardill-Kilner advancement flap m.
Wardrop m.
Warthin-Starry staining m.
Waterston m.
Watson m.
Watson-Crick m.
Weiss logarithmic m.
Welcker m.
Westergren sedimentation rate m.
Wheeler m.
Willett-Stampfer m.
Wilson-White m.
Winston-Lutz m.
Wintrobe and Landsberg m.
Wintrobe sedimentation rate m.
Wolfe m.

Woolf m.
Wroblewski m.
xenon m.
x-line m.
zeta sedimentation ratio m.
zinc-sulfate flotation m.
Methodist vascular suction tube
methohexital
m. sodium
methotrimeprazine hydrochloride
methoxamine hydrochloride
methoxyflurane
m. anesthesia
methyl
m. chloride
m. isopropyl ether anesthetic
m. methacrylate graft
methylation
methylchloroform
methylene
m. blue
m. blue dye
m. blue dye localization
methylhydroxymandelic acid (MOMA)
methylparaben free (MPF)
methylphenidate
cocaine m.
methyl-*tert*-butyl ether (MTBE)
metocurine
metopic
m. point
m. suture
metopion
metopoplasty
metoposcopy
metrectomy
metric ophthalmoscopy
metrofibroma
Metro I.V. injection
metromalacoma
metroperitoneal fistula
metroplasty
Strassman m.
metrotomy
Metubine Iodide
Metycaine
Metzer-Boyce method
Meuli arthroplasty
MEVA Probe for endovaginal scanning
Meyer
M. cartilages

M. incision
M. line
Meyerding
M. bone graft
M. method
M. spondylolisthesis classification line
Meyerding-Van Demark technique
Meyer-Schwickerath
M.-S. light coagulation
M.-S. operation
Meyers-McKeever classification of tibial fracture
Meyers quadratus muscle-pedicle bone graft
Meynert
M. decussation
M. retroflex bundle
Meyn reduction of elbow dislocation
MH
malignant hyperthermia
MHA-TP
microhemagglutination *Treponema pallidum*
MHA-TP test
Miami pouch
MIC
M. gastrostomy tube
M. jejunal tube
M. jejunostomy tube
micelle formation
Michaelson
M. counter pressure
M. operation
Michal
M. I, II procedure
M. II technique
Michel
M. anomaly
M. deformity
M. malformation
Mic-Key gastrostomy tube
Micro
M. FET isometric force dynamometer
microadenoma
pituitary m.
microadenomectomy
selective m.
microaerosol

M

NOTES

microamperage
    m. electrical nerve stimulation
    m. neural stimulation
microanastomosis
    laser-assisted m. (LAMA)
microaspiration
microatheroma
microbic dissociation
microbiliary inflammation
microbubble
microcalcification
microcavitation
microchromoendoscopy
microcirculation
    native myocardial m.
    pulp m.
microcolon
microcolpohysteroscopy
microcorneal
microcurrent therapy
microcystic disease of renal medulla
microdensitophotometric quantification
microdialysis
microdiffusion
microdiskectomy, microdiscectomy
    arthroscopic m.
    uniportal arthroscopic m.
microembolization
microfilament bundle
Microfuge tube
microgastria
microgenia
microgenitalism
microglioma
micrograms per kilogram per minute
microhamartoma
microhemagglutination *Treponema pallidum* (MHA-TP)
microincineration
microincision
microinjection
    m. method
microinvasive carcinoma classification
micro-Kjeldahl method
Microknit
    M. patch graft
    M. vascular graft
microlaryngeal endotracheal tube
microlaryngoscopy
    Thornell m.
Microlase transpupillary diode
micro liquid extraction
microlith
microlithiasis
microlumbar
    m. diskectomy
    m. disk excision

micromanipulation
    gamete m.
    oocyte m.
micrometastasis
    hematogenous m.
micromyelia
Micron bobbin ventilation tube
microneurography
    sympathetic m.
microneurolysis
microneurorrhaphy
microneurovascular anastomosis
micro-operative procedure
micro-organism
    Gram-negative m.-o.
    Gram-positive m.-o.
micropenis
microperforation
Microplate fixation
micropoint suture
microprolactinoma
microproliferation
micropuncture
microscopic
    m. epididymal sperm aspiration
    m. sphincter
microscopically controlled surgery
microscopy
    binocular m.
    cryoelectron m.
    dark-field m.
    electron m.
    fluorescence m.
    fundus m.
    immune electron m.
    immunofluorescence m.
    intravital m.
    light m.
    paraffin-section light m.
    polarization m.
    rotary shadowing electron m.
    scanning electron m.
    scanning force m.
    specular m.
    transmission electron m.
microspectrofluorometry
microspectroscopy
    Fourier transform infrared m.
microsphere
    radioactive m.
microstomia
microsurgery
    m. method
    m. procedure
    m. technique
    transanal endoscopic m. (TEM)
microsurgical
    m. diskectomy

m. epididymal sperm aspiration
m. epididymal sperm aspiration
  procedure
m. extraction of sperm from
  epididymis
m. inguinal varicocelectomy
m. tubocornual anastomosis
microsuture
microtia
microtransducer technique
micro-tubulotomy technique
microvascular
m. free flap
m. free flap transfer
m. surgical anastomosis
m. technique
Microvel double velour graft
microvillous membrane
microwave
m. coagulation
endoscopic m.
m. fixation
m. radiation injury
m. therapy
microwave-assisted streptavidin-biotin
  peroxidase method
microwelding
micrurgical
midabdominal transverse incision
midaxillary
m. line
m. line incision
midazolam
m. conscious sedation
m. HCl
m. hydrochloride
midazolam-induced excitatory reaction
midbrain reticular formation
midcarpal
m. arthroscopy
m. dislocation
midclavicular line
midcoronal plane
middle
m. axillary line
m. cardiac vein
m. cerebral artery
m. cervical cardiac nerve
m. cervical fascia
m. cervical ganglion
m. colic artery
m. colic lymph nodes

m. colic vein
m. collateral artery
m. constrictor muscle of pharynx
m. costotransverse ligament
m. cranial fossa
m. cranial fossa line
m. cuneiform bone
m. ear infection
m. extrahepatic bile duct
m. finger amputation
m. fossa approach
m. fossa exposure
m. fossa floor/petrous dissection
m. genicular artery
m. group of mesenteric lymph
  nodes
m. hemorrhoidal artery
m. hemorrhoidal plexuses
m. hemorrhoidal veins
m. hepatic veins
m. lobe branch
m. lobe of prostate
m. meatal antrostomy
m. mediastinum
m. meningeal artery
m. meningeal artery groove
m. meningeal branch of maxillary
  nerve
m. meningeal veins
m. palatine suture
m. palmar space
m. rectal artery
m. rectal lymph node
m. rectal node
m. rectal plexuses
m. rectal veins
m. sacral artery
m. sacral plexus
m. scalene muscle
m. supraclavicular nerve
m. suprarenal artery
m. temporal artery
m. temporal vein
m. thyroid vein
m. tibial shaft fracture
m. transverse rectal fold
m. trunk of brachial plexus
m. umbilical fold
m. umbilical ligament
midesophageal
midexpiratory/midinspiratory flow ratio

M

NOTES

midface
m. degloving technique
m. fracture
midfoot fracture
midforceps maneuver
midfrontal
m. plane
m. plane coronal section
midgastric transverse sphincter
midgut
m. volvulus with malrotation
midheel line
midhumeral line
midlateral approach
midline
m. disk herniation
m. exposure
m. forehead flap
m. lower abdominal incision
m. medial approach
m. myelotomy
m. oblique incision
m. position
m. spinal approach
m. upper abdominal incision
midmalleolar line
midoccipital
midpalatal suture opening
midpalmar space
midpapillary
anterior m. (AM)
lateral m.
m. longitudinal (MP-L)
septal m.
m. transverse (MP-T)
midpelvis
plane of m.
midpoint to meatal line
midriff
midsagittal
m. plane
m. section
midsection
midshaft fracture
midsigmoid sphincter
midsternal line
midsternum
midthalamic plane
midthigh amputation
MIGET
multiple inert gas elimination technique
migrating abscess
migration
m. abnormalities
calculus m.
cell m.
cellular m.
electrode m.

embolus m.
epithelial m.
gallstone m.
gastrostomy tube m.
graft m.
implant m.
instrument m.
intravesical m.
Luque rod m.
lymphocyte m.
metallic biliary stent m.
neural crest m.
neuronal m.
neutrophil m.
phagocyte m.
physiologic mesial m.
pigmentary m.
placental m.
rod m.
tooth m.
trochanteric m.
tube m.
mika operation
Mik gastrostomy tube
Mikulicz
M. colostomy
M. operation
M. pyloroplasty
Milch
M. classification of humeral fracture
M. condylar fracture classification
M. cuff resection of ulna technique
M. elbow fracture classification
M. elbow technique
mild chromic suture
Miles
M. abdominoperineal resection
M. operation
Milford mallet finger technique
miliary
m. abscess
m. aneurysm
m. granulomatous inflammation
military
m. brace position
m. tuck position
milk
m. ducts
m. gland
m. spots
milk-ejection reflex
milkmaid elbow dislocation
milkman fracture
milky ascites
Millard advancement rotation flap reconstruction

Millender arthroplasty
Millen-Read modification
Millen technique
mille pattes technique
Miller
    M. endotracheal tube
    M. flatfoot operation
    M. procedure
    M. tube
Miller-Abbott
    M.-A. double-lumen intestinal tube
    M.-A. intestinal tube
Miller-Galante knee arthroplasty
Millesi
    M. interfascicular graft
    M. modified technique
    M. nerve graft
millibar
milligram
milligram-hour
Milliknit graft
millimeters partial pressure
millimicrogram
Millin suction tube
milliosmole/kilogram
Millipore suture
Mill-Rose tube
milrinone
Milroy-Piper suction tube
Miltner-Wan calcaneus resection
mimetic muscles
mineral
    m. oil aspiration
    m. oil foreign body
mineralized tissue
Ming gastric carcinoma classification
miniature
    m. end-plate potential
    m. uterine cavity
minicholecystostomy
    surgical-radiologic m.
minification
minikeratoplasty
    Castroviejo m.
minilaparoscope cholecystectomy
minilaparotomy
minimal
    m. access general surgery
    m. air
    m. anesthetic concentration (MAC)
    m. bactericidal concentration
    m. leak technique

    m. transurethral resection of prostate
minimal-access
    m.-a. method
    m.-a. procedure
    m.-a. technique
minimal-change
    m.-c. disease
    m.-c. nephrotic syndrome
minimal-incision pubovaginal suspension
minimal-lesion nephrotic syndrome
minimally
    m. displaced fracture
    m. invasive biopsy
    m. invasive procedure
    m. invasive surgery
    m. invasive surgical technique
minimi
    extensor digiti m.
minimum
    m. alveolar anesthetic concentration (MAC)
    m. alveolar concentration (MAC)
    1-m. alveolar concentration (1-MAC)
    m. audible pressure
    m. bactericidal concentration
    m. detectable concentration
    m. effective analgesic concentration
    m. effective concentration (MEC)
    m. lethal concentration
    m. local analgesic concentration (MLAC)
minipilon fracture
Minkoff-Jaffe-Menendez posterior approach
Minkoff-Nicholas procedure
Minnesota
    M. EKG classification
    M. tube
Minocin I.V. injection
minor
    m. amputation
    m. calices
    m. duodenal papilla
    m. fissure
    justo m.
    m. operation
    m. sublingual ducts
    m. surgery
Minsky operation

M

NOTES

minute
>alveolar ventilation per m.
>micrograms per kilogram per m.
>physiological dead space ventilation
>>per m.
>m. polypoid lesion
>m. ventilation (V_E)
>m. volume

Miochol solution
Mirizzi syndrome
mirror
mirror-image
>m.-i. breast biopsy
>m.-i. interpretation
>m.-i. laryngoscopy
>m.-i. reflection

misarticulation
misdirection phenomenon
mismatch
>ventilation/perfusion m.

misoprostol protection
misregistration
>chemical shift m.
>flow m.
>oblique flow m.

missed fracture
missile injury
missionary position
mistranslation
Mital elbow release technique
Mitchell osteotomy
miter technique
mitomycin transarterial embolization
treatment
mitral
>m. balloon commissurotomy
>m. balloon valvotomy
>m. regurgitation murmur
>m. valve aneurysm
>m. valve annulus
>m. valve area
>m. valve closure index
>m. valve disorder
>m. valve gradient
>m. valve insufficiency
>m. valve leaflet
>m. valve prolapse syndrome
>m. valve replacement
>m. valve-transverse (MV-T)
>m. valve valvotomy
>m. valvuloplasty

mitralization
Mitran Oral
Mitrofanoff
>M. appendicovesicostomy
>M. conduit
>M. continent urinary diversion
>>technique

>M. principle
>M. procedure
>M. stoma

Mivacron
mivacurium
>m. chloride

mixed
>m. acid fermentation
>m. chancre
>m. connective-tissue disease
>m. connective tissue disorder
>m. fat-water density lesion
>m. nail infection
>m. nerve
>m. sclerotic and lytic bone lesion
>m. tumor of salivary gland
>m. venous-lymphatic malformation
>m. venous oxygen content
>m. venous oxygen saturation

mixed-density mass
mixillectomy
Mixter tube
mixture
>epinephrine-anesthetic m.
>Neo-Synephrine Cocaine m. 50:50
>racemic m.

Mize-Bucholz-Grogen approach
Mizuno-Hirohata-Kashiwagi technique
Mizuno technique
mks
>meter-kilogram-second

MLAC
>minimum local analgesic concentration

MLN
>mesenteric lymph node

MLR
>major liver resection

MMK
>Marshall-Marchetti-Krantz
>MMK procedure

MO
>mesio-occlusal
>MO cavity

Moberg
>M. advancement flap
>M. dowel graft
>M. key-pinch procedure

Moberg-Gedda
>M.-G. fracture
>M.-G. open reduction

mobility
>muscle tissue m.
>rotation m.
>translation m.

mobilization
>grade 1–5 m.
>grades of m.
>joint m.

lateral band m.
localized leukocyte m.
nonthrust m.
rectal m.
soft tissue m.
spinal joint m.
stapes m.
stem cell m.
m. test
m. with impulse
mobilize
Mobin-Uddin
M.-U. umbrella filter
M.-U. vena cava filter
MOD
mesio-occlusodistal
MOD cavity
model
corpectomy m.
guidance-cooperation m.
implant m.
mutual participation m.
Zimmerman-Brittin exchange m.
Model 810 axial closed-loop hydraulic mechanical testing
modeling-derivation
moderate hypothermia
moderator
m. band
modification
activator m.
Al-Ghorab m.
appliance m.
A-V nodal m.
Bloom-Raney m.
Bonfiglio m.
bracket m.
Burch m.
Burwell-Scott m. of Watson-Jones incision
C-D screw m.
Clark-Southwick-Odgen m.
Deller m.
Duncan-Lovell m.
environment m.
Fairbanks technique with Sever m.
fiber tip m.
Gesell test with Knobloch m.
glutathione m.
Gunderson-Sosin m.
Harriluque sublaminar wiring m.
interference m.

Jacobs locking-hook spinal rod instrumentation m.
Kelly-Kennedy m.
Kleinert m.
Losee m.
Mason-Likar limb lead m.
Millen-Read m.
Mullins m.
Muzsnai m.
Neer m.
Pereyra-Lebhertz m.
posttranslation m.
racemic m.
Raz m.
Rosch m.
Schoemaker m. of Billroth I
Seddon m.
Sequeira-Khanuja m.
Smith m.
Stauffer m.
Strickland m.
thiol m.
Van Herick m.
Youngwhich m.
modified
m. band lid method
m. Belsey fundoplication
m. Belsey fundoplication method
m. Belsey fundoplication procedure
m. Belsey fundoplication technique
m. brachial technique
m. Cantwell technique
m. Essed-Schroeder corporoplasty
m. flap operation
m. Gibson incision
m. Ham F-10 solution
m. Hassan open technique
m. Hoke-Miller flatfoot procedure
m. Irving-type tubal ligation
m. Kessler suture
m. Kessler-Tajima suture
m. method of Pugh
m. Minnesota tube
m. mold and surface replacement arthroplasty
m. Norfolk procedure
m. Pomeroy technique
m. radical hysterectomy
m. radical mastectomy
m. radical mastoidectomy
m. radical neck dissection
m. Raynaud phenomenon

M

NOTES

modified *(continued)*
m. Ritgen maneuver
m. Sacks-Vine push-pull technique
m. Seldinger method
m. Seldinger procedure
m. Scldinger technique
m. suction tube
m. Toupe method
m. Toupe procedure
m. Toupe technique
m. two-portal endoscopic carpal tunnel release
m. Van Lint anesthesia
m. Weber-Fergusson procedure
m. Whitehead hemorrhoidectomy
m. Wies procedure
m. Young urethroplasty

modiolus
m. labii

modulation
amplitude m.
antigenic m.
autonomic m.
biochemical m.
brightness m.
frequency m.
immune m.
obstruction-induced m.
pain m.
m. potential
pressure amplitude m.
sex steroid m.
specific m.

module
dialysate preparation m.

Modulock posterior spinal fixation
Moebius anomaly
Moe scoliosis technique
MOF
multiple organ failure

Mogensen procedure
Mohrenheim
M. fossa
M. space

Mohr syndrome
Mohs
M. fresh tissue chemosurgery technique
M. fresh-tissue technique
M. micrographic surgery
M. microsurgery technique
M. microsurgical resection

moist mucous membrane
moisture exchanger
molar
anchor m.
m. tooth fracture
m. tube

mold acetabular arthroplasty
molding
compression m.
m. of head
injection m.
polyethylene compression m.
tissue m.

molecular
m. external layer
m. lesion
m. mass
m. sieve

Molesworth-Campbell elbow approach
Molesworth osteotomy
verruca mollusciformis
Moloney line
Molteno
M. drainage
M. episcleral explant

MOMA
methylhydroxymandelic acid

Momberg tube
moment
activation m.
three-point bending m.

Monakow
M. bundle
M. tract

Mon-a-Therm
M.-a.-T. thermocouple
M.-a.-T. 6510 two-channel thermometer

Moncrieff operation
Mondini
M. anomaly
M. deformity
M. pulmonary arteriovenous malformation

Mondini-Alexander malformation
Monfort operation
monilial infection
monitor
Engstrom multigas m.

monitored
m. anesthesia care (MAC)
m. anesthesia care anesthetic technique
m. anesthesia control

monitoring
airway gas m.
anesthetic m.
anterior fontanel pressure m.
blood pressure m.
central venous pressure m.
depth of anesthesia m.
ECoG m.
electrophysiologic m.
epicardial m.

esophageal pH m.
evoked external urethral sphincter
  potential m.
external fetal m.
hemodynamic m.
intracranial pressure m.
intraoperative neurophysiologic m.
  (IOM)
intraoperative transcranial
  Doppler m.
neuromuscular blockade m.
outcome m.
posttetanic count m.
radiation m.
screw position perioperative m.
m. technique
tissue pH m.
transcutaneous oxygen m.
two-dimensional m.
vigilance m.
water vapor m.
monoamine reuptake-inhibitor
monochromatic aberration
Monocryl poliglecaprone suture
monocular
  m. fixation
  m. patch
monodermoma
monodisperse
monofilament
  m. absorbable suture
  m. clear suture
  m. green suture
  m. nylon suture
  m. polypropylene suture
  m. skin suture
  m. steel suture
  m. wire fixation
  m. wire suture
monofixation syndrome
monoinfection
Monolyth oxygenator
monomalleolar ankle fracture
mononuclear cell infiltration
monopolar
  m. coagulation
  m. electrocoagulation
monorchidic
monorchidism
monorecidive chancre
Monosof suture

**monospherical total shoulder
  arthroplasty**
monotypic lesion
monoxide
  carbon m. (CO)
  dinitrogen m.
Monro line
Monro-Richter line
mons, pl. **montes**
  m. plasty
  m. pubis
Monsel solution
Montando tube
Monte
  M. Carlo multiway sensitivity
    analysis method
  M. Carlo simulation
  M. Carlo stimulation
Montefiore tracheal tube
Monteggia
  M. dislocation
  M. equivalent lesion
  M. forearm fracture
Montercaux fracture
montes (*pl. of* mons)
Montgomery
  M. esophageal tube
  M. glands
  M. salivary bypass tube
  M. tracheal tube
  M. tracheostomy
Monticelli-Spinelli distraction technique
Moore
  M. fracture
  M. method
  M. osteotomy-osteoclasis
  M. posterior approach
  M. procedure
  M. technique
  M. tibial plateau fracture
    classification
Moran-Karaya ring
Moran operation
Morax
  M. keratoplasty
  M. operation
morbidity
  m. and mortality
morcel
morcellation
  m. operation
  Robinson m.

M

NOTES

morcellation *(continued)*
    Robinson-Chung-Farahvar m.
    Robinson-Chung-Farahvar
     clavicular m.
    m. technique
morcellement
Morch swivel tracheostomy tube
Moreland-Marder-Anspach femoral stem
  removal
Morel-Fatio-Lalardie operation
Morel-Lavele lesion
Moretz Tiny Tytan ventilation tube
Morgagni
    M. cartilage
    M. caruncle
    M. columns
    M. crypts
    M. foramen
    M. fossa
    M. fovea
    M. frenum
    M. hernia
    M. lacuna
    M. retinaculum
    M. sinus
    M. tubercle
    M. ventricle
Morgan-Casscells meniscus suturing
  technique
Morganella
    M. morganii
Morgan line
moribund
Morison
    M. incision
    M. method
    M. pouch
morning glory optic disk anomaly
morphallactic regeneration
morphea-like lesion
morphine
    m. narcotic analgesic therapy
    m. sulfate
morphologic classification
morphology
    endometrial m.
    Gram-stain m.
    lesion m.
Morrey-Bryan total elbow arthroplasty
Morrison
    M. neurovascular free flap
    M. technique
Morse
    M. head
    M. suction tube
Morse-Andrews suction tube
Morse-Ferguson suction tube

mortality
    morbidity and m.
mortar kidney
mortification
Morton plane
Moschcowitz procedure
Mose technique
Mosher
    M. intubation tube
    M. Life Saver antichoke suction
     device
    M. life-saving suction tube
    M. life-saving tracheal tube
    M. operation
Mosher-Toti operation
900 mOsmolar amino acid-glucose
  solution
Moss
    M. classification
    M. gastrostomy tube
    M. Mark IV tube
    M. operation
    M. Suction Buster tube
Motais operation
moth-eaten bone destruction
mother method
moth patch
motility
    contractile m.
motion
    angulation m.
    m. barrier
    hip extension range of m.
    limitation of joint m.
    osteokinematic m.
    pattern of m.
    range of m. (ROM)
    translation m.
motion-preserving procedure
motivating operation
motor
    m. decussation
    m. examination
    m. fusion
    m. nerve
    m. nerve of face
    m. oil peritoneal fluid
    m. perseveration
    m. point
    m. point block
    m. point block anesthetic technique
motor-evoked
    m.-e. potential (MEP)
    m.-e. response (MER)
    m.-e. response to transcranial
     stimulation (tc-MER)
Mott body
Mouchet fracture

Mould arthroplasty
Moulton lacrimal duct tube
mounted point stone
mouse
    joint m.
    peritoneal m.
Mousseau-Barbin
    M.-B. esophageal tube
    M.-B. prosthetic tube
mouth
    levator muscle of angle of m.
    m. mask
    m. preparation
mouth-to-mouth
    m.-t.-m. respiration
    m.-t.-m. resuscitation
    m.-t.-m. ventilation
movable
    m. joint
    m. kidney
    m. spleen
    m. testis
Movat pentachrome method
movement
    anterosuperior external ilium m.
    border tissue m.
    bowel m.
    dissociation m.
    external ilium m.
    extraneous m.
    extraocular m.'s
    fetal body m.
    head m.
    lateropulsion of body m.
    limitation of m.
    posteroinferior external m.
    primary rotation m.
    segmentation m.
    sound-stimulated fetal m.
moxisylyte injection
MPD
    main pancreatic duct
MPF
    methylparaben free
    MPF labeling
MPGR
    multiple planar gradient-recalled
    MPGR technique
MP-L
    midpapillary longitudinal
    MP-L image

MP-RAGE
    magnetization prepared-rapid gradient echo
    magnitude preparation-rapid acquisition gradient echo
    MP-RAGE technique
M-Prednisol injection
MP-T
    midpapillary transverse
    MP-T image
MR spectroscopy
MSB
    mediastinal shed blood
MS Contin Oral
MSI
    magnetic source imaging
    MSI nylon membrane
MSIR Oral
MTBE
    methyl-*tert*-butyl ether
    MTBE therapy
Mubarak-Hargens decompression technique
mucilaginous gland
mucinous ascites
muciparous gland
mucobuccal
    m. fold
    m. reflection
mucocele
    appendix m.
    breast m.
    frontal sinus m.
    frontoethmoidal m.
    m. of gallbladder
    maxillary sinus m.
    orbital m.
    paranasal m.
    retention m.
    sinus m.
    sphenoid m.
mucocutaneous
    m. lesion
    m. lymph node syndrome
    m. manifestation
    m. muscle
    m. pigmentation of Peutz-Jeghers syndrome
mucogingival
    m. line
    m. surgery
mucoid ascites

M

NOTES

457

mucolytic-antifoam solution
mucoperichondrial flap
mucoperiosteal
    m. periodontal flap
    m. periodontal graft
    m. sliding flap
mucopurulent exudate
mucopyelocele
mucopyocele
mucor infection
mucosa
    biopsy of gastric m.
    m. of colon
    m. of ductus deferens
    ectopic gastric m.
    endocervical m.
    m. of gallbladder
    gastric m.
    inlet patch m.
    lingual m.
    multifocal ectopic gastric m.
    pharyngeal m.
    m. of seminal vesicle
    m. of small intestine
    ulceration of oral m.
    upper respiratory tract m.
    m. of ureter
    m. of urinary bladder
    m. of uterine tube
mucosa-associated lymphoid tissue
mucosal
    m. barrier
    m. biopsy
    m. destruction
    m. esophageal ring
    m. folds of gallbladder
    m. inflammation
    m. lesion
    m. line
    m. needle aspiration
    m. neuroma syndrome
    m. patch replacement
    m. periodontal flap
    m. periodontal graft
    m. proctectomy
    m. relaxing incision technique
    m. remnant
    m. tunics
    m. ulceration
    m. vascular dilation
    m. web
mucosa-to-mucosa anastomosis
mucosectomy
    endoanal m.
    hand-sewn ileoanal anastomosis
      with m.
    rectal m.

    stapled ileoanal anastomosis
      without m.
    transabdominal m.
    transanal m.
mucositis
    radiation m.
mucous
    m. desiccation
    m. fistula
    m. gland
    m. membrane graft
    m. membrane lesion
    m. membrane of lip
    m. membranes
    m. membrane of tongue
    m. membrane ulceration
    m. patch
    m. plug syndrome
    m. sheath of tendon
mucro
    m. sterni
mucronate
mucus
    excess m.
    oyster mass of m.
mud bed
Muehrcke line
Mueller
    M. femoral supracondylar fracture
      classification
    M. hip arthroplasty
    M. intertochanteric varus osteotomy
    M. maneuver
    M. method
    M. operation
    M. patellar tendon graft
    M. suction tube
    M. technique
    M. tibial fracture classification
    M. transposition osteotomy
Mueller-Frazier suction tube
Mueller-Pool suction tube
Mueller-Pynchon suction tube
Mueller-type femoral head replacement
Mueller-Walle method
Mueller-Yankauer suction tube
Muerhrcke line
MUGA
    multigated angiogram
      MUGA exercise stress test
mulberry
    m. calculus
    m. lesion
mulberry-shaped mass
Muldoon tube
Mules
    M. graft
    M. operation

Mulholland sphincterotomy
Müller
- M. capsule
- M. duct
- M. duct body
- M. maneuver

Müller-Hillis maneuver
müllerian
- m. duct anomaly
- m. duct derivation syndrome
- m. duct fusion
- m. inhibiting substance

Mullins
- M. blade technique
- M. modification

multangular
- m. bone
- m. ridge fracture

multiaxial
- m. classification
- m. joint

multidose vial
multifetal pregnancy reduction
multifetation
multifidus muscle
multifilament steel suture
multifocal
- m. ectopic gastric mucosa
- m. enhancing lesion
- m. inflammation

multigated angiogram (MUGA)
multi-infection
multilamellar body
multilevel
- m. fracture
- m. laminectomy

multilocular cystic lesion
multiloculated renal mass
multimerization
multimodal
- m. adjuvant therapy
- m. analgesia

multimodality therapy
multiorgan
- m. hernia
- m. system failure

multiparameter sensor
multiple
- m. cancellous chip graft
- m. cone root canal filling method
- m. core biopsy
- m. endocrine neoplasia syndrome

- m. endocrinopathy
- m. exostoses
- m. fracture
- m. hamartoma syndrome
- m. hepatitis virus infection
- m. inert gas elimination technique (MIGET)
- m. inert gas exchange
- m. line scan imaging
- m. loop wiring
- MAC m.'s
- m. mechanism inhaled anesthetic
- m. mucosal neuroma syndrome
- m. myeloma staging
- m. neuroma syndrome
- m. organ failure (MOF)
- m. planar gradient-recalled (MPGR)
- m. plane imaging
- m. pterygium syndrome
- m. ray amputation
- m. sensitive point
- m. shunt levels
- m. site
- m. site inhaled anesthetic
- m. spin-echo imaging
- m. system atrophy
- m. system organ failure
- m. therapy

multiple-balloon valvuloplasty
multiple-echo imaging
multiple-point sacral fixation
multiple-port
- m.-p. incisions
- m.-p. incisions method
- m.-p. incisions procedure
- m.-p. incisions technique

multiple-punch resection
multipolar
- m. coagulation
- m. electrocoagulation

Multipulse 1000 compression pump
multipurpose breathing circuit
multiray fracture
multistaged carrier flap
Multistage Maximal Effort exercise stress test
multistrand suture
multivessel PTCA
Muma Assessment Program
Mumford
- M. procedure
- M. resection

NOTES

Mumford-Gurd arthroplasty
mummification
 m. necrosis
 pulp m.
Munro
 M. and Parker classification for
 laparoscopic hysterectomy
 M. point
Munro-Kerr maneuver
Muraco vaporizer
Mu receptor
murine
 m. graft
 m. mesangial cell line
 M. solution
murmur
 aortic regurgitation m.
 diamond ejection m.
 ejection m.
 endocardial m.
 exit block m.
 exocardial m.
 expiratory m.
 extracardiac m.
 left ventricular-right atrial
 communication m.
 mitral regurgitation m.
 reduplication m.
 systolic ejection m.
Murocel Ophthalmic solution
Murphy method
muscarinic
 m. agonist
 m. receptor
muscimol
muscle
 m.'s of abdomen
 abdominal external oblique m.
 abdominal internal oblique m.
 abductor digiti minimi m. of foot
 abductor digiti minimi m. of hand
 abductor m. of great toe
 abductor hallucis m.
 abductor m. of little finger
 abductor m. of little toe
 abductor pollicis brevis m.
 abductor pollicis longus m.
 accessory flexor m. of foot
 Aeby m.
 airway smooth m. (ASM)
 Albinus m.
 anconeus m.
 antagonistic m.'s
 anterior auricular m.
 anterior cervical
 intertransversarii m.'s
 anterior cervical intertransverse m.'s
 anterior rectus m. of head

anterior scalene m.
anterior serratus m.
anterior tibial m.
antigravity m.'s
antitragicus m.
m. of antitragus
appendicular m.
arrector pili m.
articular m. of elbow
articularis cubiti m.
articularis genu m.
articular m. of knee
aryepiglottic m.
axial m.
m.'s of the back
Bell m.
m. biopsy
bipennate m.
Bovero m.
brachial m.
brachialis m.
brachioradial m.
brachioradialis m.
branchiomeric m.'s
Braune m.
broadest m. of back
bronchoesophageal m.
buccinator m.
bulbocavernosus m.
Casser perforated m.
ceratocricoid m.
cervical iliocostal m.
cervical interspinal m.
cervical interspinales m.'s
cervical longissimus m.
cervical rotator m.'s
cheek m.
chin m.
chondroglossus m.
coccygeal m.
coccygeus m.
m.'s of coccyx
Coiter m.
compressor m. of lips
coracobrachial m.
coracobrachialis m.
corrugator cutis m. of anus
corrugator supercilii m.
cowl m.
cremaster m.
cricopharyngeus m.
cricothyroid m.
cruciate m.
cutaneomucous m.
cutaneous m.
dartos m.
deep m.'s of back

deep layer of levator palpebrae
  superioris m.
deep transverse perineal m.
deep transverse m. of perineum
deltoid m.
depressor anguli oris m.
depressor m. of epiglottis
depressor m. of eyebrow
depressor labii inferioris m.
depressor m. of lower lip
depressor septi m.
depressor m. of septum
depressor supercilii m.
detrusor m. of urinary bladder
digastric m.
dilator m. of ileocecal sphincter
dilator naris m.
dilator m. of pylorus
m. dissection
dorsal interosseous m.'s of foot
dorsal interosseous m.'s of hand
dorsal sacrococcygeal m.
dorsal sacrococcygeus m.
Duverney m.
m. dystonia
elevator m.
elevator m. of anus
elevator m. of prostate
elevator m. of rib
elevator m. of scapula
elevator m. of soft palate
elevator m. of thyroid gland
elevator m. of upper eyelid
elevator m. of upper lip
elevator m. of upper lip and wing
  of nose
m. energy technique
epicranial m.
epicranius m.
erector spinae m.'s
erector m. of spine
extensor carpi radialis brevis m.
extensor carpi radialis longus m.
extensor carpi ulnaris m.
extensor comminicus m.
extensor digiti minimi m.
extensor digiti quinti m.
extensor digitorum brevis m.
extensor digitorum communis m.
extensor digitorum longus m.
extensor hallucis brevis m.
extensor hallucis longus m.

extensor indicis proprius m.
extensor pollicis brevis m.
extensor pollicis longus m.
external anal sphincter m.
external intercostal m.'s
external intercostal m.
external oblique m.
external obturator m.
external pterygoid m.
external sphincter m. of anus
extraocular m.'s
extrinsic m.'s
m.'s of eyeball
facial m.'s
m.'s of facial expression
femoral m.
fixator m.
m. flap
frontalis m.
Gavard m.
genioglossal m.
genioglossus m.
geniohyoid m.
gluteus maximus m.
greater posterior rectus m. of head
greater psoas m.
greater rhomboid m.
greater zygomatic m.
Guthrie m.
hamstring m.'s
m.'s of head
helicis major m.
helicis minor m.
m. hernia
Horner m.
Houston m.
hyoglossal m.
hyoglossus m.
iliac m.
iliacus minor m.
iliococcygeal m.
iliococcygeus m.
iliocostal m.
iliocostalis m.
iliocostalis cervicis m.
iliocostalis lumborum m.
iliocostalis thoracis m.
iliopsoas m.
inferior constrictor m. of pharynx
inferior longitudinal m. of tongue
inferior oblique extraocular m.
inferior oblique m. of head

NOTES

M

muscle *(continued)*

inferior posterior serratus m.
inferior rectus extraocular m.
infrahyoid m.'s
innermost intercostal m.
intercostalis externus m.
intermediate great m.
intermediate vastus m.
internal intercostal m.
internal oblique m.
internal pterygoid m.
internal sphincter m. of anus
interosseous m.'s
interspinal m.'s
interspinales m.'s
intertransversarii m.'s
intertransverse m.'s
intrinsic m.'s
ischiocavernous m.
Jung m.
Klein m.
Kohlrausch m.
Krause m.
large m. of helix
m.'s of larynx
lateral great m.
lateral lumbar intertransversarii m.'s
lateral lumbar intertransverse m.'s
lateral pterygoid m.
lateral rectus extraocular m.
lateral rectus m. of the head
lateral vastus m.
latissimus dorsi m.
lesser rhomboid m.
lesser zygomatic m.
levator anguli oris m.
levator ani m.
levator costae m.
levatores costarum m.'s
levator glandulae thyroidea m.
levator labii superioris alaeque
  nasi m.
levator palati m.
levator palpebrae superioris m.
levator prostatae m.
levator scapulae m.
levator m. of thyroid gland
levator trochlear m.
levator veli palatini m.
long abductor m. of thumb
long adductor m.
long m. of head
longissimus capitis m.
longissimus cervicis m.
longissimus thoracis m.
long levatores costarum m.'s
long m. of neck
long palmar m.

longus capitis m.
longus colli m.
lumbar iliocostal m.
lumbar interspinal m.
lumbar interspinales m.'s
lumbar quadrate m.
lumbar rotator m.'s
lumbrical m. of foot
lumbrical m. of hand
Marcacci m.
mastication m.
m.'s of mastication
m. measurement
medial great m.
medial lumbar
  intertransversarii m.'s
medial lumbar intertransverse m.'s
medial pterygoid m.
medial vastus m.
mentalis m.
Merkel m.
middle constrictor m. of pharynx
middle scalene m.
mimetic m.'s
mucocutaneous m.
multifidus m.
mylohyoid m.
nasal m.
nasalis m.
m.'s of neck
m. of notch of helix
oblique arytenoid m.
oblique auricular m.
obliquus abdominis externus m.
obliquus capitis inferior m.
obliquus capitis superior m.
obturator externus m.
obturator internus m.
occipitalis m.
occipitofrontal m.
occipitofrontalis m.
ocular m.'s
omohyoid m.
orbicular m. of eye
orbicularis oculi m.
orbicularis oris m.
orbicular m. of mouth
orbital m.
orbitalis m.
palatouvularis m.
pectorodorsal m.
pectorodorsalis m.
m. pedicle bone graft
pennate m.
perineal m.'s
peroneal m.
peroneus brevis m.
peroneus longus m.

peroneus tertius m.
piriform m.
piriformis m.
plantar interosseous m.
plantaris m.
plantar quadrate m.
platysma m.
pleuroesophageal m.
popliteal m.
popliteus m.
posterior auricular m.
posterior cervical
  intertransversarii m.'s
posterior cervical
  intertransverse m.'s
posterior cricoarytenoid m.
posterior scalene m.
procerus m.
pronator quadratus m.
pronator teres m.
psoas major m.
psoas minor m.
pubococcygeal m.
pubococcygeus m.
puboprostatic m.
puborectal m.
puborectalis m.
pubovaginal m.
pubovaginalis m.
pubovesical m.
pubovesicalis m.
pyramidal m. of auricle
pyramidal auricular m.
pyramidalis m.
quadrate m.
quadrate m. of loins
quadrate m. of thigh
quadrate m. of upper lip
quadratus femoris m.
quadratus lumborum m.
quadratus plantae m.
quadriceps femoris m.
quadriceps m. of thigh
radial dilator m.
radial flexor m. of wrist
rectococcygeal m.
rectococcygeus m.
rectourethral m.
rectourethralis m.
rectouterine m.
rectovesical m.
rectovesicalis m.

rectus m. of abdomen
rectus abdominis m.
rectus capitis anterior m.
rectus capitis lateralis m.
rectus capitis posterior major m.
rectus capitis posterior minor m.
rectus femoris m.
rectus m. of thigh
red m.
Reisseisen m.'s
m. relaxant
m. repositioning
m. resection
resection of m.
rhomboideus major m.
rhomboid minor m.
ribbon m.'s
Riolan m.
risorius m.
rotator cuff m.
rotatores cervicis m.'s
rotatores lumborum m.'s
rotatores thoracis m.'s
salpingopharyngeal m.
scalenus anterior m.
scalenus medius m.
scalenus minimus m.
scalenus posterior m.
scalp m.
Sebileau m.
second tibial m.
semimembranosus m.
semispinal m.
semispinal m. of head
semispinalis capitis m.
semispinalis cervicis m.
semispinalis thoracis m.
semispinal m. of neck
semispinal m. of thorax
semitendinosus m.
serratus anterior m.
serratus posterior inferior m.
serratus posterior superior m.
shunt m.
Sibson m.
skeletal m.
m. sliding operation
smaller m. of helix
smaller posterior rectus m. of head
smaller psoas m.
smallest scalene m.
smooth m.

NOTES

M

muscle *(continued)*

Soemmerring m.
sphincter m.
sphincter m. of common bile duct
sphincter m. of pancreatic duct
sphincter m. of pylorus
sphincter m. of urethra
sphincter m. of urinary bladder
spinal m.
spinal m. of head
spinalis capitis m.
spinalis cervicis m.
spinalis thoracis m.
spinal m. of neck
spinal m. of thorax
splenius capitis m.
splenius cervicis m.
splenius m. of head
splenius m. of neck
sternal m.
sternalis m.
sternochondroscapular m.
sternoclavicular m.
sternocleidomastoid m.
sternocostalis m.
sternohyoid m.
sternomastoid m.
sternothyroid m.
strap m.'s
striated m.
styloauricular m.
styloglossus m.
stylohyoid m.
stylopharyngeal m.
stylopharyngeus m.
subclavian m.
subclavius m.
subcostal m.
suboccipital m.'s
subscapular m.
subscapularis m.
superficial back m.'s
superficial lingual m.
superficial transverse perineal m.
superficial transverse m. of
  perineum
superior constrictor m. of pharynx
superior longitudinal m. of tongue
superior oblique extraocular m.
superior oblique m. of head
superior posterior serratus m.
superior rectus extraocular m.
supinator m.
supraclavicular m.
suprahyoid m.'s
supraspinalis m.
supraspinatus m.
supraspinous m.

suspensory m. of duodenum
synergistic m.'s
temporal m.
temporalis m.
temporoparietal m.
temporoparietalis m.
tensor fascia lata m.
tensor m. of fascia lata
tensor m. of soft palate
tensor tarsi m.
tensor veli palati m.
teres major m.
Theile m.
thoracic interspinal m.
thoracic interspinales m.'s
thoracic intertransversarii m.'s
thoracic intertransverse m.'s
thoracic longissimus m.
thoracic rotator m.'s
m.'s of thorax
thyroarytenoid m.
thyroepiglottic m.
thyrohyoid m.
m. tissue mobility
Tod m.
toe extensor m.
m.'s of tongue
Toynbee m.
trachealis m.
tracheloclavicular m.
tragicus m.
m. of tragus
transverse m. of abdomen
transverse arytenoid m.
transverse m. of auricle
transverse m. of chin
transverse m. of nape
transverse rectus abdominis m.
  (TRAM)
transverse m. of thorax
transverse m. of tongue
transversospinal m.
transversospinalis m.
transversus abdominis m.
transversus menti m.
transversus nuchae m.
transversus thoracis m.
Treitz m.
triangular m.
true m.'s of back
two-bellied m.
unipennate m.
unstriated m.
m. of uvula
uvular m.
Valsalva m.
ventral sacrococcygeus m.
vertical m. of tongue

vestigial m.
visceral m.
vocal m.
vocalis m.
white m.
Wilson m.
wrinkler m. of eyebrow
zygomaticus major m.
zygomaticus minor m.

muscle-balancing procedure
muscle-periosteal flap
muscle-plasty
Speed V-Y m.-p.
muscle-sparing thoracotomy
muscle-splitting
m.-s. incision
m.-s. technique
muscle-tendon transplantation
muscular
m. anesthesia
m. artery
m. coat of bronchi
m. coat of colon
m. coat of ductus deferens
m. coat of esophagus
m. coat of female urethra
m. coat of gallbladder
m. coat of pharynx
m. coat of rectum
m. coat of small intestine
m. coat of stomach
m. coat of trachea
m. coat of ureter
m. coat of urinary bladder
m. coat of uterine tube
m. coat of uterus
m. coat of vagina
m. esophageal ring
m. fascia of extraocular muscle
m. graft
m. pulley
m. substance of prostate
m. tissue
m. triangle
m. tunic of gallbladder
m. tunics
muscularis
m. mucosae
m. tunnel closure
musculature
left erector spinae m.
right erector spinae m.

musculi (*pl. of* musculus)
musculoaponeurotic
musculocutaneous
m. free flap
m. nerve
m. nerve of leg
musculomembranous
musculophrenic
m. artery
m. veins
musculoplasty
Rambo m.
musculoskeletal
m. infection
m. tumor
musculospiral
m. groove
m. nerve
musculotendinous
m. flap
musculotubal canal
musculus, pl. musculi
musculi abdominis
m. abductor digiti minimi manus
m. abductor hallucis
m. abductor pollicis brevis
m. anconeus
m. antitragicus
m. articularis
m. articularis cubiti
m. articularis genus
m. aryepiglotticus
m. arytenoideus obliquus
m. arytenoideus transversus
m. aryvocalis
m. attollens aurem
m. attrahens aurem
m. auricularis anterior
m. auricularis posterior
m. auricularis superior
m. azygos uvulae
m. biceps brachii
m. biceps femoris
m. bipennatus
m. biventer mandibulae
m. brachialis
m. brachioradialis
m. bronchoesophageus
m. buccinator
m. buccopharyngeus
musculi bulbi
m. bulbocavernosus

M

NOTES

musculus *(continued)*
  m. bulbospongiosus
  m. caninus
  musculi capitis
  m. cephalopharyngeus
  m. ceratocricoideus
  m. ceratopharyngeus
  m. cervicalis ascendens
  m. chondroglossus
  m. chondropharyngeus
  m. cleidoepitrochlearis
  m. cleidomastoideus
  m. cleido-occipitalis
  musculi coccygei
  m. coccygeus
  musculi colli
  m. complexus
  m. complexus minor
  m. compressor naris
  m. compressor urethrae
  m. constrictor pharyngis inferior
  m. constrictor pharyngis medius
  m. constrictor pharyngis superior
  m. constrictor urethrae
  m. coracobrachialis
  m. corrugator cutis ani
  m. corrugator supercilii
  m. cremaster
  m. cricoarytenoideus lateralis
  m. cricoarytenoideus posterior
  m. cricopharyngeus
  m. cricothyroideus
  m. cruciatus
  m. cutaneomucosus
  m. cutaneus
  m. deltoideus
  m. depressor anguli oris
  m. depressor labii inferioris
  m. depressor septi
  m. depressor supercilii
  m. detrusor urinae
  m. diaphragma
  m. digastricus
  m. dilatator
  m. dilator
  m. dilator naris
  m. dilator pupilla
  m. dilator pylori gastroduodenalis
  m. dilator pylori ilealis
  musculi dorsi
  m. ejaculator seminis
  m. epicranius
  m. erector clitoridis
  m. erector penis
  m. erector spinae
  extensor indicis proprius m.
  musculi faciales
  m. frontalis

  m. genioglossus
  m. geniohyoglossus
  m. geniohyoideus
  m. glossopharyngeus
  m. helicis major
  m. helicis minor
  m. hyoglossus
  m. hypopharyngeus
  m. iliacus
  m. iliacus minor
  m. iliocapsularis
  m. iliococcygeus
  m. iliocostalis
  m. iliocostalis cervicis
  m. iliocostalis dorsi
  m. iliocostalis lumborum
  m. iliocostalis thoracis
  m. iliopsoas
  m. incisivus labii inferioris
  m. incisivus labii superioris
  m. incisurae helicis
  m. infracostalis
  musculi infrahyoidei
  m. infraspinatus
  m. intercostales externi
  m. intercostalis internus
  m. intercostalis intimus
  musculi interossei
  musculi interossei dorsalis manus
  musculi interossei dorsalis pedis
  m. interosseus palmaris
  m. interosseus plantaris
  m. interosseus volaris
  musculi interspinales
  m. interspinalis cervicis
  m. interspinalis lumborum
  m. interspinalis thoracis
  m. intertragicus
  musculi intertransversarii
  musculi intertransversarii anteriores
    cervicis
  musculi intertransversarii laterales
    lumborum
  musculi intertransversarii mediales
    lumborum
  musculi intertransversarii posteriores
    cervicis
  musculi intertransversarii thoracis
  m. ischiocavernosus
  m. ischiococcygeus
  m. keratopharyngeus
  musculi laryngis
  m. laryngopharyngeus
  m. latissimus dorsi
  m. levator alae nasi
  m. levator anguli oris
  m. levator anguli scapulae
  m. levator ani

m. levator costae
musculi levatores costarum
musculi levatores costarum breves
musculi levatores costarum longi
m. levator glandulae thyroideae
m. levator labii inferioris
m. levator labii superioris
m. levator labii superioris alaeque nasi
m. levator palati
m. levator palpebrae superioris
m. levator prostatae
m. levator scapulae
m. levator veli palatini
musculi linguae
m. longissimus
m. longissimus capitis
m. longissimus cervicis
m. longissimus dorsi
m. longissimus thoracis
m. longus capitis
m. longus colli
m. lumbricalis manus
m. lumbricalis pedis
m. masseter
m. mentalis
m. multifidus
m. multifidus spinae
m. mylohyoideus
m. mylopharyngeus
m. nasalis
m. obliquus auriculae
m. obliquus capitis inferior
m. obliquus capitis superior
m. obliquus externus abdominis
m. obliquus inferior
m. obliquus internus abdominis
m. obliquus superior
m. obturator externus
m. obturator internus
m. occipitalis
m. occipitofrontalis
m. omohyoideus
m. orbicularis oculi
m. orbicularis oris
m. orbicularis palpebrarum
m. orbitalis
m. orbitopalpebralis
musculi ossiculorum auditus
m. palatosalpingeus
m. palatostaphylinus
m. palmaris brevis

m. palmaris longus
musculi perinei
m. petropharyngeus
m. petrostaphylinus
m. piriformis
m. plantaris
m. platysma
m. platysma myoides
m. pleuroesophageus
m. popliteus
m. procerus
m. prostaticus
m. psoas major
m. psoas minor
m. pterygoideus externus
m. pterygoideus internus
m. pterygoideus lateralis
m. pterygoideus medialis
m. pterygopharyngeus
m. pterygospinosus
m. pubococcygeus
m. puboprostaticus
m. puborectalis
m. pubovaginalis
m. pubovesicalis
m. pyramidalis
m. pyramidalis auriculae
m. pyramidalis nasi
m. pyriformis
m. quadratus
m. quadratus femoris
m. quadratus labii inferioris
m. quadratus labii superioris
m. quadratus lumborum
m. quadratus menti
m. quadratus plantae
m. quadriceps extensor femoris
m. quadriceps femoris
m. rectococcygeus
m. rectourethralis
m. rectouterinus
m. rectovesicalis
m. rectus abdominis
m. rectus capitis anterior
m. rectus capitis anticus major
m. rectus capitis anticus minor
m. rectus capitis lateralis
m. rectus capitis posterior major
m. rectus capitis posterior minor
m. rectus capitis posticus major
m. rectus capitis posticus minor
m. rectus externus

NOTES

M

musculus *(continued)*
m. rectus femoris
m. rectus inferior
m. rectus internus
m. rectus lateralis
m. rectus medialis
m. rectus superior
m. rectus thoracis
m. retrahens aurem
m. rhomboatloideus
m. rhomboideus major
m. rhomboideus minor
m. risorius
musculi rotatores
musculi rotatores cervicis
musculi rotatores lumborum
musculi rotatores thoracis
m. sacrococcygeus anterior
m. sacrococcygeus dorsalis
m. sacrococcygeus posterior
m. sacrococcygeus ventralis
m. sacrolumbalis
m. sacrospinalis
m. salpingopharyngeus
m. scalenus anterior
m. scalenus anticus
m. scalenus medius
m. scalenus minimus
m. scalenus posterior
m. scalenus posticus
m. semimembranosus
m. semispinalis
m. semispinalis capitis
m. semispinalis cervicis
m. semispinalis colli
m. semispinalis dorsi
m. semispinalis thoracis
m. serratus anterior
m. serratus magnus
m. serratus posterior inferior
m. serratus posterior superior
m. skeleti
m. sphenosalpingostaphylinus
m. sphincter
m. sphincter ampullae
   hepatopancreaticae
m. sphincter ani externus
m. sphincter ani internus
m. sphincter ductus choledochi
m. sphincter ductus pancreatici
m. sphincter oris
m. sphincter pylori
m. sphincter urethrae
m. sphincter urethrae membranaceae
m. sphincter vaginae
m. sphincter vesicae
m. spinalis
m. spinalis capitis

m. spinalis cervicis
m. spinalis colli
m. spinalis dorsi
m. spinalis thoracis
m. splenius capitis
m. splenius cervicis
m. splenius colli
m. sternalis
m. sternochondroscapularis
m. sternoclavicularis
m. sternocleidomastoideus
m. sternofascialis
m. sternohyoideus
m. sternothyroideus
m. styloauricularis
m. styloglossus
m. stylohyoideus
m. stylolaryngeus
m. stylopharyngeus
m. subclavius
m. subcostalis
musculi suboccipitales
m. subscapularis
m. supinator radii brevis
m. supraclavicularis
musculi suprahyoidei
m. supraspinalis
m. supraspinatus
m. suspensorius duodeni
m. temporalis
m. temporoparietalis
m. tensor fasciae latae
m. tensor palati
m. tensor tympani
m. tensor veli palatini
m. teres major
m. teres minor
m. tetragonus
musculi thoracis
m. thyroarytenoideus
m. thyroarytenoideus externus
m. thyroarytenoideus internus
m. thyroepiglotticus
m. thyrohyoideus
m. tibialis anterior
m. tibialis anticus
m. tibialis gracilis
m. tibialis posterior
m. trachealis
m. tracheloclavicularis
m. trachelomastoideus
m. tragicus
m. transversalis abdominis
m. transversalis capitis
m. transversalis cervicis
m. transversalis nasi
m. transversospinalis
m. transversus abdominis

m. transversus auriculae
m. transversus linguae
m. transversus menti
m. transversus nuchae
m. transversus perinei profundus
m. transversus perinei superficialis
m. transversus thoracis
m. trapezius
m. triangularis
m. triangularis labii inferioris
m. triangularis labii superioris
m. triangularis sterni
m. triceps brachii
m. triceps coxae
m. triceps surae
m. unipennatus
m. uvulae
m. vastus externus
m. vastus intermedius
m. vastus internus
m. vastus lateralis
m. vastus medialis
m. ventricularis
m. verticalis linguae
m. vocalis
m. zygomaticus
m. zygomaticus major
m. zygomaticus minor
mushroom
corneal m.
m. corneal graft
mushroom-shaped mass
mussitation
Mustard
M. intra-atrial procedure
M. operation
Mustarde
Mustardé
M. graft
M. operation
M. otoplasty procedure
M. rotational cheek flap
mutation
mutilation
mutual participation model
Muzsnai modification
MV
maternal venous
MV blood
MV-T
mitral valve-transverse
MV-T image

MVV
maximum voluntary ventilation
mycelial mass
mycetoma
mycobacterial
m. infection
m. nodal infection
Mycobacterium
M. avium complex infection
M. avium-intracellulare (MAI)
M. avium-intracellulare infection
Mycoplasma **infection**
mycotic
m. aneurysm
m. club nail
m. infection
Mydfrin Ophthalmic solution
myectomy
anorectal m.
m. operation
septal m.
myectopy
myelination
nerve fiber m.
optic pathway m.
myelinization
myelinolysis
central pontine m.
pontine m.
myelitis
myeloablation
myeloblastoma
myelocele
myelocystocele
myelocystomeningocele
myelocytoma
myelodiastasis
myelodysplasia
myeloid tissue
myelolipoma
myelolysis
myeloma
myelomalacia
myelomeningocele
m. repair
myelomonocytic cell line
myelonic
myelopathy
human T cell lymphotropic virus
type 1-associated m. (HAM)
radiation m.
myelophthisic

M

NOTES

myelophthisis
myelopoiesis
    extramedullary m.
myelorrhagia
myelorrhaphy
    commissural m.
myelosarcoma
myeloschisis
myeloscopy
    flexible fiberoptic m.
myelotomy
    Bischof m.
    commissural m.
    midline m.
    T m.
myenteric
    m. plexus
    m. reflex
myenteron
Myer loop fiber
Myerson wash tube
Mylaxen
mylohyoid
    m. artery
    m. fossa
    m. groove
    m. line
    m. muscle
    m. nerve
    m. ridge
mylohyoideus
myoablative therapy
myoarchitectonic
myoblastoma
myocardial
    m. contusion
    m. hibernation
    m. inflammation
    m. mass
    m. perforation
    m. protection
    m. revascularization
    m. rupture
    m. tissue
myocardiorrhaphy
myocarditis
myocardium
    fragmentation of m.
    inferior apical aspect of the m.
    postischemic stunned m.
    stunned m.
myocele
myocutaneous flap
myocytolysis
    coagulative m.
    m. of heart
myocytoma
myodegeneration

myodermal flap
myodesis
myodiastasis
myoelastic-aerodynamic theory of
    phonation
myoepithelioma
myofascial
    m. flap
    m. manipulation
    m. pain
    m. pain syndrome
    m. trigger point
myofibroblastoma
myofibroma
myofunctional therapy
myogenic motor-evoked potential (MEP)
Myograph 2000 neuromuscular function
    analyzer
myolipoma
myolysis
    cardiotoxic m.
myoma
myomatectomy
myomectomy
    abdominal m.
    vaginal m.
myomedulloblastoma
myometrial
    m. arcuate arteries
    m. radial arteries
myometrium
myomotomy
myonecrosis
    clostridial m.
myoneural blockade
myoneurectomy
myoneuroma
myoneurotization
myopathy
myopia
    space m.
myoplastic
    m. muscle stabilization
myoplasty
myorrhaphy
myorrhexis
myosalpinx
myosarcoma
myositis
myosteoma
myotenontoplasty
myotenotomy
Myotest train-of-four nerve stimulator
myotomy
    circular m.
    cricoid m.
    cricopharyngeal m.
    diverticulectomy with m.

esophageal m.
Heller m.
Livadatis circular m.
longitudinal m.
marginal m.
m. operation
septal m.
Z m.
myotomy-myectomy-septal resection
myotonia fluctuans
myotoxicity
myovascular sphincter
myovenous sphincter
myringoplasty
myringostapediopexy
myringotomy
m. drain tube
m. with aspiration

myxadenoma
myxochondrofibrosarcoma
myxochondroma
myxofibroma
myxofibrosarcoma
myxolipoma
myxoliposarcoma
myxoma
m. sarcomatosum
myxomatosis
myxoneuroma
myxopapilloma
myxosarcoma

NOTES

M

N
newton
n1–n2 node
N2-Sargenti technique
Nachlas gastrointestinal tube
Nachlas-Linton tube
Naclerio
V-sign of N.
NaCl solution
NACS
Neurologic and Adaptive Capacity Score
nadir
Nafcil injection
Naffziger operation
Nafion dryer line
NaFrinse acidulated solution
nail
anteroposterior n.
Augustine boat n.
azure lunula of n.
Bailey-Dubow n.
Barr n.
beak n.
n. bed
n. bed graft
n. bed hematoma evacuation
bent n.
boat n.
brittle n.
Brooker-Wills n.
cannulated n.
Capener n.
centromedullary n.
n. change
Chick n.
closed n.
clubbed n.
n. clubbing
clubbing of n.
condylocephalic n.
convex n.
delta tibial n.
digital n.
n. disorder
Dooley n.
dystrophic n.
egg shell n.
n. fold
n. fold capillaroscopy
n. fold removal
geographic stippling of n.
n. groove
half-and-half n.
hooked intramedullary n.
n. horn

ingrown n.
left-sided n.
n. length gauge method
n. lesion
locking n.
n. matrix
mycotic club n.
nested n.
onychocryptosis n.
Ony-Clear N.
open-section n.
parrot-beak n.
pincer n.
n. pit
pitted n.
n. pitting
pitting of n.
n. plate fixation
n. plate removal
racket n.
ram horn n.
reamed n.
reedy n.
right-sided n.
ringworm of n.
n. root
shell n.
sliding n.
specialized n.
splitting n.
n. suture
telescoping n.
thickened n.
n. wall
yellow n.
nail-bending
nailing
intramedullary n.
tibiocalcaneal medullary n.
nail-patella-elbow syndrome
nail-patella syndrome
nail-to-nail bed angle
NaK-ATPase membrane
Nakayama
N. anastomosis
N. ring
nalbuphine hydrochloride
Nalebuff classification
Nalebuff-Millender lateral band
mobilization technique
Nallpen injection
nalmefene hydrochloride
nalorphine
naloxone
n. hydrochloride

N

naltrexone
Nance leeway space
nanogram
Nanomex
nape
    n. of neck flap
napex
napkin-ring
    n.-r. annular lesion
    n.-r. carcinoma
    n.-r. compression
    n.-r. defect
Narcan injection
narcosis
narcotic
    n. analgesic
    n. reversal
narcotic/nitrous oxide anesthesia
narcotism
naris, pl. nares
    dilator n.
Narkotest meter
Naropin
narrowed pulse pressure
narrow-field laryngectomy
narrowing
    disk space n.
    eccentric n.
    joint space n.
narrow-slit illumination
Narula method
Nasahist B injection
nasal
    n. airway
    n. antrostomy
    n. border of frontal bone
    n. canal
    n. cavity
    n. cavity cancer
    n. deformity
    n. dissection
    n. endoscopy
    n. foramen
    n. fracture
    n. height
    n. hemorrhage
    n. index
    n. intubation
    n. mucosal identification
    n. mucosal ulceration
    n. muscle
    n. part of frontal bone
    n. part of pharynx
    n. pharynx
    n. port
    n. provocation test
    n. Rae tube
    n. reconstruction

    n. respiration
    n. septal perforation
    n. suction tube
    n. surface of maxilla
    n. surface of palatine bone
    n. surgery
    n. tip
    n. tract
    n. trumpet
Nasalcrom Nasal solution
nasalis muscle
nasioiniac
nasion
    n. soft tissue
nasion-alveolar point line
Nasmyth membrane
nasobasilar line
nasobiliary tube
nasobregmatic arc
nasociliary
nasocystic drainage tube
nasoduodenal feeding tube
nasoenteric feeding tube
nasofrontal
    n. vein
nasogastric (NG)
    n. feeding tube
    n. intubation
    n. suction
    n. tonometry
nasoileal tube
nasojejunal (NJ)
    n. feeding tube
nasojugal fold
nasolabial
    n. groove
    n. line
    n. lymph node
    n. rotation flap
nasolacrimal
    n. canal
    n. sac
nasomandibular fixation
nasomaxillary suture
naso-occipital arc
naso-oral
naso-orbital fracture
nasopalatine
    n. injection
nasopharyngeal
    n. biopsy
    n. carcinoma
    n. groove
    n. hematoma
    n. passage
    n. suction
nasopharyngoscopy
nasopharynx

nasorostral
nasotracheal
>   n. intubation (NTI)
>   n. intubation anesthetic technique
>   n. suction
>   n. tube

nasovesicular catheter technique
natal cleft
nates
Nathan-Trung modification of Krukenberg hand reconstruction
National
>   N. Football Head and Neck Injury Registry
>   N. Marrow Donor Program
>   N. Surgical Adjuvant Breast and Bowel Project

native
>   n. coronary anatomy
>   n. myocardial microcirculation
>   n. renal biopsy

natriuresis
>   pressure n.

natural
>   n. focus of infection
>   n. method
>   n. suture

naturales
>   per vias n.

nature
>   n. root canal filling
>   N. Tears solution

navel
navicular
>   n. abdomen
>   n. bone
>   n. fossa of urethra
>   n. fracture
>   Kidner procedure for accessory n.

naviculocapitate
>   n. fracture
>   n. fracture syndrome

naviculocuneiform fusion
NCC Hi-Lo Jet endotracheal tube
ND-Stat injection
Nd:YAG
>   neodymium:yttrium-aluminum-garnet
>   Nd:YAG cyclophotocoagulation
>   Nd:YAG laser ablation
>   Nd:YAG laser irradiation
>   Nd:YAG laser therapy

nealbarbital

Nealon technique
near
>   n. fixation
>   n. visual point

near-infrared (NIR)
>   n.-i. measurement
>   n.-i. spectrophotometry
>   n.-i. spectroscope
>   n.-i. spectroscopy

near-point
>   n.-p. relative

near-total
>   n.-t. laryngectomy
>   n.-t. thyroidectomy

Nebcin injection
NEB hip arthroplasty
nebula
>   corneal n.

nebulization
>   continuous albuterol n.

necessity
>   fracture of n.

neck
>   n. dissection
>   n. flap
>   n. fracture
>   n. of gallbladder
>   n. of glans penis
>   implant n.
>   implant superstructure n.
>   osteotomy of condylar n.
>   potato tumor of n.
>   n. of rib
>   n. of scapula
>   surgical n.
>   n. of urinary bladder
>   n. of uterus
>   n. of womb

necrectomy
necrolysis
>   epidermal n.
>   toxic epidermal n.

necropsy
necroscopy
necrosectomy
necrosis
>   caseation n.
>   coagulation n.
>   cystic medial n.
>   electrocoagulation n.
>   ethanol-induced tumor n.
>   flap n.

N

NOTES

necrosis *(continued)*
    mummification n.
    periodontal membrane n.
    pressure n.
    radiation n.
    Ratliff classification of avascular n.
    skin flap n.
    soft-tissue n.
    strangulation n.
    tissue n.
    tumor n.

necrotic
    n. hyalinized tissue
    n. inflammation
    n. metastasis
    n. ulceration

necrotizing
    n. angiitis
    n. granulomatous inflammation
    n. infection

necrotomy
    osteoplastic n.

needle
    n. arthroscopy
    n. aspiration
    n. aspiration cytology
    n. biopsy
    21-G n. thermocouple
    22-G n. thermocouple
    Hustead epidural n.
    n. localization
    n. localization of breast lesion
    SafeTap spinal n.
    N.'s split cast method
    n. suspension procedure
    n. thermocouple
    n. thoracentesis
    n. thoracentesis method
    n. thoracentesis procedure
    n. thoracentesis technique
    n. tracheoesophageal puncture
    n. tract

needle-catheter jejunostomy
needle-free system
needle-holder
needle-knife
    n.-k. papillotomy
    n.-k. sphincterotomy
    n.-k. technique

needleless intravenous administration system
needle-point
needlestick injury
needle-through-needle single interspace technique
needle-tract seeding
Neer
    N. acromioplasty

    N. acromioplasty for rotator cuff tear
    N. capsular shift procedure
    N. femur fracture classification
    N. hemiarthroplasty
    N. modification
    N. open reduction
    N. posterior shoulder reconstruction
    N. shoulder fracture classification
    N. unconstrained shoulder arthroplasty

Neer-Horowitz classification of humeral fracture
negative
    n. aspiration
    n. control enzyme induction
    n. correlation
    n. end-expiratory pressure
    n. inotropy
    n. inspiratory breathing
    n. inspiratory pressure measurement
    n. laparotomy
    n. pressure-controlled tube
    n. pressure tube
    tumor receptor protein n.

negative-pressure
NegGram
neglected rupture
Neher operation
Nehra-Mack operation
Neill-Mooser body
neisserial infection
Nélaton
    N. ankle dislocation
    N. dislocation of ankle
    N. fibers
    N. fold
    N. line
    N. sphincter

Nellcor
    N. N-2500 capnograph
    N. N200 pulse oximeter
    N. Oxsensor II D-25 disposable adhesive pulse oximeter monitor sensors

nematode infection
Nembutal
neoadjuvant
    n. therapy
    n. total androgen ablation

neocystostomy
neodymium:YAG laser therapy
neodymium:yttrium-aluminum-garnet (Nd:YAG)
neoformation
neoglottic reconstruction
neoglottis reconstruction
neointima formation

neonatal
  n. anesthesia
  n. infection
  n. intracranial hemorrhage
  n. intraventricular hemorrhage
  n. line
  n. pulmonary transplantation
  n. resuscitation
  n. ring
  n. thymectomy
neonate
  n. examination
  n. ventilation
neoplasia
neoplasm
  n. metastasis
neoplastic
  n. fracture
  n. lesion
  n. renal mass
  n. tissue
neorectal
  n. function
neosalpingostomy
  terminal n.
Neosar injection
Neosporin ophthalmic solution
neostigmine
  n. toxicity
neostomy
Neo-Synephrine
  N.-S. Cocaine mixture 50:50
  N.-S. Ophthalmic solution
neovagina
  skin graft n.
neovascular
  n. bundle
  n. membrane
neovascularization
  choroidal n.
  corneal n.
  disk n.
  n. of disk
  disseminated asymptomatic
    unilateral n.
  interstitial n.
  iris n.
  preretinal n.
  n. of retina
  retinal quadrant n.
  stromal n.

  subretinal n.
  vitreous n.
neovasculature
  tumor n.
NeoVO-2-R volume control resuscitator
nephradenoma
nephralgia
nephralgic
nephratonia
nephrectomy
  abdominal n.
  adjuvant n.
  anterior n.
  apical polar n.
  Balkan n.
  extracorporeal partial n.
  extraperitoneal laparoscopic n.
  laparoscopic n.
  laser partial n.
  live donor n.
  lumbar n.
  paraperitoneal n.
  partial n.
  perifascial n.
  posterior n.
  radical n.
  retroperitoneoscopic n.
  transperitoneal laparoscopic n.
  transplant n.
  unilateral n.
nephredema
nephrelcosis
nephric
nephritic
  n. calculus
  n. syndrome
nephritis
nephritogenic
nephroblastoma
nephrocalcinosis
nephrocapsectomy
nephrocardiac
nephrocele
nephrogenetic
nephrogenic
  n. cord
  n. tissue
nephrogenous
nephrohydrosis
nephroid
nephrolith
nephrolithiasis

NOTES

N

nephrolithotomy
    anatrophic n.
    percutaneous n.
    simultaneous bilateral
      percutaneous n.
nephrology
nephrolysis
nephrolytic
nephroma
nephron
nephronic loop
nephron-sparing surgery
nephropathic
nephropathy
nephropexy
nephrophthisis
nephroptosis
nephropyeloplasty
nephropyosis
nephrorrhaphy
nephros
nephrosclerosis
nephroscopic fulguration
nephroscopy
    anatrophic n.
    flexible n.
    percutaneous n.
nephrosis
nephrospasia
nephrostolithotomy
    caliceal n.
    percutaneous n.
nephrostomy
    circle wire n.
    n. drainage
    percutaneous n.
    n. puncture
    n. tube
nephrotic
    n. edema
nephrotomic cavity
nephrotomy
    anatrophic n.
    n. tube
nephrotoxic
nephrotoxicity
nephrotoxin
nephrotrophic
nephrotropic
nephrotuberculosis
nephroureterectomy
    bilateral n.
    radical n.
    transperitoneal laparoscopic n.
nephroureterocystectomy
nephroureteroscopy
Neptune girdle

nerve
    abdominopelvic splanchnic n.
    aberrant degeneration of third n.
    aberrant regeneration of n.
    accelerator n.
    accessory n.
    accommodation of n.
    acoustic n.
    n. anastomosis
    Andersch n.
    anterior auricular n.
    anterior cutaneous n. of abdomen
    anterior ethmoidal n.
    anterior labial n.
    anterior scrotal n.
    anterior supraclavicular n.
    augmentor n.
    auriculotemporal n.
    autonomic n.
    axillary n.
    baroreceptor n.
    Bell respiratory n.
    n. block
    n. block anesthesia
    Bock n.
    buccal n.
    buccinator n.
    cavernous n. of clitoris
    cavernous n. of penis
    centrifugal n.
    centripetal n.
    cervical splanchnic n.
    circumflex n.
    coccygeal n.
    coloboma of optic n.
    common peroneal n.
    n. compression anesthesia
    n. compression-degeneration
      syndrome
    corneal n.
    cranial n.
    n. cross section
    cutaneous cervical n.
    n. decompression
    decussation of trochlear n.
    deep peroneal n.
    deep temporal n.
    dental n.
    descending tract of trigeminal n.
    dorsal n. of clitoris
    dorsal interosseous n.
    dorsal n. of penis
    dorsal n. of scapula
    dorsal scapular n.
    eighth cranial n.
    eleventh cranial n.
    esodic n.
    n. excitability test

excitor n.
excitoreflex n.
exodic n.
external nasal n.
external saphenous n.
external spermatic n.
facial n.
femoral n.
n. fiber bundle
n. fiber bundle layer
n. fiber myelination
fifth cranial n.
first cranial n.
fourth cranial n.
fourth lumbar n.
furcal n.
Galen n.
gangliated n.
genitocrural n.
genitofemoral n.
glossopharyngeal n.
n. graft
great auricular n.
greater occipital n.
greater petrosal n.
greater splanchnic n.
greater superficial petrosal n.
hemorrhoidal n.
hypogastric n.
iliohypogastric n.
ilioinguinal n.
n. implantation
inferior alveolar n.
inferior hemorrhoidal n.
inferior rectal n.
inferior vesical n.
infraorbital n.
infratrochlear n.
inhibitory n.
intercostal n.
intercostohumeral n.
intermediary n.
intermediate dorsal cutaneous n.
intermediate supraclavicular n.
intervaginal space of optic n.
jugular n.
lacrimal n.
Latarget n.
lateral antebrachial cutaneous n.
lateral anterior thoracic n.
lateral cutaneous n. of calf
lateral cutaneous n. of forearm

lateral cutaneous n. of thigh
lateral dorsal cutaneous n.
lateral femoral cutaneous n.
lateral pectoral n.
lateral plantar n.
lateral popliteal n.
lateral supraclavicular n.
lateral sural cutaneous n.
lesser internal cutaneous n.
lesser occipital n.
lesser splanchnic n.
long buccal n.
long subscapular n.
long thoracic n.
lowest splanchnic n.
lumbar splanchnic n.
lumboinguinal n.
masseteric n.
masticator n.
maxillary n.
medial antebrachial cutaneous n.
medial anterior thoracic n.
medial brachial cutaneous n.
medial cutaneous n. of arm
medial cutaneous n. of forearm
medial cutaneous n. of leg
medial dorsal cutaneous n.
medial plantar n.
medial popliteal n.
medial supraclavicular n.
medial sural cutaneous n.
median n.
mental n.
mesencephalic tract of trigeminal n.
middle cervical cardiac n.
middle supraclavicular n.
mixed n.
motor n.
motor n. of face
musculocutaneous n.
musculocutaneous n. of leg
musculospiral n.
mylohyoid n.
n. to mylohyoid
ninth cranial n.
obturator n.
parasympathetic n.
pelvic splanchnic n.
perineal n.
peroneal communicating n.
phrenic n.
pneumogastric n.

NOTES

nerve *(continued)*
    popliteal communicating n.
    posterior auricular n.
    posterior labial n.
    posterior scapular n.
    posterior scrotal n.
    posterior supraclavicular n.
    posterior thoracic n.
    presacral n.
    proper palmar digital n.
    proper plantar digital n.
    pterygoid n.
    n. of pterygoid canal
    pterygopalatine n.
    pudendal n.
    pudic n.
    recurrent laryngeal n.
    recurrent meningeal n.
    regeneration of n.
    n. to rhomboid
    n. root
    n. root compression
    n. root injection
    n. root lesion
    n. rootlet ablation
    sacral splanchnic n.
    second cranial n.
    secretory n.
    sensory n.
    seventh cranial n.
    sinuvertebral n.
    sixth cranial n.
    smallest splanchnic n.
    somatic n.
    spinal accessory n.
    spinal tract of trigeminal n.
    splanchnic n.
    n. stimulator
    n. stimulator anesthetic technique
    subclavian n.
    subcostal n.
    suboccipital n.
    subscapular n.
    superficial cervical n.
    superficial peroneal n.
    superior cervical cardiac n.
    superior gluteal n.
    superior laryngeal n.
    superior maxillary n.
    supraorbital n.
    suprascapular n.
    n. suture
    sympathetic n.
    temporomandibular n.
    tenth cranial n.
    third cranial n.
    third occipital n.
    thoracic cardiac n.

    thoracic spinal n.
    thoracic splanchnic n.
    thoracoabdominal n.
    thoracodorsal n.
    n. to thyrohyoid muscle
    n. tract
    transverse cervical n.
    transverse n. of neck
    trifacial n.
    trigeminal n.
    n. trunk
    tumor of optic n.
    twelfth cranial n.
    upper subscapular n.
    upper thoracic splanchnic n.
    vaginal n.
    vagus n.
    vascular n.
    vasomotor n.
    vertebral n.
    visceral n.
    zygomatic n.
nerve-point massage
nerve-sparing
    n.-s. dissection
    n.-s. radical retropubic
        prostatectomy
nervi (*pl. of* nervus)
Nervocaine
    N. with epinephrine
nervous
    n. exhaustion
    n. respiration
    n. system involvement
nervus, pl. **nervi**
    n. accessorius
    nervi anococcygei
    nervi auriculares anteriores
    n. auricularis magnus
    n. auricularis posterior
    n. auriculotemporalis
    n. axillaris
    n. buccalis
    nervi cardiaci thoracici
    nervi cavernosi clitoridis
    nervi cavernosi penis
    nervi cervicales
    n. cervicalis superficialis
    n. coccygeus
    nervi craniales
    n. cutaneus surae lateralis
    n. cutaneus surae medialis
    n. dorsalis clitoridis
    n. dorsalis penis
    n. dorsalis scapulae
    nervi erigentes
    n. ethmoidalis anterior
    n. ethmoidalis posterior

n. facialis
n. femoralis
n. furcalis
n. genitofemoralis
n. glossopharyngeus
n. hemorrhoidalis
n. hypogastricus
n. iliohypogastricus
n. ilioinguinalis
n. infraorbitalis
n. infratrochlearis
nervi intercostales
n. intermedius
n. jugularis
nervi labiales anteriores
nervi labiales posteriores
n. lacrimalis
n. massetericus
n. maxillaris
n. medianus
n. mentalis
n. musculocutaneus
n. mylohyoideus
nervi nervorum
n. occipitalis major
n. occipitalis minor
n. occipitalis tertius
n. pectoralis lateralis
n. pectoralis medialis
nervi pelvici splanchnici
nervi perineales
nervi phrenici accessorii
n. phrenicus
n. plantaris lateralis
n. plantaris medialis
n. presacralis
n. pudendus
nervi rectales inferiores
nervi sacrales
nervi scrotales anteriores
nervi scrotales posteriores
n. spermaticus externus
nervi spinales
n. spinosus
nervi splanchnici lumbales
nervi splanchnici sacrales
n. splanchnicus imus
n. splanchnicus major
n. splanchnicus minor
n. stapedius
n. subclavius
n. subcostalis

n. sublingualis
n. suboccipitalis
nervi subscapulares
n. supraclavicularis intermedius
n. supraclavicularis lateralis
n. supraclavicularis medialis
n. supraorbitalis
n. suprascapularis
nervi temporales profundi
n. thoracicus longus
n. thoracodorsalis
n. tibialis
n. transversus colli
n. trigeminus
nervi vaginales
n. vagus
n. vascularis
n. vertebralis
n. zygomaticus
Nesacaine-MPF
Nesbit
    N. operation
    N. plication
    N. tuck procedure
nesidiectomy
nesidioblastoma
nest
    Brunn n.'s
    choristoma n.
nested
    n. nail
NESTED procedure
Netromycin injection
network
    acromial arterial n.
    articular vascular n.
    calcaneal arterial n.
    lateral malleolar n.
    medial malleolar n.
    patellar n.
    Pentax EndoNet digital
      endoscopy n.
    peritarsal n.
    plantar venous n.
    Purkinje n.
    trabecular n.
Neubauer artery
Neuber bone tube
Neufeld dynamic method
Neugebauer-LeFort procedure
Neupogen injection

N

NOTES

481

neural
  n. arch
  n. arch resection technique
  n. axis vascular malformation
  n. canal
  n. crest malformation
  n. crest migration
  n. lesion
  n. spine
  n. tissue
  n. tube
  n. tube defect
neuralgia
  intercostal n.
neurapophysis
neurasthenia
  experimental n.
neurectasis
neurectomy
  adductor tenotomy and obturator n.
  cochleovestibular n.
  Cotte presacral n.
  Eggers n.
  obturator n.
  occipital n.
  opticociliary n.
  pharyngeal plexus n.
  Phelps n.
  presacral n.
  retrogasserian n.
  retrolabyrinthine/retrosigmoid
    vestibular n.
  retrolabyrinthine vestibular n.
  Sonneberg n.
  transcochlear cochleovestibular n.
  transcochlear vestibular n.
  transtympanic n.
  tympanic n.
  ulnar motor n.
  vestibular n.
neurenteric canal
neurilemmosarcoma
neurilemoma, neurilemmoma
neurilemosarcoma
neurinoma
neuritic plaque
neuritis
neuroablation
neuroablative technique
neuroadenolysis
neuroanastomosis
  autogenous cable graft interposition
    VII-VII n.
neuroanatomy
neuroanesthesia
neuroastrocytoma
neuroaugmentation
neuroaxial opioid

neuroblastoma
neurocele
neurocentral
  n. joint
  n. suture
neurochronaxic theory of phonation
neurocirculation
neurocladism
neurocranium
neurocytolysis
neurocytoma
neurodiagnostic evaluation
neuroectomy
neuroeffector junction
neuroepithelioma
neurofibroma
neurofibromatosis
neurofibrosarcoma
neuroganglion
neurogastric
neurogenic
  n. bladder
  n. fracture
  n. incontinence
  n. pulmonary edema (NPE)
neurogliomatosis
Neuroguard TCD Monitoring System
neurohypophysial
neurohypophysis
neuroleptanalgesia
  n. anesthesia
  n. anesthetic technique
neuroleptanesthesia
neuroleptic
  n. agent
  n. malignant syndrome (NMS)
neurologic
  N. and Adaptive Capacity Score
    (NACS)
  n. complication
  n. evaluation
  n. examination
  n. surgery
neurological nerve conduction velocity
  examination
neurolysis
  distal n.
  internal n.
neurolytic celiac plexus block
neuroma
  acoustic n.
neuroma-in-continuity
neuromatosis
Neurometer
  N. CPT/C quantitative sensory
    nerve function tester
  N. device

neuromuscular
- n. block
- n. blockade (NMB)
- n. blockade monitoring
- n. blocking agent
- n. electrical stimulation
- n. facilitation
- n. pedicle graft
- n. relaxant
- n. system electric induction
- n. transmission

neuron
- inspiratory bulbospinal n.
- nondopaminergic n.

neuronal
- n. cell line
- n. membrane
- n. migration
- n. regeneration

neuronephric

neuronoma

neuro-ophthalmic manifestation

neuro-ophthalmologic examination

Neuropack Four mini evoked potential measuring system

neuropathic
- n. bladder
- n. fracture
- n. pain

neuropathicum
- papilloma n.

neuropathology

neuropathophysiology
- normalization of n.

neuropathy

neuroplasticity

neuroplasty

neurorrhaphy
- epineurial n.
- perineurial n.

neurosarcocleisis

neurosarcoma

neuroschwannoma

neurostimulating procedure

neurostimulation

neurosurgeon

neurosurgery
- functional n.

neurosurgical
- n. anesthesia
- n. approach

- n. intensive care unit (NICU)
- n. suture

neurosuture

neurotendinous

neurothekeoma

neurotic excoriation

neurotization

neurotize

neurotologic examination

neurotomy
- opticociliary n.
- retrogasserian n.

neurotoxicology

neurotransmitter
- n. systems

neurotripsy

neurotrosis

neuroureterectomy

neurovaricosis

neurovascular
- n. anatomy
- n. bundle
- n. complication
- n. cross compression
- n. free flap
- n. island graft
- n. lesion
- n. sheath

neuroxanthoendothelioma

Neut injection

neutracer

neutral
- n. point
- n. position
- n. rotation

neutralization
- heparin n.
- n. plate fixation
- serum n.
- n. test

Neutrexin injection

neutron
- n. activation analysis
- n. beam therapy
- n. capture therapy

neutropenia-related bacterial infection

neutrophilic
- n. infiltration
- n. inflammation

neutrophil migration

nevi, pl. **nevi** (*pl. of* nevi) (*pl. of* nevus)

N

NOTES

Neviaser
   N. acromioclavicular technique
   N. operation
Neviaser-Wilson-Gardner technique
nevocarcinoma
nevoid
   n. anomaly
   n. basal cell carcinoma syndrome
nevolipoma
nevoxanthoendothelioma
   juvenile n.
nevus, pl. **nevi**
New
   N. Luer-type speaking tube
   N. Orleans corneal cutting block
   N. York Heart Association
     classification of heart disease
newborn
   n. anesthesia
   n. examination
   n. resuscitation
Newman classification of radial neck and head fracture
newton (N)
newtonian
   n. aberration
   n. body
NG
   nasogastric
   NG suction
   NG tube
NIBP
   noninvasive blood pressure
nicardipine
Nicholas
   N. five-in-one reconstruction
     technique
   N. ligament technique
Nichols
   N. method
   N. procedure
   N. sacrospinous fixation
Nichols-Condon bowel preparation
nickel-and-dime lesion
Nicks procedure
Nicola
   N. incision
   N. shoulder procedure
Nicoladoni suture
Nicoll
   N. cancellous bone graft
   N. cancellous insert graft
   N. classification
   N. fracture operation
   N. fracture repair procedure
nicotinic receptor
nictation
nictitating membrane

nictitation
NICU
   neurosurgical intensive care unit
Nida nicking operation
Niebauer-King technique
Niebauer trapeziometacarpal arthroplasty
Niemeier gallbladder perforation
nifedipine extended release
nightstick fracture
nigroid body
nigrostriatal tract
Nikaidoh-Bex technique
Nikiforoff method
nil disease
Nilsson suction tube
Nimbex
ninety-ninety method
ninth cranial nerve
nipple
   aortic n.
   n. aspiration cytology
   n. line
   n. stimulation test
nipple-areolar reconstruction
nippled stoma
NIR
   near-infrared
Nirschl
   N. operation
   N. technique
Nishizaki-Wakabayashi suction tube
Nissen
   N. antireflux operation
   N. 360-degree wrap fundoplication
   fundoplication of N.
   N. fundoplication method
   N. fundoplication procedure
   N. fundoplication technique
   N. fundoplication wrap
   N. repair
Nissen-Rosseti
   N.-R. fundoplication
   N.-R. fundoplication method
   N.-R. fundoplication procedure
   N.-R. fundoplication technique
nitazoxanide (NTZ)
Nitchie method
Nitinol inferior vena cava filter
nitrate-induced venodilation
nitric
   n. oxide
   n. oxide blocked sphincter
     relaxation
nitrite
   amyl n.
Nitro-Bid I.V. injection
nitrogen partial pressure

nitroglycerin
    n. transdermal patch
nitroprusside
    sodium n. (SNP)
nitrous
    n. oxide (N_2O)
    n. oxide analgesic
    n. oxide/fentanyl anesthesia
    n. oxide/isoflurane anesthesia
    n. oxide/opioid/barbiturate anesthesia
    n. oxide/opioid/barbiturate anesthetic
      technique
    n. oxide/opioid/midazolam/thiopental
      anesthesia
    n. oxide-oxygen-opioid
      (N_2O/O_2/opioid)
    n. oxide-oxygen-opioid anesthetic
      technique (N_2O/O_2/opioid anesthetic
      technique)
    n. oxide-oxygen proportioning
      device
nitrovasodilator
NIXIE tube
Nizetic operation
NJ
    nasojejunal
      NJ feeding tube
NMB
    neuromuscular blockade
NMR
    nuclear magnetic resonance
      NMR spectroscopy
NMS
    neuroleptic malignant syndrome
N_2O
    nitrous oxide
no
    no infection-no rejection
    no rejection
Noble
    N. bowel plication
    N. position
    N. surgical plication of bowel
Noble-Mengert perineal repair
nociception
nociceptive
    n. stimulation
nociceptor
    n. afferent peripheral terminal
nocturia
nocturnal enuresis

nodal
    n. extirpation
    n. metastasis
    n. plane
    n. point
    n. tissue
node
    n. of Aschoff and Tawara
    atrioventricular n.
    buccinator n.
    n. of Cloquet
    coronary n.
    cystic n.
    diaphragmatic n.'s
    n. dissection
    first echelon lymph n.
    foraminal n.
    jugulodigastric n.
    jugulo-omohyoid n.
    left gastro-omental n.'s
    malar n.
    mandibular n.'s
    mesenteric lymph n. (MLN)
    mesorectal lymph n.
    middle rectal n.
    n1–n2 n.
    parietal n.'s
    precaval lymph n.
    retroperitoneal n.
    retropyloric n.'s
    Rosenmüller n.
    n. of Rouviere
    second echelon lymph n.
    subdigastric n.
    subpyloric n.
    suprapyloric n.
    Tawara n.
    visceral n.'s
node-negative disease
node-positive disease
nodi (*pl. of* nodus)
nodi lymphatici (*pl. of* nodus
    lymphaticus)
nodo-Hisian bypass tract
nodose ganglion
nodoventricular tract
nodular
    n. hidradenoma
    n. lesion
    n. transformation of liver
nodulation
nodule

N

NOTES

nodulectomy
nodule-in-nodule lesion
nodulus, pl. **noduli**
  n. lymphaticus
  n. valvulae semilunaris
nodus, pl. **nodi**
  n. atrioventricularis
  n. buccinatorius
  n. cysticus
  n. foraminalis
  nodi lymphatici iliaci communes
    promontorii
  nodi lymphatici iliaci externi
    laterales
  n. jugulodigastricus
  n. jugulo-omohyoideus
  n. malaris
  n. mandibularis
  n. rectalis medius
  nodi retropylorici
  nodi subpylorici
  n. suprapyloricus
  nodi viscerales
nodus lymphaticus, pl. **nodi lymphatici**
  n. l. arcus venae azygos
  nodi lymphatici axillares
  nodi lymphatici axillares apicales
  nodi lymphatici axillares
    subscapulares
  nodi lymphatici brachiales
  nodi lymphatici bronchopulmonales
  nodi lymphatici cervicales anteriores
  nodi lymphatici cervicales anteriores
    profundi
  nodi lymphatici cervicales anteriores
    superficiales
  nodi lymphatici cervicales laterales
    profundi
  nodi lymphatici cervicales laterales
    superficiales
  nodi lymphatici coeliaci
  nodi lymphatici colici
  nodi lymphatici colici dextri
  nodi lymphatici colici medii
  nodi lymphatici colici sinistri
  nodi lymphatici comitantes nervi
    accessorii
  nodi lymphatici cubitales
  nodi lymphatici epigastrici
    inferiores
  nodi lymphatici faciales
  nodi lymphatici gastrici dextri
  nodi lymphatici gastrici sinistri
  nodi lymphatici gastro-omentales
    dextri
  nodi lymphatici gastro-omentales
    sinistri
  nodi lymphatici gluteales

nodi lymphatici hepatici
nodi lymphatici ileocolici
nodi lymphatici iliaci communes
nodi lymphatici iliaci externi
nodi lymphatici iliaci externi
  mediales
nodi lymphatici iliaci interni
nodi lymphatici inguinales profundi
nodi lymphatici inguinales
  superficiales
nodi lymphatici intercostales
nodi lymphatici interiliaci
nodi lymphatici interpectorales
nodi lymphatici jugulares anteriores
nodi lymphatici jugulares laterales
nodi lymphatici juxta-esophageales
  pulmonales
nodi lymphatici juxta-intestinales
nodi lymphatici lienales
nodi lymphatici linguales
nodi lymphatici lumbales dextri
nodi lymphatici lumbales intermedii
nodi lymphatici lumbales sinistri
nodi lymphatici abdominis
  viscerales
nodi lymphatici anorectales
nodi lymphatici appendiculares
nodi lymphatici mesenterici
  inferiores
nodi lymphatici mesenterici
  superiores
nodi lymphatici mastoidei
nodi lymphatici mediastinales
  anteriores
nodi lymphatici mediastinales
  posteriores
nodi lymphatici mesenterici
nodi lymphatici mesocolici
nodi lymphatici obturatorii
nodi lymphatici occipitales
nodi lymphatici pancreatici
nodi lymphatici pancreatici
  inferiores
nodi lymphatici pancreatici
  superiores
nodi lymphatici
  pancreaticoduodenales
nodi lymphatici pancreticolienales
nodi lymphatici paracolici
nodi lymphatici paramammarii
nodi lymphatici pararectales
nodi lymphatici parasternales
nodi lymphatici paratracheales
nodi lymphatici parauterini
nodi lymphatici paravaginales
nodi lymphatici paravesiculares
nodi lymphatici parietales

nodi lymphatici parotidei
    intraglandulares
nodi lymphatici parotidei profundi
nodi lymphatici parotidei profundi
    infra-auriculares
nodi lymphatici parotidei profundi
    preauriculares
nodi lymphatici parotidei
    superficiales
nodi lymphatici pericardiales
    laterales
nodi lymphatici phrenici inferiores
nodi lymphatici phrenici superiores
nodi lymphatici popliteales
nodi lymphatici postcavales
nodi lymphatici postvesiculares
nodi lymphatici prececales
nodi lymphatici prelaryngeales
nodi lymphatici prepericardiales
nodi lymphatici pretracheales
nodi lymphatici prevertebrales
nodi lymphatici prevesiculares
nodi lymphatici promontorii
nodi lymphatici pulmonales
nodi lymphatici pylorici
nodi lymphatici rectales superiores
nodi lymphatici retrocecales
nodi lymphatici retropharyngeales
nodi lymphatici sacrales
nodi lymphatici sigmoidei
nodi lymphatici splenici
nodi lymphatici subaortici
nodi lymphatici submandibulares
nodi lymphatici submentales
nodi lymphatici superiores centrales
nodi lymphatici supraclaviculares
nodi lymphatici thyroidei
nodi lymphatici tracheobronchiales
    inferiores
nodi lymphatici tracheobronchiales
    superiores
nodi lymphatici vesicales laterales

noise
    n. detection threshold
    n. exposure
no-leak technique
noma
    n. vulva
nomenclature
    linnaean system of n.

nonabsorbable
    n. ligature
    n. surgical suture
nonaccommodation
nonanatomic renal bypass
nonanesthetic gas
**nonaneurysmal perimesencephalic
    subarachnoid hemorrhage**
nonappendiceal carcinoid
nonarticular distal radial fracture
**nonbacterial thrombotic endocardial
    lesion**
nonbench surgery
**nonblanchable, abnormally colored
    lesion**
nonbullous emphysema
noncalcified nodular mass
noncardiac surgery
noncausal association
noncemented total hip arthroplasty
**noncollared Press-Fit femoral stem
    implantation**
noncontact manipulation
noncontiguous fracture
nondepolarizer
nondepolarizing
    n. block
    n. muscle relaxant
nondermatophyte fungal infection
nondismembered anastomosis
nondisplaced fracture
nondopaminergic neuron
nondysgerminoma
nonerosive gastric mucosal lesion
non-fenestrated Fontan procedure
nonfunction
    primary graft n.
non-heart-beating donor
nonhepatectomize
nonideal solution
nonimmunologic complication
noninhalation
noninvasive
    n. blood pressure (NIBP)
    n. evaluation
    lower extremity n.
    n. method
    n. procedure
    n. programmed stimulation
    n. technique
nonisometric graft
nonkeratinization

N

NOTES

nonmalignant
    chronic n.
nonmeningiomatous malignant lesion
nonnecrotizing granulomatous
    inflammation
nonneoplastic tumor-like lesion
nonopaque intraluminal mass
nonoperative closure
nonopportunistic infection
nonorganic stridor
nonparametric test
nonpenetrating
    n. keratoplasty
    n. rupture
    n. wound
nonperforative lesion
nonphyseal fracture
nonplicated appendicocystostomy
nonpulmonary route of elimination
    (NPE)
nonrebreathing
    n. anesthesia
    n. mask
    n. valve
nonresectional method
nonresorbable suture
non-rib-spreading
    n.-r.-s. thoracotomy incision
    n.-r.-s. thoracotomy incision method
    n.-r.-s. thoracotomy incision
      procedure
    n.-r.-s. thoracotomy incision
      technique
nonrotation
    n. of intestine
    n. of kidney
nonrotational burst fracture
nonsecretory sigmoid cystoplasty
nonseptate cavity
nonsevered injury
nonshivering thermogenesis
nonspecific therapy
nonstereospecific action
nonsteroidal
    n. anti-inflammatory drug (NSAID)
    n. anti-inflammatory medication
nonsurvivor
nonsympathetically mediated pain
nonthoracotomy
nonthrust mobilization
nontubed
    n. closed distant flap graft
    n. open distant flap graft
nontuberculous mycobacterial infection
nonunion
    n. fracture
    n. of fracture site

nonunited fracture
nonvariceal upper GI hemorrhage
nonventilated lung
nonviable tissue
nonvisualization
    n. of gallbladder
N$_2$O/O$_2$/opioid
    nitrous oxide-oxygen-opioid
      N$_2$O/O$_2$/opioid anesthesia
      N$_2$O/O$_2$/opioid anesthetic technique
noose
    Dormia n.
noradrenergic mechanism
Norcuron
Nordryl injection
norepinephrine
Norfolk technique
norma, pl. normae
    n. anterior
    n. basilaris
    n. facialis
    n. frontalis
    n. inferior
    n. lateralis
    n. occipitalis
    n. posterior
    n. sagittalis
    n. superior
    n. temporalis
    n. ventralis
    n. verticalis
normal
    n. anatomic position
    n. body temperature
    n. intravascular pressure
    n. ovariotomy
    n. planar MR anatomy
    n. saline solution
    n. tissue
    n. transformation zone
normalization
    assay n.
    n. of neuropathophysiology
Norman Miller vaginopexy
normocapnia
normocephalic
Normodyne injection
normolipemic xanthoma planum
normothermia
    intraoperative n.
normothermic ischemia
normoventilation
normovolemic
Northern blot technique
Norton
    N. endotracheal tube
    N. operation

Norwood
    N. operation for hypoplastic left-
        sided heart
    N. univentricular heart procedure
no-scalpel vasectomy
nose
    n. anesthesia
    artificial n.
    cleft n.
    external n.
nosocomial
    n. fungal infection
    n. pneumonia
nostril
notal
notancephalia
notch
    anacrotic n.
    angular n.
    auricular n.
    clavicular n. of sternum
    costal n.
    craniofacial n.
    ethmoidal n.
    frontal n.
    inferior thyroid n.
    interarytenoid n.
    interclavicular n.
    intercondyloid n.
    intervertebral n.
    jugular n. of occipital bone
    jugular n. of temporal bone
    Kernohan n.
    lacrimal n.
    pancreatic n.
    parietal n.
    parotid n.
    presternal n.
    pterygoid n.
    n. for round ligament of liver
    scapular n.
    sternal n.
    superior thyroid n.
    supraorbital n.
    suprascapular n.
    suprasternal n.
    tentorial n.
    umbilical n.
    vertebral n.
notch-and-roll maneuver
notchplasty
    n. procedure

notencephalocele
notochord
no-touch technique
Novametrix combination O_2/CO_2 sensor
Novocain injection
Novofil suture
noxious stimuli
Noyes flexion rotation drawer test
NPE
    neurogenic pulmonary edema
    nonpulmonary route of elimination
NSAID
    nonsteroidal anti-inflammatory drug
        NSAID analgesic
N-shaped sigmoid loop
NTI
    nasotracheal intubation
NTZ
    nitazoxanide
        NTZ Long Acting Nasal solution
nub
    fibrotic n.
nucha
nuchal
    n. fascia
    n. ligament
    n. plane
    n. region
Nuck
    N. canal
nuclear
    n. external layer
    n. magnetic resonance (NMR)
    n. tissue
nucleation time
nucleolysis
    percutaneous laser n.
nucleus, pl. nuclei
    n. ambiguus lesion
    anterior extremity of caudate n.
    external cuneate n.
    extrapyramidal n.
    head of caudate n.
    n. of the mamillary body
    n. masticatorius
    n. of medial geniculate body
    n. pulposus herniation
    n. rotator
    n. of solitary tract
Nuhn gland

NOTES

N

Nu-Hope
  N.-H. ileostomy pouch
  N.-H. Nu-Self drainable pouch
Nulicaine
null point
numbness
numerary renal anomaly
numerical cipher method
nummular lesion
nummulation
Numorphan
  N. injection
  N. Oral
Nunez ventricular ventilation tube
Nuport PEG tube
Nurolon suture
Nuromax injection
nurse anesthetist
nutcracker fracture
Nu-Tears II solution
nutmeg liver
Nutracid
nutrient
  n. arteries of humerus
  n. artery
  n. artery of femur
  n. artery of fibula
  n. artery of the tibia
  n. canal

  n. foramen
  n. vessel
nutrition
  tissue n.
  total parenteral n. (TPN)
nutritional
  n. assessment
  n. status
Nutromat Pad S feeding pump
nycturia
Nydrazid injection
Nyhus-Nelson gastric decompression and jejunal feeding tube
Nylen-Barany maneuver
nylon
  n. monofilament suture
  n. retention suture
  n. 66 suture
nympha
nymphal
nymphectomy
nymphocaruncular sulcus
nymphohymenal sulcus
nymphotomy
nystagmogram
nystagmoid-like oscillation
Nystroem abdominal suction tube
nyxis

O₂
>oxygen

Oakley-Fulthorpe technique

oat cell carcinoma

OAV
>oculoauriculovertebral dysplasia
>OAV syndrome

obcecation

O'Beirne
>O. sphincter
>O. sphincter tube

Ober
>O. incision
>O. tendon technique

Ober-Barr
>O.-B. procedure for brachioradialis transfer
>O.-B. transfer technique

Obersteiner-Redlich line

obesity-hypoventilation syndrome

object
>O. Classification Test
>fixation o.
>o. program
>o. space

objective
>O. Pain Scale
>surgical treatment o.

object-space focus

oblique
>o. aberration
>aponeurosis of external o.
>o. arytenoid muscle
>o. auricular muscle
>o. base-wedge osteotomy
>o. bundle of pons
>o. cord
>o. coronal plane
>o. displacement osteotomy
>external o.
>o. facial cleft
>o. fibers of stomach
>o. fissure of lung
>o. flap
>o. flap in mucogingival surgery
>o. flow misregistration
>o. fracture
>o. head
>o. illumination
>o. incision
>left anterior o. (LAO)
>o. line of mandible
>o. line of thyroid cartilage
>o. metacarpal line
>o. part of cricothyroid muscle

>o. projection
>o. ridge of trapezium
>right anterior o. (RAO)
>o. sagittal gradient-echo MR imaging
>o. screw insertion
>o. section
>o. vein of left atrium

obliquus
>o. abdominis externus muscle
>o. capitis inferior muscle
>o. capitis superior muscle

obliteration
>balloon-occluded retrograde transvenous o.
>endoscopic extirpation cicatricial o.
>fibrous o.
>percutaneous transhepatic o.
>subdeltoid fat plane o.
>total ear o.

obliterative inflammation

O'Brien
>O. akinesia technique
>O. anesthesia
>O. capsular shift procedure
>O. classification of radial fracture
>O. pelvic halo operation
>O. radial fracture classification

obscuration
>transient visual o.

obstetric
>o. anesthesia
>o. pain
>o. position

obstetrical
>o. complication
>o. hysterectomy
>o. operation
>o. traction injury

obstipation

obstruction
>ball-valve o.
>biliary tract o.
>catheter o.
>closed-loop intestinal o.
>clot-induced urinary tract o.
>extrahepatic bile duct o.
>extrahepatic biliary o.
>extrahepatic binary o.
>extrahepatic portal vein o.
>extramural upper airway o.
>gastrointestinal tract o.
>intermittent subclavian vein o.
>left ventricular inflow tract o.
>left ventricular outflow tract o.

O

obstruction *(continued)*
>longer-segment o.
>mechanical extrahepatic o.
>outflow tract o.
>stop-valve airway o.
>upper airway o.
>ureteropelvic o.
>ureterovesical o.
>urinary tract o.
>ventricular inflow tract o.
>ventricular outflow tract o.

obstruction-induced modulation

obstructive
>o. apnea
>o. jaundice
>o. uropathy

obstruent

obtainer space

obtundation

Obtura injectable technique

obturation
>canal o.
>intermittent self-o.
>retrograde o.
>root canal filling technique o.

obturator
>o. artery
>o. avulsion fracture
>o. canal
>o. crest
>o. externus
>o. externus muscle
>o. fascia
>o. foramen
>o. groove
>o. hernia
>o. internus
>o. internus muscle
>o. internus tendon
>o. line
>o. lymphatic chain
>o. lymph nodes
>o. nerve
>o. nerve block
>o. nerve damage
>o. nerve injury
>o. neurectomy
>o. shelf cystourethropexy
>o. test
>o. tubercle

occipital
>o. angle of parietal bone
>o. artery
>o. belly of occipitofrontalis muscle
>o. bone
>o. border
>o. border of parietal bone
>o. border of temporal bone

>o. branch
>o. cephalocele
>o. cerebral veins
>o. condyle
>o. condyle fracture
>o. emissary vein
>o. fontanel
>o. groove
>left anterior o. (LAO)
>o. lobe lesion
>o. lymph nodes
>o. malformation
>o. margin
>o. neurectomy
>o. plane
>o. plexus
>o. point
>o. region of head
>right anterior o. (RAO)
>o. sinus
>o. triangle
>o. vein

occipitalis
>o. muscle

occipitalization

occipitoanterior position

occipitoatlantal dislocation

occipitoatlantoaxial anomaly

occipitoatloid

occipitoaxial

occipitobregmatic

occipitocervical
>o. fixation
>o. fusion
>o. stabilization

occipitocollicular tract

occipitofacial

occipitofrontal
>o. muscle

occipitofrontalis
>o. muscle

occipitomastoid
>o. suture

occipitomental
>o. projection

occipitoparietal

occipitopontine tract

occipitoposterior position

occipitotectal tract

occipitotemporal

occipitothalamic radiation

occipitotransverse position

occiput

occlude

occluding
>o. centric relation record
>o. ligature
>o. relation

occlusal
- o. cavity
- o. correction
- o. equilibration
- o. plane
- o. plane angle
- o. position
- o. pressure
- o. projection
- o. registration dye
- o. relation
- o. therapy

occlusion
- angioplasty-related vessel o.
- centric relation o.
- eccentric o.
- endovascular balloon o.
- laparoscopic total o. (LTO)
- line of o.
- plane of o.
- plastic stent o.
- o. pressure
- o. therapy
- tourniquet o.
- two-plane o.

occlusive
- o. disease
- o. patch test
- o. therapy

occlusorehabilitation

occult
- o. blood
- o. cerebrovascular malformation
- o. fracture
- o. primary tumor of testis
- o. talar lesion
- o. vascular malformation

occupational
- o. therapy
- o. toxin exposure

ochre
- o. hemorrhage
- o. mass

Ochsenbein gingivectomy
Ochsenbein-Luebke flap
Ochsner
- O. gallbladder tube
- O. ring

Ochterlony gel diffusion technique
Ockerblad-Boari flap
O'Connor operation
O'Connor-Peter operation

OCR
- oculocardiac reflex

ocrylate
octanol/water coefficient
Octocaine
- O. injection

Ocu-Caine
OcuCoat PF Ophthalmic solution
ocular
- o. adnexal lesion
- o. barrier
- o. cul-de-sac
- o. inflammation
- o. manifestation
- o. metastasis
- o. muscles
- o. oscillation
- o. radiation therapy
- o. tumor

ocular-mucous membrane syndrome
oculi (*pl. of* oculus)
oculoauriculovertebral dysplasia (OAV)
oculobuccogenital syndrome
oculocardiac reflex (OCR)
oculocephalic
- o. maneuver
- o. vascular anomaly

oculofacial
oculogyration
oculomandibulofacial syndrome
oculomotor decussation
oculovertebral syndrome
oculozygomatic
oculus, pl. **oculi**
- endothelium oculi
- equator bulbi oculi

odansetron
odd-even method
Oddi sphincter
O'Donnell operation
O'Donoghue
- O. ACL reconstruction
- O. facetectomy
- O. procedure

odontectomy
odontoameloblastoma
odontoblastoma
odontocele
odontoclastoma
odontogenic infection
odontoid
- o. condyle fracture

O

NOTES

odontoid *(continued)*
  o. fracture internal fixation
  o. fracture stabilization
  o. perpendicular line
  o. process osteosynthesis
odontoidectomy
odontolysis
odontoma
  o. adamantinum
odontoplasty
odontoscopy
odontosteophyte
odontotomy
  prophylactic o.
odoriferous gland
O'Dwyer
  O. intubation
  O. tube
OEC lag screw component with keyway
OFD
  oral-facial-digital
  OFD syndrome
off-center isoperistaltic technique
off-label use
off-line
off-set V-osteotomy
Ogata
  O. method
  O. technique
Ogden
  O. classification of epiphyseal fracture
  O. knee dislocation classification
Ogilvie syndrome
O-glycosylation
Ogston-Luc operation
Ogura operation
O'Hanlon-Poole suction tube
O'Hara two-clamp method
Ohio Hope resuscitator
Ohmeda
  O. 9000 computer-cotrolled infusion pump
  O. continuous-vacuum regulator
  O. intermittent suction unit
  O. model 7000 ventilator
  O. Rascal II Raman spectroscope
  O. Sevotec 5 vaporizer
  O. thoracic suction regulator
Ohngren line
OHS
  open heart surgery
OI
  oxygenation index
oil
  o. drop lesion
  o. glands

  iodized o.
  joint o.
oil-aspiration pneumonia
oil-based facial foundation
oiled silk suture
ointment
  Biofreeze with Ilex topical analgesic o.
Okamoto method
Okamura technique
Okuda transhepatic obliteration of varix
O'Leary lesser curvature gastroplasty
olecranization
olecranon
  o. fracture
  o. process
oleogranuloma
oleoma
olfactory
  o. anesthesia
  o. bundle
  o. sulcus of nasal cavity
  o. tract
oligoastrocytoma
  recurrent vermian o.
oligodendroblastoma
oligodendroglioma
oligomerization
oligometastasis
oligosegmental correction
oligospermia
oligozoospermatism
oliguresia
oliguria
olisthesis
olivae
  siliqua o.
olivary body
olive ring
Oliver-Rosalki method
olivocerebellar tract
olivocochlear bundle
olivospinal tract
Ollier
  O. arthrodesis approach
  O. incision
  O. lateral approach
  O. method
  O. technique
  O. thick split free graft
Ollier-Thiersch graft
Olshausen
  O. procedure
  O. suspension
OLT
  orthotopic liver transplant
  orthotopic liver transplantation

OLV
    one-lung ventilation
Olympus
    O. gastrostomy
    O. One-Step Button gastrostomy
        tube
Ombrédanne operation
OmegaPort access port
omega-shaped incision
omental
    o. branches
    o. bursa
    o. enterocleisis
    o. flap
    o. J-pexy
    o. patch
    o. pedicle flap graft
    o. pouch
    o. sac
    o. tenia
    o. tuber
omentectomy
    greater o.
    lesser o.
omentitis
omentofixation
omentopexy
omentoplasty
    pedicled o.
omentorrhaphy
omentovolvulus
omentulum
omentum
    gastrocolic o.
    gastrohepatic o.
    gastrosplenic o.
    greater o.
    lesser o.
    o. majus
    o. majus flap procedure
    o. minus
omentumectomy
Omer-Capen
    O.-C. carpectomy
    O.-C. technique
Ommaya ventricular tube
Omniflex head
omniplane scan
Omni-Trak 3100 MRI vital Signs
    Monitoring System
omocervical flap

omoclavicular
    o. triangle
omohyoid
    o. muscle
omothyroid
omotracheal triangle
omphalectomy
omphalic
omphalocele
    infraumbilical o.
omphalomesenteric
omphalos
omphalospinous
omphalotomy
omphalotripsy
omphalovesical
omphalus
OMS Oral
oncho-osteodysplasia
oncocytoma
oncology
    surgical o.
oncoma
oncometric
oncotic pressure
oncotomy
Oncovin injection
ondansetron HCl
one-flight exertional dyspnea
one-handed knot
one-hour office pad test
one-inclinometer method
oneirogmus
oneiroscopy
one-lung
    o.-l. anesthesia
    o.-l. ventilation (OLV)
    o.-l. ventilation anesthetic technique
one-minute endoscopy room test
one-part fracture
one-phase subperiosteal implant
    technique
one-piece ostomy pouch
one-plane
    o.-p. deformity
    o.-p. instability
one-pour technique
one-session removal
one-sitting endodontics
one-snip punctum operation
one-stage
    o.-s. amputation

NOTES

495

one-stage *(continued)*
    o.-s. hypospadias repair
    o.-s. procedure
One-Touch electrolysis
onion
    o. scale lesion
    o. skin-like membrane
onlay
    o. bone graft
    o. cancellous iliac graft
    o. island flap
    o. island flap urethroplasty
    o. patch anastomosis
    o. technique
onlay-tube-onlay urethroplasty technique
on-line data
onset of blockade
onychectomy
onychocryptosis nail
onycholysis
onychoma
onycho-osteodysplasia
onychoplasty
onychotomy
Ony-Clear Nail
oocyte
    o. extrusion
    o. micromanipulation
oophorectomy
    prophylactic o.
oophorocystectomy
oophorohysterectomy
oophoroma
oophoropeliopexy
oophoropexy
oophoroplasty
oophororrhaphy
oophorosalpingectomy
oophorostomy
oophorotomy
ooze
opacification
opacity
opaline patch
opaque myringotomy tube
open
    o. amputation
    o. anesthesia system
    o. application test
    o. bone graft epiphysiodesis
    o. cavity
    o. circuit method
    o. colectomy
    o. cordotomy
    o. disk surgery
    o. drainage
    o. drop anesthesia
    o. drop technique

    o. flap
    o. flap technique
    o. head injury
    o. heart surgery (OHS)
    o. hemorrhoidectomy
    o. herniorrhaphy
    o. laparoscopy
    o. loop
    o. lung biopsy
    o. osteotomy
    o. palm technique
    o. patch test
    o. pinning
    o. pneumothorax
    o. pyelolithotomy
    o. pyelotomy
    o. reduction
    o. reduction and internal fixation
    o. retroperitoneal high ligation
    o. skull fracture
    o. stereotactic craniotomy
    o. surgical biopsy
    o. thoracotomy
    o. wedge
    o. wound
open-book fracture
open-break fracture
open-end ostomy pouch
opening
    appendiceal o.
    o. flap
    ileocecal o.
    internal urethral o.
    maximum mouth o.
    midpalatal suture o.
    o. of orbital cavity
    o. pressure
    saphenous o.
    tendinous o.
    urethral o.'s
    uterine o. of uterine tubes
    o. of uterus
    vaginal o.
    o. wedge manipulation
    o. wedge manipulation and
      reapplication of plaster
open-section nail
open-sky
    o.-s. cryoextraction operation
    o.-s. technique
    o.-s. trephination
    o.-s. vitrectomy
operable
opera-glass deformity
operant procedure
operate
operating room (OR)

operation

Abbé o.
Abbé-Estlander o.
Abbott-Lucas shoulder o.
ab externo filtering o.
Adams hip o.
Adler o.
Agnew o.
Agrikola o.
Alexander o.
Allen o.
Allport o.
Alsus o.
Alsus-Knapp o.
Alvis o.
Ammon o.
Amsler o.
Amussat o.
Anagnostakis o.
Anel o.
Angelucci o.
annular corneal graft o.
antireflux o.
Argyll-Robertson o.
Aries-Pitanguy o.
Arion o.
Arlt o.
Arlt-Jaesche o.
Armistead ulnar lengthening o.
Arrowhead o.
Arroyo o.
Arruga o.
Arruga-Berens o.
arterial switch o.
Ashford retracted nipple o.
atrial baffle o.
Aylett o.
Babcock o.
Bacon-Babcock o.
Badal o.
Baker patellar advancement o.
Baker translocation o.
Baldy o.
Ball o.
Ball-Hoffman o.
Band-Aid o.
Bangerter pterygium o.
Bankart o.
Bankart-Putti-Platt o.
Bardelli lid ptosis o.
bariatric o.
Barkan-Cordes linear cataract o.

Barkan double cyclodialysis o.
Barkan goniotomy o.
Barnard o.
Barraquer enzymatic zonulolysis o.
Barraquer keratomileusis o.
Barrie-Jones
 canaliculodacryorhinostomy o.
Barrio o.
Barr tendon transfer o.
Bassini o.
Basterra o.
Bateman modification of Mayer
 transfer o.
Battle o.
Baudelocque o.
Bauer-Tondra-Trusler o.
Beard o.
Beard-Cutler o.
Beck I, II o.
Beer o.
Belsey Mark IV antireflux o.
Benedict orbit o.
Berens pterygium transplant o.
Berens sclerectomy o.
Berens-Smith o.
Berger o.
Berke o.
Berke-Motais o.
Bethke o.
Bielschowsky o.
biliary-enteric anastomosis o.
Billroth I, II o.
Birch-Hirschfeld entropion o.
Blair o.
Blalock-Hanlon o.
Blalock-Taussig o.
Blasius lid flap o.
Blaskovics canthoplasty o.
Blaskovics dacryostomy o.
Blaskovics inversion of tarsus o.
Blaskovics lid o.
Blatt o.
Bloch-Paul-Mikulicz o.
bloodless o.
Böhm o.
Bonaccolto-Flieringa scleral ring o.
Bonaccolto-Flieringa vitreous o.
Bonnet enucleation o.
Bonzel o.
Bora o.
Borthen iridostasis o.
Bossalino blepharoplasty o.

O

NOTES

operation *(continued)*
  bottle o.
  Bowman o.
  Boyd o.
  Bozeman o.
  Brailey o.
  Bricker o.
  Bridge o.
  bridge pedicle flap o.
  Briggs strabismus o.
  Bristow o.
  Brock o.
  Bromley foreign body o.
  Bronson foreign body removal o.
  Brophy o.
  Brunschwig o.
  Budinger blepharoplasty o.
  Burch eye evisceration o.
  Burow flap o.
  Butler fifth toe o.
  Buzzi o.
  bypass o.
  Byron Smith ectropion o.
  Cairns o.
  Caldwell-Luc o.
  Calhoun-Hagler lens extraction o.
  Callahan o.
  Camey I, II o.
  Campodonico o.
  capital o.
  Carmody-Batson o.
  Carter o.
  Casanellas lacrimal o.
  Casey o.
  Castroviejo o.
  Castroviejo-Scheie cyclodiathermy o.
  cataract extraction o.
  cautery o.
  Cawthorne o.
  Celsus-Hotz o.
  Celsus spasmodic entropion o.
  cerclage o.
  cesarean o.
  Chandler-Verhoeff o.
  Chandler vitreous o.
  Chaput anal o.
  Cibis o.
  cinching o.
  Cleasby iridectomy o.
  Cloward o.
  Collin-Beard o.
  Collis antireflux o.
  Comberg foreign body o.
  commando o.
  comparison o.
  Conn o.
  Conrad orbital blowout fracture o.
  Cooper o.

  corneal graft o.
  Cotte o.
  Cotting toenail o.
  Counsellor-Davis artificial vagina o.
  Crawford sling o.
  crescent o.
  Crespo o.
  Critchett o.
  Crock encircling o.
  cryoextraction o.
  cryotherapy o.
  Csapody orbital repair o.
  Cupper-Faden o.
  curative o.
  Cusick o.
  Cusick-Sarrail ptosis o.
  Custodis o.
  Cutler o.
  Cutler-Beard o.
  cyclodiathermy o.
  Czermak pterygium o.
  dacryoadenectomy o.
  dacryocystectomy o.
  dacryocystorhinotomy o.
  dacryocystostomy o.
  dacryocystotomy o.
  Dailey o.
  Dalgleish o.
  Damus-Kaye-Stancel o.
  Dana o.
  Dandy o.
  Danforth fetal o.
  Daviel o.
  debulking o.
  decompression of orbit o.
  de Grandmont o.
  Deiter o.
  DeKlair o.
  de Lapersonne o.
  Delorme rectal prolapse o.
  Del Toro o.
  Denker sinus o.
  Derby o.
  Desmarres o.
  de Vincentiis o.
  DeWecker o.
  Diamond-Gould syndactyly o.
  Dianoux o.
  diathermy o.
  Dickey o.
  Dickey-Fox o.
  Dickson-Wright o.
  Dieffenbach o.
  dilation of punctum o.
  discission of lens o.
  DKS o.
  Döderlein roll-flap o.
  D'ombrain o.

Donald-Fothergill o.
Doyle o.
drainage of lacrimal gland o.
drainage of lacrimal sac o.
Duhamel colon o.
Duke-Elder o.
Dunnington o.
Dupuy-Dutemps o.
Durham flatfoot o.
Durr o.
Duverger-Velter o.
Dwyer clawfoot o.
Eaton-Malerich fracture-
  dislocation o.
Edlan-Mejchar o.
effector o.
Elliot o.
Elschnig canthorrhaphy o.
Ely o.
Emmet o.
encircling of globe o.
encircling of scleral buckle o.
enucleation of eyeball o.
equilibrating o.
Erbakan inferior fornix o.
Escapini cataract o.
Esser inlay o.
Estes o.
Estlander o.
Eversbusch o.
eversion o.
evisceration o.
Ewing o.
excision of lacrimal gland o.
excision of lacrimal sac o.
exenteration of orbital contents o.
extracapsular cataract extraction o.
Faden o.
Falk-Shukuris o.
Fanta cataract o.
Farmer o.
Fasanella o.
Fasanella-Servat ptosis o.
fascia lata sling for ptosis o.
fenestrated Fontan o.
fenestration o.
Fergus o.
Filatov o.
Filatov-Marzinkowsky o.
filtering o.
Fink o.
Finney o.

Flajani o.
flap o.
floating forehead o.
Föerster o.
Foley o.
Fontan o.
Fothergill o.
Fothergill-Donald o.
Fothergill-Hunter o.
Fould entropion o.
Fox o.
Franceschetti coreoplasty o.
Franceschetti corepraxy o.
Franceschetti deviation o.
Franceschetti keratoplasty o.
Franceschetti pupil deviation o.
Frangenheim-Goebell-Stoeckel o.
Frazier-Spiller o.
Fredet-Ramstedt o.
French supracondylar fracture o.
Freund o.
Fricke o.
Friede o.
Friedenwald o.
Friedenwald-Guyton o.
Frost-Lang o.
Fuchs canthorrhaphy o.
Fuchs iris bombe transfixation o.
Fukala o.
Furlow-Fisher modification of Virag
  1 o.
Galeazzi patellar o.
Gardner o.
Gauderer-Ponsky PEG o.
Gayet o.
Georgariou cyclodialysis o.
Gifford delimiting keratotomy o.
Gigli o.
Gilles o.
Gilliam o.
Gilliam-Doleris o.
Gillies scar correction o.
Gil-Vernet o.
Giordano o.
Girard keratoprosthesis o.
Gittes o.
Glenn o.
Goldmann-Larson foreign body o.
Goldsmith o.
gold weight and wire spring o.
Gomez-Marquez lacrimal o.
Gonin cautery o.

NOTES

499

operation *(continued)*
    goniotomy o.
    Goodall-Power o.
    Gradle keratoplasty o.
    Graefe o.
    Grant-Ward o.
    Greaves o.
    Grimsdale o.
    Grondahl-Finney o.
    Grossmann o.
    Gutzeit dacryostomy o.
    Guyton ptosis o.
    Halpin o.
    Halsted o.
    Hampton o.
    hanging hip o.
    hanging toe o.
    Harman o.
    Harms-Dannheim trabeculotomy o.
    Hartmann o.
    Hasner o.
    Haultain o.
    Heaney o.
    Heine o.
    Heisrath o.
    Heller o.
    Heller-Belsey o.
    Heller-Dor o.
    Heller-Nissen o.
    hemi-Fontan o.
    Herbert o.
    Hess eyelid o.
    Hess ptosis o.
    Hiff o.
    Hill antireflux o.
    Hinsberg o.
    Hippel o.
    Hirst o.
    Hofmeister o.
    Hogan o.
    Holth o.
    Horay o.
    Horvath o.
    Hotz-Anagnostakis o.
    Hotz entropion o.
    Huggins o.
    Hughes o.
    Hummelsheim o.
    Hunter o.
    Hunt-Transley o.
    Hutch ureteral reflux o.
    I-beam hip o.
    Iliff o.
    Iliff-Haus o.
    Imre lateral canthoplasty o.
    indentation o.
    Indian o.
    interval o.

    intracapsular cataract extraction o.
    iridectomy o.
    iridencleisis o.
    iridodialysis o.
    iridotasis o.
    iridotomy o.
    Irvinc o.
    Italian o.
    Ivalon sponge-wrap o.
    Jaboulay-Doyen-Winkleman o.
    Jaesche o.
    Jaesche-Arlt o.
    Jaime lacrimal o.
    Jameson o.
    Japanese standard o.
    Jensen o.
    Johnson o.
    Jones o.
    Kasai o.
    Katzin o.
    Kazanjian o.
    Keen o.
    Keller-Madlener o.
    Kelly o.
    Kelman o.
    Kennedy-Pacey o.
    keratectomy o.
    keratocentesis o.
    keratomileusis o.
    keratoplasty o.
    keratotomy o.
    Key o.
    kidney-sparing o.
    King o.
    Kirby o.
    Knapp o.
    Knapp-Imre o.
    Knapp-Wheeler-Reese o.
    Kocks o.
    Koerte-Ballance o.
    Koffler o.
    Kondoleon o.
    Konno o.
    Kraske o.
    Kraupa o.
    Kreiker o.
    Krempen-Silver-Sotelo nonunion o.
    Krönlein o.
    Krönlein-Berke o.
    Kropp o.
    Kuhnt eyelid o.
    Kuhnt-Helmbold o.
    Kuhnt-Szymanowski o.
    Kuhnt-Thorpe o.
    Kwitko o.
    Ladd o.
    Lagleyze o.
    Lagleyze-Trantas o.

Lagrange o.
laissez-faire lid o.
Lancaster o.
Lanchner o.
Landolt o.
Lane o.
Langenbeck o.
Laroyenne o.
laryngeal keel o.
Lash o.
Leahey o.
Le Fort o.
Le Fort-Neugebauer o.
Leriche o.
Lester-Jones o.
Lester Martin modification of
  Duhamel o.
Levine dislocation o.
Lewis o.
Lexer o.
limb-sparing o.
Lincoff o.
Lindesmith o.
Lindner o.
Lindsay o.
logical o.
Löhlein o.
Londermann o.
Longmire o.
Lopez-Enriquez o.
Löwenstein o.
Luc o.
Macewen hernia o.
Machek-Blaskovics o.
Machek-Brunswick o.
Machek-Gifford o.
Machek ptosis o.
Mack-Brunswick o.
MacNab o.
Madlener o.
Magitot keratoplasty o.
magnet o.
magnetic o.
Magnus o.
Magnuson-Stack o.
Magpi o.
Mainz pouch o.
Majewsky o.
major o.
Maladie de Graeffe o.
Malbec o.
Malbran o.

Manchester o.
Manchester-Fothergill o.
mandibular swing o.
Mann-Williamson o.
Mansson o.
Marckwald o.
Marquez-Gomez o.
Marshall-Marchetti-Krantz o.
Mason o.
mastoid obliteration o.
Matas o.
Mauksch o.
Mauksch-Maumenee-Goldberg o.
Maumenee-Goldberg o.
Maunsell-Weir o.
Mayo o.
McGavic o.
McGuire o.
McIndoe o.
McKay-Simons clubfoot o.
McLaughlin o.
McLean o.
McReynolds o.
McVay o.
Meek o.
Meller o.
Mensor-Scheck hanging hip o.
Merindino o.
Meyer-Schwickerath o.
Michaelson o.
mika o.
Mikulicz o.
Miles o.
Miller flatfoot o.
minor o.
Minsky o.
modified flap o.
Moncrieff o.
Monfort o.
Moran o.
Morax o.
morcellation o.
Morel-Fatio-Lalardic o.
Mosher o.
Mosher-Toti o.
Moss o.
Motais o.
motivating o.
Mueller o.
Mules o.
muscle sliding o.
Mustard o.

NOTES

O

501

operation *(continued)*

Mustardé o.
myectomy o.
myotomy o.
Naffziger o.
Neher o.
Nehra-Mack o.
Nesbit o.
Neviaser o.
Nicoll fracture o.
Nida nicking o.
Nirschl o.
Nissen antireflux o.
Nizetic o.
Norton o.
Norwood o. for hypoplastic left-sided heart
O'Brien pelvic halo o.
obstetrical o.
O'Connor o.
O'Connor-Peter o.
O'Donnell o.
Ogston-Luc o.
Ogura o.
Ombrédanne o.
one-snip punctum o.
open-sky cryoextraction o.
optical iridectomy o.
orbital implant o.
orthotopic hemi-Kock o.
Pagenstecher o.
palliative o.
Palma o.
Palomo o.
Panas o.
parallel o.
pars plana o.
Partsch o.
pattern cut corneal graft o.
Paufique o.
Payne o.
pedicle flap o.
Pemberton o.
peripheral iridectomy o.
Peter o.
Physick o.
Pico o.
plastic o.
plombage o.
pocket o.
Pólya o.
Polyak o.
Pomeroy o.
Porro o.
Potts o.
Poulard o.
Power o.
Preziosi o.

probing lacrimonasal duct o.
protective antireflux o.
pubovaginal o.
Puestow-Gillesby o.
pull-through o.
pulsed-mode o.
Putenney o.
Quaglino o.
radical o. for hernia
Ramstedt o.
Ransohoff o.
Rastan o.
Rastelli o.
Raverdino o.
Ray-Brunswick-Mack o.
Ray-McLean o.
reattachment of choroid o.
reattachment of retina o.
Récamier o.
recession of ocular muscle o.
Redmond-Smith o.
Reese-Cleasby o.
Reese-Jones-Cooper o.
Reese ptosis o.
removal of foreign body o.
resurfacing o.
Richet o.
Ripstein rectal prolapse o.
Rizzoli o.
Rosenburg o.
Rosengren o.
Roux-en-Y o.
Roux-Goldthwait dislocation o.
Roveda o.
Rovsing o.
Rowbotham o.
Rowinski o.
Rubbrecht o.
Ruedemann o.
Rycroft o.
sacrofixation o.
Saemisch o.
Saenger o.
Safar o.
Sanders o.
Sato o.
Savin o.
Sawyer o.
Sayoc o.
Schauta vaginal o.
Scheie o.
Schepens o.
Schimek o.
Schirmer o.
Schmalz o.
Schönbein o.
Schroeder o.
Schuchardt o.

scleral buckling o.
scleral fistulectomy o.
scleral shortening o.
scleroplasty o.
sclerotomy o.
Scott o.
scrotal pouch o.
Scudder o.
second-look o.
sector iridectomy o.
Selinger o.
Senning o.
sensor o.
serial o.
seton o.
sex change o.
Shaffer o.
Shirodkar o.
Shugrue o.
Sichi o.
Silva-Costa o.
Silver-Hildreth o.
slant muscle o.
Smith-Boyce o.
Smith eyelid o.
Smith-Indian o.
Smith-Kuhnt-Szymanowski o.
Smith-Robinson o.
Snellen ptosis o.
Soave o.
Soria o.
Soriano o.
Sorrin o.
Sourdille keratoplasty o.
Sourdille ptosis o.
Spaeth cystic bleb o.
Spaeth ptosis o.
Speas o.
Spencer-Watson Z-plasty o.
Spinelli o.
splitting lacrimal papilla o.
staging o.
Stallard eyelid o.
Stallard flap o.
Stallard-Liegard o.
Stamey o.
step graft o.
stereotactic o.
Stock o.
Stocker o.
Stoffel o.
Stookey-Scarff o.

Straith eyelid o.
Strampelli-Valvo o.
Strap o.
Streatfield o.
Streatfield-Fox o.
Streatfield-Snellen o.
Sturmdorf o.
Suarez-Villafranca o.
subcutaneous o.
Sugarbaker o.
Summerskill o.
suprapubic urethrovesical
  suspension o.
suspensory sling o.
suture of cornea o.
suture of eyeball o.
suture of iris o.
suture of muscle o.
suture of sclera o.
switch o.
symmetry o.
synchrocyclotron o.
Szymanowski o.
Szymanowski-Kuhnt o.
tagliacotian o.
talc o.
Tanner o.
Tansley o.
Tasia o.
tattoo of cornea o.
Teale-Knapp o.
TeLinde o.
tenotomy o.
Terson o.
Tessier craniofacial o.
Thal fundic patch o.
Thiersch anal incontinence o.
Thiersch graft o.
Thomas o.
three-snip punctum o.
Tillett o.
tongue-in-groove o.
Torek o.
total excisional o.
Toti o.
Toti-Mosher o.
Townley-Paton o.
trabeculectomy o.
Trainor o.
Trainor-Nida o.
transection and devascularization o.
transfixion of iris o.

NOTES

operation *(continued)*
    transplantation of muscle o.
    transsphenoidal o.
    Trantas o.
    trap-door scleral buckle o.
    Trendelenburg o.
    Tripier o.
    Troutman o.
    Truc o.
    Tudor-Thomas o.
    tumbling technique o.
    Turnbull multiple ostomy o.
    Ulloa o.
    unattended laboratory o.
    Urban o.
    Uyemura o.
    Van Milligen o.
    Vecchietti o.
    Verhoeff o.
    Verhoeff-Chandler o.
    Verwey eyelid o.
    Viers o.
    Virag o.
    Vogt o.
    Von Ammon o.
    von Blaskovics-Doyen o.
    von Graefe o.
    von Hippel o.
    Waldhauer o.
    Walter Reed o.
    Waters o.
    Waterston o.
    Watzke o.
    Way o.
    Webster o.
    Weeker o.
    Weeks o.
    Weir o.
    Weisinger o.
    Wendell Hughes o.
    Werb o.
    Wertheim o.
    Wertheim-Schauta o.
    West o.
    Weve o.
    Wharton-Jones o.
    Wheeler o.
    Wheeler-Reese o.
    Wheelhouse o.
    Whipple o.
    Whitehead o.
    Whitnall sling o.
    Wicherkiewicz eyelid o.
    Wiener o.
    Wies o.
    Williams copulating pouch o.
    Wilmer o.
    Wolfe ptosis o.
    Worst o.
    Worth ptosis o.
    Wright o.
    Young o.
    Young-Dees o.
    Young-Dees-Leadbetter o.
    Zickel subtrochanteric fracture o.
    Ziegler o.
    Zylik o.

operative
    o. approach
    o. arthroscopy
    o. arthrotomy
    o. choledochoscopy
    o. débridement
    o. laparoscopy
    o. management
    o. perforation
    o. site complication
    o. stress
    o. technique

operatively stabilized
operator
    o. exposure
operculectomy
operculum, pl. **opercula**
    o. ilei
O'Phelan technique
ophryon
ophryospinal angle
ophthalmectomy
ophthalmic
    o. anesthesia
    o. cul-de-sac
    o. examination
    o. solution
ophthalmocarcinoma
ophthalmocele
ophthalmologic anesthesia
ophthalmomyotomy
ophthalmopathy
ophthalmophlebotomy
ophthalmoplasty
ophthalmoplegia
ophthalmoscopy
    binocular indirect o.
    direct o.
    indirect o.
    medical o.
    metric o.
    slit-lamp o.
ophthalmospectroscopy
ophthalmostasis
ophthalmotomy
Ophthalon suture
opioid
    o. agonist
    o. analgesia

o. analgesic
o. anesthesia
o. anesthetic
endogenous o.
epidural o.
esterase-metabolized o.
lipophilic o.
neuroaxial o.
o. receptor
opioid/nitrous oxide/oxygen anesthesia
opioid-sparing drug
opisthion
opisthionasial
opisthotonus, opisthotonos
opium
opponensplasty
abductor digiti minimi o.
abductor digiti quinti o.
Bunnell o.
Huber adductor digiti quinti o.
Manske-McCarroll o.
opportunistic
o. complication
o. systemic fungal infection
opposition respiration
opposure
opsonization
optic
o. canal
o. chiasm compression
o. cul-de-sac
o. cup-to-disk ratio
o. decussation
o. disk
o. evagination
o. foramen
o. iridectomy
o. keratoplasty
o. nerve head
o. nerve lesion
o. nerve tumor
o. papilla cavity
o. pathway myelination
o. radiation
o. tract
o. tract compression
o. tract lesion
o. tract syndrome
optical
o. aberration
o. correction
o. density method

o. iridectomy
o. iridectomy operation
o. keratoplasty
o. nodal point
o. rotation
optici
excavatio papillae nervi o.
vaginae externa nervi o.
opticociliary
o. neurectomy
o. neurotomy
Optimal Observation Score
OptiMed glaucoma pressure regulator
Opti-Soft
optode
fluorescent o.
OR
operating room
ora, pl. **orae**
Orabase with benzocaine
orad
orae (*pl. of* ora)
O'Rahilly limb deficiency classification
oral
o. administration
o. analgesic
o. anesthetic
o. anesthetic technique
o. anomaly
o. cavity
o. cavity abnormality
o. cavity cytology
o. cavity tumor
o. cephalocele
Compazine O.
o. complication
o. condyloma planus
Demerol O.
o. endotracheal intubation
o. fissure
o. infection
o. iron preparation
o. irrigation
Levo-Dromoran O.
o. lighted-stylet intubation
o. manifestation
o. and maxillofacial surgery
Mitran O.
MS Contin O.
MSIR O.
Numorphan O.
OMS O.

NOTES

505

oral *(continued)*
  Oramorph SR O.
  o. part of pharynx
  o. peripheral examination
  o. pharyngeal airway
  o. pharynx
  o. region
  Reposans-10 O.
  o. respiration
  Roxanol SR O.
  o. tissue
  Toradol dO.
  o. transmucosal fentanyl citrate
    (OTFC)
  o. ulceration
  Valium O.
  Valrelease O.
oral-aural method
Oralet
  Fentanyl O.
  O. lozenge
oral-facial-digital (OFD)
Oraminic II injection
Oramorph SR Oral
Orandi technique
orbicular
  o. muscle of eye
  o. muscle of mouth
  o. zone
orbiculare
orbicularis
  o. oculi muscle
  o. oris muscle
orbit
  blow-out fracture of o.
  fracture of o.
  lesion of o.
orbita, pl. **orbitae**
  exenteratio orbitae
orbital
  o. adipose tissue
  o. anesthesia
  o. angioma
  o. arteriovenous malformation
  o. blow-out fracture
  o. branch of middle meningeal
    artery
  o. branch of pterygopalatine
    ganglion
  o. canal
  o. cavity
  o. decompression
  o. eminence of zygomatic bone
  o. exenteration
  o. exenteration gastroscopic access
    technique
  o. extension
  o. fasciae

  o. fat pad
  o. floor fracture
  o. height
  o. hematoma
  o. hernia
  o. implant operation
  o. index
  o. infection
  o. lamina of ethmoid bone
  o. layer of ethmoid bone
  o. lesion
  o. line
  o. metastasis
  o. mucocele
  o. muscle
  o. plane
  o. plane of frontal bone
  o. plate of ethmoid bone
  o. plate of frontal bone
  o. region
  o. rim fracture
  o. rim reconstruction
  o. section
  o. surface
  o. surgery
  o. tubercle of zygomatic bone
  o. tumor
  o. wall fracture
orbitale
orbitalis muscle
orbitofrontal artery
orbitomaxillectomy
orbitomeatal line
orbitonasal
  o. index
  o. tissue
orbitosphenoid
orbitotomy
  Berke-Krönlein o.
  Krönlein o.
orbitozygomatic
  o. mandibular osteotomy
  o. temporopolar approach
orchectomy
orchialgia
orchichorea
orchidectomy
  partial o.
  radical o.
orchidic
orchiditis
orchidoblastoma
orchidoptosis
orchidorraphy
orchiectomy
  prophylactic o.
  radical o.
  radical inguinal o.

orchiepididymitis
orchioblastoma
orchiocele
orchiodynia
orchioneuralgia
orchiopathy
orchiopexy
> Bevan o.
> Cabot-Nesbit o.
> eversion o.
> Fowler-Stephens o.
> laparoscopic o.
> Prentiss o.
> scrotal pouch o.
> staged o.
> Torek o.
> transseptal o.
> two-step o.

orchioplasty
orchiorrhaphy
orchiotherapy
orchiotomy
orchis
orchitic
orchitis
orchotomy
ordinal classification
organ
> o. ablation
> o. allograft
> effector o.
> external female genital o.'s
> external male genital o.'s
> floating o.
> genital o.'s
> o. harvest
> internal female genital o.'s
> internal male genital o.'s
> intromittent o.
> o. perfusion
> O. Procurement Program
> ptotic o.
> o. of Rosenmüller
> secondary retroperitoneal o.
> supernumerary o.'s
> o. transplantation
> urinary o.'s
> wandering o.
> Weber o.

organa (*pl. of* organum)

organic
> o. articulation disorder
> o. lesion

organism
organized hematoma
organizing inflammation
organoaxial rotation
organology
organopexy
organoscopy
organum, pl. **organa**
> organa genitalia
> organa genitalia feminina externa
> organa genitalia feminina interna
> organa genitalia masculina externa
> organa genitalia masculina interna
> organa urinaria

orientation
> angle of o.
> limbal parallel o.
> phalangeal articular o.
> temporal o.
> visual o.

orifice
> anal o.
> appendiceal o.
> esophagogastric o.
> eustachian tube o.
> exocranial o.
> external urethral o.
> gastroduodenal o.
> golf-hole ureteral o.
> ileocecal o.
> o. of inferior vena cava
> internal urethral o.
> pulmonary o.
> pyloric o.
> root canal o.
> ureteric o.
> vaginal o.

orificium, pl. **orificia**
> o. externum uteri
> o. internum uteri
> o. ureteris
> o. urethrae externum
> o. vaginae

origin
> ectal o.
> flexor-pronator o.

Ormond disease
Ornidyl injection
oroantral fistula

O

NOTES

orocutaneous fistula
oroendotracheal tube
orofacial
    o. carcinoma
    o. fistula
orofaciodigital syndrome
orogastric
    o. Ewald tube
    o. pathway
oromandibular
    o. defect
    o. reconstruction
oronasal fistula
oropharyngeal
    o. approach
    o. carcinoma
    o. passage
    o. tube
oropharynx
oro-respiratory tract
orostoma
orotracheal
    o. intubation
    o. tube
Orr-Loygue transabdominal proctopexy
Orsi-Grocco method
orthocaine
orthodontia
    surgical o.
orthodontic
    o. maintainer space
    o. procedure
    o. therapy
orthodontics
    surgical o.
orthodox procedure
OrthoFrame external fixation
OrthoGen implantable stimulator for
  nonunion of fracture
orthognathic
    o. surgery
orthogonal
    o. plane
    o. projection
orthokeratinization
Ortho-mesh
Orthopaedic Trauma Association
  classification
orthopedic, orthopaedic
    o. anesthesia
    o. surgery
orthoptic transplantation
orthoscopy
orthosis drop-lock ring
OrthoSorb pin fixation
orthotopic
    o. appendicocystostomy
    o. graft

    o. hemi-Kock operation
    o. liver transplant (OLT)
    o. liver transplantation (OLT)
    o. transplantation
    o. ureterocele
Orticochea
    O. procedure
    O. scalping technique
Ortolani maneuver
os, pl. ossa
    o. basilare
    o. breve
    o. calcis
    o. calcis osteotomy
    o. capitatum
    o. centrale tarsi
    o. clitoridis
    o. costale
    ossa cranii
    o. cuboideum
    o. cuneiforme intermedium
    o. cuneiforme laterale
    o. cuneiforme mediale
    ossa digitorum
    o. ethmoidale
    external o.
    external o. of uterus
    ossa faciei
    o. frontale
    o. hamatum
    o. hyoideum
    o. iliacum
    o. ilium
    o. incae
    o. intermedium
    o. interparietale
    o. ischii
    o. lacrimale
    o. longum
    o. lunatum
    o. magnum
    o. malare
    o. nasale
    o. naviculare
    o. naviculare manus
    o. occipitale
    o. odontoideum
    o. palatinum
    o. parietale
    o. pisiforme
    o. planum
    o. pneumaticum
    o. pubis
    o. pyramidale
    o. scaphoideum
    o. sesamoideum
    o. suprasternale
    ossa suturarum

ossa tarsi
o. temporale
o. tibiale externum
o. tibiale posterius
o. trapezium
o. trapezoideum
o. triangulare
o. tribasilare
o. trigonum
o. triquetrum
o. unguis
o. uteri externum
o. uteri internum
o. zygomaticum
Osbon pressure-point tension ring
Osborne-Cotterill
O.-C. elbow technique
O.-C. procedure
Osborne posterior approach
oscheal
oscheltis
oschelephantiasis
oscheohydrocele
oscheoplasty
oscillation
grade I, II o.
high-frequency o. (HFO)
laryngeal o.
nystagmoid-like o.
ocular o.
oscillatory ventilation
oscillometric
o. blood pressure cuff
o. calibration
oscillometry
Osgood
O. modified technique
O. rotational osteotomy
Osgood-Schlatter lesion
osmication
osmification
Osmitrol injection
Osmond-Clarke technique
osmotic pressure
ossa (*pl. of* os)
osseointegration
osseoligamentous ring
osseous
o. anomaly
o. fixation
o. labyrinth
o. lesion

o. metastasis
o. part of skeletal system
o. ring of Lacroix
o. spiral lamina
o. surgery
o. tissue
ossicle
ossicula (*pl. of* ossiculum)
ossicular
o. chain reconstruction
ossiculectomy
ossiculoplasty
tympanoplasty o.
ossiculum, pl. **ossicula**
ossification
o. of cartilaginous structure
o. of the posterior longitudinal
ligament
ossifying
o. epiphysis
o. inflammation
Ossoff-Karlan laser suction tube
ostectomy
buccal o.
fibular o.
partial o.
periodontal o.
osteoaneurysm
osteoarthritis
o. disease
osteoarthropathy
osteoarticular
o. allograft
o. allograft transplantation
o. defect
o. graft
osteoblast
osteoblastic
o. bone regeneration
o. lesion
o. metastasis
osteoblastoma
osteobunionectomy
osteocachexia
osteocarcinoma
osteocartilaginous
o. loose body
osteocementum
osteochondral
o. allograft
o. defect
o. fragment

O

NOTES

osteochondral *(continued)*
    o. graft
    o. injury
    o. lesion
    o. loose body
    o. prominence
    o. ridge
osteochondritis
osteochondrodesmodysplasia
osteochondrodysplasia
osteochondrodystrophy
    familial o.
osteochondrofibroma
osteochondrolysis
osteochondroma
osteochondromatosis
osteochondropathy
osteochondrophyte
osteochondrosarcoma
osteochondrosis
osteochrondral slice fracture
osteoclasia
osteoclasis
    Blount technique for o.
    o. maneuver
osteoclastic
osteoclastoma
osteoconduction
osteocranium
osteocutaneous flap
osteocystoma
osteocyte
osteocytic
    o. lacuna
osteocytoma
osteodentin
osteodentinoma
osteodermatopoikilosis
osteodermatous
osteodermia
osteodiastasis
osteodysplasty
osteodystrophia
osteodystrophy
osteoectasia
osteoectomy
osteoenchondroma
osteoepiphysis
osteofibrochondrosarcoma
osteofibroma
osteofibromatosis
osteofibrosis
osteogenesis
    o. imperfecta
    o. imperfecta congenita syndrome
osteogenetic fibers
osteogenic
osteohalisteresis

osteohypertrophy
osteoid
osteoinduction
osteokinematic motion
osteokinematics
osteolathyrism
osteolipochondroma
osteolipoma
Osteolock
osteologia
osteologist
osteology
osteolysis
osteolytic
    o. bone lesion
osteoma
osteomalacia
osteomalacic
    o. pelvis
Osteomark agent
osteomatoid
osteomatosis
Osteomeasure computer-assisted image analyzer
osteomeatal
osteomere
osteomesopyknosis
osteometry
osteomized
osteomusculocutaneous flap
osteomyelitic sinus
osteomyelitis
osteomyelodysplasia
osteomyelofibrosis
osteomyelofibrotic syndrome
osteomyelosclerosis
osteomyocutaneous flap
osteon
osteonal
    o. bone union
    o. lamellar bone
osteoncus
osteonecrosis
osteonectin
osteoneuralgia
osteo-onychodysostosis
osteo-onychodysplasia
osteopathia
    o. striata syndrome
osteopathic
    o. lesion
osteopathy
osteopedion
osteopenia
osteoperiosteal
    o. bone graft
    o. flap
osteoperiostitis

osteopetrosis
    o. acro-osteolytica
    cranial o.
osteopetrotic
    o. scar
osteophlebitis
osteophyma
osteophyte
    o. formation
osteophytosis
osteoplastic
    o. bone flap
    o. craniotomy
    o. frontal sinus procedure
    o. necrotomy
    o. reconstruction
osteoplasty
    Maquet anteromedial o.
osteopoikilosis
osteopontin
osteoporosis
    o. pseudoglioma syndrome
osteoporotic
    o. bone
    o. fracture
    o. spine
osteopsathyrosis
osteopulmonary arthropathy
osteoradionecrosis
osteosarcoma
osteosarcomatosis
osteosclerosis
    o. fragilis
osteosclerotic
    o. lesion
osteosis
osteospongioma
osteosteatoma
osteosynovitis
osteosynthesis
    anterior column o.
    cranial o.
    facial o.
    lumbar spine vertebral o.
    odontoid process o.
    plate-screw o.
    posterior column o.
    thoracic spine vertebral o.
    thoracolumbar spine vertebral o.
    vertebral o.
    wire o.
osteotabes

osteotelangiectasia
osteothrombophlebitis
osteothrombosis
osteotomize
osteotomy
    Abbott-Gill o.
    abduction o.
    abductor o.
    abductory wedge o.
    adduction o.
    Agliette supracondylar o.
    Akin proximal phalangeal o.
    Amspacher-Messenbaugh closing wedge o.
    Amstutz-Wilson o.
    Anderson-Fowler calcaneal displacement o.
    angular o.
    angulation o.
    anterior calcaneal o.
    anterior innominate o.
    Austin o.
    Axer lateral opening wedge o.
    Axer varus derotational o.
    Bailey-Dubow o.
    Baker-Hill o.
    Balacescu closing wedge o.
    ball-and-socket trochanteric o.
    base-of-the-neck o.
    base wedge o.
    basilar o.
    Bellemore-Barrett closing wedge o.
    Berman-Gartland metatarsal o.
    bifurcation o.
    biplane trochanteric o.
    blind o.
    block o.
    Blount displacement o.
    Brackett o.
    Brett-Campbell tibial o.
    calcaneal L o.
    Campbell o.
    Canale o.
    canal innominate o.
    Carstan reverse wedge o.
    Cartam-Treander reverse wedge o.
    cervical o.
    C-form o.
    Chambers o.
    chevron o.
    Chiari innominate o.
    Chiari-Salter-Steel pelvic o.

NOTES

O

osteotomy *(continued)*

closed intramedullary o.
closed wedge o.
closing abductory wedge o.
closing base wedge o.
Cole o.
Cole o. for midfoot deformity
compensatory basilar o.
o. of condylar neck
controlled rotational o.
Conventry proximal tibial o.
countersinking o.
Coventry distal femoral o.
Coventry femoral o.
Coventry vagal o.
craniofacial o.
Crego femoral o.
crescentic calcaneal o.
C sliding o.
cuneiform o.
cup-and-ball o.
cylindrical o.
Dega pelvic o.
delayed femoral o.
Derosa-Graziano step-cut o.
derotational o.
dial pelvic o.
dial periacetabular o.
diaphyseal o.
Dickinson-Coutts-Woodward-
  Handler o.
Dickson geometric o.
Diebold-Bejjani o.
Dillwyn-Evans o.
Dimon-Hughston intertrochanteric o.
displacement o.
distal metatarsal o.
distal oblique sliding o.
dome o.
dome-shaped o.
dorsal closing wedge o.
dorsal proximal metatarsal o.
dorsal-V o.
dorsiflexory wedge o.
double o.
Dunn o.
Dunn-Hess trochanteric o.
Dwyer o.
Elizabethtown o.
Emmon o.
epiphyseal-metaphyseal o.
Eppright dial o.
Estersohn o.
ethmoidal o.
Evans anterior calcaneal o.
eversion o.
extension o.
failed femoral o.

femoral o.
Ferguson-Thompson-King two-
  stage o.
Fernandez o.
flexion o.
Fowler o.
French lateral closing wedge o.
frontonasomaxillary o.
fronto-orbital o.
Gant o.
geometric supracondylar
  extension o.
Gerbert o.
Giannestras oblique metatarsal o.
Gibson-Piggott o.
glabellar exposure o.
Gleich o.
glenoid o.
Golden closing wedge o.
Grant-Small-Lehman supracondylar
  extension o.
Greenfield o.
Green-Reverdin o.
greenstick dorsal proximal
  metatarsal o.
Green-Watermann o.
Gudas scarf Z-plasty o.
Haber-Kraft o.
Haddad metatarsal o.
Herman-Gartland o.
high tibial o.
hinge o.
Hirayma o.
horizontal o.
iliac o.
Ingram-Canle-Beaty epiphyseal-
  metaphyseal o.
innominate o.
intertrochanteric varus o.
intra-articular o.
intracapsular o.
intraepiphyseal o.
inverted L-form o.
Irwin o.
Japas o.
Johnson chevron o.
Kalish o.
Kaplan o.
Kawamura dome o.
Kawamura pelvic o.
Kelly-Keck o.
Kempf-Grosse-Abalo Z-step o.
Kessel-Bonney extension o.
Kitaoka-Leventen medial
  displacement metatarsal o.
Koutsogiannis calcaneal
  displacement o.
Koutsogiannis-Fowler-Anderson o.

Kramer-Craig-Noel basilar femoral
neck o.
Lambrinudi o.
lateral closing wedge o.
lateral displacement o.
lateral opening wedge o.
Leach-Igou step-cut medial o.
Le Fort o.
Lelièvre o.
Lichtblau o.
Lindseth o.
linear o.
Ludloff o.
Macewen-Shands o.
malleolar o.
o. of mandible
mandibular ramus o.
Maquet dome o.
Marquardt angulation o.
Martin o.
Mau o.
maxillary o.
medial displacement o.
medial opening wedge o.
metacarpal o.
metaphyseal o.
metatarsal neck o.
metatarsal oblique o.
metatarsal proximal dome o.
metatarsal Reverdin o.
metatarsal V-shaped o.
Mitchell o.
Molesworth o.
Mueller intertochanteric varus o.
Mueller transposition o.
oblique base-wedge o.
oblique displacement o.
open o.
orbitozygomatic mandibular o.
os calcis o.
Osgood rotational o.
Pauwels proximal o.
Pauwels valgus o.
peg-in-hole o.
Peimer reduction o.
pelvic o.
Pemberton pericapsular o.
perforation o.
pericapsular o.
phalangeal o.
Platou o.
Pol Le Coueur o.

posterior iliac o.
posterior spinal wedge o.
Pott eversion o.
proximal dome o.
proximal femoral o.
proximal metatarsal o.
proximal phalangeal o.
proximal tibial o.
radial wedge o.
Ranawat-DeFiore-Straub o.
Rappaport o.
reduction o.
Reverdin o.
Reverdin-Laird o.
reverse Dillwyn-Evans calcaneal o.
reverse wedge o.
Root-Siegal varus derotational o.
rotational o.
sagittal split mandibular o.
Sakoff o.
Salter innominate o.
Salter pelvic o.
Samilson crescentic calcaneal o.
Sarmiento intertrochanteric o.
Scanz o.
scarf o.
Schanz angulation o.
Schanz femoral o.
Schwartz dorsiflexory o.
segmental alveolar o.
Siffert intraepiphyseal o.
Siffert-Storen intraepiphyseal o.
Simmonds-Menelaus metatarsal o.
Simmonds-Menelaus proximal
phalangeal o.
Simmons o.
sliding oblique o.
Smith-Petersen o.
Sofield o.
Southwick biplane trochanteric o.
spinal o.
Sponsel oblique o.
Stamm metatarsal o.
Steel triple innominate o.
step-cut o.
step-down o.
Stren intraepiphyseal o.
subcapital o.
subcondylar oblique o.
subtrochanteric o.
Sugioka transtrochanteric
rotational o.

O

NOTES

osteotomy *(continued)*
    supracondylar varus o.
    supramalleolar varus derotation o.
    Sutherland-Greenfield o.
    tarsal wedge o.
    Tessier o.
    Thompson telescoping V o.
    through-and-through V-shaped
      horizontal o.
    tibial tuberosity o.
    transtrochanteric rotational o.
    transverse diaphyseal o.
    transverse metatarsal o.
    transverse supracondylar o.
    trapezoidal o.
    Trethowan metatarsal o.
    triplane o.
    triple innominate o.
    trochanteric o.
    tubercle o.
    unplanned valgus o.
    valgus extension o.
    valgus high tibial o.
    valgus intertrochanteric-wedge o.
    valgus subtrochanteric o.
    valgus wedge-prop o.
    valgus Y-shaped prop o.
    varus rotational o.
    varus rotation shortening o.
    varus supramalleolar o.
    vertical o.
    V-shaped o.
    Waterman o.
    Weber humeral o.
    Weber subcapital o.
    wedge o.
    wedge-shaped o.
    Whitman o.
    Wilson oblique displacement o.
    Wiltse ankle o.
    Wiltse varus supramalleolar o.
    Yancey o.
    Yu o.
osteotomy/bunionectomy
    scarf o.
osteotomy-osteoclasis
    Moore o.-o.
osteotribe
osteotripsy
osteotrite
osteotympanic
    o. bone conduction
ostial
    o. lesion
    o. sphincter
ostium, pl. **ostia**
    o. abdominale tubae uterinae
    abdominal o. of uterine tube

    o. appendicis vermiformis
    o. ileocecale
    o. internum
    o. pyloricum
    o. ureteris
    o. urethrae externum
    o. urethrae internum
    o. uteri
    o. uteri externum
    o. uteri internum
    uterine o. of uterine tubes
    o. uterinum tubae
    o. vaginae
    o. of vermiform appendix
ostomate
ostomy
    ConvaTec Durahesive Wafer o.
    o. loop
    o. skin
Ostrum-Furst syndrome
Ostrup
    O. harvesting technique
    O. vascularized rib graft
Osypka rotational angioplasty
OTFC
    oral transmucosal fentanyl citrate
otic
    o. ganglion
    o. periotic shunt procedure
otitis
otolaryngologic manifestation
otolithic membrane
otomandibular syndrome
otomicrosurgical transtemporal approach
otopharyngeal tube
otoplasty
    mattress suture o.
otorhinolaryngology
otoscopy
    pneumatic o.
Ott insufflator filter tubing
Otto pelvis dislocation
ouabain
Ouchterlony
    O. method
    O. technique
Oudard procedure
outcome monitoring
outer
    o. limiting membrane
    o. table of skull
Outerbridge classification
outflow
    o. tract
    o. tract obstruction
outlet
    pelvic plane of o.
    o. strut fracture

out-of-phase endometrial biopsy
outpatient
    o. anesthesia
    o. biopsy
    o. endoscopy
    o. physical therapy
output
    cardiac o. (CO)
    pacemaker o.
    radiation o.
    saturation o.
    thermodilution cardiac o. (TDCO)
outside-to-outside arthroscopy technique
outward rotation
ova (pl. of ovum)
oval
    o. cup erysiphake
    o. window
ovarian
    o. ablation
    o. artery
    o. branch of uterine artery
    o. bursa
    o. cancer metastasis
    o. carcinoma
    o. carcinoma debulking
    o. clear cell adenocarcinoma
    o. cystectomy
    o. fimbria
    o. follicle exhaustion
    o. hyperstimulation syndrome
    o. masculinization
    o. mass
    o. overstimulation syndrome
    o. plexus
    o. thecoma
    o. tumor
    O. Tumor Registry
    o. veins
    o. vein syndrome
    o. wedge resection
ovariectomy
ovarii
    mesoblastoma o.
    stroma o.
ovariocele
ovariohysterectomy
ovariosalpingectomy
ovariostomy
ovariotomy
    Beatson o.
    normal o.

ovary
overall sound level
over-and-over suture
overangulation
overbite
overcirculation
    pulmonary o.
overcompensation
overcorrection
overdetermination
overdilation
overfilled canal
overflow incontinence
overgrafting
overgrowth
overhang
overhanging restoration
Overhauser technique
Overholt procedure
overinflation
overinstrumentation
overlap
overlay restoration
overload
    compression o.
    pressure o.
overprojecting nasal tip
overriding of fracture fragments
overrotation
oversedation
overshoot
    calibration o.
overstimulation
over-the-counter medication
over-the-wire technique
Overton dowel graft
overventilation
overwhelming postsplenectomy infection
oviducal
oviduct
    angiomyoma of o.
oviductal
ovoid mass
ovotestis
ovular transmigration
ovulation
    estimated time of o. (ETO)
    o. induction
    o. rate
    o. stimulation
ovum, pl. ova

NOTES

O

Owen
  contour line of O.
  interglobular space of O.
  O. line
  line of O.
owl eye inclusion body
oxalate calculus
Oxford
  O. miniature vaporizer inhaler
  O. nonkinking cuffed tube
  O. technique
oxidation
  o. of solution
  o. state
β-oxidation pathway
oxidation-reducing potential
oxide
  ethyl o.
  nitric o.
  nitrous o. (N_2O)
oxide-oxygen-opioid
  nitrous o.-o.-o. (N_2O/O_2/opioid)
oximeter
  Datex model CH-S-23 pulse o.
  Masimo SET pulse o.
  Nellcor N200 pulse o.
  pulse o.
  Satellite Plus pulse o.
oximetry
  oxygen saturation as measured
    using pulse o.
  pulse o.
oxophenarsine hydrochloride
oxybarbiturates
oxycardiorespirogram
oxycephalia
oxycephalic
oxycephaly
oxygen (O_2)
  o. administration
  o. in air
  o. analyzer
  o. concentration in pulmonary
    capillary blood
  o. consumption
  o. desaturation
  o. dissociation curve
  o. effect
  o. extraction rate
  hyperbaric o.
  partial pressure of o. (PO_2)
  partial pressure of alveolar o.
  partial pressure of arterial o.
  o. poisoning
  rapid recompression - high
    pressure o.
  o. reduction product
  o. saturation

  o. saturation as measured using
    pulse oximetry
  o. saturation of the hemoglobin of
    arterial blood
  o. saturation indices
  o. saturation measurement
  o. step-up method
  supplementary o.
  o. supply line
  o. tank
  o. tent
  o. therapy
  o. toxicity
  transcutaneous partial pressure
    of o.
  o. under high pressure
oxygenation
  apneic o.
  bubble o.
  cell o.
  disk o.
  extracorporeal membrane o.
    (ECMO)
  fetal scalp o.
  film o.
  hyperbaric o.
  o. index (OI)
  medullary o.
  pump o.
  rotating disk o.
  screen o.
  splanchnic o.
  tissue o.
  tumor o.
oxygenator
  Bentley o.
  bubble o.
  Capiox-E bypass system o.
  Capiox hollow flow o.
  CML o.
  Cobe CML o.
  Cobe Optima hollow-fiber
    membrane o.
  DeBakey heart pump o.
  Digi-Dyne cardiopulmonary
    bypass o.
  disk o.
  extracorporeal membrane o.
  extracorporeal pump o.
  Gambro o.
  High Flex D 700 S bubble o.
  intravascular o.
  Lilliput neonatal o.
  Maxima Plus plasma resistant
    fiber o.
  membrane o.
  Monolyth o.
  Oxy-Hood o.

   plasma-resistant fiber o.
   pump o.
   Sarnes Turbo membrane o.
oxygen-hemoglobin dissociation curve
oxyhemoglobin dissociation curve
oxyhemogram
Oxy-Hood oxygenator

oxymorphone hydrochloride
oxytocin
   o. augmentation
Oyloidin suture
oyster mass of mucus
ozonization
ozonolysis

NOTES

O

P2 prolongation
P32 intraperitoneal treatment
p53 tumor suppressor gene analysis
PA
    PA filling pressure
    PA projection
pacchionian granulation
pacemaker
    p. adaptive rate
    p. artifact
    p. burst pacing
    p. capture
    p. escape interval
    p. failure
    p. impedance
    p. lead fracture
    p. malfunction
    P. Nafeen solution
    p. output
    p. pocket
    p. potential
    p. syndrome
    p. threshold
    P. topical fluoride solution
    p. undersensing
pacemaker-mediated tachycardia
Pacey technique
Pachon
    P. method
    P. test
pachydermatocele
pachymeningitis
pachyperitonitis
pachyvaginalitis
pacing
    p. esophageal stethoscope (PES)
    implantable cardioverter-
      defibrillator/atrial tachycardia p.
    pacemaker burst p.
    p. system analyzer
    transesophageal atrial p. (TEAP)
    transesophageal echocardiography
      with p.
    transesophageal ventricular p.
      (TEVP)
packed red blood cells (PRBC)
Pack-Ehrlich deep iliac dissection
Pack technique
PaCO₂
    partial pressure of arterial carbon dioxide
Pacquin ureterolysis
PACU
    postanesthesia care unit
PAD
    percutaneous abscess drainage

pad
    abdominal fat p.
    adenoidal p.
    antimesenteric fat p.
    artificial fat p.
    Bichat fat p.
    branch p.
    buccal fat p.
    buccal fat p.
    bulbocavernosus fat p.
    buttocks p.
    digital p.
    epicardial fat p.
    esophagogastric fat p.
    fat p.
    felt p.
    heel fat p.
    herniated presacral fat p.
    Hoffa fat p.
    ileocecal fat p.
    infrapatellar fat p.
    infrapatellar fat p.
    ischiorectal fat p.
    labial p.
    malar fat p.
    masticatory fat p.
    metatarsal p.
    orbital fat p.
    patellar fat p.
    pericardial fat p.
    pubic p.
    retrodiskal p.
    retromolar p.
    retropatellar fat p.
Padgett mesh skin graft
Padua bladder urinary pouch
PAF
    paroxysmal atrial fibrillation
    pulmonary arteriovenous fistula
Pagenstecher
    P. circle
    P. linen thread suture
    P. operation
    P. suture technique
Paget-Eccleston stain
Paget extramammary disease
Paget-von Schrötter syndrome
PAH
    pulmonary artery hypertension
pain
    burning p.
    cancer p.
    central p.
    chronic p.
    colorectal distention p.

P

pain *(continued)*
> deafferentation p.
> exacerbation of p.
> existential p.
> experimental p.
> expulsive p.
> exquisite p.
> herpes zoster p.
> p. induction
> inflammatory p.
> intractable p.
> joint line p.
> labor p.
> limb ischemia p.
> p. management
> P. Management Provider
> P. Management Provider IV-PCA
> p. modulation
> myofascial p.
> neuropathic p.
> nonsympathetically mediated p.
> obstetric p.
> palliation of p.
> pancreatic cancer p.
> pediatric p.
> phantom foot p.
> phantom limb p.
> postoperative cesarean section p.
> postthoracotomy p.
> referred trigger point p.
> P. Relief Scoring System
> somatic p.
> spinal cord injury p.
> sympathetically maintained p.
> sympathetically mediated p.
> thalamic p.
> p. threshold reduction
> tourniquet-induced p.
> tourniquet ischemic p.
> visceral p.

painful
> p. anesthesia
> p. point

paired electrical stimulation
Pais fracture
Pajot maneuver
Paladon graft
palatal
> p. expansion
> p. flap
> p. index
> p. lengthening procedure

palate
> Byzantine arch p.
> classification of cleft p.
> cleft p.
> hard p.
> itchy soft p.

> longitudinal ridge of hard p.
> longitudinal suture of p.
> pillar of soft p.
> p. reconstruction
> soft p.

palatine
> p. canal
> p. suture
> vertical plate of p.

palatini
> levator veli p.

palatization
palatoethmoidal suture
palatomaxillary
> p. canal
> p. index
> p. suture

palato-occipital line
palatopharyngeal
> p. closure
> p. ring
> p. sphincter

palatopharyngoplasty
palatopharyngorrhaphy
palatoplasty
palatorrhaphy
palatouvularis muscle
palatovaginal
> p. canal
> p. groove

Paley classification
Palfyn
> P. sinus
> P. suture technique

Pall
> P. Biomedical heat- and moisture-exchanging filter
> P. ELD-series filter
> P. ELD-96 Set Saver filter
> P. filter PL100KL/50K
> P. leukocyte removal filter
> P. PL-series filter
> P. RC-series filter
> P. SP 3840 arterial line filter
> P. transfusion filter

palliation
> p. of pain

palliative
> p. esophagostomy
> p. exeresis
> p. gastrostomy
> p. intent
> p. operation
> p. resection
> p. surgery
> p. therapy
> p. total gastrectomy

pallidectomy

pallidoamygdalotomy
pallidoansotomy
pallidotomy
    posteroventral p.
    VPL p.
pallor
Palma operation
palmar
    p. advancement flap
    p. angulation
    p. approach
    p. branch of median nerve
    p. branch of ulnar nerve
    p. crease
    p. cross-finger flap
    p. interosseous artery
    p. synovectomy
palmate folds
Palmer
    P. method
    P. technique
    P. transscaphoid perilunar
    dislocation
Palmer-Dobyns-Linscheid ligament repair
Palmer-Widen shoulder technique
palmoscopy
palm space
Palomo
    P. operation
    P. procedure
    P. technique
palpable
    p. mass
    p. rib diastasis
palpation
    p. of anterior superior iliac spine
    p. of iliac crest
    p. of posterior superior iliac spine
    p. testing
palpatory examination
palpebra, pl. **palpebrae**
    p. inferior
    levator palpebrae
    p. superior
palpebral
    p. branches of infratrochlear nerve
    p. fissure
palpebralis
palpebration
palpebronasal fold

palpitation
    paroxysmal p.
    premonitory p.
palsy
PAM
    Potential Acuity Meter
pampiniform
    p. body
    p. plexus
pampinocele
PAM procedure
Panas operation
panclavicular dislocation
Pancoast suture
pancolectomy
pancolonoscopy
pancreas
    p. accessorium
    accessory p.
    Aselli p.
    ectopic p.
    head of p.
    lesser p.
    p. minus
    small p.
    uncinate p.
    Willis p.
    Winslow p.
pancreatectomy
    Child radical p.
    distal p.
    en bloc distal p.
    left-to-right subtotal p.
    partial p.
    subtotal distal p.
    total p.
    Whipple p.
pancreatemphraxis
pancreatic
    p. abscess
    p. adenocarcinoma
    p. biopsy
    p. branches
    p. calculus
    p. cancer pain
    p. carcinoma
    p. cutaneous fistula
    p. cystoduodenostomy
    p. duct
    p. duct dilatation
    p. duct manipulation
    p. duct sphincterotomy

NOTES

P

521

pancreatic *(continued)*
    p. ducts pressure
    p. extract
    p. fluid collection
    p. head
    p. intraluminal radiation therapy
    p. lesion
    p. lithiasis
    p. lymph nodcs
    p. notch
    p. plexus
    p. pseudocystogastrostomy
    p. sphincter
    p. sphincteroplasty
    p. tail resection
    p. tumor localization
    p. veins
pancreaticobiliary
    p. endoscopy
    p. junction
    p. tract
pancreaticoblastoma
pancreaticocystostomy
pancreaticoduodenal
    p. allograft
    p. arterial arcades
    p. lymph nodes
    p. transplantation
    p. veins
pancreaticoduodenectomy
    pylorus-preserving p.
    Whipple p.
pancreaticoduodenostomy
    Child p.
    Dennis-Varco p.
    Waugh-Clagett p.
    Whipple p.
pancreaticogastrointestinal anastomosis
pancreaticogastrostomy
pancreaticojejunostomy
    caudal p.
    Duval p.
    lateral p.
    longitudinal p.
    Puestow p.
    Roux-en-Y p.
pancreaticopleural fistula
pancreaticosplenectomy
pancreaticosplenic lymph nodes
pancreatitis
pancreatitis-related hemorrhage
pancreatobiliary canal
pancreatoblastoma
pancreatocholecystostomy
pancreatoduodenectomy
pancreatoduodenostomy
pancreatogastrostomy

pancreatojejunostomy
    cystolateral p.
    retrocolic end-to-end p.
pancreatolith
pancreatolithectomy
pancreatolithiasis
pancreatolithotomy
pancreatolysis
pancrcatolytic
pancreatomy
pancreatoscopy
    peroral p.
pancreatotomy
pancrecctomy
pancreolith
pancreoprivic
pancreoscopy
    infragastric p.
pancuronium
    p. bromide
Panda
    P. gastrostomy tube
    P. nasoenteric feeding tube
pandiculation
panendoscopy
    fiberoptic p.
    lower p.
    primary p.
    upper gastrointestinal p.
panhysterectomy
Panje tube
PAN membrane
panmetatarsal head resection
panmucosal inflammatory cell infiltration
pannicular hernia
panniculectomy
panniculus
pannus
    p. formation
panoramic surface projection
PANP
    pelvic autonomic nerve preservation
panphotocoagulation
panproctocolectomy
panretinal
    p. ablation
    p. argon laser photocoagulation
pantalar fusion
pantaloon
    p. hernia
    p. patch
pants-over-vest
    p.-o.-v. capsulorrhaphy
    p.-o.-v. hernial repair
    p.-o.-v. herniorrhaphy
    p.-o.-v. technique
Panum fusion area

PAO$_2$
> alveolar oxygen partial pressure

PaO$_2$
> arterial oxygen partial pressure

PAOD
> popliteal artery occlusive disease

PAOP
> pulmonary artery occlusion pressure

PAP
> positive airway pressure
> pulmonary artery pressure

Papanicolaou
> P. method
> P. solution

papaphysis

Paparella
> P. myringotomy tube
> P. ventilation tube

Paparella-Frazier suction tube

Papavasiliou classification of olecranon fracture

papaveretum

papaverine
> p. injection

paper point

papilla, pl. papillae
> balloon dilation of the p.
> bile p.
> p. of breast
> p. duodeni major
> p. duodeni minor
> p. graft
> lacrimal p.
> p. lacrimalis
> lenticular papillae
> major duodenal p.
> p. mammae
> minor duodenal p.
> renal p.
> p. renalis
> urethral p.
> p. of Vater

papillary
> p. adenoma of large intestine
> p. ducts
> p. ectasia
> p. foramina of kidney
> p. hidradenoma
> p. lesion
> p. muscle rupture
> p. muscle tip
> p. pedicle graft

> p. process
> p. projection
> p. reconstruction
> p. tip

papillectomy

papillitis

papilloadenocystoma

papillocarcinoma

papillogram

papilloma
> p. neuropathicum

papillomacular nerve fiber bundle

papillomavirus infection

Papillon-Léage and Psaume syndrome

papillotomy
> accessory p.
> endoscopic p.
> needle-knife p.
> precut p.

Papineau
> P. bone graft
> P. technique

papulation

papulopustular lesion

papulosis

papulosquamous lesion

papulovesicular lesion

Paquin technique

par

para-aortic
> p.-a. hematoma
> p.-a. lymphadenectomy
> p.-a. lymph node dissection
> p.-a. node irradiation

para-appendicitis

parabiosis

parabiotic
> p. flap

paracancerous tissue

paracanthoma

paracardiac metastasis

paracentesis

paracentetic

paracentral nerve fiber bundle

paracervical
> p. block
> p. block anesthesia
> p. injection

paracervix

paracetaldehyde

parachroma

NOTES

parachute
    p. deformity
    p. jumper dislocation
paraclavicular thoracic outlet
  decompression
paracoagulation
paracolic
    p. gutters
    p. recesses
paracollicular biopsy
paracolpium
paracystic
    p. pouch
paracystitis
paracystium
paradidymal
paradidymis
paradoxical
    p. embolism
    p. extensor reflex
    p. incontinence
    p. reaction
    p. respiration
    p. technique
paraduodenal
    p. fossa
    p. hernia
    p. recess
paraesophageal
    p. diaphragmatic hernia
    p. hiatal hernia
paraesophagogastric devascularization
para-exstrophy skin flap
paraffin graft
paraffinoma
paraffin-section light microscopy
paraganglioma
paragenital
    p. tubules
paraglenoid groove
paraglottic space
paragranuloma
parahepatic
parahiatal hernia
parahypophysis
paraileostomal hernia
parainfluenza virus infection
parajejunal fossa
parakeratinization
parakeratosis
paralaryngeal space
paraldehyde
parallel
    p. operation
    p. technique
paralleling
    p. cone position
    p. technique

paralysis
    compression p.
    hernia p.
    pharmacologically induced p.
    pressure p.
    soft palate p.
    tourniquet p.
paralyzant
paramagnetic
    p. contrast injection
    p. enhancement accentuation by
      chemical shift imaging
    p. relaxation
    p. shift relaxation
paramammary lymph nodes
paramedial incision
paramedian
    p. approach
    p. incision
    p. pontine reticular formation
    p. sagittal plane
paramesonephric duct
parameter
    canonical univariate p.
parametrectomy
    radical p.
parametrial
parametric
    p. test
parametrium
paranalgesia
paranasal
    p. mucocele
    p. sinuses
paraneoplastic ectopic ACTH production
paranephric
    p. abscess
    p. body
paranephros
paranesthesia
paraneural infiltration
paraomphalic
paraoperative
paraoral tissue
paraorbital lesion
paraovarian
parapancreatic
paraparesis
parapatellar
    p. arthrotomy
    p. incision
paraperitoneal
    p. hernia
    p. nephrectomy
parapharyngeal
    p. space
    p. space abscess

paraphasia
    extended jargon p.
paraphimosis
paraphysis
parapineal
paraplegia
    p. in extension
paraproctium
paraprostatitis
parapubic hernia
pararectal
    p. fistula
    p. fossa
    p. line
    p. lymph nodes
    p. pouch
pararectus
    p. approach
    p. incision
pararenal
    p. space
parasaccular hernia
parasacral
parasagittal
    p. lesion
    p. plane
    p. section
parascapular flap
parasellar
    p. mass
    p. metastasis
parasinoidal
parasitic
    p. castration
    p. flap
    p. infection
paraspinal
    p. approach
    p. line
    p. rod application
paraspinous aspect
parasternal
    p. examination
    p. line
    p. lymph nodes
parastomal hernia
parasympathectomy
    sinoatrial nodal p.
parasympathetic
    p. ganglia
    p. nerve

    p. part
    p. projection
paraterminal body
parathyroid
    p. adenoma
    p. biopsy
    p. carcinoma
    p. extract
    p. gland
    p. tumor ablation
parathyroidectomy
paratracheal
    p. lymph node
    p. tissue stripe
paratrachoma
paratransplantal tissue
Paratrend 7 fiberoptic PCO$_2$ sensor
paratrooper fracture
paraumbilical
    p. veins
paraurethral
    p. ducts
    p. glands
parauterine lymph nodes
paravaccinia virus infection
paravaginal
    p. defect repair
    p. hysterectomy
    p. lymph nodes
    p. soft tissue
paravariceal
    p. injection
    p. sclerotherapy
paravertebral
    p. anesthesia
    p. ganglia
    p. gutter
    p. line
    p. lumbar sympathetic block
paravesical
    p. fossa
    p. lymph nodes
    p. pouch
parectasis
parencephalia
parencephalocele
parencephalous
parenchyma
    p. testis
parenchymal
    p. brain metastasis
    p. hematoma

NOTES

P

parenchymal *(continued)*
    p. laceration
    p. sparing surgery
    p. tissue
parenchymatous
    p. intracerebral hemorrhage
parenteral
    p. administration
    p. analgesia
    p. anesthesia
    p. medication
    p. therapy
parepicele
parepididymis
Pare reduction of elbow dislocation
paresis
    elevation p.
paresthesia
    p. anesthetic technique
paresthetica
    meralgia p.
Paré suture
paries, pl. parietes
    p. anterior gastris
    p. anterior vaginae
    p. membranaceus tracheae
    p. posterior gastris
    p. posterior vaginae
parietal
    p. angle
    p. arteries
    p. bone
    p. border
    p. border of frontal bone
    p. border of sphenoid bone
    p. border of temporal bone
    p. branch
    p. branch of medial occipital artery
    p. branch of middle meningeal artery
    p. branch of superficial temporal artery
    p. cell vagotomy
    p. eminence
    p. emissary vein
    p. fistula
    p. foramen
    p. hernia
    p. layer of leptomeninges
    p. layer of tunica vaginalis
    p. lymph nodes
    p. margin
    p. nodes
    p. notch
    p. pelvic fascia
    p. pericardiectomy
    p. peritoneum
    p. pleura
    p. region
    p. tuber
    p. wall
parietofrontal
parietography
parietomastoid suture
parietooccipital
    p. artery
parietopontine tract
parietosphenoid
parietosplanchnic
parietosquamosal
parietotemporal
parietovisceral
Paris
    P. classification
    P. method
    P. method for radium therapy
park-bench position
Parker
    P. incision
    P. tube
Parker-Kerr
    P.-K. closed method
    P.-K. enteroenterostomy
    P.-K. suture
Parks
    P. ileoanal anastomosis
    P. ileostomy pouch
    P. method of anal fistulotomy
    P. partial sphincterotomy
    P. staged fistulotomy
Parks-Bielschowsky three-step head-tilt test
paroccipital
    p. process
parolivary
paromphalocele
Parona space
paronychial infection
parorchidium
parorchis
parosteal
parotic
parotid
    p. bed
    p. branches
    p. carcinoma
    p. dissection
    p. duct
    p. duct ligation
    p. fascia
    p. gland
    p. notch
    p. recess
    p. resection
    p. sheath

p. space
p. veins
parotidectomy
facial nerve-preserving p.
lateral p.
superficial p.
parotideomasseteric fascia
parotidoauricularis
parovarian
p. mass
parovariotomy
parovarium
paroxysmal
p. atrial fibrillation (PAF)
p. palpitation
Parrish-Mann hammertoe technique
Parrish procedure
parrot-beak nail
Parry-Jones vulvectomy
pars, pl. **partes**
p. abdominalis aortae
p. abdominalis ductus thoracici
p. abdominalis esophagi
p. abdominalis ureteris
p. annularis vaginae fibrosae
p. anterior commissurae anterioris
cerebri
p. anterior commissurae rostralis
p. anterior faciei diaphragmatis
hepatis
p. anterior fornicis vaginae
p. ascendens duodeni
p. atlantica
p. basilaris ossis occipitalis
p. cardiaca gastris
p. cardiaca ventriculi
p. cartilaginosa systematis skeletalis
p. cavernosa
p. cavernosa arteriae carotidis
internae
p. centralis
p. cerebralis arteriae carotidis
internae
p. cervicalis arteriae carotidis
internae
p. cervicalis ductus thoracici
p. cervicalis esophagi
p. cervicalis medullae spinalis
p. clavicularis musculi pectoralis
majoris
p. coccygea medullae spinalis
p. convoluta lobuli corticalis renis

p. corticalis arteriae cerebralis
mediae
p. costalis diaphragmatis
p. cruciformis vaginae fibrosae
p. descendens duodeni
p. dextra faciei diaphragmaticae
hepatis
p. endocrina pancreatis
p. exocrina pancreatis
partes genitales femininae externae
partes genitales masculinae externae
p. horizontalis duodeni
p. inferior duodeni
p. inferior rami lingularis
p. infraclavicularis plexus brachialis
p. interarticularis fracture
p. intracranialis arteriae vertebralis
p. intraocularis nervi optici
p. laryngea pharyngis
p. lateralis fornicis vaginae
p. lateralis ossis occipitalis
p. lateralis ossis sacri
p. lumbalis diaphragmatis
p. lumbalis medullae spinalis
p. mastoidea ossis temporalis
p. medialis arcus pedis
longitudinalis
p. mediastinalis pulmonis
p. membranacea urethrae
masculinae
p. nasalis ossis frontalis
p. nasalis pharyngis
p. obliqua musculi cricothyroidei
p. oralis pharyngis
p. ossea systematis skeletalis
p. pelvica
p. pelvica ureteris
p. peripherica
p. perpendicularis
p. petrosa ossis temporalis
p. pharyngea hypophyseos
p. plana approach
p. plana operation
p. plana vitrectomy
p. postcommunicalis arteria cerebri
anterior
p. posterior commissurae anterioris
p. posterior faciei diaphragmatis
hepatis
p. posterior fornicis vaginae
p. precommunicalis arteriae cerebri
anterior

NOTES

P

527

pars *(continued)*

    p. profunda musculi masseteri
    p. profunda musculi sphincteri ani externi
    p. prostatica urethrae
    p. pylorica gastris
    p. pylorica ventriculi
    p. quadrata hepatis
    p. radiata lobuli corticalis renis
    p. recta musculi cricothyroidei
    p. sacralis medullae spinalis
    p. sphenoidalis arteriae cerebralis mediae
    p. spinalis nervi accessorii
    p. spongiosa urethrae masculinae
    p. squamosa ossis temporalis
    p. sternalis diaphragmatis
    p. subcutanea musculi sphincteri ani externi
    p. superficialis musculi masseteri
    p. superficialis musculi sphincteri ani externi
    p. superior duodeni
    p. superior faciei diaphragmaticae hepatis
    p. superior ganglii vestibularis
    p. supraclavicularis plexus brachialis
    p. sympathica
    p. tecta
    p. terminalis
    p. thoracica aortae
    p. thoracica ductus thoracici
    p. thoracica esophagi
    p. thoracica medullae spinalis
    p. tibiocalcanea ligamenti medialis
    p. tibionavicularis ligamenti medialis
    p. tibiotalaris anterior ligamenti medialis
    p. tibiotalaris posterior ligamenti medialis
    p. transversa rami sinistri venae portae hepatis
    p. transversaria arteriae vertebralis
    p. umbilicalis rami sinistri venae portae hepatis
    p. uterina placentae
    p. uterina tubae uterinae
    p. vagalis nervi accessorii

Parsonnet pulse generator pouch

part

    abdominal p. of aorta
    abdominal p. of esophagus
    abdominal p. of thoracic duct
    abdominal p. of ureter
    anterior p. of anterior commissure of brain

anterior p. of diaphragmatic surface of liver
anterior p. of fornix of vagina
ascending p. of duodenum
atlantic p. of vertebral artery
basal p. of occipital bone
basilar p. of the occipital bone
cardiac p. of stomach
cartilaginous p. of skeletal system
cavernous p. of internal carotid artery
cerebral p. of arachnoid
cerebral p. of dura mater
cerebral p. of internal carotid artery
cervical p. of esophagus
cervical p. of internal carotid artery
cervical p. of spinal cord
cervical p. of thoracic duct
clavicular p. of pectoralis major muscle
coccygeal p. of spinal cord
convoluted p. of kidney lobule
cortical p.
cortical p. of middle cerebral artery
costal p. of diaphragm
deep p. of external anal sphincter
deep p. of flexor retinaculum
deep p. of masseter muscle
deep p. of parotid gland
descending p. of duodenum
descending p. of facial canal
endocrine p. of pancreas
exocrine p. of pancreas
hidden p.
horizontal p. of duodenum
horizontal p. of facial canal
inferior p. of duodenum
infraclavicular p. of brachial plexus
intracranial p. of vertebral artery
intraocular p. of optic nerve
laryngeal p. of pharynx
lateral p. of occipital bone
lateral p. of sacrum
lateral p. of vaginal fornix
lumbar p. of diaphragm
lumbar p. of spinal cord
mastoid p. of the temporal bone
medial p. of longitudinal arch of foot
mediastinal p. of lung
membranous p. of male urethra
nasal p. of frontal bone
nasal p. of pharynx
oblique p. of cricothyroid muscle
oral p. of pharynx

osseous p. of skeletal system
parasympathetic p.
pelvic p.
pelvic p. of ureter
petrous p. of temporal bone
postcommunical p. of anterior
  cerebral artery
posterior tibiotalar p. of deltoid
  ligament
postsulcal p. of tongue
precommunical p. of anterior
  cerebral artery
presulcal p. of tongue
pyloric p. of stomach
quadrate p. of liver
right p. of diaphragmatic surface
  of liver
sacral p. of spinal cord
soft p.'s
sphenoidal p. of middle cerebral
  artery
spinal p. of accessory nerve
spinal p. of arachnoid
spongy p. of the male urethra
squamous p. of frontal bone
squamous p. of occipital bone
squamous p. of temporal bone
sternal p. of diaphragm
straight p. of cricothyroid muscle
subcutaneous p. of external anal
  sphincter
suboccipital p. of vertebral artery
superficial p. of external anal
  sphincter
superficial p. of masseter muscle
superior p. of diaphragmatic
  surface of liver
superior p. of duodenum
superior p. of vestibular ganglion
supraclavicular p. of brachial
  plexus
sympathetic p.
terminal p.
thoracic p. of aorta
thoracic p. of esophagus
thoracic p. of spinal cord
thoracic p. of thoracic duct
tibiocalcaneal p. of deltoid
  ligament
tibionavicular p. of deltoid
  ligament

transverse p. of left branch of
  portal vein
tympanic p. of temporal bone
umbilical p. of left branch of
  portal vein
uterine p. of uterine tube
vagal p. of accessory nerve
vertebral p. of the costal surface
  of the lungs
vertebral p. of diaphragm
partes (*pl. of* pars)
partial
  p. alveolectomy
  p. atrioventricular canal
  p. breech extraction
  p. central hypophysectomy
  p. cystectomy
  p. diskectomy
  p. dislocation
  p. duplication
  p. encircling endocardial
    ventriculotomy
  p. ethmoidectomy
  p. facetectomy
  p. fasciectomy
  p. fibulectomy
  p. gastrectomy
  p. glossectomy
  p. hemilaminectomy
  p. hepatectomy
  p. ileal bypass
  p. inferior retrocolic end-to-side
    gastrojejunostomy
  p. internal hemipelvectomy
  p. keratoplasty
  p. laryngopharyngectomy
  p. liquid ventilation
  p. matrixectomy
  p. meniscectomy
  p. nephrectomy
  p. orchidectomy
  p. ossicular replacement prosthesis
    (PORP)
  p. ostectomy
  p. pancreatectomy
  p. patellectomy
  p. pressure
  p. pressure of alveolar oxygen
  p. pressure of arterial carbon
    dioxide ($PaCO_2$)
  p. pressure of arterial oxygen

NOTES

P

partial *(continued)*
p. pressure of carbon dioxide (PCO_2)
p. pressure of CO_2 gas
p. pressure of intramuscular carbon dioxide ($PiCO_2$)
p. pressure of mesenteric venous carbon dioxide ($PmvCO_2$)
p. pressure of oxygen (PO_2)
p. pressure of water vapor
p. pulpectomy
p. pulpotomy
p. resection of the acetabulum
p. saturation
p. saturation spin-echo (PSSE)
p. superior retrocolic end-to-side gastrojejunostomy
p. zonal dissection

partial-thickness
p.-t. burn
p.-t. craniectomy
p.-t. flap
p.-t. periodontal graft
p.-t. skin graft

partial-throw surgeon knot
particle beam radiation therapy
particulate cancellous bone graft
Partipilo gastrostomy
Partsch operation
parturient
p. canal

parumbilical
paruresis
Parvin
P. gravity technique
P. reduction

PAS
peripheral access system
PAS port
PAS technique

pascal unit of pressure measurement
passage
nasopharyngeal p.
oropharyngeal p.
p. pressure
transforaminal p.
transperineurial p.
wire p.

passé
coma dé p.

passive
p. gliding technique
p. incontinence
p. joint manipulation
p. reciprocation
p. tissue cooling

Pastia line

patch
p. amnesia
aortic p.
ash leaf p.
autologous pericardial p.
binocular eye p.
blood p.
Bowen p.
butterfly p.
cardiac p.
Carrel aortic p.
p. clamp electrophysiology
colic p.
colonic p.
cotton-wool p.
Dacron intracardiac p.
defibrillation p.
Donaldson eye p.
eczematous p.
electrodispersive skin p.
epicardial defibrillator p.
epidural blood p.
estradiol transderm p.
eye p.
glue p.
Gore-Tex cardiovascular p.
Gore-Tex soft tissue p.
p. graft
gray p.
herald p.
histoacryl glue p.
Hutchinson p.
Ionescu-Shiley pericardial p.
p. lesion
lyophilized dural p.
MacCallum p.
monocular p.
moth p.
mucous p.
nitroglycerin transdermal p.
omental p.
opaline p.
pantaloon p.
pericardial p.
peritoneal p.
Peyer p.
pigskin p.
polypropylene intracardiac p.
prosthetic p.
pruritic erythematous p.
salmon p.
sandwich p.
sclerotic calvarial p.
smoker p.
soldier p.
p. stage
subcutaneous defibrillator p.
p. technique

p. testing
p. test scarring
transdermal medication p.
vein p.
venous sheath p.
white p.
wicking glue p.

patch-clamp

patch-graft
p.-g. angioplasty
Dacron onlay p.-g.

patchplasty

patchy
p. colonic ulceration
p. infiltration

patefaction

patella
patellae
p. turndown approach

patellapexy

patellar
p. affection
p. fat pad
p. intra-articular dislocation
p. network
p. retinaculum
p. sleeve fracture
p. tendon graft
p. tendon graft donor site
(PTGDS)
p. tendon repair

patellectomy
partial p.
total p.
West-Soto-Hall p.

patelliform

patellofemoral articulation

Patel medial meniscectomy

patency
biliary stent p.
catheter p.
stent p.
valve p.

patent
p. ductus arteriosus (PDA)
p. iridectomy
p. processus vaginalis
p. vein

Paterson
P. procedure
P. technique

Patey modified radical mastectomy

path
p. of insertion
p. of removal

pathetic

pathologic
p. amputation
p. barrier
p. dislocation
p. fracture
p. perforation
p. retraction ring
p. sphincter

pathological anatomy

pathology
experimental p.
surgical p.

pathomechanics
kyphotic deformity p.
spinal fusion p.

pathostimulation

pathway
coagulation p.
coagulation p.
effector p.
extrapyramidal p.
extrinsic p.
orogastric p.
β-oxidation p.
receptor-mediated endocytosis p.
shunt p.
somatosensory p.

patient
brain-dead p.
endoscopically normal p.
poor-risk p.
p. self-administration device
tube-fed p.

patient-controlled
p.-c. analgesia (PCA)
p.-c. analgesia anesthetic technique
p.-c. anesthesia pump
p.-c. epidural analgesia (PCEA,
PEA)
p.-c. epidural anesthesia
p.-c. intranasal analgesia (PCINA)
p.-c. intravenous anesthesia

Patil-Syracuse mask

patrilineal

pattern
p. arborization
p. of breathing
p. cut corneal graft operation

NOTES

531

pattern *(continued)*
  p. of distribution
  p. of motion
  p. recognition
  p. of staining
pattern-cut corneal graft
patulous
Pauchet procedure
Paufique
  P. keratoplasty
  P. operation
  P. synechiotomy
Pauli exclusion principle
Pauling theory of antibody formation
Paul intestinal drainage tube
Paul-Mikulicz resection
Paul-Mixter tube
Paulos ligament technique
Pauly point
pause-squeeze method
Pauwels
  P. femoral neck fracture
  classification
  P. fracture
  P. proximal osteotomy
  P. technique
  P. valgus osteotomy
  P. Y-osteotomy
Pavlov method
Pavulon
Payne operation
Payr
  P. clamp method
  P. membrane
PBG
  porphobilinogen
PCA
  patient-controlled analgesia
  PCA pump
PCA-plus infusion device
PCEA
  patient-controlled epidural analgesia
PCINA
  patient-controlled intranasal analgesia
PCO$_2$
  partial pressure of carbon dioxide
PC Polygraf HR
PDA
  patent ductus arteriosus
PDPH
  postdural puncture headache
PD root canal post
PDS Vicryl suture
PEA
  patient-controlled epidural analgesia
Peabody-Mitchell bunionectomy
Peabody procedure
PEACH approach

Peacock transposing technique
peak
  p. exercise oxygen consumption
  p. expiratory flow
  p. expiratory flow rate
  p. flowmeter
  p. inspiratory ventilator pressure
  p. pressure analysis
  p. systolic aortic pressure
  p. systolic gradient (PSG)
  p. systolic gradient pressure
  p. transaortic valve gradient
pearl
  cholesteatoma p.
  perineal p.
Pearsall
  P. Chinese twisted suture
  P. silk suture
Pearson product-moment coefficient of correlation
Pecquet
  P. cistern
  P. duct
pecten
  anal p.
  p. analis
  p. band
  p. ossis pubis
  p. pubis
pectinate
  p. body
  p. line
  p. zone
pectineal
  p. ligament
  p. line of pubis
pectineus
pectiniform
  p. septum
pectoral
  p. branch of thoracoacromial artery
  p. fascia
  p. group of axillary lymph nodes
pectoralis
  p. major flap
  p. major myocutaneous flap
  p. myofascial flap
pectorodorsalis muscle
pectorodorsal muscle
pectus
  p. carinatum deformity
  p. excavatum
  p. excavatum deformity
pedes (*pl. of* pes)
Pedialyte
  P. oral electrolyte maintenance solution
  P. RS electrolyte solution

pediatric
- p. airway
- p. analgesic
- p. anesthesia system
- p. anesthetic
- p. circle
- p. colonoscopy
- p. endoscopy
- p. esophagogastroduodenoscopy
- p. feeding tube
- p. hypothermia
- p. mass
- p. nasogastric tube
- p. pain
- p. Racine adapter
- p. radiotherapy anesthesia
- p. surgery
- p. vaginoscopy

pedicel

pedicellation

pedicle
- p. anatomy
- p. of arch of vertebra
- p. bone graft
- p. entrance point
- p. evaluation
- p. fat graft
- Filatov-Gillies tubed p.
- p. flap in mucogingival surgery
- p. flap operation
- p. flap urethroplasty
- p. fracture
- p. groin flap
- p. landmark
- p. localization
- p. method
- portal p.
- p. screw chord length
- p. screw construct
- p. screw hardware prominence
- p. screw insertion
- p. screw path length
- p. screw plating
- p. screw pull-out strength
- p. screw-rod fixation
- vascular p.

pedicled
- p. jejunal reconstruction
- p. myocutaneous flap
- p. omentoplasty

pedicolaminar fracture-dislocation

pedicular fixation

pediculation

pediculus
- p. arcus vertebrae

Pedi PEG tube

pediphalanx

pedodontic endodontics

peduncle
- p. of mamillary body

peduncular loop

pedunculated loose body

pedunculation

pedunculotomy

pedunculus of pineal body

peeling
- membrane p.

PEEP
- positive end-expiratory pressure

PEEP/CPAP
- positive end-expiratory pressure/continuous positive airway pressure

PEEPi
- intrinsic positive end-expiratory pressure

Peet
- P. splanchnic resection
- P. Z-plasty

Pee Wee low-profile gastrostomy tube

PEG
- percutaneous endoscopic gastrostomy
  - PEG insertion
  - PEG tube

peg
- p. bone graft
- fixation p.
- p. flap
- p. and socket technique

PEG-400 tube

peg-and-socket
- p.-a.-s. articulation
- p.-a.-s. joint

peg-in-hole osteotomy

PEI
- percutaneous ethanol injection
  - PEI therapy

Peimer reduction osteotomy

PEJ
- percutaneous endoscopic jejunostomy
  - PEJ tube

pelidnoma

pelioma

peliosis hepatitis

Pell and Gregory classification

NOTES

P

pelma
pelmatic
peltation
pelves (*pl. of* pelvis)
pelvic
    p. abscess
    p. adhesive disease
    p. aspiration biopsy
    p. autonomic nerve preservation
      (PANP)
    p. autonomic plexus
    p. avulsion fracture
    p. axis
    p. brim
    p. canal
    p. cavity
    p. colonic surgery
    p. diaphragm
    p. direction
    p. examination
    p. exenteration
    p. fascia
    p. fixation
    p. floor dysfunction
    p. ganglia
    p. girdle
    p. hematocele
    p. ileal reservoir construction
    p. inclination
    p. infection
    p. inflammation
    p. irradiation
    p. kidney
    p. laparoscopy
    p. limb
    p. lymphadenectomy
    p. lymph node dissection (PLND)
    p. lymphocelectomy
    p. mass
    p. node dissection
    p. osteotomy
    p. part
    p. part of ureter
    p. peritonectomy
    p. peritonectomy with resection of
      sigmoid colon
    p. plane
    p. plane of greatest dimensions
    p. plane of inlet
    p. plane of least dimensions
    p. plane of outlet
    p. plexus
    p. pouch
    p. pouchoscopy
    p. pouch procedure
    p. promontory
    p. relaxation
    p. ring

    p. ring fracture
    p. rotation
    p. sidewall
    p. splanchnic nerve
    p. stimulation
    p. straddle fracture
pelvicaliceal
pelvic-floor surgery
pelvifixation
pelvilithotomy
pelviolithotomy
pelvioplasty
pelvioscopy
pelviotomy
pelvirectal sphincter
pelvis, pl. **pelves**
    android p.
    anthropoid p.
    assimilation p.
    brachypellic p.
    contracted p.
    cordate p.
    Deventer p.
    dolichopellic p.
    dwarf p.
    extrarenal renal p.
    false p.
    flat p.
    funnel-shaped p.
    p. of gallbladder
    greater p.
    gynecoid p.
    heart-shaped p.
    inverted p.
    p. justo major
    p. justo minor
    juvenile p.
    large p.
    lesser p.
    longitudinal oval p.
    p. major
    masculine p.
    mesatipellic p.
    p. minor
    p. nana
    osteomalacic p.
    p. plana
    platypellic p.
    platypelloid p.
    pseudo-osteomalacic p.
    renal p.
    p. renalis
    reniform p.
    Robert p.
    round p.
    small p.
    spider p.
    p. spuria

transverse oval p.
true p.
ureteric p.
p. vera
pelvisacral
pelviscopic
    p. clip ligation technique
    p. intrafascial hysterectomy
pelviscopy
pelvitherm
pelvitomy
pelvivertebral angle
pelvoscopy
Pemberton
    P. acetabuloplasty
    P. operation
    P. pericapsular osteotomy
PEMF
    pulsed electromagnetic field
    PEMF therapy
pemphigoid
pemphigus
penalization
Penaz volume-clamp method
pencil-in-cup deformity
pendemoma
pendulous abdomen
pendulum
    fibroma p.
penectomy
penes (*pl. of* penis)
penetrate
penetrating
    p. corneal transplant
    p. fracture
    p. full-thickness corneal graft
    p. keratoplasty
    p. rupture
    p. trauma
    p. wound
penetration
    p. test
Penfield method
penial
penicillary
penicillate
penicillin G procaine
penicillus
penile
    p. amputation
    p. block
    p. carcinoma

p. deformity
p. erection
p. extensibility
p. incarceration
p. injection testing
p. injection therapy
p. island flap
p. lesion
p. raphe
p. revascularization
p. rupture
p. urethra
p. vein occlusion therapy
p. venous ligation surgery
penile-brachial pressure index
penis, pl. **penes**
    bifid p.
    buried p.
    clubbed p.
    concealed p.
    p. femineus
    p. lunatus
    p. muliebris
    p. palmatus
    webbed p.
penischisis
peniscopy
penitis
Penlon
    P. infant resuscitator
    P. vaporizer
Penn
    P. method
    P. pouch
Pennal classification
pennate muscle
penoid tissue
penoplasty
penoscrotal
    p. transposition
penotomy
Pentacarinat injection
pentadactyl
pentagonal block excision
Pentam-300 injection
pentane excretion level
pentastarch
Pentax EndoNet digital endoscopy network
pentazocine
Penthrane
    P. analgizer

NOTES

pentobarbital
Pentothal
    P. Sodium
pentoxifylline
Peptavlon stimulation test
peptic
    p. aspiration pneumonitis
    p. gland
peptide
    atrial natriuretic p.
    brain natriuretic p. (BNP)
    connective tissue activating p.
    endogenous opioid p.
    fusion p.
per
    p. anum
    p. contiguum
    p. continuum
    p. primam
    p. vias naturales
peraxillary
perceived exertion
perceptual expansion
percolation
Percoll technique
percussion
    hard p.
    p. therapy
percutaneous
    p. abscess drainage (PAD)
    p. access
    p. alcohol injection
    p. anesthetic loss
    p. arterial cannulation
    p. aspiration thromboembolectomy
    p. balloon angioplasty
    p. balloon aortic valvuloplasty
    p. balloon aspiration
    p. balloon dilation
    p. balloon mitral valvuloplasty
    p. balloon pericardiotomy
    p. balloon pulmonic valvuloplasty
    p. bone marrow infection
    p. catheter cecostomy
    p. catheter drainage
    p. catheter insertion
    p. cholecystectomy
    p. cholecystolithotomy
    p. cholecystostomy
    p. cordotomy
    p. coronary rotational atherectomy
    p. corticotomy
    p. CT-guided aspiration
    p. dilatation of biliary duct
    p. dilational tracheostomy
    p. embolization therapy
    p. endofluoroscopy
    p. endopyeloureterotomy

p. endoscopic gastrostomy (PEG)
p. endoscopic gastrostomy tube
p. endoscopic jejunostomy (PEJ)
p. endoscopic placement of jejunal
    tube
p. endoscopic removal
p. endoscopy
p. enterostomy
p. epididymal sperm aspiration
p. ethanol ablation
p. ethanol injection (PEI)
p. ethanol injection therapy
p. fetal cystoscopy
p. fetal tissue sampling
p. fine-needle aspiration
p. fine-needle aspiration biopsy
p. fine-needle pancreatic biopsy
p. fixation
p. gastroenterostomy
p. glycerol rhizolysis
p. injury (PI)
p. intra-aortic balloon
    counterpulsation
p. laser nucleolysis
p. line
p. liver biopsy
p. localization
p. low-stress angioplasty
p. lumbar diskectomy
p. microwave coagulation therapy
p. mitral balloon commissurotomy
p. mitral balloon valvotomy
p. native renal biopsy
p. needle biopsy
p. needle puncture
p. nephrolithotomy
p. nephroscopy
p. nephrostolithotomy
p. nephrostomy
p. nephrostomy tube placement
p. pancreas biopsy
p. patent ductus arteriosus closure
p. pin insertion
p. pinning
p. plantar fasciotomy
p. portocaval anastomosis
p. pressure ureteral perfusion test
p. radical cryosurgical ablation of
    prostate
p. radiofrequency catheter ablation
p. radiofrequency gangliolysis
p. radiofrequency rhizolysis
p. radiofrequency rhizotomy
p. reduction
p. renal puncture
p. retrogasserian glycerol
    chemoneurolysis
p. retrogasserian glycerol rhizolysis

p. rotational thrombectomy
p. sampling method
p. stimulation
p. stone removal
p. technique
p. tenotomy
p. transatrial mitral commissurotomy
p. transcatheter therapy
p. transhepatic approach
p. transhepatic biliary procedure
p. transhepatic cardiac catheterization
p. transhepatic cholangioscopy
p. transhepatic cholecystoscopy
p. transhepatic obliteration
p. transhepatic obliteration of esophageal varix
p. transluminal angioscopy
p. transluminal balloon valvuloplasty
p. transluminal coronary angioplasty (PTCA)
p. transluminal coronary revascularization
p. transluminal renal angioplasty
p. transtracheal jet ventilation (PTV)
p. transvenous mitral commissurotomy
p. tumor ablation
p. venoablation

Pereyra
P. bladder neck suspension
P. needle suspension
P. procedure

Pereyra-Lebhertz modification
Pereyra-Raz cystourethropexy
perflation
perfluorochemical (PFC)
perforans
perforated space
perforating
p. abscess
p. arteries of internal mammary
p. branches of internal thoracic artery
p. canal of Zuckerkandl
p. keratoplasty
p. wound
perforation
appendiceal p.

bladder p.
bowel p.
cardiac p.
p. of colon
colon p.
colonic p.
corneal p.
cortical p.
ductal system p.
duodenal p.
esophageal p.
gallbladder p.
p. of gallbladder
gastric p.
guidewire p.
ileal p.
inflammatory p.
intestinal p.
intraperitoneal p.
lateral p.
mechanical p.
myocardial p.
nasal septal p.
Niemeier gallbladder p.
operative p.
p. osteotomy
pathologic p.
peritoneal p.
prepyloric p.
retroduodenal p.
retroperitoneal p.
root p.
sealing p.
septal p.
strip p.
sublabial p.
tooth p.
ureteral p.
uterine p.
vascular p.
ventricular p.
perforative lesion
perfrigeration
perfusate
p. solution
perfusion
cerebral p.
continuous hyperthermic peritoneal p.
distal p.
extracorporeal liver p.
ex vivo p.

NOTES

P

perfusion *(continued)*
    p. flow rate
    p. hypothermia technique
    hypothermic p.
    intraperitoneal hyperthermic p.
    isolated limb p. (ILP)
    Langendorff p.
    p. measurement technique
    organ p.
    p. O ring
    p. pressure
    superficial renal cortical p. (SRCP)
    p. therapy
    tissue p.
perfusion/ventilation
pergolide dopaminergic medication
periadvential tissue
periampullary
    p. carcinoma
    p. mass
perianal
    p. anorectal space
    p. condyloma
    p. fistula
    p. fistula abscess
    p. hematoma
    p. infection
    p. lesion
perianesthetic thermoregulation
perianeurysmal hemorrhage
periangiocholitis
periaortic mediastinal hematoma
periaortitis
periapical
    p. curettage
    p. infection
    p. pressure
    p. surgery
    p. tissue
    p. tooth repair
periappendiceal abscess
periappendicitis
periappendicular
periarterial
    p. plexus
    p. plexus of maxillary artery
    p. plexus of vertebral artery
    p. sympathectomy
periarticular
    p. fluid collection
    p. fracture
    p. tissue
periauricular
periaxial
periaxillary
peribronchial
peribronchiolar
    p. lymphocyte infiltration

peribuccal
peribulbar
    p. anesthesia
    p. anesthetic technique
    p. injection
peribursal
pericallosal artery
pericanalicular
    p. connective tissue
pericapsular
    p. fat infiltration
    p. osteotomy
pericardectomy
pericardiacophrenic
    p. artery
    p. veins
pericardial
    p. biopsy
    p. branch of phrenic nerve
    p. branch of thoracic aorta
    p. decompression
    p. fat pad
    p. flap
    p. fluid examination
    p. hematoma
    p. patch
    p. pressure
    p. puncture
    p. reflex
    p. sac
    p. veins
    p. window
pericardiectomy
    parietal p.
    thoracoscopic p.
    visceral p.
pericardiocentesis
pericardioplasty in pectus excavatum repair
pericardiorrhaphy
pericardioscopy
pericardiostomy
pericardiotomy
    percutaneous balloon p.
    subxiphoid limited p.
    p. syndrome
pericarditis
pericardium externum
pericardotomy
pericecal
pericholecystic fluid collection
perichondral
    p. circulation
    p. ring
perichondrium
perichoroidal
    p. space

pericolic
 p. membrane syndrome
pericolonitis
pericolostomy area
pericorneal plexus
pericoronal flap
pericostal suture
pericranial
 p. temporalis flap
pericranium
pericystic
pericystitis
pericystium
peridectomy
peridental
 p. ligament
 p. membrane
 p. space
peridentinoblastic space
peridesmic
peridesmium
peridiaphragmatic hematoma
perididymis
perididymitis
peridural
 p. anesthesia
perienteric
periependymal
periesophageal
periesophagogastric lymph node
 metastasis
perifascial nephrectomy
Periflux 3 laser-Doppler flowmetry
periganglionic
perigastric
perigenicular vascular injury
perigraft hematoma
Peri-Guard vascular graft
perihepatic
 p. space
perihernial
peri-implant
 p.-i. space
 p.-i. tissue
peri-implantation
perilaryngeal
periligamentous
perilimbal suction
perilobular connective tissue
perilunar transscaphoid dislocation

perilunate
 p. carpal dislocation
 p. fracture-dislocation
perilymphatic
 p. duct
 p. fistula
 p. space
perilymph fistula
perimesencephalic cistern
perimeter
 p. corneal reflex test
 p. projection
perimetric
perimetrium
perimyelis
perimylolysis
perinatal
 p. infection
 p. torsion
perineal
 p. abscess
 p. analgesia
 p. anesthesia
 p. artery
 p. body
 p. defect
 p. flap
 p. flexure of rectum
 p. hernia
 p. impact trauma
 p. incision
 p. infection
 p. laceration
 p. lithotomy
 p. membrane
 p. muscles
 p. nerve
 p. nerve terminal motor latency
  test
 p. pearl
 p. polyp
 p. post
 p. prostatectomy
 p. raphe
 p. region
 p. repair
 p. scar
 p. section
 p. sinus
 p. sinus tract
 p. spaces
 p. urethrostomy

NOTES

P

539

perineal *(continued)*
    p. urethrotomy
    p. urinary fistula
perineocele
perineoplasty
perineorrhaphy
    vaginal p.
perineoscrotal
perineostomy
perineosynthesis
perineotomy
perineovaginal
    p. fistula
perinephrial
perinephric
    p. abscess
    p. fluid collection
    p. hematoma
    p. space hemorrhage
    p. tissue
perinephritis
perinephrium
perineum
perineural
    p. anesthesia
    p. infiltration
    p. invasion
    p. tissue
perineurial neurorrhaphy
perineurium
perinodal tissue
perinuclear
    p. cisterna
    p. space
periocular
    p. injection
periodic respiration
periodontal
    p. flap
    p. inflammation
    p. lesion
    p. ligament
    p. ligament anesthesia
    p. membrane
    p. membrane necrosis
    p. ostectomy
    p. therapy
periodontolysis
periomphalic
perioperative
    p. antibiotic therapy
    p. corneal abrasion
    p. reduction
perioptic subarachnoid space
periorbital
    p. infection
    p. membrane
periost

periostea (*pl. of* periosteum)
periosteal
    p. elevation
    p. flap
    p. graft
    p. implantation
    p. layer of dura mater
    p. new bone formation
    p. tissue
periosteoma
periosteophyte
periosteotomy
periosteous
periosteum, pl. periostea
    p. cranii
periostoma
periotic bone
peripartum endoscopy
peripenial
peripharyngeal
    p. space
peripheral
    p. access system (PAS)
    p. aneurysm
    p. arterial aneurysmal disease
    p. arterial line
    p. balloon angioplasty
    p. capillary filtration slit length
    p. cavity wall
    p. chemoreflex loop
    p. circulation
    p. extremity edema
    p. fusion
    p. intravenous alimentation
    p. iridectomy
    p. iridectomy operation
    p. laser angioplasty
    p. lesion
    p. lymphoid tissue
    p. nerve block
    p. nerve block anesthesia
    p. nerve block anesthetic technique
    p. panretinal ablation
    p. pressure
    p. segment of lung tissue resection
    p. tissue
    p. vascular surgery
    p. venous cannulation
peripherally inserted central catheter (PICC)
periporoma
periportal
    p. sinusoidal dilation
periproctic
periprostatic
    p. tissue
periprostatitis
periprosthetic fracture

peripylephlebitis
peripylic
peripyloric
perirectal
    p. abscess
    p. inflammation
    p. mass
    p. pelvic dissection
perirenal
    p. fascia
    p. hematoma
    p. insufflation
    p. space
perisalpinx
periscleral space
perisellar vascular lesion
perisinusoidal space
perisplanchnic
perisplenic
perispondylic
peristasis
peristomal infection
peritarsal network
peritectomy
peritendineum
perithelioma
perithoracic
peritomist
peritomy
peritoneal
    p. access
    p. adenocarcinoma
    p. adhesion
    p. anatomy
    p. aspiration
    p. band
    p. biopsy
    p. cancer
    p. carcinomatosis
    p. cavity
    p. cavity abscess
    p. cavity fluid
    p. cytology
    p. defect
    p. dialysis
    p. encapsulation
    p. envelope
    p. equilibration test
    p. fluid examination
    p. fossae
    p. friction rub
    p. fungal infection

    p. hernia
    p. insufflation
    p. lavage
    p. membrane permeability
    p. metastasis
    p. mouse
    p. patch
    p. perforation
    p. reconstruction
    p. reflection
    p. sac
    p. seeding
    p. soilage
    p. space
    p. spill
    p. studding
    p. tap
    p. toilet
    p. transfusion
    p. tuberculosis
    p. vein
    p. villi
    p. washing
    p. washout
    p. window
peritonectomy
    left upper quadrant p.
    pelvic p.
    right upper quadrant p.
peritoneocentesis
peritoneoclysis
peritoneopericardial
    p. diaphragmatic hernia
peritoneopexy
peritoneoplasty
peritoneoscopy
peritoneotomy
    inverted-V p.
peritoneovenous shunt patency scan
peritoneum
    parietal p.
    p. parietale
    visceral p.
    p. viscerale
peritonitis
    adhesive p.
peritonsillar
    p. space
peritracheal
peritrochanteric
    p. fracture
perityphlic

NOTES

periumbilical
    p. incision
    p. port
periureteral
    p. abscess
periureteric venous ring
periurethral
    p. abscess
periurethritis
periuterine
perivascular
    p. canal
    p. mass
    p. space
peri-Vaterian therapeutic endoscopic procedure
periventricular
    p. hyperintense lesion
    p. white matter lesion
periventricular-intraventricular hemorrhage
perivertebral
perivesical
perivisceral
perivitelline space
Perkins vertical line
Per-Lee
    P.-L. equalizing tube
    P.-L. myringotomy tube
    P.-L. ventilation tube
Perlon suture
Perma-Flow coronary graft
Perma-Hand braided silk suture
permanent
    p. end colostomy
    p. loop ileostomy
    p. pacemaker placement
    p. pedicle flap
    p. restoration
    p. section
    p. stoma
Permapen injection
permeability
    membrane p.
    peritoneal membrane p.
permeation
    analgesia p.
    lymphatic p.
permissive hypercapnia
permutation
perone
peroneal
    p. artery
    p. brevis tendon
    p. communicating nerve
    p. compartment syndrome
    p. dislocation
    p. groove

p. longus tendon
p. muscle
p. muscle atrophy
p. nerve entrapment
p. nerve injury
p. phenomenon
p. pulley
p. retinaculum
p. somatosensory evoked potential
p. spastic flatfoot
p. tendon
p. tendon sheath injection
p. vein
peroncus
    p. brevis muscle
    p. longus muscle
    p. tertius muscle
peroral
    p. approach
    p. cholangiopancreatoscopy
    p. cholangioscopy
    p. endoscopy
    p. esophageal dilation
    p. intestinal biopsy
    p. maneuver
    p. pancreatoscopy
perpendicular plane
Perry
    P. extensile anterior approach
    P. technique
Perry-Nickel technique
Perry-O'Brien-Hodgson technique
Perry-Robinson cervical technique
perseveration
    infantile p.
    motor p.
persistent
    p. anovulation
    p. common atrioventricular canal
    p. fetal circulation
    p. müllerian duct syndrome
    p. occiput posterior position
    p. ovarian mass
    p. tolerant infection
personality formation
personal space
perspective
    surgical p.
perspiratory glands
Perthes
    P. incision
    P. lesion
    P. procedure
    P. test
Pertrach percutaneous tracheostomy tube
pertubation
    hemodynamic p.

PES
pacing esophageal stethoscope
pes, pl. **pedes**
p. planus deformity
pessary
Blair modification of Gellhorn p.
blue ring p.
cup p.
prolapse ring p.
ring p.
PET
positron emission tomography
PETCO$_2$
extrapolated end-tidal carbon dioxide tension
petechia, pl. **petechiae**
petechial hemorrhage
Peter operation
Peters anomaly
PET-guided biopsy
Petit
P. aponeurosis
P. canal
P. hernia
P. herniotomy
P. ligament
P. lumbar triangle
petroccipital
petromastoid
petro-occipital
p.-o. fissure
p.-o. joint
petropharyngeus
petrosa
petrosal
p. approach
p. bone
p. branch of middle meningeal artery
p. foramen
p. fossa
p. fossula
p. ganglion
p. sinus
p. vein
petrosalpingostaphylinus
petrositis
petrosomastoid
petrosphenoid
petrosquamosal

petrosquamous
p. fissure
p. suture
petrostaphylinus
petrotympanic
p. fissure
p. suture
petrous
p. carotid-to-intradural carotid saphenous vein graft
p. part of temporal bone
p. pyramid
p. pyramid air cell exploration
p. pyramid exenteration
p. pyramid fracture
petrousitis
Peustow procedure
Peyer
P. glands
P. patch
Peyeyra-Lebhertz modification of Frangenheim-Stoeckel procedure
Peyman
P. full-thickness eye-wall resection
P. iridocyclochoroidectomy
Peyronie disease
Peyrot thorax
Pfannenstiel
P. incision
P. transverse approach
PFC
perfluorochemical
Pfeiffer-Comberg method
Pfiffner and Myers method
Pfizerpen-AS injection
Pfizerpen injection
PGE2
exogenous P.
PGE1 injection
pH
p. electrode placement
esophageal p.
intramural p.
phacocele
phacocystectomy
phacoemulsification
Alcon p.
phacoexcavation
phacofragmentation
phacoglaucoma
phacolysis
phacoma

NOTES

P

phacomatosis
phacoscopy
phagocyte migration
phagolysis
phako-anaphylactic-endophthalmitis
phakoemulsification
phakoma
phakomatosis
phalangeal
    p. articular orientation
    p. diaphyseal fracture
    p. dislocation
    p. fracture fixation
    p. malunion correction
    p. osteotomy
phalangealization
phalangectomy
    intermediate p.
phalangization
phalanx, pl. phalanges
Phalen
    P. maneuver
    P. position
phallalgia
phallectomy
phallic
phalliform
phallitis
phallocampsis
phallocrypsis
phallodynia
phalloid
phalloncus
phalloplasty
phallotomy
phallus
Phaneuf-Graves repair
phantasmoscopia, phantasmoscopy
phantasmoscopy
    phantasmoscopia, p.
phantom
    p. aneurysm
    p. foot pain
    p. limb
    p. limb pain
pharmacodynamics
pharmacologic
    p. manipulation
    p. method of purging
pharmacologically
    p. induced erection
    p. induced paralysis
pharyngeal
    p. airway
    p. anesthesia
    p. branch of descending palatine artery
    p. branches

    p. branch of glossopharyngeal nerve
    p. branch of inferior thyroid artery
    p. branch of pterygopalatine ganglion
    p. branch of vagus nerve
    p. canal
    p. exudate
    p. flap
    p. fornix
    p. glands
    p. gonococcal infection
    p. hypophysis
    p. mucosa
    p. plexus
    p. plexus neurectomy
    p. pouch
    p. pouch syndrome
    p. raphe
    p. ridge
    p. space
    p. tissue
    p. tubercle
    p. veins
    p. wall carcinoma
pharyngectomy
pharyngei
pharynges (pl. of pharynx)
pharyngeus
pharyngobasilar fascia
pharyngocutaneous fistula
pharyngoepiglottic
    p. fold
pharyngoesophageal
    p. diverticulectomy
    p. reconstruction
pharyngoesophagogastroduodenoscopy
pharyngoesophagoplasty
pharyngoglossal
pharyngoglossus
pharyngolaryngeal
pharyngolaryngectomy
pharyngomaxillary
    p. space
pharyngonasal
    p. cavity
pharyngo-oral
pharyngopalatine
pharyngopalatinus
pharyngoplasty
    Hynes p.
    Wardill p.
pharyngoscleroma
pharyngoscopy
pharyngostaphylinus
pharyngostoma
pharyngotomy
    transhyoid p.

pharyngotympanic
>p. groove
>p. tube

pharynx, pl. **pharynges**
>laryngeal p.
>nasal p.
>oral p.

phase
>eclipse p.
>ejection p.
>end-expiratory p.
>excitement p.
>exponential p.
>extradural p.
>granulation p.
>p. I, II block
>implantation p.
>maturation p.
>presensitization p.
>prolonged expiratory p.
>reservoir p.
>transverse magnetization p.
>vector p.

phase-encoding direction
phase-sensitive gradient-echo MR
imaging
PHCA
>profoundly hypothermic circulatory arrest

Pheasant elbow technique
Phelps
>P. neurectomy
>P. partial resection
>P. scapulectomy

Phemister
>P. acromioclavicular pin fixation
>P. medial approach to tibia
>P. onlay bone graft
>P. onlay bone graft technique

Phemister-Bonfiglio technique
phenacaine
>p. hydrochloride

Phenazine injection
phenazopyridine hydrochloride
Phenergan injection
phenobarbital
phenol
>camphorated p.
>p. cauterization
>2,6-diisopropyl p.
>p. matrixectomy

phenol-preserved extract

phenomenon
>Ascher glass-rod p.
>common cavity p.
>declamping p.
>doll's head p.
>entry p.
>extinction p.
>extravasation p.
>glass-rod negative p.
>glass-rod positive p.
>Goldblatt p.
>hesitation p.
>identification p.
>misdirection p.
>modified Raynaud p.
>peroneal p.
>referred trigger point p.
>relaxation p.
>steal p.
>temporary cavity p.
>tip-of-the-tongue p.
>truncation p.
>yo-yo weight fluctuation p.

phenozygous
phenylcarbinol
phenylephrine
phenylethylbarbituric acid
phenylethylmalonylurea
pheochromoblastoma
pheochromocytoma
phimosis
phimotic
phlebectomy
>greater saphenous p.

phlebitis
phlebolite
phlebolith
phlebophlebostomy
phlebophthalmotomy
phleboplasty
phleborrhagia
phleborrhaphy
phleborrhexis
phlebostasis
phlebostrepsis
phlebotomy
>bloodless p.
>therapeutic p.

phlegmon
phlegmonous
>p. abscess
>p. mass

NOTES

P

Phocas syndrome
phonation
    hypervalvular p.
    maximum duration of p.
    myoelastic-aerodynamic theory of p.
    neurochronaxic theory of p.
    reverse p.
    ventricular p.
    voice disorders of p.
phonoscopy
phorbol dibutyrate
phosphate
    p. buffered saline solution
    p. excretion index
phosphotope oral solution
phosphotungstic acid-magnesium chloride
  precipitation method
photic stimulation
photoablation
    laser p.
photoactivation
photocarbonization
photocoagulation
    argon laser p.
    infrared p.
    laser p.
    macular p.
    panretinal argon laser p.
    retinal scatter p.
    scatter p.
    in situ p.
    transendoscopic laser p.
    p. treatment
    xenon arc p.
photocoreoplasty
photodisintegration
photodissociation
photodocumentation
photoexcitation
photography
    cross-polarization p.
    endoscopic p.
    laparoscopic p.
photoinactivation
photoirradiation
photolysis
    flash p.
photon-deficient bone lesion
photo-onycholysis
photo-patch
photophore
photo-protection
photoradiation therapy
photorefractive
    p. keratectomy
    p. keratoplasty
photoresection

photoscopy
phototherapeutic keratectomy
photothermolysis
    selective p.
photovaporization
    laser p.
phren
phrencctomy
phrenemphraxis
phrenic
    p. ganglia
    p. nerve
    p. nerve block
    p. nerve block anesthetic technique
    p. pleura
    p. plexus
    p. veins
phrenicectomy
phreniclasia
phrenicoabdominal branch of phrenic
  nerve
phrenicocolic
    p. ligament
phrenicocostal sinus
phrenicoexeresis
phrenicogastric
phrenicoglottic
phrenicohepatic
phrenicolienal ligament
phrenicomediastinal recess
phreniconeurectomy
phrenicopleural fascia
phrenicosplenic
    p. ligament
phrenicotomy
phrenicotripsy
phrenocolic
phrenocolopexy
phrenoesophageal membrane
phrenogastric
    p. ligament
phrenohepatic
phrenosplenic ligament
phrictopathic
phrygian
    p. cap
    p. cap deformity
physeal
    p. fracture
    p. line
physical
    p. barrier
    p. capacity evaluation
    p. examination
    p. manipulation
    p. restoration
    p. therapy

Physick
P. operation
P. pouch
physicochemical basis of gallstone formation
physiologic
p. barrier
p. excavation
p. mesial migration
p. pattern release
p. position of rest
p. rest position
p. retraction ring
p. saline solution
p. salt solution
physiological
p. dead space
p. dead space ventilation per minute
p. sphincter
physiology
exercise p.
physiolysis
central p.
physis
physocele
PI
percutaneous injury
pial-glial membrane
piano-wire adhesion
PICC
peripherally inserted central catheter
PICC line
Pichlmayer
P. method
P. procedure
P. technique
Pick bundle
Pickerill
P. imbrication line
imbrication lines of P.
pickling solution
pickup spatula suture
PiCO$_2$
partial pressure of intramuscular carbon dioxide
Pico operation
Picot incision
picrotoxin
picture frame vertebra
pie-crusting skin graft
Piedmont fracture

Pierce antrum wash tube
Pierrot-Murphy
P.-M. advancement insertion
P.-M. tendon technique
Piersol point
piezoelectric lithotripsy
pigeon-breast deformity
piggyback liver transplantation
pigment
p. cell transplantation
p. epithelial lesion
p. induration of lung
pigmentary
p. demarcation line
p. migration
pigmented
p. layer of ciliary body
p. lesion
p. line of cornea
pigskin
p. graft
p. patch
pigtail
p. fixation
p. nephrostomy tube
pileus
pili (*pl. of* pilus)
pilimiction
pillar of soft palate
Pilling duralite tube
pillion fracture
pillow fracture
pilocarpine iontophoresis method
piloerection
pilojection
piloleiomyoma
pilomatricoma
pilomatrixoma
pilon ankle fracture
pilonidal
p. cystectomy
p. fistula
pilot application
pilus, pl. pili
arrector p.
pimobendan
pin
cranial p.'s
p. and plaster fixation
p. and plaster method
p. retention
p. site

NOTES

P

547

pin *(continued)*
　　p. suture
　　p. track
　　p. tract infection
Pinard maneuver
pin-bone interface
pincer nail
pinch
　　p. biopsy
　　p. restoration
　　p. skin graft
pin-cushion distortion
pineal
　　p. body
　　p. eye
　　p. gland
　　p. recess
　　p. region
　　p. teratocarcinoma
pinealcytoma
pinealectomy
pinealoblastoma
pinealocytoma
pinealoma
pineoblastoma
pineocytoma
ping-pong
　　p.-p. ball deformity
　　p.-p. fracture
piniform
pin-index safety system
pink
　　p. frothy sputum
　　p. twisted cotton suture
pinning
　　closed p.
　　hip p.
　　Knowles p.
　　open p.
　　percutaneous p.
　　Sherk-Probst percutaneous p.
　　Sofield p.
　　Wagner closed p.
pinpoint electrocoagulation
pinprick
　　p. method
pin-supported
　　p.-s. restoration
pinworm preparation
Pin-X
pipe bone
pipecuronium
　　p. bromide
Pipelle biopsy
piperocaine hydrochloride
pipette
Pipkin
　　P. classification of femoral fracture

　　P. posterior hip dislocation
　　　classification
　　P. subclassification of Epstein-
　　　Thomas classification
Pirie bone
piriform
　　p. fossa
　　p. muscle
　　p. recess
　　p. sinus
piriformis muscle
piritramide
Pirogoff
　　P. amputation
　　P. angle
　　P. triangle
piroxicam
pisiform
　　p. bone
　　p. fracture
pit
　　p. of atlas for dens
　　costal p. of transverse process
　　p. and fissure cavity
　　gastric p.
　　granular p.'s
　　herniation p.
　　inferior articular p. of atlas
　　inferior costal p.
　　nail p.
　　pterygoid p.
　　p. of stomach
　　sublingual p.
　　superior costal p.
　　suprameatal p.
Pitocin
　　P. augmentation
　　P. induction
Pitressin injection
pitted
　　p. keratolysis
　　p. nail
pitting
　　p. of nail
　　nail p.
Pitt talking tracheostomy tube
pituicytoma
pituitary
　　p. ablation
　　p. adenoma
　　p. body
　　p. endocrine disorder
　　p. fossa
　　p. gland
　　p. gland transplantation
　　p. microadenoma
　　p. stalk section
　　p. tumor

pituitous
pivot
    p. joint
    p. point
Pizzolato peroxide-silver method
place
    p. of articulation
    4-p. laminectomy
placebo therapy
placement
    bone graft p.
    clip p.
    dilator p.
    electrode p.
    endoscopic biliary stent p.
    endotracheal tube p.
    feeding tube p.
    five-port "fan" p.
    four-port "diamond" p.
    graft p.
    implant p.
    Kirschner wire p.
    K-wire p.
    long-term central venous access
      catheter p.
    percutaneous nephrostomy tube p.
    permanent pacemaker p.
    pH electrode p.
    plate p.
    posterolateral bone graft p.
    radiologic biliary stent p.
    rod p.
    sacral screw p.
    temporary pacemaker p.
    tube p.
    ureteral stent p.
    variable screw p.
    wire-guided p.
placenta, pl. **placentae**
    endotheliochorial p.
    endothelio-endothelial p.
    extrachorial p.
    premature separation of p.
placental
    p. barrier
    p. circulation
    p. extrusion
    p. fragment
    p. hemangioma syndrome
    p. hemorrhage
    p. implantation
    p. localization

    p. membrane
    p. metastasis
    p. migration
    p. respiration
    p. tissue
    p. tissue transplant
    p. transfer
    p. uptake
placentation bleeding
placentoma
placido ring
placoid pigmentation of epithelium
pladaroma
plafond fracture
plagiocephaly
plain
    p. catgut suture
    Citanest P.
    p. collagen suture
    p. gut suture
plana (*pl. of* planum)
plane
    Aeby p.
    alveolar point-meatus p.
    anatomic p.
    auriculo-infraorbital p.
    axial p.
    axiobuccolingual p.
    axiolabiolingual p.
    axiomesiodistal p.
    base p.
    bite p.
    Broca visual p.
    buccolingual p.
    Camper p.
    cleavage p.
    coronal p.
    cove p.
    cusp p.
    datum p.
    Daubenton p.
    diffuse p.
    p. of dissection
    equatorial p.
    equivalent refracting p.
    eye-ear p.
    facet p.
    facial p.
    fascial p.
    fat p.
    first parallel pelvic p.
    flexion-extension p.

NOTES

P

549

plane *(continued)*
  focal p.
  fourth parallel pelvic p.
  Frankfort horizontal p.
  French p.
  frontal p.
  guide p.
  guiding p.
  Hensen p.
  His p.
  Hodge p.
  horizontal p.
  p. of incidence
  p. of inlet
  internervous p.
  interspinal p.
  intertubercular p.
  ischiorectal fossa p.
  p. joint
  labiolingual p.
  p. of least pelvic dimensions
  lens p.
  Listing p.
  Ludwig p.
  mandibular p.
  mean foundation p.
  median sagittal p.
  mesiodistal p.
  midcoronal p.
  midfrontal p.
  p. of midpelvis
  midsagittal p.
  midthalamic p.
  Morton p.
  nodal p.
  nuchal p.
  oblique coronal p.
  occipital p.
  occlusal p.
  p. of occlusion
  orbital p.
  orthogonal p.
  p. of outlet
  paramedian sagittal p.
  parasagittal p.
  pelvic p.
  p. of pelvic canal
  pelvic p. of greatest dimensions
  pelvic p. of inlet
  pelvic p. of least dimensions
  pelvic p. of outlet
  perpendicular p.
  preglenoid p.
  primary movement p.
  principal p.
  sagittal p.
  scan p.

  second parallel pelvic p.
  sensitive p.
  short-axis p.
  slant of occlusal p.
  spectacle p.
  spinous p.
  sternal p.
  sternoxiphoid p.
  subcostal p.
  subpectoral p.
  supracrestal p.
  supracristal p.
  suprasternal p.
  p. suture
  symmetry p.
  temporal p.
  terminal p.
  thalamic p.
  third parallel pelvic p.
  thoracic p.
  tooth p.
  transaxial scan p.
  transpyloric p.
  transtubercular p.
  transverse p.
  varus-valgus p.
  vertical p.
  visual p.
  wide p.
planimetry
planithorax
planned
  p. awakening
  p. extracapsular cataract extraction
planning
  image-integrated surgery
  treatment p.
planta, pl. **plantae**
  p. pedis
plantar
  p. angulation
  p. approach
  p. aspect
  p. compartmental anatomy
  p. condylectomy
  p. fasciotomy
  p. flexion-inversion deformity
  p. interosseous muscle
  p. longitudinal incision
  p. plate release
  p. pressure
  p. quadrate muscle
  p. space
  p. tendon sheath of peroneus
    longus muscle
  p. venous network
plantar-hindfoot-midfoot bony mass

plantaris
  p. muscle
  p. tendon graft
planum, pl. **plana**
  p. interspinale
  p. intertuberculare
  normolipemic xanthoma p.
  p. occipitale
  p. sphenoidale
  p. sternale
  p. subcostale
  p. supracristale
  p. temporale
  p. transpyloricum
  xanthoma p.
planuria
planus
  Anderson-Fowler anterior calcaneal
    osteotomy for pes p.
  condyloma p.
  Gleich osteotomy for pes valgo p.
  oral condyloma p.
  Selakovich procedure for pes
    valgo p.
plaque
  atheromatous p.
  augmentation p.
  echogenic p.
  echolucent p.
  eczematoid pruritic p.
  p. fracture
  p. incision
  neuritic p.
  Randall p.'s
  p. rupture
  senile p.
  p. technique
plaque-like lesion
plaquing
plasma
  p. cell portal infiltration
  p. colloid osmotic pressure
  p. exchange
  expanded p.
  extracellular p.
  p. gastrin concentration
  p. iron concentration
  p. membrane
  p. norepinephrine concentration
  p. oncotic pressure
  p. renin concentration

  p. TFE vascular graft
  p. thrombin clot method
  p. urea concentration
  p. volume expansion
plasmacytoma
Plasmalyte
  P. A
  P. solution
plasma-resistant fiber oxygenator
plasmin coagulation
plasmocytoma
plasmolysis
plaster
  p. cast application burn
  closing wedge manipulation and
    reapplication of p.
  opening wedge manipulation and
    reapplication of p.
plastic
  p. bowing fracture
  p. induration
  p. matrix technique
  p. operation
  p. repair
  p. repair of eyelid
  p. section
  p. sewing ring
  p. stent occlusion
  p. surgery
  p. suture
  p. wedge
plastic-cuffed tracheostomy tube
plasticity
  connective tissue p.
plastron
plasty
  Coleman p.
  Durham p.
  endoventricular circular patch p.
  Foley Y-V p.
  mons p.
  posterior bladder flap p.
  rotation p.
  skin p.
  sliding p.
  V-Y p.
  Y-V p.
plate
  p. fixation
  p. placement
  p. spacer washer

NOTES

P

plateau
    alveolar p.
    p. method
platelet concentrates
plate-screw
    p.-s. fixation
    p.-s. osteosynthesis
plating
    compression p.
    pedicle screw p.
Platou osteotomy
platybasia
platycephaly
platycrania
platyhieric
platymeric
platyopia
platyopic
platypellic
    p. pelvis
platypelloid
    p. pelvis
platyrrhine
platyrrhiny
platysma
    p. muscle
    p. myocutaneous flap
platyspondylia
platystencephaly
Pleatman
    P. pouch
    P. sac
pledgeted
    p. Ethibond suture
    p. mattress suture
pledget suture
pleoptics
    Bangerter method of p.
    Cüppers method of p.
plethysmograph
plethysmography
    forearm p.
    impedance p.
    Respitrace p.
    venous-occlusion volume p.
    volume p.
pleura, pl. pleurae
    cervical p.
    costal p.
    p. costalis
    diaphragmatic p.
    p. diaphragmatica
    mediastinal p.
    p. mediastinalis
    parietal p.
    p. parietalis
    p. pericardiaca
    phrenic p.

    p. phrenica
    p. pulmonalis
    pulmonary p.
    visceral p.
    p. visceralis
pleuracentesis
pleuracotomy
pleurae (*pl. of* pleura)
pleural
    p. biopsy
    p. calculus
    p. cavity
    p. cupula
    p. fluid
    p. fluid aspiration
    p. fluid collection
    p. fluid examination
    p. lines
    p. mass
    p. recesses
    p. sac
    p. sinuses
    p. space
    p. symphysis
    p. tube
    p. villi
pleurapophysis
pleurectomy
    thorascopic apical p.
Pleur-evac
    P.-e. suction
    P.-e. suction tube
pleurisy
pleurobiliary fistula
pleurocele
pleurocentesis
pleurocentrum
pleuroclysis
pleurodesis
    talc p.
pleuroesophageal
    p. fistula
    p. line
    p. muscle
pleurolith
pleuroparietopexy
pleuropericardial
pleuropericarditis
pleuroperitoneal
    p. canal
    p. fold
    p. foramen
    p. hernia
    p. hiatus
    p. shunting
pleuropneumonectomy
pleuropulmonary
pleuroscopy

pleurotomy
pleurovisceral
plexectomy
plexiform
 p. external layer
 p. lesion
Plexiglas graft
plexus, pl. **plexuses**
 abdominal aortic p.
 p. of anterior cerebral artery
 p. aorticus abdominalis
 p. aorticus thoracicus
 p. arteriae cerebri anterioris
 p. arteriae cerebri mediae
 ascending pharyngeal p.
 Auerbach p.
 p. auricularis posterior
 autonomic plexuses
 p. autonomici
 p. axillaris
 axillary p.
 basilar p.
 p. basilaris
 Batson p.
 brachial p.
 p. brachialis
 cardiac p.
 p. cardiacus
 p. cardiacus profundus
 p. cardiacus superficialis
 p. caroticus communis
 p. caroticus externus
 p. caroticus internus
 p. cavernosi concharum
 p. cavernosus
 cavernous p. of clitoris
 cavernous p. of penis
 celiac (lymphatic) p.
 celiac (nervous) p.
 p. celiacus
 cervical p.
 p. cervicalis
 choroid p.
 p. of choroid artery
 p. choroideus
 coccygeal p.
 p. coccygeus
 common carotid p.
 p. coronarius cordis
 coronary p.
 Cruveilhier p.
 deep cardiac p.

deferential p.
p. deferentialis
enteric p.
p. entericus
esophageal p.
p. esophageus
Exner p.
external carotid p.
external iliac p.
external maxillary p.
extrapancreatic nerve p.
facial p.
femoral p.
p. femoralis
gastric plexuses of autonomic
 system
p. gastrici systematis autonomici
gastroesophageal variceal p.
p. gulae
Haller p.
Heller p.
hemorrhoidal p.
hepatic p.
p. hepaticus
p. hypogastricus inferior
p. hypogastricus superior
iliac p.
p. iliaci
p. iliacus externus
inferior hemorrhoidal plexuses
inferior hypogastric p.
inferior mesenteric p.
inferior rectal plexuses
inferior thyroid p.
inferior vesical p.
inguinal p.
p. inguinalis
intermesenteric p.
p. intermesentericus
internal carotid (nervous) p.
internal carotid venous p.
internal mammary p.
internal maxillary p.
internal thoracic p.
internal thoracic lymphatic p.
intracavernous p.
p. intraparotideus
intraparotid p. of facial nerve
ischiadic p.
Jacques p.
jugular p.
p. jugularis

NOTES

P

plexus *(continued)*
  p. lesion
  p. lienalis
  lingual p.
  p. lingualis
  p. lumbalis
  lumbar p.
  lumbosacral p.
  p. lumbosacralis
  lymphatic p.
  p. lymphaticus
  p. mammarius
  p. mammarius internus
  mammary p.
  p. maxillaris externus
  Meissner p.
  meningeal p.
  p. meningeus
  p. mesentericus inferior
  p. mesentericus superior
  p. of middle cerebral artery
  middle hemorrhoidal plexuses
  middle rectal plexuses
  middle sacral p.
  myenteric p.
  p. myentericus
  p. nervorum spinalium
  p. nervosus
  occipital p.
  p. occipitalis
  ovarian p.
  p. ovaricus
  pampiniform p.
  p. pampiniformis
  pancreatic p.
  p. pancreaticus
  pelvic p.
  pelvic autonomic p.
  p. pelvinus
  periarterial p.
  p. periarterialis
  periarterial p. of maxillary artery
  periarterial p. of vertebral artery
  pericorneal p.
  pharyngeal p.
  p. pharyngeus
  p. pharyngeus ascendens
  phrenic p.
  popliteal p.
  posterior auricular p.
  posterior coronary p.
  prostatic p.
  prostaticovesical p.
  p. prostaticovesicalis
  p. prostaticus
  prostatic venous p.
  pterygoid p.
  p. pterygoideus

p. pudendalis
p. pudendus nervosus
p. pulmonalis
pulmonary p.
Quénu hemorrhoidal p.
rectal plexuses
p. rectales inferiores
p. rectales medii
p. rectalis superior
rectal venous p.
Remak p.
renal p.
p. renalis
sacral p.
p. sacralis
p. sacralis medius
sacral venous p.
Santorini p.
Sappey p.
sciatic p.
solar p.
spermatic p.
p. of spinal nerves
splenic p.
p. splenicus
stroma p.
subclavian p.
subclavian periarterial p.
p. subclavius
submucosal p.
p. submucosus
suboccipital venous p.
superficial cardiac p.
superficial temporal p.
superior hemorrhoidal p.
superior hypogastric p.
superior mesenteric p.
superior rectal p.
superior thyroid p.
suprarenal p.
p. suprarenalis
p. temporalis superficialis
testicular p.
p. testicularis
thoracic aortic p.
p. thyroideus impar
p. thyroideus inferior
p. thyroideus superior
ureteric p.
p. uretericus
uterine venous p.
uterovaginal p.
vaginal venous p.
vascular p.
p. vasculosus
p. venosus
p. venosus areolaris
p. venosus foraminis ovalis

p. venosus prostaticus
p. venosus rectalis
p. venosus sacralis
p. venosus suboccipitalis
p. venosus uterinus
p. venosus vaginalis
p. venosus vertebralis
p. venosus vesicalis
venous p.
venous p. of bladder
venous p. of foramen ovale
vertebral p.
p. vertebralis
vertebral venous p.
vesical p.
p. vesicalis
p. vesicalis inferior
vesicular venous p.
Walther p.
plica, pl. **plicae**
plicae alares
p. aryepiglottica
p. axillaris
plicae cecales
p. cecalis vascularis
p. chordae tympani
plicae circulares
p. duodenalis inferior
p. duodenalis superior
p. duodenojejunalis
p. duodenomesocolica
p. epigastrica
plicae gastricae
plicae gastropancreaticae
p. glossoepiglottica lateralis
p. glossoepiglottica mediana
p. hypogastrica
p. ileocecalis
p. incudis
p. interureterica
p. lacrimalis
p. longitudinalis duodeni
p. nervi laryngei
p. palatina transversa
p. palpebronasalis
p. paraduodenalis
plicae recti
p. rectouterina
p. rectovaginalis
p. semilunaris of colon
p. sigmoidea
p. spiralis ductus cystici

p. synovialis
plicae transversales recti
plicae tunicae mucosae vesicae felleae
p. umbilicalis lateralis
p. umbilicalis media
p. umbilicalis medialis
p. umbilicalis mediana
p. urachi
p. ureterica
p. uterovesicalis
p. ventricularis
p. vesicalis transversa
p. vesicouterina
p. vestibularis
p. vestibuli
p. villosa
plicated appendicocystostomy
plication
buccinator p.
Child-Phillips bowel p.
disk p.
fundal p.
Graham p.
Kelly p.
Nesbit p.
Noble bowel p.
Rehne-Delorme p.
retractor p.
soft tissue p.
suture p.
p. suture
tongue p.
transgastric p.
transmesenteric p.
plicectomy
plicotomy
PLIF
posterior lumbar interbody fusion
PLIF procedure
PL100KL/50K
Pall filter P.
PLND
pelvic lymph node dissection
ploidy
tumor p.
plombage operation
plop
cardiac tumor p.
tumor p.
plosive-injection method

NOTES

plot
    load-displacement p.
    pressure-flow p.
plug flow
plumb line
plume
    laser p.
Pluronic F-68
Plystan graft
PMP pump
PmvCO$_2$
    partial pressure of mesenteric venous carbon dioxide
pneumatic
    p. bag dilation of esophagus
    p. bag esophageal dilation
    p. balloon catheter dilation
    p. bone
    p. compression
    p. compression stocking
    p. dilatation
    p. otoscopy
    p. reduction
    p. retinopexy
    p. space
pneumatinuria
pneumatization
pneumatocele
pneumatorrhachis
pneumaturia
pneumectomy
pneumobulbar
pneumocardial
pneumocele
pneumocentesis
pneumocephalus
pneumococcal infection
pneumococcolysis
pneumoconiosis
pneumocystography
pneumocystosis
pneumodissection
    laparoscopic p.
pneumoencephalos
pneumogastric
    p. nerve
pneumography
    impedance p.
    retroperitoneal p.
pneumohydroperitoneum
pneumolysis
pneumonectomy
    p. chest
pneumonia
    aspiration p.
    congenital aspiration p.
    endogenous lipid p.
    extensive bilateral p.

    Gram-negative p.
    inhalation p.
    nosocomial p.
    oil-aspiration p.
    postoperative p.
    ventilator-associated p.
pneumonic
pneumonitis
    acute radiation p.
    aspiration p.
    peptic aspiration p.
    radiation p.
pneumonocele
pneumonocentesis
pneumonopexy
pneumonoresection
pneumonorrhaphy
pneumonotomy
pneumo-orbitography
pneumopericardium
    ventilator-induced p.
pneumoperitoneum
    CO$_2$ p.
    stent-induced p.
pneumopexy
pneumopleuroparietopexy
pneumopyelography
pneumoresection
pneumoretroperitoneum
    unilateral p.
pneumostatic dilation
pneumotachogram
pneumotachograph
    Fleish No. 2 p.
    Gould Godard p.
pneumotachograph/pressure transducer system
pneumotachometer
    hot-wire p.
pneumothorax
    extrapleural p.
    iatrogenic tension p.
    open p.
    pressure p.
    p. simplex
    ventilator-induced p.
pneumotomy
Pneumo-Wrap
pneuPAC resuscitator
PNF
    proprioceptive neuromuscular facilitation
    PNF technique
PNPB
    positive-negative pressure breathing
PO$_2$
    partial pressure of oxygen
pocket
    elimination p.

ionization chamber p.
p. operation
pacemaker p.
subpectoral p.
pocketed calculus
podalic extraction
podofilox solution
Pog
point P.
pogonion
Pogrund lateral approach
point
A p.
p. A, B
abrasive p.
p. of abscess
absorbent p.
Addison p.
alveolar p.
anchoring p.
p. angle
anterior focal p.
APACHE-II p.
apophysary p.
apophysial p.
p. of Arrhigi
p. of articulation
associated myofascial trigger p.
auricular p.
axial p.
p. B
B p.
bleeding p.
blur p.
Boas p.
Bolton p.
bounce p.
Boyd p.
break p.
Brinell hardness indenter p.
Broadbent registration p.
p. B, supramentale
Cannon p.
Capuron p.'s
cardinal p.
Castellani p.
central-bearing p.
central yellow p.
p. centric
change p.
Chauffard p.
choroid p.

Clado p.
colliculocentral p.
condenser p.
conjugate p.
contact area p.
convenience p.
convergence p.
copular p.
corresponding p.
craniometric p.'s
Crowe pilot p.
cut p.
D p.
de Mussy p.
Desjardins p.
disparate p.
dorsal p.
E p.
electrodesiccated bleeding p.
end p.
entry p.
equivalence p.
Erb p.
ethmoid registration p.
Excell polishing p.
exit p.
eye p.
far p.
faulty contact p.
F2 focal p.
fibromyalgia trigger p.
fixation p.
p. of fixation
fixed p.
focal bleeding p.
focal image p.
freezing p.
fusing p.
gingival p.
glenoid p.
growing p.
Guéneau de Mussy p.
gutta-percha p.
Halle p.
Hartmann p.
3-p. head rest
hinge-axis p.
ice p.
identical p.
p. IdI
p. IdS
ignition p.

NOTES

P

point *(continued)*
 image p.
 p. imaging
 impaction p.
 incident p.
 incisal p.
 p. incisor
 incisor p.
 p. of inflection
 isoelectric p.
 isometric p.
 isosbestic p.
 J p.
 jugal p.
 jugomaxillary p.
 Keen p.
 Knoop hardness indenter p.
 Kocher p.
 Krackow p.
 lacrimal p.
 Lanz p.
 Legat p.
 loss of contact p.
 lustrous central yellow p.
 Mackenzie p.
 material failure break p.
 p. of maximum impulse
 maximum occipital p.
 McBurney p.
 median mandibular p.
 melting p.
 mental p.
 metopic p.
 motor p.
 multiple sensitive p.
 Munro p.
 myofascial trigger p.
 near visual p.
 neutral p.
 nodal p.
 null p.
 occipital p.
 optical nodal p.
 p. of ossification
 painful p.
 paper p.
 Pauly p.
 pedicle entrance p.
 Piersol p.
 pivot p.
 p. Pog
 posterior focal p.
 power p.
 preauricular p.
 pressure inversion p.
 primary myofascial trigger p.
 primary p. of ossification
 principal p.

 purchase p.
 radix p.
 Ramond p.
 referred p.
 respiratory inversion p.
 restoration p.
 retention p.
 retromandibular p.
 Robson p.
 root canal p.
 rotary mounted p.
 sacral brim target p.
 satellite myofascial trigger p.
 p. scanning
 secondary focal p.
 secondary myofascial trigger p.
 secondary p. of ossification
 sensitive p.
 separation p.
 set p.
 p. source
 spinal p.
 Starlite p.
 Steinmann pin with Crowe pilot p.
 stereo-identical p.
 subspinale p. A
 Sudeck critical p.
 sulfur and silver p.
 supra-auricular p.
 supraorbital p.
 sylvian p.
 tender p.
 thermal death p.
 trial p.
 trigger p.
 triple p.
 Trousseau p.
 Valleix p.
 virtual p.
 visual p.
 Weber p.
 white p.
 William Dixon Cratex p.
 wood p.
 yellow p.
 Z p.
 zygomaxillary p.
point-counting image
pointed condyloma
Poirier
 P. gland
 P. line
 space of P.
Poiseuille space
poisoning
 oxygen p.
 radiation p.

Poland
  P. anomaly
  P. classification of epiphyseal fracture
  P. classification of physeal injury
polar
  P. Bair forced-air active cooling device
  P. wrap therapy
polariscopy
polarization microscopy
polarographic method
pole
  inferior p.
  inferior p. of kidney
  inferior p. of testis
  lateral p.
  p. ligation
  medial p. of ovary
  superior p.
  superior p. of kidney
  superior p. of testis
poli (*pl. of* polus)
polidocanol injection
poliomyelitis
Polisar-Lyons adapted tracheal tube
Politano-Leadbetter
  P.-L. anastomosis
  P.-L. tunnel creation
  P.-L. ureterolysis
  P.-L. ureteroneocystostomy
Politzer method
pollakiuria
Pol Le Coueur osteotomy
pollex
  p. pedis
pollicization
  Buck-Gramcko p.
  Riordan p.
pollination
Polmedco endotracheal tube cuff
Polocaine
  P. injection
polus, pl. poli
  poli lienalis inferior et superior
  poli renalis inferior et superior
Pólya
  P. anastomosis
  P. gastrectomy
  P. gastroenterostomy
  P. method
  P. operation

  P. procedure
  P. technique
polyacrylonitrile
  p. membrane
polyadenous
polyadenylation
polyagglutination
Polyak operation
polyamide suture
polyaxial joint
polybutester suture
polycentric rotation
polycystic liver
polydactylous
polydactyly
Polydek suture
polydioxanone suture
polydysplasia
polyembryoma
polyester fiber suture
polyethylene
  ArCom compression-molded p.
  p. compression molding
  p. glycol electrolyte lavage solution
  p. glycol electrolyte solution
  p. graft
  p. suture
  p. tube
  p. tubing
polyfilament suture
polygalactic acid suture
polygalactide suture
polygalactin 910 suture
polyganglionic
polyglandular
polyglecaprone 25 suture
polyglycolic acid suture
polyglycol suture
polyglyconate suture
polymer anesthetic
polymicrobial infection
polyorchism
polyp
  adenomatous p.
  endocervical p.
  endometrial p.
  hyperplastic p.
  juvenile p.
  perineal p.
polypapilloma
polypectomy
  colonoscopic p.

NOTES

P

polypectomy *(continued)*
  duodenal endoscopic p.
  electrosurgical snare p.
  endoscopic sessile p.
  gastric p.
  incomplete p.
  intranasal p.
Poly-Plus Dacron vascular graft
polypoid
  p. degeneration of the true fold
  p. lesion
  p. mass
polypoidal lesion
polyposis
polypropylene
  p. button suture
  p. intracardiac patch
polyradiculopathy
polysinusectomy
Polysorb suture
polyspermia
polysyndactyly
polytetrafluoroethylene (PTFE)
  expanded p. (EPTFE)
  p. graft
  p. paste injection
polythelia
polyurethane graft
polyuria
polyvinyl
  p. alcohol (PVA)
  p. alcohol fixative method
  p. alcohol sponge hysterosacropexy
  p. chloride tube
  p. graft
Pomeroy
  P. operation
  P. tubal ligation
POMS 20/50 oxygen conservation device
Poncet perineal urethrostomy
pond fracture
Ponka
  P. herniorrhaphy
  P. technique for local anesthesia
pons, pl. **pontes**
  p. hepatis
  oblique bundle of p.
Ponsky
  P. PEG tube
  P. pull or guidewire insertion
    technique
Ponsky-Gauderer PEG tube
Pontén fasciocutaneous flap
pontes (*pl. of* pons)
ponticulus
  p. hepatis
pontile

pontine
  p. arteries
  p. cistern
  p. hemorrhage
  p. myelinolysis
  p. paramedian reticular formation
  p. tractotomy
pontis
  cisterna p.
Pontocaine
  P. injection
  P. Topical
PONV
  postoperative nausea and vomiting
Poole
  P. abdominal suction tube
  P. suction tube
pool therapy
poorly compliant bladder
poor-risk patient
poples
popliteal
  p. artery
  p. artery occlusive disease (PAOD)
  p. artery trifurcation
  p. communicating nerve
  p. fascia
  p. fossa
  p. groove
  p. lymph nodes
  p. muscle
  p. plexus
  p. region
  p. space
  p. web syndrome
popliteus
  p. muscle
pop-off
  p.-o. suture
  p.-o. valve
Poppen suction tube
population-based registry
population sample
porcelain
  p. cervical contact and single bake
    technique
  p. cervical ditching technique
  p. condensation
  p. fracture
  p. gallbladder
  p. jacket restoration
porcelain-bonded restoration
porcelain-fused-to-metal restoration
porcine skin graft
pore
porocarcinoma
porocele
poroid hidradenoma

poroma
porotomy
porous
    p. filter membrane
    p. ingrowth fixation
    p. polyethylene graft
PORP
    partial ossicular replacement prosthesis
porphobilinogen (PBG)
porphyria
    acute intermittent p.
Porro
    P. cesarean section
    P. hysterectomy
    P. operation
Porstmann technique
port
    Arrow percutaneous sheath introducer with integral side p.
    Berkeley Bioengineering infusion terminal p.
    Celsite implanted p.
    chest p.
    Gills-Welsh guillotine p.
    Hasson blunt p.
    implantable infusion p.
    p. incision
    Infuse-A-Port p.
    infusion p.
    inlet p.
    Luer-Lok p.
    lumbar p.
    MCL p.
    nasal p.
    OmegaPort access p.
    PAS p.
    periumbilical p.
    SEA p.
    side p.
    subcostal p.
    subcutaneous implanted injection p.
    suprapubic p.
    Thora-Port p.
    umbilical p.
    velopharyngeal p.
    p. vitrectomy
porta, pl. **portae**
    p. hepatis
    p. lienis
    p. pulmonis
    p. renis

portable C-arm image intensifier fluoroscopy
portacaval
    p. anastomosis
    p. H graft
port-access
    p.-a. coronary artery bypass grafting
portae (*pl. of* porta)
portal
    arthroscopic entry p.
    aspiration p.
    p. eosinophilic inflammation
    p. fissure
    p. pedicle
    p. shunt index
    p. space
    p. tract
    p. tract inflammation
    p. triad
    p. vein
    p. vein resection
    p. venous pressure
portal-collateral circulation
portal-hypophysial circulation
portal-systemic
    p.-s. anastomoses
    p.-s. shunt surgery
Porter fascia
Porter-Richardson-Vainio
    P.-R.-V. synovectomy
    P.-R.-V. technique
Portex
    P. bacterial filter
    P. Per-Fit tracheostomy tube
    P. preformed blue line tracheal tube
    P. SS endotracheal tube cuff
    P. ThermoVent heat and moisture exchanger
    P. XL endotracheal tube cuff
portio, pl. **portiones**
    p. intermedia
    p. major nervi trigemini
    p. minor nervi trigemini
    p. supravaginalis
    p. vaginalis
portion
    accessory p. of spinal accessory nerve
    mesenteric p. of small intestine

NOTES

P

portion *(continued)*
    subcutaneous p. of external anal
      sphincter
    supravaginal p. of cervix
    vaginal p. of cervix
portiplexus
portmanteau procedure
portobilioarterial
portoenterostomy
    Kasai p.
portoportal anastomosis
portopulmonary venous anastomosis
portosystemic
    p. anastomosis
    p. collateral circulation
Porto-Vac suction tube
port-wine
    p.-w. hemangioma
    p.-w. mark
    p.-w. stain
porus
    p. crotaphytico-buccinatorius
Posada fracture
position
    p. ametropia
    anatomical p.
    angular p.
    antero-oblique p.
    antiembolic p.
    "arch and slouch" p.
    arm p.
    asynclitic p.
    back-up p.
    backward p.
    barber chair p.
    batrachian p.
    bayonet fracture p.
    beach chair p.
    Bertel p.
    bisecting angle cone p.
    body p.
    Bonner p.
    Boyce p.
    Bozeman p.
    Brickner p.
    brow p.
    brow-anterior p.
    brow-down p.
    brow-posterior p.
    brow-up p.
    Buie p.
    cardiac p.
    cardinal p.
    Casselberry p.
    catheter p.
    centric p.
    cervical p.
    chin p.

condylar hinge p.
consonant p.
convergence p.
cottonloader p.
curved flank p.
cuspid-molar p.
decubitus p.
dissociated p.
distoangular p.
dorsal birthing p.
dorsal lithotomy p.
dorsal recumbent p.
dorsosacral p.
Duncan p.
eccentric jaw p.
Edebohls p.
electrical heart p.
Elliot p.
en face p.
English p.
equinus p.
exaggerated sniffing p.
face-down p.
face-to-pubes p.
Feist-Mankin p.
fetal head p.
Fick p.
figure-four p.
final cone p.
final consonant p.
first cone p.
flank p.
flexed p.
forehead-nose p.
Fowler p.
frog-leg p.
frontoanterior p.
frontoposterior p.
frontotransverse p.
Fuchs p.
fusion-free p.
Gaynor-Hart p.
genucubital p.
genupectoral p.
gingival p.
greater curve p.
head-up tilt p.
heart p.
heterophoric p.
hinge p.
horizontal p.
initial consonant p.
intercuspal p.
intrinsic minus p.
jackknife p.
James p.
jaw-to-jaw p.
Jones p.

jumper-knee p.
knee-chest p.
knee-elbow p.
kneeling p.
Kraske p.
LAO p.
lateral decubitus p.
lateral occlusal p.
lateral recumbent p.
leapfrog p.
left anterior oblique p.
left decubitus p.
left frontoanterior p.
left frontoposterior p.
left frontotransverse p.
left lateral decubitus p.
left lateral Sims p.
left mentoanterior p.
left mentoposterior p.
left mentotransverse p.
left occipitoanterior p.
left occipitoposterior p.
left occipitotransverse p.
left sacroanterior p.
left sacroposterior p.
left sacrotransverse p.
left scapuloanterior p.
left scapuloposterior p.
left-side-down p.
levo-transposed p.
lithotomy p.
lotus p.
mandibular hinge p.
mandibular rest p.
maternal birthing p.
Mayo-Robson p.
median occlusal p.
mentoanterior p.
mentoposterior p.
mentotransverse p.
mentum anterior p.
mentum posterior p.
mentum transverse p.
mesioangular p.
midline p.
military brace p.
military tuck p.
missionary p.
neutral p.
Noble p.
normal anatomic p.
obstetric p.

occipitoanterior p.
occipitoposterior p.
occipitotransverse p.
occlusal p.
paralleling cone p.
park-bench p.
persistent occiput posterior p.
Phalen p.
physiologic rest p.
posterior border p.
postural resting p.
prayer p.
primary p.
prone split-leg p.
protrusive p.
protrusive occlusal p.
pterygoid p.
quasistatic stressed p.
RAO p.
reclining p.
rectus p.
recumbent p.
rest p.
p. of rest
retruded p.
reverse Trendelenburg p.
Rhese p.
right acromiodorsoposterior p.
right anterior oblique p.
right antero-oblique p.
right frontoanterior p.
right frontoposterior p.
right frontotransverse p.
right mentoanterior p.
right mentoposterior p.
right mentotransverse p.
right occipitoanterior p.
right occipitoposterior p.
right occipitotransverse p.
right sacroanterior p.
right sacroposterior p.
right sacrotransverse p.
right scapuloanterior p.
right scapuloposterior p.
right-side-down p.
Robson p.
Rose p.
sacroanterior p.
sacroposterior p.
sacrotransverse p.
scissor-leg p.
Scultetus p.

NOTES

P

position *(continued)*
    semi-Fowler p.
    semilateral p.
    semioblique p.
    semiprone p.
    semirecumbent p.
    semiupright p.
    shock p.
    Simon p.
    Sims p.
    sitting p.
    ski p.
    sniffing p.
    p. in space
    spinal fusion p.
    steep Trendelenburg p.
    sulcus fixated p.
    superior labrum anterior p. (SLAP)
    supine p.
    terminal hinge p.
    tooth p.
    tooth-to-tooth p.
    translational p.
    Trendelenburg p.
    tricuspid p.
    tuck p.
    upright p.
    Valentine p.
    vertex p.
    vertical divergence p.
    Walcher p.
positional release therapy
positioning
    automated endoscopic system for
      optimal p.
    surgical p.
positive
    p. airway pressure (PAP)
    p. control enzyme induction
    p. correlation
    p. end-airway pressure
    p. end-expiratory pressure (PEEP)
    p. end-expiratory pressure/continuous
      positive airway pressure
      (PEEP/CPAP)
    p. expiratory pressure
    extradomain A p.
    p. inspiratory pressure
    p. pressure ventilation (PPV)
**positive-negative pressure breathing
  (PNPB)**
positive-pressure ventilation
positron emission tomography (PET)
post
    extrinsic rearfoot p.
    Hahnenkratt root canal p.
    implant p.
    Isola spinal implant system iliac p.
    PD root canal p.
    perineal p.
    screw p.
    split-shank screw p.
    Stalite root canal p.
    surgical instrument p.
    P. total shoulder arthroplasty
postactivation
    p. exhaustion
    p. facilitation
postadrenalectomy syndrome
postage stamp skin graft
postanal
    p. repair
postanesthesia care unit (PACU)
postanesthetic
    p. central nervous system
      dysfunction
postangioplasty
    p. intimal flap
    p. restenosis
postaugmentation
postauricular incision
post-autoclave contamination
postaxial
postaxillary line
post-balloon angioplasty restenosis
postbiopsy
    p. renal AV fistula
    p. vascular complication
postbrachial
postbulbar ulceration
postburn
postcardiotomy
    p. syndrome
postcatheterization
postcaval ureter
postcementation
postcentral sulcal artery
post-cesarean anesthesia
postcholecystectomy
    p. flatulent dyspepsia
    p. syndrome
postclavicular
postcolonoscopy distention syndrome
postcommissurotomy syndrome
**postcommunical part of anterior
  cerebral artery**
postcondensation
postcordial
postcore restoration
postcostal
postcricoid web
postdischarge
postdrug latency
postductal coarctation of aorta
postdural puncture headache (PDPH)

postembolization
    p. syndrome
postendoscopy
posterior
    p. alveolar artery
    p. antebrachial region
    anterior and p. (A&P)
    p. anterior jugular vein
    p. arch of atlas
    p. arch fracture
    p. atlanto-occipital membrane
    p. auricular groove
    p. auricular muscle
    p. auricular nerve
    p. auricular plexus
    p. auricular vein
    p. axillary line
    p. basal branch
    p. basal segment
    p. belly of digastric muscle
    p. bladder flap plasty
    p. bone graft
    p. border jaw relation
    p. border of petrous part of
    temporal bone
    p. border position
    p. border of radius
    p. border of testis
    p. border of ulna
    p. brachial region
    p. branch of great auricular nerve
    p. branch of lateral cerebral sulcus
    p. branch of obturator artery
    p. branch of obturator nerve
    p. branch of recurrent ulnar artery
    p. branch of renal artery
    p. branch of right branch of portal
    vein
    p. branch of right hepatic duct
    p. branch of spinal nerves
    p. branch of superior thyroid
    artery
    p. canal line
    p. capsular zonular barrier
    p. capsulorrhaphy
    p. capsulotomy
    p. cecal artery
    p. cerebral artery
    p. cervical fixation
    p. cervical fusion
    p. cervical intertransversarii muscles
    p. cervical intertransverse muscles

    p. cervical line
    p. cervical space
    p. choroidal artery
    p. circumflex humeral artery
    p. column
    p. column cordotomy
    p. column fracture
    p. column osteosynthesis
    p. communicating artery
    p. condyloid foramen
    p. cord of brachial plexus
    p. coronary plexus
    p. costotransversectomy approach
    p. costotransverse ligament
    p. cranial fossa
    p. cricoarytenoid muscle
    p. cruciate ligament graft
    p. crus of stapes
    p. element fracture
    p. explant
    p. facial vein
    p. fixation suture
    p. flap
    p. flap technique
    p. flap vaginoplasty
    p. focal point
    p. fontanel
    p. fossa circulation
    p. fracture-dislocation
    p. fundoplasty
    p. glenoplasty
    p. group of axillary lymph nodes
    p. hip dislocation
    p. humeral circumflex artery
    p. hyaloid membrane
    p. iliac osteotomy
    p. inferior cerebellar artery
    p. inferior iliac spine
    p. innominate rotation
    p. intercostal arteries 1–2
    p. intercostal arteries 3-11
    p. intercostal veins
    p. interosseous artery
    p. interosseous nerve compression
    syndrome
    p. intraoccipital joint
    p. intraoccipital synchondrosis
    p. inverted U approach
    p. junction line
    p. knee region
    p. labial arteries
    p. labial commissure

NOTES

P

posterior *(continued)*
- p. labial nerve
- p. labial veins
- p. layer of rectus abdominis sheath
- p. limb of stapes
- p. limiting ring
- p. lip of uterine os
- p. lobe of hypophysis
- p. longitudinal bundle
- p. longitudinal ligament
- p. lower cervical spine stabilization
- p. lower cervical spine surgery
- p. lumbar approach
- p. lumbar interbody fusion (PLIF)
- p. lumbar interbody fusion procedure
- p. lumbar interbody fusion surgery
- p. lumbar spine and sacrum surgery
- p. median line
- p. mediastinal arteries
- p. mediastinal lymph nodes
- p. mediastinal mass
- p. mediastinum
- p. meningeal artery
- p. midline approach
- p. mitral valve leaflet
- p. neck region
- p. nephrectomy
- p. occipitoaxial ligament
- p. occipitocervical approach
- p. pancreaticoduodenal artery
- p. parietal artery
- p. parotid veins
- p. pelvic exenteration
- p. Pólya procedure
- p. primary division
- p. process of septal cartilage
- p. process of talus
- p. proctotomy
- p. rectopexy
- p. region of arm
- p. region of forearm
- p. region of leg
- p. region of neck
- p. region of thigh
- p. repair
- p. rhizotomy
- p. ring fracture
- p. root
- p. sacroiliac ligaments
- p. sacrosciatic ligament
- p. scalene muscle
- p. scapular nerve
- p. sclerotomy
- p. screw fixation
- p. scrotal nerve
- p. scrotal veins

- p. segmental artery of kidney
- p. segmental fixation
- p. shoulder dislocation
- p. spinal artery
- p. spinal fusion
- p. spinal wedge osteotomy
- p. spinocerebellar tract
- p. sternoclavicular ligament
- p. superior alveolar artery
- p. superior iliac spine
- p. supraclavicular nerve
- p. surface of arytenoid cartilage
- p. surface of cornea
- p. surface of eyelids
- p. surface of kidney
- p. surface of pancreas
- p. surface of petrous part of temporal bone
- p. surface of prostate
- p. surface of suprarenal gland
- p. synechia formation
- p. talar articular surface of calcaneus
- p. temporal artery
- p. thermal sclerostomy
- p. thoracic nerve
- p. tibial artery
- p. tibial lymph node
- p. tibial recurrent artery
- p. tibiotalar part of deltoid ligament
- p. translation
- p. transolecranon approach
- p. transthoracic incision
- p. triangle of neck
- p. truncal vagotomy
- p. tubercle of atlas
- p. tubercle of cervical vertebrae
- p. upper cervical spine surgery
- p. urethra
- p. vaginal hernia
- p. vein of left ventricle
- p. vertical canal
- p. vitrectomy
- p. wall fracture
- p. wall of stomach
- p. wall of vagina

posterior-anterior pressure
posterior-interbody lumbar spinal fusion
posterior-lateral lumbar spinal fusion
posterior-superior oblique projection
posteroanterior projection
posteroinferior
- p. external
- p. external movement

posterolateral
- p. approach
- p. aspect

   p. bone graft
   p. bone graft placement
   p. bundle
   p. central arteries
   p. costotransversectomy incision
   p. costotransversectomy technique
   p. fontanel
   p. herniation
   p. interbody fusion
   p. lumbosacral fusion

posteromedial
   p. approach
   p. central arteries
   p. dislocation

posteroventral pallidotomy
postesophageal
postevacuation
postextraction hemorrhage
postextubation laryngospasm
postfracture lesion
postfundoplication
   p. syndrome

postgastrectomy
   p. bleed
   p. cancer
   p. dysfunction
   p. hemorrhage
   p. syndrome

posthemorrhagic
posthepatic
posthetomy
posthioplasty
posthitis
postholith
posthyoid
posthyperventilation apnea
posticum
   staphyloma p.
   tibiale p.

postinfection lipoatrophy
postinflammatory hypopigmentation
postinsufflation
postintervention
postirradiation
   p. fracture
   p. study
   p. syndrome

postischemic stunned myocardium
postischial
postkeratoplasty

postlaminectomy
   p. kyphosis
   p. syndrome

postlumpectomy
   p. skin thickening

postmastoid
postmedian
postmediastinal
postmediastinum
postmembrane
   p. pressure
   p. rupture

postmenopausal body mass
postmortem
   p. examination
   p. hypostasis
   p. suggillation

postnatal therapy
postocular
postoperative
   p. analgesia
   p. analgesic
   p. anesthesia
   p. anisocoria
   p. anticoagulation therapy
   p. apnea
   p. cesarean section pain
   p. choledochoscopy
   p. complication
   p. extubation
   p. fracture
   p. immobilization
   p. infection
   p. irrigation-suction
   p. irrigation-suction drainage
   p. nausea and vomiting (PONV)
   p. pelvic radiation
   p. pleurobiliary fistula
   p. pneumonia
   p. radiation
   p. regimen for oral early feeding (PROEF)
   p. repair
   p. tetany

postpartum
   p. hemorrhage
   p. infection

postpericardiotomy syndrome
postpharyngeal
   p. space

postphlebitic syndrome

NOTES

P

postpneumonectomy tuberculous
empyema
postpolypectomy
    p. bleed
    p. coagulation syndrome
    p. hemorrhage
postprostatectomy incontinence
postpyloric
    p. feeding tube
    p. sphincter
postradiation
    p. fistula
    p. kyphosis
    p. therapy
postradical neck dissection
postreduction
    p. mammaplasty
postrema
    area p. (AP)
postresection
    p. defect
    p. filling
    p. filling technique
postsacral
postscapular
postsensation
postsphenoid bone
postsphincterotomy
    p. ERCP cannulation
postsplenectomy infection
postsplenic
poststenotic
    p. dilatation
    p. dilation
postsulcal part of tongue
postsurgical endoscopy
postsynaptic membrane
posttecta
posttetanic
    p. count
    p. count monitoring
    p. facilitation
postthoracotomy
    p. change
    p. pain
posttranslation modification
posttransplant
    p. antiglomerular basement
      membrane
    p. immunosuppression therapy
posttransplantation
    p. lymphoproliferative disorder
posttransverse
posttraumatic
    p. autotransplantation
    p. chondrolysis
    p. hemorrhage
    p. intradiploic pseudomeningocele

    p. pancreatic-cutaneous fistula
    p. spinal deformity
    p. subcapsular hepatic fluid
      collection
posttubal ligation syndrome
postural
    p. deformity
    p. drainage
    p. fixation back maneuver
    p. reduction
    p. resting position
posture
    compensatory head p.
    forward head p.
    head p.
postureteral ligation
postureteroscopic manipulation
postuterine
postvagotomy
    p. dysphagia
    p. gastroparesis
    p. syndrome
postvalvar
postvasectomy change in epididymis
postvitrectomy fibrin
postzygomatic space
potassium space
potato
    p. tumor of neck
potency
    anesthetic p.
    sphincteric p.
potent
potential
    compound muscle action p.
      (CMAP)
    demarcation p.
    denervation p.
    electrode p.
    endogenous event-related p.
    excitatory junction p.
    excitatory postsynaptic p.
    extreme somatosensory evoked p.
    fasciculation p.
    fibrillation p.
    membrane p.
    miniature end-plate p.
    modulation p.
    motor-evoked p. (MEP)
    myogenic motor-evoked p. (MEP)
    oxidation-reducing p.
    pacemaker p.
    peroneal somatosensory evoked p.
    reduction p.
    regeneration motor unit p.
    resting membrane p.
    somatosensory evoked p. (SEP,
      SSEP)

standard electrode p.
standard reduction p.
Potential Acuity Meter (PAM)
potentially lethal x-ray damage repair
potentiation
potentiometric titration
Pott
    P. aneurysm
    P. ankle fracture
    P. eversion osteotomy
Potter
    P. classification
    P. facies
Potts
    P. anastomosis
    P. operation
    P. procedure
Potts-Smith anastomosis
pouch
    anal p.
    antibiotic bead p.
    arachnoid retrocerebellar p.
    Bard Extra Ileo B p.
    Bard Integrale p.
    bead p.
    Benchekroun p.
    p. biopsy
    bladder replacement urinary p.
    Blake p.
    blind upper esophageal p.
    Bongort urinary diversion p.
    Bricker p.
    Broca p.
    Camcy urinary p.
    Cardio-Cool myocardial
      protection p.
    closed-end ostomy p.
    Coloplast Flange p.
    Coloplast mini p.
    coloplasty p.
    continent ileal p.
    continent urinary p.
    ConvaTec colostomy p.
    ConvaTec Little One Sur-Fit p.
    ConvaTec ostomy p.
    ConvaTec Sur-Fit two-piece p.
    ConvaTec urostomy p.
    copulating p.
    Cymed Micro Skin one-piece
      drainage p.
    Dansac Karaya Seal one-piece
      drainage p.

Dansac Standard Ileo p.
deep perineal p.
Denis Browne p.
dermal p.
double loop p.
Douglas p.
p. of Douglas
drainable ostomy p.
Duke p.
endorectal ileal p.
Florida urinary p.
gastric p.
Greer EZ Access drainage p.
Hartmann p.
haustral p.
heat-seal p.
hepatorenal p.
hernia p.
Hollister First Choice p.
Hollister Holligard p.
Hollister Karaya 5 ostomy p.
Hollister Karaya Seal p.
Hollister Premium p.
Hunt-Lawrence p.
ileal neobladder urinary p.
p. ileitis
ileoanal p.
ileocecal p.
ileocolonic p.
Indiana urinary p.
inflamed synovial p.
intraluminal p.
intravaginal p.
inverted-U p.
jejunal p.
J-shaped ileal p.
J versus S versus W pelvic
  ileal p.
kangaroo p.
Kock urinary p.
labioperineal p.
laryngeal p.
lateral-lateral p.
Le Bag ileocolonic p.
Le Bag urinary p.
Mainz urinary p.
ManHood absorbent p.
Mansson urinary p.
Marlen Gas Relief drainage p.
Marlen Odor-Ban ileostomy p.
Marlen Solo ileostomy p.
Marlen Zip Klosed p.

NOTES

P

pouch *(continued)*
Miami p.
Morison p.
Nu-Hope ileostomy p.
Nu-Hope Nu-Self drainable p.
omental p.
one-piece ostomy p.
open-end ostomy p.
Padua bladder urinary p.
paracystic p.
pararectal p.
paravesical p.
Parks ileostomy p.
Parsonnet pulse generator p.
pelvic p.
Penn p.
pharyngeal p.
Physick p.
Pleatman p.
Rathke p.
Reality vaginal p.
p. reconstruction
rectal p.
rectouterine p.
rectovaginal p.
rectovaginouterine p.
rectovesical p.
renal p.
Rowland p.
Seessel p.
self-seal p.
sigma rectum p.
sigmoid rectum p.
Squibb urostomy p.
S-shaped p.
superficial inguinal p.
superficial perineal p.
suprapatellar p.
Sur-Fit Mini p.
Sur-Fit urostomy p.
Tena p.
terminal ileal p.
three-loop ileal p.
triple loop p.
two-loop J-shaped ileal p.
two-piece ostomy p.
U p.
United Bongort Life-style p.
United Max-E drainable p.
United Surgical Bongort Life-style p.
United Surgical Featherlite ileostomy p.
United Surgical Shear Plus drainable p.
United Surgical Soft & Secure p.
uterovesical p.
VBG p.
vertical banded gastroplasty p.
vesicouterine p.
visceral p.
VPI nonadhesive open-end p.
wallaby p.
Willis p.
W-shaped p.
Zenker p.

pouched ileostomy
pouchitis
pouchoscopy
pelvic p.
Poulard operation
Poupart
P. ligament
P. line
povidone-iodine solution
power
P. operation
p. point
p. spectral analysis
Pozzi procedure
PPH
primary pulmonary hypertension
PPT
pressure pain threshold
PPV
positive pressure ventilation
Prague maneuver
pramoxine hydrochloride
Pratt
P. open reduction
P. technique
prayer position
PRBC
packed red blood cells
preadaptation
preadventitial dissection
preanal
preanesthetic
p. medication
p. skin-surface warming
preantiseptic
preaortic
preaseptic
preauricular
p. deep parotid lymph nodes
p. fistula
p. groove
p. incision
p. point
p. sulcus
preaxial
preaxillary line
precancerous
p. lesion
precapillary
p. anastomosis

precatheterization
precaution
    radiation p.
precaval lymph node
prececal lymph nodes
precentral
    p. artery
    p. sulcal artery
prechiasmal
    p. compression
    p. optic nerve lesion
precipitate in solution
Precision Osteolock hip
preclotted graft
Preclude
    P. pericardial membrane
    P. peritoneal membrane
precommissural bundle
precommunical part of anterior
    cerebral artery
preconditioning
    ischemic p.
precordial
precordium, pl. precordia
precorneal
precostal
precuneal
    p. artery
precursor lesion
precut
    p. incision
    p. papillotomy
Predaject injection
Predalone injection
Predcor injection
predental space
Predent disclosing solution
predialysis plasma phosphate
    concentration
Predicort-50 injection
Prednisol TBA injection
predorsal bundle
preeclamptic liver disease
preemergence
preemptive
    p. analgesia
    p. anesthesia
preendoscopy
preepiglottic soft tissue
preepiglottic space

preexcitation
    p. syndrome
    ventricular p.
prefabrication
preformed polyvinyl chloride
    endotracheal tube
Prefrin ophthalmic solution
prefrontal
    p. leukotomy
    p. lobotomy
preganglionic
    p. cardiac sympathetic blockade
    p. sympathectomy
    p. sympathetic block
    p. sympathetic denervation
preglenoid plane
pregnancy
    p. complication
    p. luteoma
pregnancy-induced anesthesia
prehelicine
prehospital
prehyoid
    p. gland
preimplantation
    p. embryo
preinduction
preinsufflation
preinterparietal bone
preintervention
prelabor membrane rupture
prelaryngeal
    p. lymph nodes
prelimbic
preliminary iridectomy
preload reduction
premalignant lesion
premasseteric
    p. space
    p. space abscess
premature
    p. airway closure
    p. amnion rupture
    p. ductus arteriosis closure
    p. membrane rupture
    p. separation of placenta
premaxilla
premaxillary suture
premedicate
premedication

NOTES

P

premembrane
    p. pressure
    p. rupture
premicturition pressure
premonitory palpitation
prenalterol
prenatal
    p. diethylstilbestrol exposure
    p. dislocation
    p. therapy
Prentiss
    P. maneuver
    P. orchiopexy
preoperative
    p. analgesia
    p. anesthetic
    p. evaluation
    p. fasting
    p. lesion
    p. preparation
    p. skin-surface warming
    p. staging
preoperatively donated autologous blood
preoxygenation
prepapillary sphincter
preparation
    access p.
    biomechanical p.
    bone-patellar tendon-bone p.
    bowel p.
    Brown dietary method for colon p.
    cavity p.
    chamfer p.
    corrosion p.
    crush p.
    Debrun latex balloon p.
    facet joint p.
    facial butt joint p.
    figure-eight p.
    fortified topical p.
    full shoulder p.
    galenic p.
    graft p.
    heart-lung p.
    impression p.
    incisal p.
    initial p.
    insulin p.
    intermediate-acting insulin p.
    KOH p.
    lactobacilli p.
    Langendorff heart p.
    lavage bowel p.
    liposomal p.
    long-acting insulin p.
    lupus erythematosus p.
    Matsura p.
    medicinal p.

    mouth p.
    Nichols-Condon bowel p.
    oral iron p.
    pinworm p.
    preoperative p.
    renal proximal tubule p.
    rod contour p.
    short-acting insulin p.
    shoulder with bevel p.
    skin p.
    slice p.
    slot p.
    slot-type p.
    Spälteholz p.
    step p.
    surgical p.
    tar p.
    vertical vs. horizontal p.
    wire contour p.
preparatory iridectomy
prepared
    p. cavity
    p. cavity impression
prepatellar
    p. bursa
    p. bursa inflammation
prepericardiac lymph nodes
preperitoneal
    p. anesthesia
    p. approach
    p. fat
    p. space
preplacental hemorrhage
prepontine
    p. cistern
    p. white epidermoidoma
preprostate urethral sphincter
preprosthetic surgery
prepuce
preputial
    p. calculus
    p. continent vesicostomy
    p. glands
    p. sac
preputiotomy
preputium
    p. clitoridis
prepyloric
    p. perforation
    p. sphincter
    p. vein
prepyramidal tract
prerecruitment
prerectal
    p. lithotomy
prerenal
prerepair

preretinal
    p. hemorrhage
    p. membrane
    p. neovascularization
pre-Rolandic artery
presacral
    p. anesthesia
    p. anomaly
    p. cystic lesion
    p. fascia
    p. insufflation
    p. mass
    p. nerve
    p. neurectomy
    p. rectopexy
    p. space
    p. sympathectomy
presaturation technique
presensitization phase
presentation
    p. of cord
    p. of fetus
presenting clinical manifestation
preseptal space
preservation
    autonomic nerve p. (ANP)
    breast p.
    cadaver renal p.
    carotid p.
    extracorporeal renal p.
    extremity p.
    lordosis p.
    lumbar lordosis p.
    pelvic autonomic nerve p. (PANP)
    renal p.
    simple cold storage p.
    p. technique
    p. time
    tissue p.
    visual p.
preservatives in solution
presigmoid-transtransversarium
    intradural approach
presphenoid
    p. bone
prespinal
presplenic fold
Press-Fit
    P.-F. collared femoral stem
      implantation
    P.-F. condylar knee arthroplasty
    P.-F. fixation

    P.-F. noncollared femoral stem
      implantation
pressor
    p. medication
pressoreceptor
pressure
    abdominal p.
    acoustic p.
    airway p.
    Alladin InfantFlow nasal continuous
      positive air p.
    p. alopecia
    alveolar carbon dioxide p.
    alveolar oxygen partial p. (PAO_2)
    alveolar partial p.
    p. amaurosis
    p. amplitude modulation
    anal sphincter squeeze p.
    p. anesthesia
    aortic blood p.
    aortic dicrotic notch p.
    aortic pullback p.
    applanation p.
    p. area
    arterial blood p.
    arterial carbon dioxide p.
    arterial dicrotic notch p.
    arterial oxygen partial p. (PaO_2)
    arterial partial p.
    ascending aortic p.
    atmospheres of p.
    atrial filling p.
    p. atrophy
    average mean p.
    barometric p.
    basal anal canal p.
    basal anal sphincter p.
    bile duct p.
    bi-level positive airway p. (BiPAP)
    biliary tract p.
    BiPAP nasal continuous positive
      airway p.
    biting p.
    bladder p.
    p. blister
    blood p.
    bone marrow p.
    capillary wedge p.
    carbon dioxide p.
    cardiovascular p.
    central posterior-anterior p.
    central venous p. (CVP)

NOTES

P

pressure *(continued)*
  cerebral perfusion p.
  cerebrospinal fluid p. (CSFP)
  choledochal basal p.
  closing p.
  closure p.
  coaxial p.
  colloidal osmotic p.
  colloid osmotic p. (COP)
  compartmental p.
  compliance, rate, oxygenation, and p.
  p. condensation
  continuous distending airway p.
  continuous negative airway p.
  continuous positive airway p. (CPAP)
  p. conversion
  coronary perfusion p.
  coronary venous p.
  cricoid p.
  critical closing p.
  CSF p.
  detrusor p.
  diastolic blood p. (DBP)
  diastolic filling p.
  differential blood p.
  digital p.
  disk p.
  Donders p.
  downstream venous p.
  dynamic closure p.
  elastic recoil p.
  end-diastolic left ventricular p.
  end-expiratory intragastric p.
  end-systolic left ventricular p.
  p. epiphysis
  esophageal peristaltic p.
  exophthalmos due to p.
  expiratory positive airway p.
  eye restored to normotensive p.
  free hepatic venous p.
  p. gangrene
  gastric p.
  glomerular capillary p.
  p. gradient
  group p.
  p. half-time technique
  hepatic vein wedge p.
  hepatic venous p.
  hepatic wedge p.
  high blood p.
  high-frequency positive p. (HFPP)
  high intraluminal p.
  hydrostatic p.
  hyperbaric p.
  increased p.
  p. increment rate

inferior vena cava p. (IVCP)
inspiratory occlusion p.
inspiratory positive airway p.
insufflation p.
interesophageal variceal p.
intermittent positive p.
intra-abdominal p. (IAP)
intra-anal p.
intracardiac p.
intracholedochal p.
intracranial p. (ICP)
intradiscal p.
intraductal p.
intraesophageal peristaltic p.
intragastric p.
intraglomerular p.
intraluminal esophageal p.
intraluminal urethral p.
intramyocardial p.
intrancural p.
intraocular p.
intraoral p.
intraperiapical p.
intrapericardial p.
intrapleural p.
intrapulpal p.
intrathoracic p.
intraurethral p.
intravariceal p.
intravascular p.
intravesical p.
intrinsic end-expiratory p.
intrinsic positive end-expiratory p. (PEEPi)
p. inversion point
jugular venous p.
juxtacardiac pleural p.
labile blood p.
lateral root p.
leak point p.
left atrial p.
left ventricular end-diastolic p.
left ventricular filling p.
left ventricular systolic p.
LES p.
lower body negative p.
lower esophageal sphincter p.
manual p.
maternal abdominal p.
maximum urethral closure p.
mean arterial p. (MAP)
mean arterial blood p. (MABP)
mean diastolic left ventricular p.
mean pulmonary artery p.
mean pulmonary artery wedge p.
mean systolic left ventricular p.
p. measurement
mercury p.

Michaelson counter p.
millimeters partial p.
minimum audible p.
narrowed pulse p.
p. natriuresis
p. necrosis
negative end-expiratory p.
nitrogen partial p.
noninvasive blood p. (NIBP)
normal intravascular p.
occlusal p.
occlusion p.
oncotic p.
opening p.
osmotic p.
p. overload
oxygen under high p.
PA filling p.
p. pain threshold (PPT)
pancreatic ducts p.
p. paralysis
partial p.
passage p.
peak inspiratory ventilator p.
peak systolic aortic p.
peak systolic gradient p.
perfusion p.
periapical p.
pericardial p.
peripheral p.
plantar p.
plasma colloid osmotic p.
plasma oncotic p.
p. pneumothorax
portal venous p.
positive airway p. (PAP)
positive end-airway p.
positive end-expiratory p. (PEEP)
positive end-expiratory
  pressure/continuous positive
  airway p. (PEEP/CPAP)
positive expiratory p.
positive inspiratory p.
posterior-anterior p.
postmembrane p.
premembrane p.
premicturition p.
proximal p.
PSG p.
pullback p.
pulmonary artery p. (PAP)

pulmonary artery occlusion p.
  (PAOP)
pulmonary artery occlusive
  wedge p.
pulmonary capillary wedge p.
pulmonary hypertension p.
pulmonary vascular p.
pulmonary wedge p.
pulp p.
pulse p.
p. rate quotient
p. receptor
p. recovery
p. regulated electrohydraulic
  lithotripsy
resting anal sphincter p.
p. reversal
p. reversal of anesthesia
right atrial p.
right ventricular end-diastolic p.
right ventricular systolic p.
p. ring
screen filtration p.
selection p.
shock wave p.
sinusoidal capillary p.
p. sore
sphincter of Oddi p.
spinal cord perfusion p. (SCPP)
splanchnic capillary p.
squeeze p.
standard temperature and p.
static closure p.
p. study
stump p.
subglottic p.
p. support ventilation
systemic mean arterial p.
systolic blood p. (SBP)
systolic left ventricular p.
p. technique filling
tentorial p.
time p.
tissue p.
p. tolerance
tongue p.
torr p.
tourniquet p.
transglomerular hydrostatic
  filtration p.
transmembrane hydraulic p.
p. transmission

NOTES

P

pressure *(continued)*
>p. transmission ratio
>transmural p.
>transmyocardial perfusion p.
>ureteral p.
>urethral p.
>vapor p.
>variable positive airway p.
>variceal p.
>vascular p.
>venous p.
>ventilation peak p.
>ventricular diastolic p.
>ventricular filling p.
>p. waveform
>wedge p.
>wedged hepatic venous p.
>p. welding
>white without p.
>zero end-expiratory p. (ZEEP)
>zero end-inspiratory p.
>z point p.

pressure-controlled inverse ratio ventilation
pressure-flow
>p.-f. electromyography study
>p.-f. plot
>p.-f. relation
>p.-f. relationship

pressure-natriuresis curve
pressure-point tension ring
pressure-regulated volume control ventilation
pressure-sensitive
>p.-s. area
>p.-s. tissue

pressure-separator tubing
pressure-tolerant tissue
pressure-volume
>p.-v. analysis
>p.-v. curve
>p.-v. index
>p.-v. relation

prestandardization
prestenotic dilatation
presternal
>p. notch
>p. region

presternum
presulcal part of tongue
presurgical medical evaluation
presynaptic membrane
presystolic pressure and volume
pretecta
pretemporal space
prethyroid
pretracheal
>p. fascia

>p. layer
>p. lymph nodes

pretransplant evaluation
pretreatment evaluation
pretympanic
prevention
>extension for p.
>heterotopic ossification p.
>infection p.
>rod rotation p.

preventive intravesical therapy
prevertebral
>p. fascia
>p. ganglia
>p. layer
>p. lymph nodes
>p. soft tissue
>p. space
>p. space abscess

prevesical
prewarming
Preziosi operation
prezonular space
priapus
Pribram suction tube
prick
>p. puncture test
>p. test concentration

prick-test method
Pridie incision
Pridie-Koutsogiannis procedure
prilocaine
>p. hydrochloride
>lidocaine and p.

primam
>per p.

primary
>p. adhesion
>p. amputation
>p. anesthetic
>p. cesarean section
>p. closure
>p. diagnostic endoscopy
>p. end-to-end anastomosis
>p. fibrinolysis
>p. gastric lymphoma staging
>p. glomerular lesion
>p. graft nonfunction
>p. healing after radiation therapy
>p. hemorrhage
>p. herpes simplex infection
>p. movement plane
>p. myofascial trigger point
>p. panendoscopy
>p. perineal hypospadias surgery
>p. pigmentary degeneration of retina
>p. point of ossification

p. position
p. procedure
p. pulmonary hypertension (PPH)
p. radiation
p. rejection
p. renal calculus
p. repair
p. rotation movement
p. shock
p. skin graft
p. sodium phosphate
p. suture
p. tumor
p. union
p. yolk sac

primer
Bowen cavity p.
cavity p.

priming dose

primitive
p. dislocation
p. knot
p. yolk sac

primordial catheter tube

princeps
p. cervicis artery
p. pollicis artery

Princeteau tubercle

principal
p. artery of thumb
p. fiber bundle
p. line
p. line of direction
p. plane
p. point
p. visual direction

principle
anatomic fracture reduction p.
axial compression p.
closure p.
Fick p.
Goodwin cup-patch p.
image formation p.
Le Chatelier p.
line focus p.
Mitrofanoff p.
Pauli exclusion p.

Pringle
P. maneuver
P. vascular control
P. vascular control method

P. vascular control procedure
P. vascular control technique

prior drug exposure
Priscoline injection
prism
p. adaptation test
p. method

proactive hemostasis
proatlas
probability
bone cyst fracture p.

probenecid-containing solution
probing lacrimonasal duct operation
procaine
p. hydrochloride
penicillin G p.

procallus formation
procedure
Abbé-McIndoe p.
Abbé-McIndoe-Williams p.
Abbé-Wharton-McIndoe p.
abdominal p.
ablative p.
Adams p.
advancement p.
Akin p.
Albee-Delbert p.
Aldridge sling p.
Al-Ghorab p.
Alliston p.
anchovy p.
Anderson p.
Anderson-Fowler p.
anecdotal p.
antegrade continence enema p.
antenna p.
anterior Pólya p.
anterior stabilization p.
anti-incontinence p.
antireflux p.
AO p.
arterial switch p.
articulatory p.
Axer-Clark p.
Baden p.
Badgley combination p.
Baldy-Webster p.
Bandi p.
Bankart p.
Barsky p.
Bartlett p.
Bassini p.

NOTES

P

577

procedure *(continued)*

Bastiaanse-Chiricuta p.
Baxter-D'Astous p.
Bell-Tawse p.
Belsey fundoplication p.
Bentall p.
Berman-Gartland p.
B.H. Moore p.
Bick p.
Bickel-Moe p.
bilateral inguinal hernia repair p.
Bilhaut-Cloquet p.
Billroth I, II p.
Bing-Taussig heart p.
Björk method of Fontan p.
bladder chimney p.
Blair-Brown p.
Blalock-Hanlon p.
Blalock-Taussig p.
Blatt p.
Blatt-Ashworth p.
blocking p.
Boari bladder flap p.
bone block p.
bony p.
Bose p.
bowel refashioning p.
Boyce-Vest p.
Boyd-Bosworth p.
Boyd-McLeod p.
Boyd-Sisk p.
Boytchev p.
Brahms p.
Brantigan p.
Brantigan-Voshell p.
Braun p.
breast-conserving p.
Bricker p.
Bridle p.
Bristow-Helfet p.
Bristow-May p.
Brock p.
Brockman p.
Broström p.
Bryan p.
Bunnell-Williams p.
Burch bladder suspension p.
burn-out p.
bypass p.
Calandriello p.
Caldwell-Luc window p.
Camey p.
Campbell-Akbarnia p.
Campbell-Goldthwait p.
canalith repositioning p.
capsular shift p.
carotid ablative p.
Castaneda p.

Castle p.
catheter-directed interventional p.
Cawthorne-Day p.
cecal imbrication p.
Cecil p.
cervical spine stabilization p.
Chamberlain p.
Chambers p.
Charles p.
Chassar Moir-Sims p.
Chassar Moir sling p.
checkrein p.
Cherry-Crandall p.
cherry-picking p.
Chester-Winter p.
Chrisman-Snook p.
Cibis liquid silicone p.
ciliary p.
Clayton p.
Cleveland p.
Cloward p.
Cockett p.
Cohen antireflux p.
Cole intubation p.
Collis-Nissen fundoplication p.
colon p.
commando p.
compartment p.
composite pelvic resection p.
concentration p.
Connolly p.
core drilling p.
coronary artery revascularization p.
corporeal rotation p.
corridor p.
Cox Maze III p.
Cracchiolo p.
Custodis nondraining p.
cyclodestructive p.
Cyclops p.
Damian graft p.
Damus-Kaye-Stancel p.
Damus-Kaye-Stancel p. for single
  ventricle physiology
Damus-Stancel-Kaye p.
Danus-Fontan p.
Darrach p.
dartos pouch p.
Das Gupta p.
Datta p.
Davis-Kitlowski p.
Davydov p.
DAWG p.
de-airing p.
debubbling p.
debulking p.
degloving p.
dental prosthetic laboratory p.

Devine-Devine p.
Dewar posterior cervical fixation p.
diagnostic p.
Dickson-Diveley p.
domino p.
Donald p.
Donders p.
Dor fundoplication p.
Dorrance p.
dot-blot p.
double-stapled ileoanal reservoir p.
Downey-McGlamery p.
DREZ p.
Duckett p.
Dukes p.
Duval p.
Dwyer p.
Ebbehoj p.
Eden-Hybbinette p.
Eden-Lange p.
Edwards p.
Effler-Groves mode of Allison p.
elimination p.
Elmslie p.
Elmslie-Cholmely p.
Elmslie-Trillat patellar p.
endorectal ileoanal pull-through p.
endoscopic mucosal resection p.
endoscopy p.
end-to-end reconstruction p.
enucleation p.
esophageal sling p.
Estes p.
evacuation p.
Evans p.
Evans-Steptoe p.
Everard Williams p.
excisional biopsy p.
ex situ in vivo p.
extended Ross p.
extra-anatomic bypass p.
extra-articular p.
extracorporeal p.
Faden p.
failed p.
Fairbanks-Sever p.
Fasanella-Servat p.
fascial sling p.
fiberoptic intubation p.
Ficat p.
filtering p.
Fired-Hendel p.

five-incision p.
flip-flap p.
floppy Nissen fundoplication p.
Fontan-Baudet p.
Fontan-Kreutzer p.
Fontan modification of Norwood p.
forage p.
four-incision p.
four-port p.
Fowler p.
Fowler-Stephens p.
Fox-Blazina p.
Frank p.
Fredet-Ramstedt p.
Fried-Green foot p.
Froimson p.
Frost p.
Fulford p.
Gallie p.
Gartland p.
gaseous laparoscopy p.
gasless laparoscopy p.
gastric bypass p.
gastric emptying p. (GEP)
gastric pull-through p.
gastric valve tightening p.
Gelman p.
Gepfert p.
Gilchrist p.
Gill p.
Gill-Jonas modification of
  Norwood p.
Gillquist p.
Gil-Vernet p.
Girard p.
Girdlestone hip p.
Girdlestone-Taylor p.
Gittes p.
Gittes-Loughlin p.
Glenn p.
Goebell p.
Goebell-Stoeckel-Frangenheim p.
Goldner-Hayes p.
Goldthwait-Hauser p.
Gould p.
Goulding p.
gracilis p.
Green p.
Gregoir-Lich p.
Grice p.
Gurd p.
Halban p.

NOTES

P

579

procedure *(continued)*
  hallux valgus p.
  Hambly p.
  Hammon p.
  hamular p.
  Hancock p.
  Hanley rectal bladder p.
  Harada-Ito p.
  Harewood suspension p.
  Hark p.
  Harmon p.
  Hartmann p.
  Hass p.
  Hauser patellar tendon p.
  Hawkins p.
  Hedley p.
  Heifetz p.
  Heller myotomy with Dor fundoplication p.
  hemi-Fontan p.
  hemi-Kock p.
  heparinization p.
  hepatic vascular exclusion and in situ perfusion p.
  hex p.
  Heyman p.
  Heyman-Herndon clubfoot p.
  Hibbs p.
  Hill p.
  Hinman p.
  His-Haas p.
  Hodgson technique of modified Lich p.
  Hodor-Dobbs p.
  Hoffmann-Clayton p.
  Hofmeister p.
  Hohmann p.
  Hoke p.
  Hoke-Miller p.
  Hood p.
  Hovanian p.
  Howorth p.
  Howorth-Keillor p.
  Hughston p.
  Hughston-Hauser p.
  Hui-Linscheid p.
  Hummelsheim p.
  hypoglossal facial transfer p.
  hypophysis staining p.
  ileoanal pouch p.
  ileoanal pull-through p.
  iliac buttressing p.
  Ilizarov p.
  Inclan-Ober p.
  infrarenal template p.
  Ingelman-Sundberg gracilis muscle p.
  inner ear tack p.
  Insall p.
  installation p.
  intercalary allograft p.
  interventional p.
  intestinal bypass p.
  intra-articular p.
  intraparavariceal p.
  intraperitoneal p.
  island flap p.
  Ito p.
  Jacobaeus p.
  Jaeger-Hamby p.
  Jaffe p.
  Jahss p.
  Jannetta microvascular decompression p.
  Jansey p.
  Jatene arterial switch p.
  jejunoileal bypass reversal p.
  Jensen transposition p.
  Jobe-Glousman capsular shift p.
  Johnson p.
  Johnson-Spiegl p.
  Johnston buttonhole p.
  Jonas modification of Norwood p.
  Jones tube p.
  J. R. Moore p.
  Junod p.
  Juvara p.
  Kaliscinski ureteral p.
  Karakousis-Vezeridis p.
  Karhunen-Loeve p.
  Karlsson p.
  Kasai p.
  Kawaii-Yamamoto p.
  Kelikian p.
  Kelikian-McFarland p.
  Keller p.
  Kelling-Madlener p.
  Kelly plication p.
  Kendrick p.
  Kennedy p.
  Kessel-Bonney p.
  Kestenbaum p.
  Kidner foot p.
  Kiehn-Earle-DesPrez p.
  Killian frontoethmoidectomy p.
  Knapp p.
  Knobby-Clark p.
  Ko-Airan bleeding control p.
  Kocher ureterosigmoidostomy p.
  Kolmogorov-Smirnov p.
  Kondoleon-Sistrunk elephantiasis p.
  Konno p.
  Kortzeborn p.
  Koutsogiannis p.
  Krönlein p.
  Kropp p.

Krukenberg p.
Kuhnt-Szymanowski p.
Ladd p.
Lam p.
Lane p.
Lange p.
Langenskiöld p.
Langevin updating p.
laparoscopic lymph node
  dissection p.
laparoscopic Nissen
  fundoplication p.
laparoscopic para-aortic lymph node
  sampling p.
laparoscopic tubal banding p.
Larmon forefoot p.
Lash p.
Latarjet p.
lateral sling p.
lathing p.
latissimus dorsi p.
Lauenstein p.
Leadbetter p.
Leadbetter-Politano p.
Lee p.
Le Fort p.
left atrial isolation p.
Lepird p.
L'Episcopo-Zachary p.
Lewis-Tanner p.
Lich p.
limb-lengthening p.
limb-salvage p.
limb-saving p.
limb-sparing p.
Lindeman p.
Linton p.
Lipscomb p.
Lipscomb-Anderson p.
Localio p.
loop electrocautery excision p.
  (LEEP)
loop electrosurgical excision p.
loop gastric bypass p.
loose knee p.
Lorenz p.
Lothrop frontoethmoidectomy p.
lower cervical spine p.
lower lid sling p.
Lowman p.
Luke p.
LVR p.

Lynch frontoethmoidectomy p.
Lyon-Horgan p.
MacAusland p.
MacCarthy p.
Magnuson-Stack p.
Mahan p.
Manktelow transfer p.
Mann p.
Mann-Coughlin p.
Maquet p.
Marshall-Marchetti p.
Marshall-Marchetti-Krantz p.
Martius p.
Mathieu p.
Matsen p.
Mauck p.
Maydl p.
Mayo-Fueth inversion p.
Maze III p.
McBride p.
McCall-Schumann p.
McCarroll-Baker p.
McCormick-Blount p.
McDonald p.
McElvenny-Caldwell p.
McGlamry-Downey p.
McIndoe p.
McIndoe-Hayes p.
McKeever p.
McLaughlin p.
McVay p.
medial rotation p.
Meigs-Okabayashi p.
Michal I, II p.
micro-operative p.
microsurgery p.
microsurgical epididymal sperm
  aspiration p.
Miller p.
minimal-access p.
minimally invasive p.
Minkoff-Nicholas p.
Mitrofanoff p.
MMK p.
Moberg key-pinch p.
modified Belsey fundoplication p.
modified Hoke-Miller flatfoot p.
modified Norfolk p.
modified Seldinger p.
modified Toupe p.
modified Weber-Fergusson p.
modified Wies p.

NOTES

P

procedure *(continued)*
    Mogensen p.
    Moore p.
    Moschcowitz p.
    motion-preserving p.
    multiple-port incisions p.
    Mumford p.
    muscle-balancing p.
    Mustardé otoplasty p.
    Mustard intra-atrial p.
    needle suspension p.
    needle thoracentesis p.
    Neer capsular shift p.
    Nesbit tuck p.
    NESTED p.
    Neugebauer-LeFort p.
    neurostimulating p.
    Nichols p.
    Nicks p.
    Nicola shoulder p.
    Nicoll fracture repair p.
    Nissen fundoplication p.
    Nissen-Rosseti fundoplication p.
    non-fenestrated Fontan p.
    noninvasive p.
    non-rib-spreading thoracotomy
      incision p.
    Norwood univentricular heart p.
    notchplasty p.
    O'Brien capsular shift p.
    O'Donoghue p.
    Olshausen p.
    omentum majus flap p.
    one-stage p.
    operant p.
    orthodontic p.
    orthodox p.
    Orticochea p.
    Osborne-Cotterill p.
    osteoplastic frontal sinus p.
    otic periotic shunt p.
    Oudard p.
    Overholt p.
    palatal lengthening p.
    Palomo p.
    PAM p.
    Parrish p.
    Paterson p.
    Pauchet p.
    Peabody p.
    pelvic pouch p.
    percutaneous transhepatic biliary p.
    Pereyra p.
    peri-Vaterian therapeutic
      endoscopic p.
    Perthes p.
    Peustow p.

Peyeyra-Lebhertz modification of
    Frangenheim-Stoeckel p.
Pichlmayer p.
PLIF p.
Pólya p.
portmanteau p.
posterior lumbar interbody
    fusion p.
postcrior Pólya p.
Potts p.
Pozzi p.
Pridie-Koutsogiannis p.
primary p.
Pringle vascular control p.
psoas hitch p.
Puestow p.
Puestow-Gillesby p.
pull-through p.
push-back p.
Putti-Platt shoulder p.
Quaegebeur p.
Quickert p.
Ramstedt p.
Ransley p.
Rashkind p.
Rastan-Konno p.
Rastelli p.
Raz p.
Raz-Leach p.
realignment p.
Récamier p.
reconstruction p.
reefing p.
Reichel-Pólya p.
Reichenheim-King p.
repeat p.
restorative p.
resurfacing p.
retrogasserian p.
revascularization p.
Reverdin-Green p.
reverse filling p.
reverse Mauck p.
reverse Putti-Platt p.
revision p.
Richardson p.
Richter and Albrich p.
Ridlon p.
Riedel frontoethmoidectomy p.
Righini p.
Ripstein p.
Rockwood p.
Rockwood-Matsen capsular shift p.
Rose p.
Ross p.
Roux-en-Y p.
Roux-Goldthwait p.
Ruiz p.

Ruiz-Mora p.
Ryerson p.
sacroiliac buttressing p.
Sade modification of Norwood p.
Saha p.
Salle p.
salting-out p.
Samilson p.
sartorial slide p.
Sato p.
Sauve-Kapandji p.
Savin p.
Sayoc p.
Schauffler p.
Schenk-Eichelter vena cava plastic
    filter p.
Schoemaker p.
Schonander p.
Schrock p.
scleral buckling p.
Scudder p.
Scuderi p.
Selakovich p.
Seldinger p.
semitendinosus p.
Senning transposition p.
septation p.
Shauta-Aumreich p.
Shea p.
Shirodkar p.
short lever specific contact p.
Silfverskiöld p.
Silver p.
Simplate p.
Sistrunk p.
in situ p.
sling p.
SLURPIE p.
Smith-Robinson p.
Snow p.
Soave p.
Somerville p.
Sondergaard p.
Southwick slide p.
spatial localization p.
Spence p.
sphincter-saving p.
sphincter-sparing p.
spinal-locking p.
Spira p.
Spittler p.
SPLATT p.

split anterior tibial tendon p.
Stack shoulder p.
Staheli shelf p.
Stamey-Martius p.
Stamey modification of Pereyra p.
Stamm p.
Stancel p.
Stanley Way p.
stapled reconstruction p.
Steindler p.
stereotactic needle core biopsy p.
Steytler-Van Der Walt p.
Stone p.
Strayer p.
strip p.
Studer pouch p.
suburethral rectus fascial sling p.
Sugiura p.
surgical enucleation p.
Swenson pull-through p.
switch p.
Syme p.
Tachdjian p.
takedown of pelvic sling p.
tarsal strip p.
Taylor p.
terminal Syme p.
Thal fundoplication p.
Thiersch p.
Thiersch-Duplay proximal tube p.
Thomas p.
Thompson p.
Tikhoff-Linberg p.
p. time
TIPS p.
total fundoplication p.
Toti p.
touch-up p.
Toupe p.
transendoscopic p.
transhepatic antegrade biliary
    drainage p.
transvaginal Burch p.
Trillat p.
triple-wire p.
Tsai-Stillwell p.
tuck p.
tumbling p.
two-stage p.
two-step p.
uncinate p.

NOTES

P

procedure *(continued)*
 uncut Collis-Nissen
  fundoplication p.
 unilateral inguinal hernia repair p.
 untethering p.
 up-and-down staircases p.
 upper cervical spine p.
 ureteral patch p.
 urethral vesicle suspension p.
 vaginal needle suspension p.
 vaginal wall sling p.
 Valpius-Compere p.
 valvulotomy p.
 Van de Kramer fecal fat p.
 Van Ness p.
 VATS p.
 video-assisted p.
 video-assisted thoracic surgical p.
 Vineberg p.
 Vulpius p.
 Vulpius-Stoffel p.
 V-Y p.
 W p.
 Waldhausen p.
 Wardill-Kilner p.
 Waterhouse transpubic p.
 Waterston-Cooley p.
 Watson-Cheyne-Burghard p.
 Watson-Jones p.
 Weaver-Dunn p.
 Weber p.
 Weber-Fergusson p.
 Wheeler p.
 Whipple p.
 White slide p.
 Whitman talectomy p.
 Whitman-Thompson p.
 Wies p.
 Williams p.
 Wilson p. for extra-articular fusion
  of elbow
 Winter p.
 Womack p.
 Woodward p.
 Yoke transposition p.
 York-Mason p.
 Young p.
 Young-Dees p.
 Yount p.
 Z p.
 Zancolli-Lasso p.
 Zancolli static lock p.
 Zarins-Rowe p.
 Zoellner-Clancy p.
 Z-plasty p.
proceedings
 care and protection p.
procelia

procephalic
procerus
 p. muscle
process
 accessory p.
 acromial p.
 articular p.
 basilar p. of occipital bone
 calcaneal p. of cuboid bone
 caudate p.
 Civinini p.
 clinoid p.
 condylar p.
 condyloid p.
 conoid p.
 coracoid p.
 coronoid p.
 costal p.
 cribriform plate of alveolar p.
 ensiform p.
 exocrinopathic p.
 falciform p.
 fenestration of alveolar p.
 frontal p. of zygomatic bone
 frontosphenoidal p.
 funicular p.
 intrajugular p.
 jugular p.
 lateral p. of calcaneal tuberosity
 lateral p. of talus
 lenticular p. of incus
 mamillary p.
 medial p. of calcaneal tuberosity
 mental p.
 olecranon p.
 papillary p.
 paroccipital p.
 posterior p. of septal cartilage
 posterior p. of talus
 pterygoid p.
 pterygospinous p.
 sheath p. of sphenoid bone
 space-occupying p.
 sphenoid p.
 sphenoid p. of palatine bone
 sphenoid p. of septal cartilage
 spinous p.
 spinous p. of tibia
 Stieda p.
 styloid p. of temporal bone
 superior articular p. of sacrum
 supracondylar p.
 supraepicondylar p.
 temporal p.
 transverse p.
 trochlear p.
 uncinate p. of pancreas
 vaginal p.

vaginal p. of peritoneum
vaginal p. of sphenoid bone
vaginal p. of testis
vermiform p.
vocal p.
vocal p. of arytenoid cartilage
xiphoid p.
zygomatic p. of frontal bone
zygomatic p. of maxilla
zygomatic p. of temporal bone

processus
    p. accessorius
    p. articularis
    p. articularis superior ossis sacri
    p. calcaneus ossis cuboidei
    p. caudatus
    p. clinoideus
    p. condylaris
    p. coracoideus
    p. coronoideus
    p. costalis
    p. falciformis
    p. ferreini
    p. frontalis ossis zygomatici
    p. intrajugularis
    p. jugularis
    p. lateralis tali
    p. lateralis tuberis calcanei
    p. lenticularis incudis
    p. mamillaris
    p. medialis tuberis calcanei
    p. papillaris
    p. posterior cartilaginis septi nasi
    p. posterior tali
    p. pterygoideus
    p. pterygospinosus
    p. sphenoidalis
    p. spinosus
    p. styloideus ossis temporalis
    p. supraepicondylaris humeri
    p. temporalis
    p. transversus
    p. trochleariformis
    p. trochlearis
    p. uncinatus pancreatis
    p. vaginalis ossis sphenoidalis
    p. vaginalis peritonei
    p. vaginalis of peritoneum
    p. vermiformis
    p. vocalis cartilaginis arytenoidei
    p. xiphoideus
    p. zygomaticus maxillae

    p. zygomaticus ossis frontalis
    p. zygomaticus ossis temporalis
procheilon
prochlorperazine
prochordal
Prochownick method
procidentia
procreate
procreation
    assisted medical p.
procreative
proctagra
proctalgia
proctectasia
proctectomy
    mucosal p.
    stapled ileal pouch-anal anastomosis
        without proctomucosal p.
proctencleisis
Procter-Livingstone tube
procteurynter
proctitis
    radiation p.
proctocele
proctoclysis
proctococcypexy
proctocolectomy
    restorative p.
    single-stage total p.
    subtotal p.
    total p.
    totally stapled restorative p.
    total p. with ileoanal anastomosis
        and J pouch
    p. with preservation of anal
        sphincter function
proctocolitis
    radiation p.
proctocolonoscopy
proctocolpoplasty
proctocystocele
proctocystoplasty
proctocystotomy
proctodynia
proctoelytroplasty
proctography
    evacuation p.
proctologic
proctologist
proctology
proctoperineoplasty
proctoperineorrhaphy

NOTES

P

585

proctopexy
    Orr-Loygue transabdominal p.
proctoplasty
proctoptosia
proctorrhagia
proctorrhaphy
proctorrhea
Proctor suction tube
proctoscopic examination
proctoscopy
    rigid p.
proctosigmoid disposable suction tube
proctosigmoidectomy
proctosigmoidoscopy
    rigid p.
proctospasm
proctostasis
proctostat
proctostenosis
proctostomy
proctotomy
    posterior p.
proctotresia
proctovalvotomy
procumbent
procurement
procurvation
Pro-Depo injection
α-prodine hydrochloride
Prodrox injection
product
    contact activation p.
    degradation p.
    Exact skin p.
    fibrin degradation p.
    fibrinogen degradation p.
    fibrinogen-fibrin degradation p.
    lipid peroxidation p.
    oxygen reduction p.
    pyrolysis p.
    rate pressure p.
    tumor-cell p.
    vector p.
production
    ectopic parathormone p.
    excessive heat p.
    metabolic heat p.
    paraneoplastic ectopic ACTH p.
productive inflammation
PROEF
    postoperative regimen for oral early
    feeding
Proetz
    P. displacement technique
    P. maneuver
profile
    aortic valve velocity p.
    coagulation p.

    extraoral radiographic
      examination p.
    facial p.
    projection p.
    resting urethral pressure p.
    stress urethral pressure p.
    urethral closure pressure p.
    vector p.
profound hypothermia
profoundly hypothermic circulatory
  arrest (PHCA)
profunda
    p. brachii artery
    p. femoris artery
profundaplasty
profundus
    p. artery fracture
progenitalis
progestational
    p. protection
    p. therapy
progestogen support therapy
prognosticator
progonoma
prograde
    p. technique
program
    aquatic stabilization p.
    Cancer Surveillance P.
    CAPRI p.
    conditioning p.
    diagnostic p.
    Expedited Recovery P.
    four-star exercise p.
    home p.
    independent exercise p.
    Linde Walker Oxygen P.
    Muma Assessment P.
    National Marrow Donor P.
    object p.
    Organ Procurement P.
    Rothman Institute total hip p.
    safety p.
    Sedlachek p.
    Solid Tumor Autologous Marrow
      Transplant P.
    source p.
    standard bone algorithm p.
    STANPUMP p.
    Starkey matrix p.
    stripping p.
    survey p.
    P. 2 syringe pump
    WALK p.
    walking p.
    Westcott Pyramid P.
    work hardening p.

programmed
>p. electrical stimulation
>p. therapy

programming

progression
>tumor p.

progressive
>P. Ambulation Scale
>p. extraction
>p. spin saturation

Project
>Breast Cancer Detection
>Demonstration P.
>National Surgical Adjuvant Breast
>and Bowel P.

projection
>afferent p.
>anterior oblique p.
>anteroposterior p.
>A&P p.
>apical lordotic p.
>axial calcaneal p.
>axial sesamoid p.
>back p.
>base p.
>bony p.
>bregma-mentum p.
>bursal p.
>Caldwell p.
>cephaloscapular p.
>convergence p.
>coronal oblique p.
>cross-sectional p.
>cross-table lateral p.
>Didiee p.
>divergent ray p.
>dorsoplantar p.
>enamel p.
>erroneous p.
>extradental p.
>false p.
>fan beam p.
>p. fiber
>p. fiber damage
>filtered-back p.
>Fischer p.
>frog-leg lateral p.
>frontal p.
>Granger p.
>half-axial p.
>Harris-Beath p.
>Hermodsson tangential p.

>horizontal p.
>Isherwood p.
>lateral jaw p.
>left anterior oblique p.
>left lateral p.
>light p.
>maximum-intensity p.
>mental p.
>Mercator p.
>oblique p.
>occipitomental p.
>occlusal p.
>orthogonal p.
>PA p.
>panoramic surface p.
>papillary p.
>parasympathetic p.
>perimeter p.
>posterior-superior oblique p.
>posteroanterior p.
>p. profile
>reverse topographic p.
>Rhese p.
>right anterior oblique p.
>Rungstrom p.
>sagittal p.
>Schüller p.
>spider p.
>Stenvers p.
>stress dorsiflexion p.
>submental vertex p.
>submentovertical p.
>surface p.
>sympathetic p.
>tangential p.
>topographic p.
>Towne p.
>p. tract imaging
>transmandibular p.
>transorbital p.
>transverse p.
>visual p.
>Waters p.

projection-reconstruction
>p.-r. imaging
>p.-r. technique

projective technique

prolabial

prolabium

prolapsed
>p. mitral valve syndrome
>p. stoma

NOTES

prolapse ring pessary
Prolene polypropylene suture
proliferation
    p. area
    p. of the gastric epithelium
    p. zone
proliferative
    p. inflammation
    p. lesion
prolongation
    p. of expiration
    expiratory p.
    P2 p.
    pulse repetition time p.
prolonged
    p. expiratory phase
    p. rupture
promethazine hydrochloride
Prometh injection
prominence
    p. of facial canal
    hypothenar p.
    laryngeal p.
    osteochondral p.
    pedicle screw hardware p.
    styloid p.
    thenar p.
    p. of venous valvular sinus
prominens
prominent
    p. indentation
    p. Schwalbe ring
prominentia, pl. prominentiae
    p. canalis facialis
    p. laryngea
    p. styloidea
promontorium
    p. ossis sacri
promontory
    p. common iliac lymph nodes
    pelvic p.
    sacral p.
    p. of the sacrum
    p. stimulation test
promoter
    tumor p.
pronate
pronation
    p. control
    p. injury
pronation-abduction
    p.-a. fracture
    p.-a. injury
pronation-eversion
    p.-e. fracture
    p.-e. injury
pronation-eversion-external
    p.-e.-e. rotation

p.-e.-e. rotation injury
p.-e.-e. rotation injury of ankle
pronation-supination
pronator
    p. quadratus
    p. quadratus muscle
    p. reflex
    p. teres
    p. teres muscle
    p. teres release
    p. teres syndrome
    p. teres tendon
prone
    p. extension test
    p. reduction
    p. split-leg position
pronephric duct
pronglike excementosis
pronograde
pronuclear stage transfer (PROST)
ProOsteon Implant 500 granule
prootic
propagate
propagation
propagative
propanidid
proparacaine
    p. HCl
    p. hydrochloride
proper
    p. hepatic artery
    p. palmar digital artery
    p. palmar digital nerve
    p. plantar digital artery
    p. plantar digital nerve
properitoneal
    p. fat
    p. fat line
    p. flank stripe
    p. inguinal hernia
prophylactic
    p. antibiotic therapy
    p. anticoagulation
    p. bone graft
    p. cholecystectomy
    p. colectomy
    p. fasciotomy
    p. irradiation
    p. lymphadenectomy
    p. medication
    p. membrane
    p. odontotomy
    p. oophorectomy
    p. operative stabilization
    p. orchiectomy
    p. resection
    p. skeletal fixation

prophylaxis
    aspiration p.
    stricture p.
propiomazine hydrochloride
propitocaine hydrochloride
Proplast graft
propofol
    p. rescue
propofol/nitrous oxide anesthesia
proportional assist ventilation
propoxycaine
propoxyphene hydrochloride
proprioceptive
    p. head-turning reflex
    p. neuromuscular facilitation (PNF)
    p. neuromuscular facilitation
      approach
proprius
    extensor indicis p.
Prorex injection
prosection
prosector tubercle
prospective
    p. evaluation of radial keratomy
    p. study
prospermia
PROST
    pronuclear stage transfer
    laparoscopic PROST
prostacyclin
    aerosolized p.
prostaglandin
    renal vasodilator p.
prostanoid
Prostaphlin injection
prostata
prostatalgia
prostate
    carcinoma of p.
    coagulation and hemostatic
      resection of the p.
    contact laser ablation of p.
      (CLAP)
    female p.
    p. gland
    minimal transurethral resection
      of p.
    percutaneous radical cryosurgical
      ablation of p.
    total transurethral resection of p.
    transurethral evaporation of p.

    transurethral laser incision of
      the p.
    transurethral resection of p.
    transurethral vaporization of p.
    visual laser ablation of p.
prostatectomy
    anatomical radical retropubic p.
    cavernous nerve-sparing p.
    nerve-sparing radical retropubic p.
    perineal p.
    radical perineal p.
    radical retropubic p.
    radical transcoccygeal p.
    salvage p.
    Stanford radical retropubic p.
    suprapubic p.
    total perineal p.
    transurethral ablative p.
    transurethral ultrasound-guided laser-
      induced p.
    visual laser assisted p.
    Walsh radical retropubic p.
prostatic
    p. adenocarcinoma
    p. adenoma
    p. calculus
    p. carcinoma
    p. ducts
    p. ductules
    p. fluid
    p. massage
    p. plexus
    p. sheath
    p. sinus
    p. urethra
    p. urethroplasty
    p. utricle
    p. venous plexus
prostaticovesical
    p. plexus
prostatism
prostatitis
prostatocystitis
prostatocystotomy
prostatodynia
prostatolith
prostatolithotomy
prostatomegaly
prostatomy
prostatorrhea
prostatoseminal vesiculectomy
prostatotomy

NOTES

P

prostatovesiculectomy
prostatovesiculitis
prosthesis
    partial ossicular replacement p. (PORP)
    total ossicular replacement p. (TORP)
prosthesis-cement interface
prosthesis interface
prosthetic
    p. arterial graft
    p. arthroplasty
    p. hemiarthroplasty
    p. patch
    p. restoration
    p. ring annuloplasty
    p. valve sewing ring
prosthetics
prosthetist
prosthokeratoplasty
Prostin VR Pediatric injection
prosyncopal medication
protamine correction
protection
    airway p.
    automated boundary p.
    barrier p.
    cerebral p.
    digital artery p.
    gastroduodenal mucosal p.
    misoprostol p.
    myocardial p.
    progestational p.
    radiation p.
    regions of p.
    p. test
    venous/arterial management p. (VAMP)
protective antireflux operation
proteinaceous aqueous exudation
protein shock therapy
proteolysis
Prothazine injection
protocol
    exsanguination p.
    fractionation p.
    reinjection p.
protoduodenum
proton
    p. pump
    p. pump inhibition therapy
protopianoma
protoplasmolysis
protozoal infection
protractor
protruded disk

protrusio
    p. deformity
    p. ring
protrusion
    corneal p.
protrusive
    p. excursion
    p. jaw relation
    p. line
    p. occlusal position
    p. position
protuberance
    external occipital p.
    internal occipital p.
protuberant abdomen
protuberantia
    p. occipitalis externa
    p. occipitalis interna
Proust space
Provector
Provider
    Pain Management P.
    P. 5500 patient-controlled analgesia device
provisional
    p. fixation
    p. ligature
    p. restoration
    p. stabilization
provocation
    p. test
provocative
    p. chelation test
    p. food thyroidectomy
Prowazek-Greeff body
proximad
proximal
    p. cavity
    p. centriole
    p. dome osteotomy
    p. femoral epiphysiolysis
    p. femoral fracture
    p. femoral osteotomy
    p. femoral resection
    p. gastrectomy
    p. gastric vagotomy
    p. humeral fracture
    p. interphalangeal joint approach
    p. loop syndrome
    p. metatarsal osteotomy
    p. nail matrix
    p. phalangeal osteotomy
    p. pressure
    p. radioulnar articulation
    p. space
    p. tendon rupture
    p. tibial metaphyseal fracture
    p. tibial osteotomy

p. tibiofibular joint dislocation
p. urethral sphincter
proximalis
proximal-row carpectomy
proximal-to-distal ring
proximate
p. space
Proxi-Strip suture
proxymetacaine hydrochloride
prune
prune-belly syndrome
prune-juice
p.-j. expectoration
p.-j. peritoneal fluid
pruritic
p. erythematous patch
p. lesion
Prussak space
PRx Endotak-Sub-Q array
psammocarcinoma
psammoma
p. body
psammomatous
psammosarcoma
pseudarthrosis
p. repair
pseudesthesia
pseudinoma
pseudoagglutination
pseudoaneurysm
p. formation
pseudoangiosarcoma
pseudoankylosis
pseudoarthrosis
p. repair
pseudoarticulation
pseudobiopsy technique
pseudo-blind loop syndrome
pseudoboutonnière deformity
pseudocalcification
pseudocancerous lesion
pseudocarcinoma
pseudocavitation
pseudocele
pseudocephalocele
pseudocholesteatoma
pseudochylous ascites
pseudoclaudication
pseudocoarctation
p. of aorta
pseudocoloboma
pseudocoma

pseudocryptorchism
pseudocyst
endosonography-guided drainage of
pancreatic p.
pseudocystobiliary fistula
pseudocystogastrostomy
pancreatic p.
pseudodefecation
pseudodislocation
pseudoepiphysis
pseudoepithelioma
pseudoexfoliation
p. of lens capsule
p. syndrome
pseudofacilitation
pseudogestational sac
pseudoglioma
pseudohernia
pseudohydrocephaly
pseudoinfection
pseudolipoma
pseudolymphoma
p. syndrome
pseudomasturbation
**pseudomedial longitudinal fasciculus
lesion**
pseudomelanoma
pseudomembranous acute inflammation
pseudomeningocele
posttraumatic intradiploic p.
traumatic p.
pseudomigration
Pseudomonas **infection**
pseudomyxoma
pseudoneurogenic bladder
pseudoneuroma
pseudo-omphalocele
pseudo-osteomalacia
pseudo-osteomalacic
p.-o. pelvis
pseudo-ovulation
pseudopod formation
pseudoprolactinoma
pseudoretinoblastoma
pseudosacculation
pseudosarcoma
pseudoserous membrane
pseudostoma
pseudosubluxation
pseudotrachoma
pseudoureterocele

NOTES

P

591

pseudoxanthoma
 p. elasticum syndrome
PSG
 peak systolic gradient
 PSG pressure
psoas
 p. hitch procedure
 p. line
 p. major muscle
 p. margin
 p. minor muscle
psoralens, ultraviolet A (PUVA)
PSSE
 partial saturation spin-echo
 PSSE technique
psychomotor retardation
psychopharmacologic medication
psychorelaxation
psychosedation
 dental p.
psychosis
psychosurgery
psychotropic medication
psychrophore
PTCA
 percutaneous transluminal coronary
  angioplasty
  multivessel PTCA
PTE
 pulmonary thromboendarterectomy
pterional
 p. approach
 p. craniotomy
pterygial tissue
pterygoid
 p. branch of maxillary artery
 p. canal
 p. fissure
 p. fossa
 p. fovea
 p. hamulus
 p. laminae
 p. nerve
 p. notch
 p. pit
 p. plexus
 p. position
 p. process
 p. ridge of sphenoid bone
 p. tubercle
 p. tuberosity
pterygomandibular
 p. ligament
 p. raphe
 p. space
 p. space abscess
pterygomaxillare

pterygomaxillary
 p. fissure
 p. fossa
 p. space
pterygopalatine
 p. canal
 p. fossa
 p. ganglion
 p. groove
 p. nerve
 p. space
pterygospinal ligament
pterygospinous
 p. ligament
 p. process
PTFE
 polytetrafluoroethylene
 PTFE Gore-Tex graft
PTGDS
 patellar tendon graft donor site
ptosed
ptosis
ptotic
 p. organ
PTV
 percutaneous transtracheal jet ventilation
ptyalocele
pubes
pubic
 p. angle
 p. arch
 p. arteries
 p. body
 p. bone
 p. branch of inferior epigastric
  artery
 p. branch of obturator artery
 p. crest
 p. diastasis
 p. fixation
 p. hair line
 p. pad
 p. ramus
 p. region
 p. spine
 p. symphysis
 p. tubercle
pubiotomy
pubocapsular
pubococcygeal
 p. line
 p. muscle
pubococcygeus muscle
pubofemoral
puboprostatic
 p. ligament
 p. muscle

puborectal
  p. muscle
puborectalis
  p. loop
  p. muscle
pubourethral triangle
pubovaginal
  p. muscle
  p. operation
pubovaginalis muscle
pubovesical
  p. muscle
pubovesicalis muscle
Puchtler
  P. alkaline Congo red method
  P. Sirius red method
Puddu tendon technique
pudenda
pudendal
  p. anesthesia
  p. canal
  p. cleft
  p. hematocele
  p. hernia
  p. nerve
  p. sac
  p. slit
  p. veins
pudendum
  p. femininum
  p. muliebre
pudic
  p. nerve
puerile respiration
puerperal
  p. hematoma
  p. infection
Puestow
  P. pancreaticojejunostomy
  P. procedure
Puestow-Gillesby
  P.-G. operation
  P.-G. procedure
Puestow-Olander gastrointestinal tube
Pugh
  P. classification
  modified method of P.
Puig
  P. Massana annuloplasty ring
  P. Massana-Shiley annuloplasty ring
Pulec and Freedman classification

pullback
  p. pressure
  p. pressure gradient
pull-enteroscopy
pulley
  muscular p.
  peroneal p.
  p. reconstruction
  p. of talus
pull maneuver
pull-out wire suture
pull-through
  endorectal ileal p.-t.
  endorectal ileoanal p.-t.
  ileoanal endorectal p.-t.
  p.-t. operation
  p.-t. procedure
  rapid p.-t. (RPT)
  sacroabdominoperineal p.-t.
  Soave endorectal p.-t.
  station p.-t.
  p.-t. technique
pulmo, pl. **pulmones**
  p. dexter
  p. sinister
pulmoaortic
  p. canal
pulmonary
  p. acid aspiration syndrome
  p. alveolar hemorrhage
  p. angioma
  p. arborization
  p. arterial malformation
  p. arterial web
  p. arteriovenous fistula (PAF)
  p. arteriovenous malformation
  p. artery catheterization
  p. artery catheterization anesthetic
    technique
  p. artery hemorrhage
  p. artery hypertension (PAH)
  p. artery occlusion pressure
    (PAOP)
  p. artery occlusive wedge pressure
  p. artery pressure (PAP)
  p. artery wedge
  p. aspiration
  p. bacterial infection
  p. blastoma
  p. capillary wedge pressure
  p. cavitation
  p. cavity

NOTES

P

pulmonary (continued)
- p. circulation
- p. compliance
- p. complication
- p. embolectomy
- p. fungal infection
- p. glomangiosis
- p. hypertension pressure
- p. hypostasis
- p. lesion
- p. ligament
- p. lymph nodes
- p. mass
- p. metastasectomy
- p. metastasis
- p. orifice
- p. outflow tract
- p. overcirculation
- p. parenchymal infection
- p. pleura
- p. plexus
- p. resection
- p. sinuses
- p. stenosis repair
- p. sulcus
- p. suppuration
- p. surface of heart
- p. sympathetic blockade
- p. thromboendarterectomy (PTE)
- p. toilet
- p. trunk
- p. tumor
- p. valve anomaly
- p. valve area
- p. valve disease
- p. valve gradient
- p. valve insufficiency
- p. valve replacement
- p. valve restenosis
- p. valve stenosis
- p. valvuloplasty
- p. vascular pressure
- p. vascular resistance
- p. vascular resistance index (PVRI)
- p. veins
- p. venous connection anomaly
- p. venous return anomaly
- p. ventilation
- p. ventilation scan
- p. wedge pressure

pulmonary-gas exchange
pulmones (pl. of pulmo)
pulmonic
- p. valve stenosis

pulp
- p. amputation
- p. approach
- p. canal

- p. canal therapy
- p. cavity
- p. devitalization
- digital p.
- exposed p.
- p. extirpation
- p. of finger
- p. flap
- p. microcirculation
- p. mummification
- p. pressure
- red p.
- splenic p.
- white p.

pulpa
- p. lienis
- p. splenica

pulpal wall
pulpation
pulpectomy
- complete p.
- partial p.

pulpifaction
pulpiform
pulpify
pulpodentinal membrane
pulpoma
pulpoperiapical lesion
pulposus
pulpotomy
- complete p.
- formocresol p.
- partial p.
- total p.

pulsatile
- p. hematoma
- p. hypothermic perfusion with University of Wisconsin solution
- p. mass
- p. pressure lavage

pulsation
pulse
- p. oximeter
- p. oximetry
- p. pressure
- p. repetition time prolongation
- p. trisection
- p. value recording (PVR)
- p. width

pulsed
- p. electromagnetic field (PEMF)
- p. irrigation
- p. laser ablation

pulsed-mode operation
pulse-echo distance measurement
pulsing current for nonunion of fracture
pulsion

pultaceous
pulverization
Pulvertaft
    P. end-to-end suture
    P. fish-mouth stitch
    P. interweave suture
    P. weave technique
pump
    angle port p.
    Bard Infus OR syringe-type
      infusion p.
    Bard PCA p.
    Baxter PCA p.
    Baxter volumetric infusion p.
    Bio-Medicus centrifugal p.
    calf p.
    computer-controlled infusion p.
    constant infusion p.
    Datascope system 90 intra-aortic
      balloon p.
    DeVilbiss suction p.
    ECMO p.
    Elmed peristaltic irrigation p.
    Endolav lavage p.
    extracorporeal p.
    Frenta System II feeding p.
    Graseby 3300 p.
    Graseby anesthesia p.
    Hakim valve and p.
    IMED infusion p.
    Infuse-A-Port p.
    Jobst extremity p.
    p. lung
    Multipulse 1000 compression p.
    Nutromat Pad S feeding p.
    Ohmeda 9000 computer-cotrolled
      infusion p.
    p. oxygenation
    p. oxygenator
    patient-controlled anesthesia p.
    PCA p.
    PMP p.
    Program 2 syringe p.
    proton p.
    roller head perfusion p.
    Sage Instruments syringe p.
    Sarns 7000 MDX p.
    servocontrolled ventilation p.
    suction p.
    syringe-type infusion p.
    volumetric infusion p.

punch
    p. biopsy
    p. grafts
    p. resection of vocal cord
punched-out lesion
puncta (*pl. of* punctum)
punctate
    p. epithelial keratoplasty
    p. hemorrhage
punctation
punctoplasty
punctum, pl. puncta
    p. coxale
    dilation of p.
    p. ossificationis
    p. ossificationis primarium
    p. ossificationis secundarium
puncture
    antegrade p.
    anterior p.
    apical p.
    apical left ventricular p.
    Bernard p.
    bone marrow p.
    brain p.
    calix p.
    cisternal p.
    cystic p.
    dental p.
    diabetic p.
    diathermy p.
    direct cardiac p.
    direct cautery p.
    direct needle p.
    dural p.
    endoscopic fine-needle p.
    femoral p.
    left ventricular p.
    lumbar p.
    needle tracheoesophageal p.
    nephrostomy p.
    percutaneous needle p.
    percutaneous renal p.
    pericardial p.
    Quincke p.
    retrograde nephrostomy p.
    self-sealing scleral p.
    skin p.
    spinal p.
    stereotactic p.
    sternal p.
    subdural p.

NOTES

P

puncture *(continued)*
    suprapubic p.
    tracheoesophageal p.
    transseptal p.
    ultrasound-guided nephrostomy p.
    venous p.
    ventricular p.
    p. wound
    Ziegler p,
pupil
    p. dilation
    dilator muscle of p.
    exclusion of p.
    exit p.
pupilla, pl. **pupillae**
    dilator pupillae
    musculus dilator p.
pupillary
    p. dilatation
    p. line
    p. margin of iris
    p. membrane
    p. membrane remnant
    p. zone
pupilloscopy
pupil-to-root iridectomy
Puralube Tears solution
purchase point
pure
    p. rotation
    p. translation
purgation
purging
    immunologic method of p.
    pharmacologic method of p.
    tumor cell p.
Purkinje network
Purlon suture
Purmann method
purpuric lesion
purpurogenous membrane
pursestring
    p. atriotomy
    p. suture
purulence
purulent
    p. exudate
    p. exudation
    p. inflammation
pus
    p. collection
    p. tube
push
    p. enteroscopy
    p. maneuver
    p. plus refraction technique

push-back
    p.-b. procedure
    p.-b. technique
push-pull T technique
push-type enteroscopy
pustular
    p. inflammation
    p. lesion
    p. patch-test reaction
pustulation
Putenney operation
Putti-Platt
    P.-P. arthroplasty
    P.-P. shoulder procedure
Putti posterior approach
putty kidney
PUVA
    psoralens, ultraviolet A
    PUVA radiation
Puzo method
PVA
    polyvinyl alcohol
    PVA fixative method
PVB suture
PVR
    pulse value recording
PVRI
    pulmonary vascular resistance index
pyelectasis
pyelitic
pyelitis
pyelocaliceal
pyelocaliectasis
pyelocalyceal
pyelocalycotomy
pyelocystitis
pyelolithotomy
    coagulum p.
    open p.
pyelolymphatic
pyelolysis
pyelonephritic kidney
pyelonephritis
    p. in exenteration
pyelonephrosis
pyeloplasty
    Anderson-Hynes p.
    capsular flap p.
    Culp spiral flap p.
    disjoined p.
    dismembered p.
    Foley Y-plasty p.
    laparoscopic dismembered p.
    Scardino vertical flap p.
    Thompson capsule flap p.
pyeloplication
pyeloscopy
pyelostomy

pyelotomy
    extended p.
    open p.
pyeloureterectasis
pyeloureterography
pyeloureterostomy
pyelovenous
    p. backflow
pyelovesicostomy
pyencephalus
pyesis
pygal
pyknic
pyknotic body
pylemphraxis
pylephlebectasis
pylethrombosis
pylorectomy
    Kocher p.
pyloric
    p. antrum
    p. artery
    p. autotransplantation
    p. canal
    p. constriction
    p. dilation
    p. glands
    p. intubation
    p. lymph nodes
    p. orifice
    p. part of stomach
    p. ring
    p. sphincter
    p. vein
pyloristenosis
pylorodilator
pylorodiosis
pylorogastrectomy
pyloromyotomy
    Ramstedt p.
    Ramstedt-Fredet p.
pyloroplasty
    double p.
    Finney p.
    Heineke-Mikulicz p.
    Jaboulay p.
    Mikulicz p.
    Ramstedt p.
    reconstructive p.
    truncal vagotomy and p.
    vagotomy and p.
    Weinberg modification of p.

pyloroptosis
pylorostenosis
pylorostomy
pylorotomy
pylorus-preserving
    pancreaticoduodenectomy
Pynchon suction tube
pyocele
pyocelia
pyocephalus
pyocolpocele
pyocystis
pyodermatous
    p. infection
    p. skin lesion
pyogen
pyogenesis
pyogenic
    p. membrane
    p. spinal infection
pyoktanin catgut suture
pyomyoma
pyonephritis
pyonephrolithiasis
pyonephrosis
pyoperitoneum
pyoperitonitis
pyopneumothorax
pyopoiesis
pyopyelectasis
pyorrhea
pyosemia
pyosis
pyospermia
pyothorax
pyoureter
    p. ectopic ureterocele
pyramid
    Ferrein p.
    Lallouette p.
    malpighian p.
    medullary p.
    p. method
    petrous p.
    renal p.
    p. of thyroid
    p. of vestibule
pyramidal
    p. auricular muscle
    p. bone
    p. decussation
    p. fracture

NOTES

P

pyramidal *(continued)*
    p. lobe of thyroid gland
    p. muscle of auricle
    p. radiation
    p. tip
    p. tract
    p. tractotomy
pyramidale
pyramidalis
    p. muscle
pyramidotomy
    medullary p.
    spinal p.

pyramis
    p. renalis
    p. vestibuli
pyretic therapy
Pyrex tube
pyridostigmine
pyriform
pyrogen
    endogenous p.
pyroglycolic acid suture
pyrolysis
    p. product
pyuria

Q-tip test
quadrangular
  q. membrane
  q. space
  q. therapy
quadrangulation of Frouin
quadrantectomy
  q., axillary dissection, radiation
    therapy
quadrant sampling technique
quadraparesis
quadrate
  q. muscle
  q. muscle of loins
  q. muscle of thigh
  q. muscle of upper lip
  q. part of liver
quadratus
  q. femoris muscle
  q. lumborum muscle
  q. plantae muscle
  pronator q.
quadriceps
  q. femoris muscle
  q. muscle of thigh
quadricepsplasty
  Judet q.
  Thompson q.
  V-Y q.
quadrigeminal cistern
quadrilateral
  q. space
  q. space syndrome
quadripedal extensor reflex
quadripolar
quadruple
  q. amputation
  q. therapy
Quaegebeur procedure
Quaglino operation
quantification
  acoustic q.

microdensitophotometric q.
  shunt q.
quantitative
  q. evaluation
  q. stool collection
quantity
  q. not sufficient for evaluation
  sound q.
  vector q.
Quartey technique
quasistatic stressed position
Quatrefages angle
quatro therapy
Quelicin injection
Quénu
  Q. hemorrhoidal plexus
  Q. nail plate removal technique
Quénu-Küss tarsometatarsal injury
  classification
quenuthoracoplasty
Questek laser tube
quick
  q. angulation technique
  q. connector
  Q. method
Quickert
  Q. procedure
  Q. suture
  Q. three-suture technique
Quickert-Dryden tube
quilted suture
Quinby classification of pelvic fracture
Quincke puncture
Quinones
  method of Q.
quinti
  extensor digiti q.
Quinton tube
quotient
  pressure rate q.
  ventilation/perfusion q.

RA
    regional anesthesia
racemate
racemic
    r. mixture
    r. modification
racemization
Racestyptine retraction ring
rachial
rachidial
rachidian
rachiotomy
rachis
rachitic metaphysis
rachitomy
racket nail
racket-shaped flap
Rackley
    R. method
    method of R.
racquet incision
racquet-shaped incision
radectomy
radiad
radial
    r. arterial line
    r. border of forearm
    r. bursa
    r. collateral artery
    r. dilator muscle
    r. eminence of wrist
    r. flexor muscle of wrist
    r. forearm flap
    r. fossa of humerus
    r. fracture reduction
    r. head
    r. head dislocation
    r. head fracture
    r. index artery
    r. iridotomy
    r. keratotomy
    r. laminectomy
    r. neck fracture
    r. recurrent artery
    r. sclerosing lesion
    r. styloid fracture
    r. suture track
    r. wedge osteotomy
    r. wrist extensor
radial-based flap
radialis
    r. indicis artery
radiate
    r. ligament of head of rib
    r. sternocostal ligaments

radiation
    r. angiopathy
    braking r.
    r. burn
    r. cataract
    characteristic r.
    r. chimera
    r. damage
    diagnostic r.
    r. enteritis
    r. enteropathy
    r. exposure
    general r.
    geniculocalcarine r.
    Goldmann coherent r.
    Gratiolet r.
    r. hepatitis
    r. hepatopathy
    homogenous r.
    r. injury
    intraoperative r.
    involved-field r.
    r. lung disease
    r. monitoring
    r. mucositis
    r. myelopathy
    r. necrosis
    occipitothalamic r.
    optic r.
    r. output
    r. pneumonitis
    r. poisoning
    postoperative r.
    postoperative pelvic r.
    r. precaution
    primary r.
    r. proctitis
    r. proctocolitis
    r. protection
    PUVA r.
    pyramidal r.
    rectosigmoid r.
    r. response
    r. risk
    superficial r.
    r. survey
    temporal lobe r.
    r. therapy
    Wernicke r.
    whole abdominal r.
    whole body r.
radiation-induced
    r.-i. carcinoma
    r.-i. colitis
    r.-i. disease

R

radiation-induced *(continued)*
    r.-i. ischemia
    r.-i. leukoencephalopathy
    r.-i. pulmonary toxicity
    r.-i. ulceration
radical
    r. abdominal hysterectomy
    r. axillary dissection
    r. compartmental excision
    r. cystectomy
    r. en bloc removal
    r. gastrectomy
    r. hemorrhoidectomy
    r. inguinal orchiectomy
    r. lymph node dissection
    r. mastectomy
    r. mastoidectomy
    r. neck dissection
    r. nephrectomy
    r. nephroureterectomy
    r. operation for hernia
    r. orchidectomy
    r. orchiectomy
    r. palmar fasciectomy
    r. parametrectomy
    r. perineal prostatectomy
    r. prefrontal lobotomy
    r. retropubic prostatectomy
    r. subtotal resection
    r. surgery
    r. transcoccygeal prostatectomy
    r. vaginal hysterectomy
    r. vulvectomy
radices *(pl. of* radix)
radicle
radicotomy
radicula
radicular
    r. arteries
    r. canal
radiculectomy
radiculomedullary fistula
radiculomeningeal spinal vascular malformation
radiectomy
radii *(pl. of* radius)
radioactive
    r. concentration
    r. microsphere
    r. seed implantation
radiobicipital
radiocapitellar
    r. articulation
    r. line
radiocarpal
    r. arthroscopy
    r. articulation
    r. dislocation

radiodense lesion
radiodigital
radiofluoroscopy
    televised r.
radiofrequency (RF)
    r. catheter ablation (RFCA)
    r. electrophrenic respiration
    r. lesion
    r. rhizotomy
radiographic
    r. technique
    r. tooth repair
radiohumeral
radioimmunoglobulin therapy
radioimmunoguided surgery
radioimmunoscintimetry
radioiodination
    lactoperoxidase r.
radiological
    r. examination
    r. sphincter
radiologic biliary stent placement
radiolucent
    r. crescent line
    r. lesion
    r. line
    r. operating room table extension
radiolunate fusion
radiolus
radiolysis
Radiometer ABL 500 blood gas analyzer
radiomuscular
radiomutation
radionuclide technique
radiopalmar
radiopaque
    r. foreign body
    r. lesion
radiopharmaceutical therapy
radiopotentiation
radioprotector
radioscaphoid fusion
radiosensitization
radio signal line
radioulnar
    r. articulation
    r. dissociation
radisectomy
radius, pl. **radii**
    r. of angulation
    r. fixus
radix, pl. **radices**
    r. anterior
    r. arcus vertebrae
    r. dorsalis
    r. facialis
    r. lateralis nervi mediani

r. linguae
r. mesenterii
r. penis
r. point
r. posterior
r. pulmonis
r. sensoria
radices spinales nervi accessorii
r. ventralis
Radley-Liebig-Brown resection
radon seed implantation
Radpour-House suction tube
RAE endotracheal tube
RAE-Flex tracheal tube
Raff-Glantz derivative method
Rafluor topical solution
rag-wheel method
Rai classification
Rainville technique
raising
straight leg r. (SLR)
rale
Ralston-Thompson pseudoarthrosis
technique
Raman spectroscopy
Rambo musculoplasty
ramex
ram horn nail
rami (*pl. of* ramus)
ramicotomy
ramification
apical r.
ramisection
Ramond point
Ramon flocculation
ramotomy
superior pubic r.
Ramsey County pyoktanin catgut suture
Ramstedt
R. operation
R. procedure
R. pyloromyotomy
R. pyloroplasty
Ramstedt-Fredet pyloromyotomy
ramus, pl. **rami**
r. acromialis arteriae suprascapularis
r. acromialis arteriae
thoracoacromialis
r. alveolaris superior medius nervi
infraorbitalis
r. anastomoticus
r. anterior

rami articulares
rami articulares arteriae
descendentis genicularis
rami atriales
r. auricularis arteriae occipitalis
r. auricularis nervi vagi
r. basalis anterior
r. basalis lateralis
r. basalis medialis
r. basalis posterior
r. basalis tentorii arteriae carotidis
internae
rami bronchiales
rami bronchiales segmentorum
rami buccales nervi facialis
rami calcanei
rami calcanei laterales nervi suralis
rami calcanei mediales nervi
tibialis
r. calcarinus arteriae occipitalis
medialis
rami capsulares arteriae renalis
rami cardiaci cervicales inferiores
nervi vagi
rami cardiaci cervicales superiores
nervi vagi
rami cardiaci thoracici nervi vagi
r. cardiacus
rami caudati
rami celiaci nervi vagi
cephalic arterial rami
r. cervicalis nervi facialis
r. clavicularis arteriae
thoracoacromialis
r. colli nervi facialis
r. communicans
r. communicans arteriae peroneae
r. communicans cum nervo
glossopharyngeo
r. communicans nervi mediani cum
nervo ulnari
r. communicans peroneus nervi
peronei communis
r. communicans ulnaris nervi
radialis
communicating rami of spinal
nerves
communicating rami of sympathetic
trunk
r. cricothyroideus
rami cutanei anteriores nervi
femoralis

NOTES

ramus *(continued)*

rami cutanei cruris mediales nervi sapheni

r. cutaneus anterior nervi iliohypogastrici

r. cutaneus lateralis

r. cutaneus lateralis nervi iliohypogastrici

r. cutaneus medialis

r. cutaneus rami anterioris nervi obturatorii

r. deltoideus

r. descendens arteriae occipitalis

r. dexter arteriae hepaticae propriae

r. dexter venae portac hepatis

r. digastricus nervi facialis

rami dorsales arteriae intercostalis supremae

rami dorsales arteriae subcostalis

rami dorsales linguae arteriae lingualis

rami dorsales nervi ulnaris

r. dorsalis arteriae lumbalium

r. dorsalis nervorum spinalium

dorsal primary r. of spinal nerve

rami epiploicae

rami esophageales

rami esophageales aortae thoracicae

rami esophageales arteriae gastricae sinistrae

rami esophageales arteriae thyroideae inferioris

rami esophagei

rami esophagei nervi laryngei recurrentis

rami csophagei nervi vagi

r. externus nervi accessorii

r. externus nervi laryngei superioris

rami fauciales nervi lingualis

r. femoralis nervi genitofemoralis

r. frame

r. frontalis arteriae temporalis superficialis

rami ganglii submandibularis

r. ganglii trigeminalis

rami ganglionares

rami ganglionici nervi maxillaris

rami gastrici anteriores nervi vagi

rami gastrici posteriores nervi vagi

r. genitalis nervi genitofemoralis

rami glandulares

rami glandulares arteriae facialis

rami glandulares arteriae thyroideae inferioris

rami glandulares ganglii submandibularis

gray rami communicantes

rami hepatici nervi vagi

r. iliacus arteriae iliolumbalis

rami inferiores nervi transversi cervicalis [colli]

r. inferior ossis pubis

r. infrahyoideus arteriae thyroidea superioris

r. infrapatellaris nervi sapheni

rami inguinales arteriae pudendae externae

rami intercostales anteriores

rami interganglionares

interganglionic rami

internal r. of accessory nerve

r. internus nervi accessorii

r. internus nervi laryngei superioris

rami interventriculares septales

ischial r.

ischiopubic r.

rami isthmi faucium nervi lingualis

rami labiales inferiores nervi mentalis

rami labiales superiores nervi infraorbitalis

rami laryngopharyngei ganglii cervicalis superioris

rami laterales rami sinistri venae portae hepatis

r. lateralis ductus hepatici sinistri

r. lateralis nervi supraorbitalis

rami lienales arteriae lienalis

rami linguales

rami linguales nervi glossopharyngei

rami linguales nervi hypoglossi

rami linguales nervi lingualis

r. lingualis

r. lingularis inferior

r. lingularis nervi facialis

r. lingularis superior

r. lobi medii

r. lobi medii arteriae pulmonalis dextrae

r. lumbalis arteriae iliolumbalis

rami mammarii

rami mammarii laterales

rami mammarii laterales nervorum intercostalium

rami mammarii mediales

r. of mandible

r. mandibulae

r. marginalis mandibulae nervi facialis

r. mastoideus arteriae occipitalis

r. meatus acustici interni

rami mediales arteriarum centralium anterolateralium

rami mediales rami sinistri venae portae hepatis

r. medialis ductus hepatici sinistri
r. medialis nervi supraorbitalis
rami mediastinales aortae thoracicae
rami mediastinales arteriae
  thoracicae internae
rami meningei
r. meningeus anterior arteriae
  vertebralis
r. meningeus arteriae carotidis
  internae
r. meningeus arteriae occipitalis
r. meningeus medius nervi
  maxillaris
r. meningeus nervi mandibularis
r. meningeus nervi vagi
r. meningeus nervorum spinalium
rami mentales nervi mentalis
r. musculi stylopharyngei nervi
  glossopharyngei
r. mylohyoideus arteriae alveolaris
  inferioris
rami nasales externi nervi
  infraorbitalis
rami communicantes nervorum
  spinalium
r. nodi atrioventricularis
r. nodi sinuatrialis arteriae
  coronaria dextra
r. obturatorius arteriae epigastricae
  inferioris
rami occipitales arteriae auricularis
  posterioris
rami occipitales arteriae occipitis
rami occipitales nervi auricularis
  posterioris
r. occipitalis
rami omentales
r. orbitalis arteriae meningeae
  mediae
r. orbitalis ganglii pterygopalatini
r. ossis ischii
r. palmaris nervi mediani
r. palmaris nervi ulnaris
r. palmaris profundus arteriae
  ulnaris
r. palmaris superficialis arteriae
  radialis
rami parietales
r. parietalis arteriae meningeae
  mediae
r. parietalis arteriae occipitalis
  medialis

r. parietalis arteriae temporalis
  superficialis
rami parotidei
r. parotidei arteriae temporalis
  superficialis
rami parotidei nervi
  auriculotemporalis
rami parotidei venae facialis
rami pectorales arteriae
  thoracoacromialis
r. perforans
r. perforans arteriae fibularis
r. perforantes arteriae thoracicae
  internae
rami pericardiaci aortae thoracicae
rami perineales nervi cutanei
  femoris posterioris
r. petrosus arteriae meningeae
  mediae
rami phrenicoabdominales nervi
  phrenici
r. plantaris profundus arteriae
  dorsalis pedis
r. posterior arteriae obturatoriae
r. posterior arteriae recurrentis
  ulnaris
r. posterior arteriae renalis
r. posterior arteriae thyroideae
  superioris
r. posterior ascendens
r. posterior descendens
rami posteriores nervorum
  spinalium
r. posterior nervi obturatorii
r. posterior rami dextri venae
  portae hepatis
r. posterior sulci lateralis cerebri
rami profundi arteriae circumflexae
  femoris medialis
r. profundus arteriae transversae
  colli
r. profundus arteria scapularis
  descendens
rami pterygoidei arteriae maxillaris
pubic r.
r. pubicus arteriae epigastricae
  inferioris
r. pubicus arteriae obturatoriae
rami pulmonales systematis
  autonomici
rami renales nervi vagi
r. renalis nervi splanchnici minoris

NOTES

ramus *(continued)*
r. sinister arteriae hepaticae propriae
r. sinister venae portae hepatis
r. sinus carotici
r. sinus cavernosi
r. sinus cavernosi arteriae carotidis arteriae
rami spinales
rami splenici arteriae splenicae
rami sternales arteriae thoracicae internae
rami sternocleidomastoidei arteriae occipitalis
r. stylohyoideus nervi facialis
rami subscapulares arteriae axillaris
r. superficialis arteriae gluteae superioris
r. superficialis arteriae plantaris medialis
r. superficialis nervi plantaris lateralis
r. superficialis nervi radialis
r. superficialis nervi ulnaris
r. superior arteriae gluteae superioris
r. superior nervi oculomotorii
r. superior nervi transversalis cervicalis (colli)
r. superior ossis pubis
superior pubic r.
r. suprahyoideus arteriae lingualis
rami temporales nervi facialis
r. tentorii
rami thymici
r. thyrohyoideus ansae cervicalis
rami tonsillares nervi glossopharyngei
r. tonsillaris arteriae facialis
rami tracheales
rami tracheales arteriae thyroideae inferioris
rami tracheales nervi laryngei recurrentis
r. tubarius arteriae uterinae
r. ulnaris nervi cutanei antebrachii medialis
rami ureterici
rami ureterici arteriae ovaricae
rami ureterici arteriae renalis
rami ureterici arteriae testicularis
rami ventrales nervorum cervicalium
rami ventrales nervorum lumbalium
rami ventrales nervorum sacralium
r. ventralis nervi spinalis
ventral primary rami of cervical spinal nerves
ventral primary rami of lumbar spinal nerves
ventral primary rami of sacral spinal nerves
ventral primary r. of spinal nerve
rami zygomatici nervi facialis
r. zygomaticofacialis nervi zygomatici
r. zygomaticotemporalis nervi zygomatici

Ranawat
R. classification
R. triangle method

Ranawat-DeFiore-Straub
R.-D.-S. osteotomy
R.-D.-S. technique

Ranawat-Dorr-Inglis method

Randall plaques

Rand-House suction tube

random
r. bladder biopsy
r. cutaneous flap
r. pattern flap

randomization

Rand-Radpour suction tube

range
r. of excursion
r. of motion (ROM)
r. of motion therapy

Ransley-Cantwell repair

Ransley procedure

Ransohoff operation

Ranson acute pancreatitis classification

RAO
right anterior oblique
right anterior occipital
RAO angulation
RAO position

raphe
r. anococcygea
anogenital r.
r. linguae
median longitudinal r. of tongue
penile r.
r. penis
perineal r.
r. perinei
pharyngeal r.
r. pharyngis
pterygomandibular r.
r. pterygomandibularis
scrotal r.
r. scroti

rapid
r. acquisition radiofrequency-echo-steady state imaging
r. maxillary expansion
r. pull-through (RPT)

r. pull-through esophageal
manometry technique
r. recompression - high pressure
oxygen
r. scan fluoroscopy
r. scan technique
r. sequence induction (RSI)
r. sequence induction of anesthesia
r. tumor lysis syndrome
**rapid-sequence induction anesthetic
technique**
Rapoport test
Rappaport
R. classification
R. osteotomy
rare system reaction
rasceta
rash
Rashkind
R. balloon technique
R. procedure
Rastan-Konno procedure
Rastan operation
Rastelli
R. conduit
R. graft
R. operation
R. procedure
R. repair
rate
average flow r.
beat-to-beat variation of fetal
heart r.
circulation r.
complication r.
dipole-dipole relaxation r.
disintegration r.
ejection r.
expiratory flow r.
flotation r.
r. of fluid filtration
fusion nonunion r.
gallbladder ejection r.
glomerular filtration r.
heart r. (HR)
implant survival r.
load-deflection r.
maximal expiratory flow r.
maximal ventilation r.
mean normalized systolic
ejection r.
metabolic r.

ovulation r.
oxygen extraction r.
pacemaker adaptive r.
peak expiratory flow r.
perfusion flow r.
pressure increment r.
r. pressure product
relaxation r.
Solomon-Bloembergen theory of
dipole-dipole relaxation r.
stroke ejection r.
systolic ejection r.
transverse relaxation r.
T2 relaxation r.
vertebral osteosynthesis fusion r.
voiding flow r.
rated perceived exertion
Rathke
R. bundles
R. pouch
rating of perceived exertion
ratio
adenoma-hyperplastic polyp r.
adenoma-nonadenoma r.
ankle-brachial blood pressure r.
body hematocrit-venous
hematocrit r.
common mode rejection r.
cough-pressure transmission r.
cup-to-disk r.
dead space:tidal volume r.
external/internal rotation r.
fetal head:abdominal
circumference r.
forced expiratory volume in 1
second to forced vital capacity r.
forced expiratory volume timed to
forced vital capacity r.
hand r.
head:body r.
head circumference/abdominal
circumference r.
inspiratory-to-expiratory r.
intrapulmonary shunt r.
MAC r.
MAC-Awake r.
MAC-intubation r.
MAC-Skin incision r.
MAC-Surgical incision r.
mean UV/MV r.
midexpiratory/midinspiratory flow r.
optic cup-to-disk r.

NOTES

ratio *(continued)*
    pressure transmission r.
    right-to-left shunt r.
    shunt r.
    tumor:cerebellum r.
    UV/MV r.
    ventilation/perfusion r.
rationalization
Ratliff classification of avascular necrosis
rat-tail deformity
Rauwolfia extract
rave
    fracture en r.
Raverdino operation
Ravocaine
ray
    r. amputation
    medullary r.
    r. resection
Ray-Brunswick-Mack operation
Ray-Clancy-Lemon technique
Rayhack technique
Ray-McLean operation
Raz
    R. bladder neck suspension
    R. four-quadrant suspension
    R. modification
    R. needle suspension
    R. procedure
    R. urethral suspension
Raz-Leach procedure
RD1000 resuscitator
RDS
    respiratory distress syndrome
reabsorbable suture
reaction
    anaphylactoid-type r.
    compensation r.
    cutaneous graft-versus-host r.
    eczematous r.
    elimination r.
    exergonic r.
    extrapyramidal r.
    foreign-body r.
    r. formation
    general adaptation r.
    graft-versus-host disease r.
    homograft r.
    immediate asthmatic r. (IAR)
    implant r.
    inflammation r.
    irritant patch-test r.
    lid closure r.
    litigation r.
    local anesthetic r.
    midazolam-induced excitatory r.
    paradoxical r.

    pustular patch-test r.
    rare system r.
    scar tissue r.
    whitegraft r.
reactivation tuberculosis
reactive
    r. dilation
    r. lymphoid lesion
reactivity
    airway r.
Read rebreathing method
realignment procedure
Reality vaginal pouch
real reconstruction
real-time
    r.-t. acquisition and velocity evaluation
    r.-t. 3-D biplanar transperineal prostate implantation
    r.-t. echo-planar image
    r.-t. endoscopic ultrasound-guided fine-needle aspiration
    r.-t. sector scanning
reamed nail
reamputation
reanastomosis
    r. of blood supply to bone graft
    laparoscopic ureteral r.
reanimation
    facial r.
reanneal
rear-entry
reattachment
    r. of choroid operation
    four-wire trochanter r.
    Harris four-wire trochanter r.
    r. of retina operation
reattribution technique
reauditorization
rebreathing
    r. anesthesia
    r. bag
    intentional r.
    r. technique
Rebuck skin window technique
recalcification
    r. time
recall
    memory r.
Récamier
    R. operation
    R. procedure
recanalization
    balloon occlusive intravascular lysis enhanced r.
    excimer vascular r.
    laser r.
    TCD r.

r. technique
umbilical vein r.
r. vs. recannulization
recannulization
recanalization vs. r.
receiver saturation
recent dislocation
receptaculum
r. chyli
r. ganglii petrosi
r. pecqueti
receptoma
receptor
acetylcholine r.
β-adrenergic r.
α-adrenergic r.
$β_2$-adrenergic r.
$α_2$-adrenergic r.
β-r. agonist
β-r. antagonist
dopamine r.
endogenous opiate r.
endometrial r.
endothelin A, B r.
Mu r.
muscarinic r.
nicotinic r.
opioid r.
pressure r.
up-regulation of the r.
receptor-mediated endocytosis pathway
recess
azygoesophageal r.
cecal r.
costodiaphragmatic r.
costomediastinal r.
duodenojejunal r.
hepatorenal r.
inferior duodenal r.
inferior ileocecal r.
inferior omental r.
intersigmoid r.
Jacquemet r.
mesentericoparietal r.
paracolic r.'s
paraduodenal r.
parotid r.
phrenicomediastinal r.
pineal r.
piriform r.
pleural r.'s
retrocecal r.

retroduodenal r.
Rosenmüller r.
sacciform r.
sphenoethmoidal r.
splenic r.
subhepatic r.
subphrenic r.'s
subpopliteal r.
superior azygoesophageal r.
superior duodenal r.
superior ileocecal r.
superior omental r.
suprapineal r.
supratonsillar r.
recession
clitoral r.
lateral rectus r.
r. of ocular muscle operation
recessional line
recession-resection
recessus
r. costodiaphragmaticus
r. costomediastinalis
r. duodenalis inferior
r. duodenalis superior
r. ellipticus
r. hepatorenalis
r. ileocecalis inferior
r. ileocecalis superior
r. inferior omentalis
r. infundiformis
r. intersigmoideus
r. lienalis
r. paraduodenalis
r. parotideus
r. pharyngeus
r. phrenicomediastinalis
r. piriformis
r. pleurales
r. retrocecalis
r. retroduodenalis
r. sacciformis
r. sphenoethmoidalis
r. sphericus
r. splenicus
r. subhepaticus
r. subphrenici
r. superior omentalis
recidivation
recipient
r. hepatectomy
reciprocal relaxation

NOTES

reciprocation
    active r.
    passive r.
recirculation
    instrument r.
Recklinghausen disease type I
reclamping
reclination
recline
reclining position
Reclus I syndrome
recoarctation of aorta
recognition
    pattern r.
    within-list r. (WLR)
recombinant
    r. DNA technique
    r. tissue-type plasminogen activator
    (rtPA)
recommendation
    FDA Anesthesia Apparatus
    Checkout R.'s
    screening r.
reconciliation
reconstruction
    Abbé-McIndoe vaginal r.
    ACL r.
    alar r.
    anal sphincter r.
    analytic r.
    Andrews iliotibial band r.
    anterior capsulolabral r.
    aortic root r.
    arthroscopic anterior cruciate
    ligament r. (AACLR)
    Bankart r.
    bifurcated vein graft for
    vascular r.
    Billroth I, II r.
    bladder outlet r.
    breast r.
    Brown knee joint r.
    Cabral coronary r.
    Cho anterior cruciate ligament r.
    Chrisman-Snook r.
    circumferential esophageal r.
    Clancy cruciate ligament r.
    columellar r.
    constrained r.
    coronal r.
    corporeal r.
    craniofacial r.
    cruciate ligament r.
    d'Aubigne femoral r.
    d'Aubigne resection r.
    3-D computer r.
    dermal pouch r.
    Dibbell cleft lip-nasal r.

    dural patch r.
    Eaton-Littler ligament r.
    Ellison lateral knee r.
    Elmslie r.
    endoscopic anterior cruciate
    ligament r.
    end-to-end r.
    epiglottic r.
    Eriksson r.
    Evans r.
    exogenous r.
    extra-articular r.
    r. of eyelid
    five-one r.
    genital r.
    Goldner r.
    hand r.
    Harmon hip r.
    hemimandible r.
    House r.
    Hughston-Degenhardt r.
    Hughston-Jacobson lateral
    compartment r.
    index metacarpophalangeal joint r.
    Insall anterior cruciate ligament r.
    intra-articular r.
    iterative r.
    joint r.
    juxtacubital r.
    Krukenberg hand r.
    Kugelberg r.
    Larson ligament r.
    lateral compartment r.
    Lee r.
    L'Episcopo hip r.
    ligament r.
    MacIntosh over-the-top ACL r.
    mandibular r.
    r. method
    Millard advancement rotation
    flap r.
    nasal r.
    Nathan-Trung modification of
    Krukenberg hand r.
    Neer posterior shoulder r.
    neoglottic r.
    neoglottis r.
    nipple-areolar r.
    O'Donoghue ACL r.
    orbital rim r.
    oromandibular r.
    ossicular chain r.
    osteoplastic r.
    palate r.
    papillary r.
    pedicled jejunal r.
    peritoneal r.
    pharyngoesophageal r.

pouch r.
r. procedure
pulley r.
real r.
Rosenberg endoscopic anterior
  cruciate ligament r.
Roux-en-Y r.
sagittal r.
septal r.
Sheen airway r.
socket r.
sphincter r.
staged r.
stapled r.
sternoclavicular joint r.
Swanson r.
synchronous bladder r.
Tanagho bladder neck r.
r. technique
tenoplastic r.
three-dimensional r.
thumb r.
Torg knee r.
tracheal r.
tubular r.
tubularized bladder neck r.
two-stage tendon graft r.
Verdan osteoplastic thumb r.
Watson-Jones r.
Whitman femoral neck r.
Wookey r.
Young-Dees bladder neck r.
Young-Dees-Leadbetter bladder
  neck r.
Zancolli r.

reconstructive
r. mammaplasty
r. preprosthetic surgery
r. pyloroplasty

reconstructor
dynamic spatial r.

record
anesthesia r.
anesthetic r.
automated anesthesia r.
centric occluding relation r.
eccentric interocclusal r.
eccentric maxillomandibular r.
jaw relation r.
medical r.
occluding centric relation r.
terminal jaw relation r.

recorder
Gould-Brush 481 eight-channel r.
Gould ES 1000 r.

recording
continuous on-line r.
pulse value r. (PVR)
segmental limb pressure r.
whole-cell patch clamp r.

record-keeper
ARKIVE automated anesthesia r.-k.

recovery
anesthetic immediate r.
pressure r.
r. and reorganization
r. room
saturation r.
selective saturation r.
short tau inversion r. (STIR)
short TI inversion r. (STIR)
time to r.

recruitment maneuver

rectal
r. alimentation
r. ampulla
r. anesthesia
r. anesthetic
r. anesthetic technique
r. biopsy
r. carcinoma
r. columns
r. dilation
r. evacuation
r. examination
r. fistula
r. folds
r. foreign body
r. laceration
r. mass
r. mobilization
r. mucosectomy
r. plexuses
r. pouch
r. probe electroejaculation
r. pulsed irrigation
r. sheath hematoma
r. shelf
r. sinuses
r. tip
r. tube
r. ulceration
r. valvotomy
r. venous plexus

NOTES

611

rectalgia
rectangular amputation
rectectomy
recti
 diastasis r.
recticulum
 endoplasmic r.
rectification
 anomalous r.
 inward-going r.
rectifier tube
rectify
rectocele
 r. repair
rectoclysis
rectococcygeal
 r. muscle
rectococcygeus muscle
rectococcypexy
rectolabial fistula
rectoperineal
rectoperineorrhaphy
rectopexy
 abdominal r.
 anterior r.
 Ivalon sponge r.
 Marlex mesh abdominal r.
 posterior r.
 presacral r.
 Ripstein anterior sling r.
 Teflon sling r.
 Wells posterior r.
rectoplasty
rectorrhaphy
rectoscopic endometrial ablation
rectoscopy
rectosigmoid
 r. anastomosis
 r. junction
 r. radiation
 r. sphincter
rectosigmoidoscopy
rectostenosis
rectostomy
rectotomy
rectourethral
 r. fistula
 r. muscle
rectourethralis muscle
rectourinary fistula
rectouterina
 excavatio r.
rectouterine
 r. cul-de-sac
 r. fold
 r. muscle
 r. pouch

rectovaginal
 r. examination
 r. fistula
 r. pouch
 r. septum
 r. surgery
 r. surgical treatment
rectovaginouterine pouch
rectovesical
 r. fascia
 r. fistula
 r. fold
 r. muscle
 r. pouch
 r. septum
rectovesicalis muscle
rectovestibular
 r. fistula
rectovulvar fistula
rectum
 r. irrigation
rectus
 r. abdominis free flap
 r. abdominis muscle
 r. abdominis muscle flap
 r. abdominis musculocutaneous flap
 r. abdominis myocutaneous flap
 r. capitis anterior muscle
 r. capitis lateralis muscle
 r. capitis posterior major muscle
 r. capitis posterior minor muscle
 r. diastasis
 r. fascial wrap
 r. femoris flap
 r. femoris muscle
 r. muscle of abdomen
 r. muscle of thigh
 r. position
 r. sheath
 r. sheath hematoma
recumbent
 r. position
recurrence
 local r.
recurrent
 r. aspiration
 r. corneal erosion
 r. exophthalmos
 r. infection
 r. inflammation
 r. interosseous artery
 r. laryngeal nerve
 r. meningeal branch of spinal
  nerves
 r. meningeal nerve
 r. patellar dislocation
 r. radial artery
 r. tumor

R

r. ulnar artery
r. upper respiratory tract infection
r. vermian oligoastrocytoma
recurvation
recurvatum angulation deformity
red
r. blood cell mass
r. desaturation
r. granulation
r. hepatization
r. induration
r. muscle
r. pulp
Reddick-Saye method
red-eyed shunt syndrome
red-filter therapy
redilation
redintegration
redistribution
r. hypothermia
Redivac suction tube
Redman approach
Redmond-Smith operation
redo
r. CABG
redox indicator
redressement forcé
reduce
reduced liver transplant (RLT)
reduced-size graft
reducible
r. hernia
reduction
afterload r.
Agee force-couple splint r.
alar base r.
Allen r.
Aries-Pitanguy breast r.
Barsky macrodactyly r.
Becton open r.
Boitzy open r.
calcaneal fracture r.
closed r.
cluster r.
concentric r.
Cooper r.
Cotton r. of elbow dislocation
Crosby r.
Cubbins open r.
delayed open r.
Dias-Giegerich open r.
r. division

Eaton closed r.
Eaton-Malerich r.
embryo r.
r. en masse
Essex-Lopresti open r.
femoral neck fracture r.
fetal r.
Flynn femoral neck fracture r.
force-couple splint r.
Fowles open r.
fracture r.
r. of fracture
fracture-dislocation r.
funic r.
Hankin r.
Hastings open r.
hip r.
Houghton-Akroyd open r.
incomplete r.
indirect r.
internal fixation, closed r.
interproximal r.
Kaplan open r.
Kinast indirect r.
King open r.
Lavine r.
limb r.
Lloyd-Roberts open r. of
    Monteggia fracture
Lowell r.
lung volume r. (LVR)
r. mammaplasty
McKeever open r.
r. method
Meyn r. of elbow dislocation
Moberg-Gedda open r.
multifetal pregnancy r.
Neer open r.
open r.
r. osteotomy
pain threshold r.
Pare r. of elbow dislocation
Parvin r.
percutaneous r.
perioperative r.
pneumatic r.
postural r.
r. potential
Pratt open r.
preload r.
prone r.
radial fracture r.

NOTES

reduction *(continued)*
    r. ring
    shoulder r.
    side posture r.
    sigmoid loop r.
    Speed-Boyd open r.
    Speed open r.
    spondylolisthesis r.
    stable r.
    stapled lung r.
    sternoclavicular joint r.
    surgical r.
    swan-neck deformity r.
    r. syndactyly
    r. technique
    trial r.
    tuberosity r.
    r. tuberosity
    volvulus r.
    Wayne County r.
    Weber-Brunner-Freuler open r.
    weight r.
reduction-stabilization
redundant sac tissue
reduplication
    r. cataract
    r. murmur
reedy nail
reefing
    r. procedure
    stomach r.
reendothelialization
reentry
    bundle branch r.
reepithelialization
Rees-Ecker
    R.-E. fluid
    R.-E. method
Reese-Cleasby operation
Reese-Jones-Cooper operation
Reese ptosis operation
reexpansion maneuver
reexploration
reexplore
reference method
referred
    r. point
    r. trigger point pain
    r. trigger point phenomenon
refired
refixation
ReFix noninvasive fixation
reflectance
    endoscopic r.
reflected inguinal ligament
reflection
    angle of r.
    Campbell triceps r.

    corneal r.
    diffuse r.
    guidewire r.
    hepatoduodenal r.
    hepatoduodenal-peritoneal r.
    mirror-image r.
    mucobuccal r.
    peritoneal r.
    shiny cellophane r.
    specular r.
    total internal r.
reflectometry
    acoustic r.
reflex
    accommodation r.
    Bezold-Jarisch r.
    body righting r.
    Breuer-Hering inflation r.
    cardiopressor r.
    celiac plexus r.
    copper-wire r.
    corneal light r.
    cremasteric r.
    crossed extension r.
    crossed extensor r.
    Cushing r.
    r. erection
    erector-spinal r.
    r. examination
    extensor thrust r.
    external oblique r.
    eyeball compression r.
    eye-closure r.
    eyelash r.
    eyelid-closure r.
    fixation r.
    flexion-extension r.
    fusion r.
    grasp r.
    Head paradoxical r.
    head-turning r.
    Hering-Breuer r.
    r. incontinence
    inflation r.
    lacrimation r.
    r. ligament
    mass r.
    milk-ejection r.
    myenteric r.
    r. neurogenic bladder
    oculocardiac r. (OCR)
    paradoxical extensor r.
    pericardial r.
    pronator r.
    proprioceptive head-turning r.
    quadripedal extensor r.
    renal r.
    silver-wire r.

R

supination r.
supinator longus r.
r. sympathetic dystrophy
sympathoexcitation r.
r. sympathoexcitation
r. therapy
vagovagal r.
r. venoconstriction
vertical suspension r.
visceral traction r.
reflexogenic erection
reflux
reformation
DentaScan multiplanar r.
fornix r.
inferior fornix r.
reformulation
refractile body
refractive
r. keratoplasty
r. keratotomy
refractory variceal hemorrhage
refresh
R. Plus ophthalmic solution
refrigeration anesthesia
regainer space
regenerate
regeneration
aberrant r.
r. aberration
atypical r.
axonal r.
carbon tetrachloride-induced liver r.
compensatory r.
epimorphic r.
incomplete r.
morphallactic r.
r. motor unit potential
r. of nerve
neuronal r.
osteoblastic bone r.
tibial bone defect r.
tissue r.
tubular r.
regimen
regio, pl. **regiones**
regiones abdominis
r. analis
r. antebrachialis anterior
r. antebrachialis posterior
r. axillaris
r. brachialis anterior

r. brachialis posterior
r. calcanea
regiones capitis
regiones cervicales
r. cervicalis anterior
r. cervicalis lateralis
r. cervicalis posterior
regiones corporis
r. deltoidea
regiones dorsales
r. epigastrica
regiones faciales
r. femoralis
r. femoralis anterior
r. femoralis posterior
r. frontalis capitis
r. genus anterior
r. genus posterior
r. hypochondriaca
r. infraclavicularis
r. inframammaria
r. infraorbitalis
r. infrascapularis
r. inguinalis
r. lateralis
r. lumbalis
r. mammaria
regiones membri inferioris
regiones membri superioris
r. mentalis
r. nuchalis
r. occipitalis capitis
r. oralis
r. orbitalis
r. parietalis capitis
r. perinealis
r. plantaris
r. presternalis
r. pubica
r. respiratoria tunicae mucosae nasi
r. sacralis
r. scapularis
r. sternocleidomastoidea
r. suralis
r. temporalis capitis
r. umbilicalis
r. urogenitalis
r. vertebralis
r. zygomatica
region
abdominal r.'s
anal r.

NOTES

region (*continued*)
    ankle r.
    anterior antebrachial r.
    anterior r. of arm
    anterior brachial r.
    anterior r. of forearm
    anterior knee r.
    anterior r. of leg
    anterior r. of neck
    anterior r. of thigh
    argyrophilic nucleolar organizer r.
    axillary r.
    r.'s of back
    calcaneal r.
    r.'s of chest
    epigastric r.
    r.'s of face
    femoral r.
    frontal r. of head
    gastric pacemaker r.
    gluteal r.
    r.'s of head
    hilar r.
    hypochondriac r.
    iliac r.
    inframammary r.
    infraorbital r.
    infrascapular r.
    inguinal r.
    lateral r. of neck
    lumbar r.
    mammary r.
    mental r.
    r.'s of neck
    nuchal r.
    occipital r. of head
    oral r.
    orbital r.
    parietal r.
    perineal r.
    pineal r.
    popliteal r.
    posterior antebrachial r.
    posterior r. of arm
    posterior brachial r.
    posterior r. of forearm
    posterior knee r.
    posterior r. of leg
    posterior r. of neck
    posterior neck r.
    posterior r. of thigh
    presternal r.
    r.'s of protection
    pubic r.
    r. of respiratory mucosa
    retroperitoneal r.
    sacral r.
    scapular r.

    sternocleidomastoid r.
    suboccipital r.
    sural r.
    temporal r. of head
    umbilical r.
    urogenital r.
    vertebral r.
    zygomatic r.

regional
    r. anesthesia (RA)
    r. anesthetic
    r. anesthetic technique
    r. block
    r. flap
    r. hypothermia
    r. wall motion abnormality
      (RWMA)

regiones (*pl. of* regio)
registration
registry
    Acoustic Neuroma R.
    Balloon Valvuloplasty R.
    Brain Tumor R.
    Kiel Pediatric Tumor R.
    Mansfield Valvuloplasty R.
    National Football Head and Neck
      Injury R.
    Ovarian Tumor R.
    population-based r.
    St. Mark polyposis r.
    tumor r.
regression
    tumor r.
regressive-reconstructive approach
Regugauge suction regulator
regulator
    current r.
    cystic fibrosis transmembrane
      conductance r.
    high-flow r.
    low-flow r.
    Medela membrane r.
    Ohmeda continuous-vacuum r.
    Ohmeda thoracic suction r.
    OptiMed glaucoma pressure r.
    Regugauge suction r.
    Regu-Vac r.
    suction Regugauge r.
    Vacutron suction r.
    voltage r.
regurgitant lesion
regurgitation
    r. jaundice
    r. test
Regu-Vac regulator
rehabilitation
    r. stage
rehalation

Rehfuss
R. duodenal tube
R. method
R. stomach tube
Rehne-Delorme plication
rehydrating solution
rehydration
r. therapy
Reichel-Pólya
R.-P. method
R.-P. procedure
R.-P. stomach resection
R.-P. technique
Reichenheim-King procedure
Reichenheim technique
Reichert membrane
Reid base line
Reifenstein syndrome
Reilly body
reimplantation
aortorenal r.
Cohen cross-trigonal r.
end-to-side r.
intentional tooth r.
Leadbetter-Politano r.
ureteral r.
Reinecke-Carroll lacrimal tube
Reinert acetabular extensile approach
reinfection
r. tuberculosis
reinforced tracheostomy tube
reinforcing suture
reinjection protocol
Reinke
R. crystalloids
R. space
reinnervation
reinoculation
reinsemination
reintegration
reintubation
reinversion
reirrigation
Reisseisen muscles
Reissner membrane
Reis-Wertheim vaginal hysterectomy
Reiter
R. disease
R. syndrome
rejection
accelerated transplant r.
acute allograft r.

acute cellular r.
acute lung r.
acute vascular r.
allograft corneal r.
r. cardiomyopathy transplant
chronic allograft r.
chronic transplant r.
delayed hyperacute transplant r.
ductopenic r.
fetal r.
first-set graft r.
graft r.
homograft r.
hyperacute r.
interstitial r.
r. line
marrow graft r.
maternal r.
no r.
no infection-no r.
primary r.
renal allograft r.
second-set graft r.
total graft area r.
transplant r.
vascular r.
rejuvenation
relation
acentric r.
acquired centric r.
acquired eccentric jaw r.
buccolingual r.
centric jaw r.
centric occluding r.
concentration-effect r.
convenience jaw r.
cusp-fossa r.
diastolic pressure-volume r.
Duane-Hunt r.
dynamic r.
eccentric jaw r.
end-systolic pressure-volume r.
end-systolic stress-dimension r.
equivalence r.
force-frequency r.
force-length r.
force-velocity r.
force-velocity-length r.
force-velocity-volume r.
Frank-Starling r.
intermaxillary r.
interval-strength r.

NOTES

relation *(continued)*
  jaw r.
  jaw-to-jaw r.
  lateral occlusion r.
  length-resting tension r.
  length-tension r.
  mandibular centric r.
  maxillomandibular r.
  median jaw r.
  median retruded r.
  occluding r.
  occlusal r.
  posterior border jaw r.
  pressure-flow r.
  pressure-volume r.
  protrusive jaw r.
  resting length-tension r.
  rest jaw r.
  retruded jaw r.
  ridge r.
  static r.
  tension-length r.
  unstrained jaw r.
  ventilation/perfusion r.
  ventricular end-systolic pressure-
    volume r.
  vertical r.
  working bite r.
relationship
  cause-effect r.
  endoscope-body position r.
  end-systolic pressure-length r.
    (ESPLR)
  intraluminal pH-pressure r.
  pressure-flow r.
  tissue-base r.
  tumor cell-host bone r.
  ventilation/perfusion r.
relative
  r. curative resection
  near-point r.
  r. noncurative resection
  r. response attributable to the
    maneuver
  r. spectacle magnification
relaxant
  depolarizing r.
  muscle r.
  neuromuscular r.
  nondepolarizing muscle r.
  r. reversal
  smooth muscle r.
relaxation
  adaptive r.
  cardioesophageal r.
  diastolic r.
  differential r.
  dipole-dipole r.

dynamic r.
endothelial-dependent r.
endothelium-mediated r.
esophageal sphincter r.
incomplete r.
intraoperative stress r.
isovolumetric r.
isovolumic r.
left ventricular diastolic r.
longitudinal r.
nitric oxide blocked sphincter r.
paramagnetic r.
paramagnetic shift r.
pelvic r.
r. phenomenon
r. rate
reciprocal r.
r. response
sinusoidal r.
smooth muscle r.
stress r.
r. suture
r. technique
r. time
r. time index
transverse r.
T1, T2 r.
upper esophageal sphincter r.
uterine r.
ventricular r.
relaxing
  r. incision
  r. solution
release
  de Quervain stenosing
    tenosynovitis r.
  endoscopic carpal tunnel r. (ECTR)
  Endotrac endoscopic carpal
    tunnel r.
  flexor-pronator origin r.
  lateral extensor r.
  modified two-portal endoscopic
    carpal tunnel r.
  nifedipine extended r.
  physiologic pattern r.
  plantar plate r.
  pronator teres r.
  soft tissue r.
  sustained r. (SR)
relief
  r. incision
  R. ophthalmic solution
  r. space
relieving incision
Remak
  R. ganglia
  R. plexus
remargination

R

remifentanil
remission induction
remnant
    Cloquet canal r.
    mucosal r.
    pupillary membrane r.
remobilization
remodeling
    extracellular matrix r.
    tissue r.
remote pedicle flap
remotivation
removable maintainer space
removal
    Cameron femoral component r.
    cast r.
    cement r.
    Collis-Dubrul femoral stem r.
    colonoscopic r.
    endoscopic r.
    excisional r.
    extracorporeal CO_2 r. (ECOR)
    forceps r.
    r. of foreign body
    foreign body r.
    r. of foreign body operation
    gastric coin r.
    Harris femoral component r.
    hump r.
    implant r.
    lens r.
    metastatic tumor r.
    Moreland-Marder-Anspach femoral
      stem r.
    nail fold r.
    nail plate r.
    one-session r.
    path of r.
    percutaneous endoscopic r.
    percutaneous stone r.
    radical en bloc r.
    rib r.
    small polyp r.
    stem r.
    through-the-scope balloon r.
    transsphenoidal r.
    tube r.
    ureteral stoma r.
    Winograd nail plate r.
remyelination
remyelinization
ren

Renacidin irrigation
renal
    r. adenocarcinoma
    r. adenoma
    r. allograft rejection
    r. allograft rupture
    r. angioplasty
    r. anomalies
    r. artery
    r. artery bypass graft
    r. autotransplantation
    r. biopsy
    r. branch of lesser splanchnic
      nerve
    r. branch of vagus nerve
    r. calculus
    r. capsulotomy
    r. carcinoma
    r. cell carcinoma
    r. columns
    r. complication
    r. cortex
    r. cortical lobule
    r. crush syndrome
    r. cyst ablation
    r. cyst decortication
    r. cyst hemorrhage
    r. cyst infection
    r cyst marsupialization
    r. duplication
    r. ectopia
    r. fascia
    r. fistula
    r. fungal infection
    r. ganglia
    r. hematoma
    r. hyperfiltration
    r. hypertension
    r. impression
    r. infusion therapy
    r. injury repair
    r. labyrinth
    r. lobe
    r. malrotation
    r. manifestation
    r. mass
    r. medulla
    r. papilla
    r. pelvis
    r. pelvis carcinoma
    r. plexus
    r. pouch

NOTES

renal *(continued)*
    r. preservation
    r. proximal tubule preparation
    r. pyramid
    r. reflex
    r. replacement therapy
    r. revascularization
    r. segments
    r. sinus
    r. surface of spleen
    r. surface of suprarenal gland
    r. surface of the suprarenal gland
    r. thromboendarterectomy
    r. transplantation
    r. tumor
    r. vasodilator prostaglandin
    r. vein renin concentration
    r. veins
renal-splanchnic steal
renaturation
renculus
Rendell-Baker Soucek mask
renewal
    tissue r.
renicapsule
renicardiac
reniculus
reniform
    r. pelvis
reninoma
reniportal
renis
    ectopia r.
renocutaneous
renogastric
    r. fistula
renointestinal
renomegaly
renopathy
renoprival
renopulmonary
renorrhaphy
renovascular
    r. hypertension
Rentrop classification
renunculus
Reo Macrodex suture
reoperation
reoperative
    r. aesthetic surgery
    r. bariatric surgery
    r. blepharoplasty
    r. ureteroneocystostomy
reorganization
    recovery and r.
reoxygenation

repair
    Abraham-Pankovich tendo
      calcaneus r.
    ACL r.
    acromioclavicular joint r.
    all-inside r.
    Allison gastroesophageal reflux r.
    Allison hiatal hernia r.
    anal sphincter r.
    anatomic r.
    Anson-McVay hernia r.
    anterior-posterior r.
    anterior and posterior r.
    aortic valve r.
    A&P r.
    Arlt epicanthus r.
    Arlt eyelid r.
    Atasoy-type flap for nail injury r.
    Bankart shoulder r.
    Barnhart r.
    Bassini inguinal hernia r.
    Belsey Mark IV r.
    Belt-Fuqua hypospadias r.
    bilateral inguinal hernia r.
    Black r.
    Blair epicanthus r.
    blepharochalasis r.
    blepharoptosis r.
    Boari ureteral flap r.
    Boerema hernia r.
    bone graft r.
    Bosworth tendo calcaneus r.
    Boyd-Anderson biceps tendon r.
    brachial plexus r.
    Brom r.
    Bunnell tendon r.
    Cantwell-Ransley epispadias r.
    Caspari r.
    cemental r.
    Collis r.
    columellar r.
    cross-trigonal r.
    cystocele r.
    Danus-Stanzel r.
    DeBakey-Creech aneurysm r.
    delayed primary r.
    density-dependent r.
    Devine hypospadias r.
    diaphragmatic crural r.
    dog-ear r.
    dural r.
    DuVries hammertoe r.
    dynamic r.
    Ecker-Lotke-Glazer patellar
      tendon r.
    Effler hiatal hernia r.
    end-to-end tendon r.
    end-to-side r.

R

epineural r.
episiotomy r.
extensor tendon r.
exteriorized uterine r.
extracorporeal r.
extraperitoneal endoscopic hernia r.
fascicular r.
fibrous r.
first-stage r.
five-one knee ligament r.
flexor tendon r.
Fontan r.
fracture r.
Froimson-Oh r.
functional r.
Gardner meningocele r.
glenohumeral dislocation r.
group fascicular r.
Halsted-Bassini hernia r.
Harrington-Allison r.
Harrington hernia r.
Hatafuku fundus onlay patch
  esophageal r.
hernia r.
hernial r.
Hill hiatus hernia r.
Hill median arcuate r.
histologic tooth r.
Hoguet pantaloon hernia r.
Jones first-toe r.
Kelikian-Riashi-Gleason patellar
  tendon r.
Kessler r.
Kleinert r.
r. of the knee for rotatory
  instability
Konno r.
Kuhnt-Junius r.
lacrimal gland r.
Lange tendon lengthening and r.
laparoscopic varicocele r.
Le Fort-Wehrbein-Duplay
  hypospadias r.
levator aponeurosis r.
Lich-Gregoire r.
Lichtenstein hernial r.
Lindholm tendo calcaneus r.
Lotheissen hernia r.
Lynn tendo calcaneous r.
MacIntosh over-the-top r.
MacNab shoulder r.
Madden r.

Magpi hypospadius r.
Ma-Griffith tendo calcaneus r.
Mandelbaum-Nartolozzi-Carney
  patellar tendon r.
Marlex hernial r.
McVay inguinal hernial r.
medial r.
medial canthal r.
meniscal r.
myelomeningocele r.
Nissen r.
Noble-Mengert perineal r.
one-stage hypospadias r.
Palmer-Dobyns-Linscheid ligament r.
pants-over-vest hernial r.
paravaginal defect r.
patellar tendon r.
periapical tooth r.
pericardioplasty in pectus
  excavatum r.
perineal r.
Phaneuf-Graves r.
plastic r.
postanal r.
posterior r.
postoperative r.
potentially lethal x-ray damage r.
primary r.
pseudarthrosis r.
pseudoarthrosis r.
pulmonary stenosis r.
radiographic tooth r.
Ransley-Cantwell r.
Rastelli r.
rectocele r.
renal injury r.
reverse sigma penoscrotal
  transposition r.
rod fracture r.
Rodney Smith biliary stricture r.
rotator cuff r.
Scuderi r.
secondary r.
Senning r.
Sever-L'Episcopo r.
shoulder r.
Shouldice hernia r.
in situ uterine r.
slipped Nissen r.
Speed sternoclavicular r.
sphincter r.
staged abdominal r.

NOTES

repair *(continued)*
 stage 2, 3 hypoplastic left heart r.
 Staples r.
 Staples-Black-Broström ligament r.
 Strickland tendon r.
 sublethal x-ray damage r.
 surgical r.
 suture r.
 Talesnick scapholunate r.
 tendon r.
 Teuffer tendo calcaneus r.
 Thal esophageal stricture r.
 Theirsch-Duplay r.
 tight Nissen r.
 tissue r.
 transabdominal preperitoneal r.
 triad knee r.
 trichiasis r.
 tricuspid valve r.
 triple ligamentous r.
 Turco-Spinella tendo calcaneus r.
 two-stage r.
 unilateral inguinal hernia r.
 in utero r.
 vaginal wall r.
 vascular laceration r.
 Veirs canaliculus r.
 vesicovaginal r.
 vest-over-pants hernial r.
 volar plate r.
 Watson-Jones fracture r.
 Wheeler halving r.
 York-Mason r.
 Young type epispadias r.
 Zancolli clawhand deformity r.
reparative cardiac surgery
repeat
 r. balloon mitral valvotomy
 r. cesarean section
 r. procedure
 r. revascularization
repeated
 r. exposure
 r. respiratory infection
 r. tissue expansion
reperfusion
reperfusion-induced hemorrhage
reperitonealization
repetitive nerve stimulation
rephasing
 echo r.
 even-echo r.
replacement
 aortic valve r.
 r. collection bag
 Cosgrove mitral valve r.
 heart valve r.
 homograft aortic valve r.

 mitral valve r.
 mucosal patch r.
 Mueller-type femoral head r.
 pulmonary valve r.
 supra-annular mitral valve r.
 tile plate facet r.
 total hip r.
 tube r.
 valve r.
replant
replantation
 intentional r.
 limb r.
Replogle tube
repolarization
Reposans-10 Oral
reposition
repositioning
 muscle r.
repreparation
reproductive
 r. tract
 r. tract abnormality
rerouting insertion
rescue
 r. analgesia
 r. angioplasty
 r. antiemetic
 propofol r.
 r. technique
 r. therapy
resect
resectable
resection
 abdominoperineal r. (APR)
 abdominosacral r.
 absolute curative r.
 absolute noncurative r.
 activation map-guided surgical r.
 anterior r.
 r. arthrodesis
 r. arthroplasty
 atrial septal r.
 Badgley iliac wing r.
 bar r.
 bleb r.
 bone r.
 bony bridge r.
 bowel r.
 bronchial sleeve r.
 calcaneonavicular bar r.
 Carrell r.
 caudal lamina r.
 cesarean r.
 Clayton procedure with
  panmetatarsal head r.
 cold-cup r.
 coloanal r.

colon r.
colosigmoid r.
combined organ r.
composite pelvic r.
condyle r.
conservative r.
craniofacial r.
cuff r.
curative r.
Darrach r.
r. dermodesis
diathermic r.
Dillwyn-Evans r.
Dwar-Barrington r.
electrocautery r.
en bloc r.
endocardial r.
endometrial r.
endoscopic mucosal r. (EMR)
endoscopic snare r.
end-to-end ileo-anal anastomosis
  without mucosal r.
epidermoid r.
epiphyseal bar r.
esophageal r.
esophagogastric r.
extended r.
extra-articular r.
femoral r.
Girdlestone r.
Guller r.
gum r.
Gurd r.
Henry r.
hepatic r.
Hoffmann panmetatarsal head r.
hyoid bone r.
ileal r.
ileocolic r.
ileocolonic r.
iliac crest r.
iliac wing r.
incomplete r.
infundibular wedge r.
Ingram bony bridge r.
innominate bone r.
intercalary r.
interdental r.
Janecki-Nelson shoulder girdle r.
Karakousis-Vezeridis r.
Kashiwagi r.
kyphos r.

Langenskiöld bony bridge r.
laparoscopic multiple-punch r.
lateral rectus r.
lateral temporal r.
lesser r.
levator r.
Lewis-Chekofsky r.
Lewis intercalary r.
limited r.
liver r.
Localio-Francis-Rossano r.
local radical r.
low anterior r. (LAR)
low rectal r.
major liver r. (MLR)
Malawer r.
Mankin r.
Marcove-Lewis-Huvos shoulder
  girdle r.
marginal r.
medial malleolus r.
r. of meniscus
metatarsal head r.
Miles abdominoperineal r.
Miltner-Wan calcaneus r.
Mohs microsurgical r.
multiple-punch r.
Mumford r.
r. of muscle
muscle r.
myotomy-myectomy-septal r.
ovarian wedge r.
palliative r.
pancreatic tail r.
panmetatarsal head r.
parotid r.
Paul-Mikulicz r.
Peet splanchnic r.
peripheral segment of lung
  tissue r.
Peyman full-thickness eye-wall r.
Phelps partial r.
portal vein r.
prophylactic r.
proximal femoral r.
pulmonary r.
radical subtotal r.
Radley-Liebig-Brown r.
ray r.
Reichel-Pólya stomach r.
relative curative r.
relative noncurative r.

NOTES

resection *(continued)*
   rim r.
   Rockwood r.
   root end r.
   scleral r.
   segmental colonic r.
   segmental lung r.
   segmental pulmonary r.
   septal r.
   skull base tumor r.
   sleeve r.
   small-bowel r.
   sphincter-sparing r.
   Stener-Gunterberg r.
   strip r.
   submucous r.
   subtotal gastric r.
   surgical r.
   terminal ileal r.
   Thompson r.
   Tikhoff-Linberg shoulder girdle r.
   Torpin cul-de-sac r.
   transanal endoscopic
     microsurgical r.
   transcervical r.
   transoral odontoid r.
   transsphenoidal microsurgical r.
   transsphenoidal pituitary r. (TPR)
   transthoracic vertebral body r.
   transurethral r.
   transverse r.
   tumor r.
   UICC-RO r.
   vertebral r.
   Weaver-Dunn r.
   wedge r.
   Whipple r.
resection-arthrodesis
   Enneking r.-a.
resection-realignment
Resectisol Irrigation solution
resective
   r. colostomy
   r. surgery
resectoscopy
resedation
reservoir
   r. bag
   r. face mask
   r. host
   r. of infection
   r. mucosal absorption
   r. phase
residual
   r. abscess
   r. body
   r. cleft
   r. ductal tissue

   r. foci
   r. fragment
   r. mesorectum
residue
resin
   r. condensation
   r. restoration
resistance
   alkylation r.
   aortic valve r.
   drug r.
   increased systemic vascular r.
   loss of r.
   mean airway r.
   pulmonary vascular r.
   tissue r.
Resol electrolyte solution
resolution
resolve
resolvent
resonance
   nuclear magnetic r. (NMR)
resonance line
resorption
respirable
   r. aerosol
respiration
   abdominal r.
   absent r.
   accelerated r.
   accessory muscles of r.
   aerobic r.
   agonal r.
   amphoric r.
   anaerobic r.
   apneustic r.
   artificial r.
   assisted r.
   asthmoid r.
   Austin-Flint r.
   Biot r.
   Bouchut r.
   bronchial r.
   bronchocavernous r.
   bronchovesicular r.
   cavernous r.
   central r.
   cerebral r.
   Cheyne-Stokes r.
   cogwheel r.
   collateral r.
   controlled diaphragmatic r.
   Corrigan r.
   cortical r.
   costal r.
   cyclic r.
   decreased r.
   diaphragmatic r.

diaphragmatic-abdominal r.
diffusion r.
direct r.
divided r.
electrophrenic r.
external r.
forced r.
granular r.
grunting r.
harsh r.
internal r.
interrupted r.
intrauterine r.
jerky r.
Kussmaul r.
Kussmaul-Kien r.
labored r.
laryngeal r.
meningitic r.
metamorphosing r.
mouth-to-mouth r.
nasal r.
nervous r.
opposition r.
oral r.
paradoxical r.
periodic r.
placental r.
puerile r.
radiofrequency electrophrenic r.
rude r.
Schäfer method of artificial r.
Seitz metamorphosing r.
shallow r.
sighing r.
slow r.
sonorous r.
stertorous r.
stridulous r.
supplementary r.
suppressed r.
temperature, pulse, and r.
thoracic r.
tissue r.
transitional r.
tubular r.
ventilator-assisted r.
vesiculocavernous r.
vicarious r.
wavy r.

R

respirator
　　r. brain
　　r. lung
respiratory
　　r. ataxia
　　r. bronchioles
　　r. complication
　　r. depression
　　r. distress syndrome (RDS)
　　r. exchange
　　r. excursion
　　r. inversion point
　　r. minute volume
　　r. syncytial virus conduit
　　r. syncytial virus infection
　　r. tract
　　r. tract fluid
　　r. tract infection
respiratory-esophageal fistula
respirometer
　　hot wire r.
Respitrace plethysmography
response
　　auditory middle-latency r. (AMLR)
　　baroreflex r.
　　brain stem evoked r.
　　canal resonance r.
　　carbon dioxide r.
　　central carbon dioxide ventilatory r.
　　Cushing pressure r.
　　deconditioned exercise r.
　　detector r.
　　foreign body r.
　　hemodynamic r.
　　hypercapnic ventilatory r.
　　hypercontractile external sphincter r.
　　hypnotic r.
　　hypoxic ventilatory r.
　　implantation r.
　　irritant patch-test r.
　　lactation letdown r.
　　motor-evoked r. (MER)
　　radiation r.
　　relaxation r.
　　sensitization r.
　　skin potential r.
　　snout r.
　　steady-state auditory evoked r.
　　　(SSAER)
　　steady-state ventilatory r.
　　stress r.
　　sympathoadrenal r.

NOTES

response *(continued)*
    sympathoexcitatory r.
    transient auditory evoked r.
      (TAER)
    twitch r.
    ventilatory r.
    white line r.
responsiveness
    airway r.
rest
    auxiliary implant r.
    Cedar anesthesia face r.
    head r.
    r. jaw relation
    physiologic position of r.
    3-point head r.
    r. position
    position of r.
restenosis
    aortic valve r.
    r. lesion
    postangioplasty r.
    post-balloon angioplasty r.
    pulmonary valve r.
restiform body
resting
    r. anal sphincter pressure
    r. energy expenditure
    r. length-tension relation
    r. line
    r. membrane potential
    r. urethral pressure profile
restoration
    acid-etched r.
    adhesive resin bonded cast r.
    after-root amputation r.
    alloy r.
    amalgam r.
    Berens-Smith cul-de-sac r.
    bonded cast r.
    buccal r.
    ceramic r.
    ceramometal r.
    combination r.
    composite resin r.
    compound r.
    r. contour
    contour r.
    crown r.
    cusp r.
    dental r.
    direct acrylic r.
    direct composite resin r.
    direct gold r.
    direct resin r.
    distal extension r.
    esthetic r.
    facial r.

    facilitating r.
    faulty r.
    foreskin r.
    full cast r.
    implant r.
    IMZ type r.
    inlay r.
    intermediate r.
    Interpore IMZ r.
    intrinsic r.
    large r.
    maxillary r.
    metal-ceramic r.
    metallic r.
    r. of normal anatomic alignment
    overhanging r.
    overlay r.
    permanent r.
    physical r.
    pinch r.
    pin-supported r.
    r. point
    porcelain-bonded r.
    porcelain-fused-to-metal r.
    porcelain jacket r.
    postcore r.
    prosthetic r.
    provisional r.
    resin r.
    root canal r.
    silicate r.
    silver amalgam r.
    temporary r.
    voice r.
restorative
    r. fixation
    r. procedure
    r. proctocolectomy
restriction
    r. endonuclease analysis
    extension r.
    r. fragment length
    soft tissue r.
resurfacing
    r. operation
    r. procedure
resuscitate
resuscitation
    cardiac r.
    cardiopulmonary r. (CPR)
    fluid r.
    heart-lung r.
    hypertonic/hyperoncotic fluid r.
    intrauterine r.
    mouth-to-mouth r.
    neonatal r.
    newborn r.
resuscitative thoracotomy

R

resuscitator
    ACD r.
    Ambu infant r.
    BagEasy disposable manual r.
    bag-valve r.
    First Response manual r.
    Fisher-Paykel RD1000 r.
    High Oxygen PRM r.
    Hope r.
    Hudson Lifesaver r.
    infant Ambu r.
    Laerdal infant r.
    Laerdal silicone r.
    Lifemask infant r.
    NeoVO-2-R volume control r.
    Ohio Hope r.
    Penlon infant r.
    pneuPAC r.
    RD1000 r.
    Robertshaw bag r.
    Safe Response manual r.
    SureGrip manual r.
retained
    r. foreign body
    r. papilla technique
    r. placental fragment
retainer
    r. closure
    r. ring
retaining ring
retard
    expiratory r.
retardation
    developmental r.
    fetal growth r.
    growth r.
    healing r.
    intrauterine growth r.
    psychomotor r.
retching
rete, pl. retia
    r. acromiale
    r. articulare cubiti
    r. articulare genus
    r. calcaneum
    r. cords
    r. foraminis ovalis
    Haller r.
    r. malleolare laterale
    r. malleolare mediale
    r. mirabile
    r. testis

    r. vasculosum articulare
    r. venosum dorsale manus
    r. venosum dorsale pedis
    r. venosum plantare
retention
    extracoronal r.
    intracoronal-extracoronal r.
    r. mucocele
    pin r.
    r. point
    r. ring
    surgical r.
    r. suture
    r. suture bridge
    viscera r.
retentive fulcrum line
retia (*pl. of* rete)
retial
reticula (*pl. of* reticulum)
reticular
    r. formation
    r. lesion
reticulate pigmented anomaly
reticulation
reticuloendothelioma
reticulogranuloma
reticulohistiocytoma
reticulospinal tract
reticulotomy
reticulum, pl. reticula
    Ebner r.
    extraconal fat r.
retina, pl. retinae
    coloboma retinae
    coloboma of r.
    demarcation line of r.
    disciform degeneration of r.
    glioma of r.
    lattice degeneration of r.
    neovascularization of r.
    primary pigmentary degeneration
        of r.
    rod cell of r.
    separation of r.
    stratum nucleare externum retinae
    stratum nucleare externum et
        internum retinae
    stratum plexiforme externum et
        internum retinae
retinaculum, pl. retinacula
    antebrachial flexor r.
    r. of articular capsule of hip

NOTES

retinaculum *(continued)*
  r. capsulae articularis coxae
  caudal r.
  r. caudale
  extensor r.
  lateral patellar r.
  medial patellar r.
  Morgagni r.
  retinacula of nail
  r. patellae laterale
  r. patellae mediale
  patellar r.
  peroneal r.
  r. of skin
  superior peroneal r.
  r. tendinum
  retinacula unguis
retinal
  r. arteriovenous malformation
  r. circulation
  r. examination
  r. excavation
  r. exudate
  r. flap
  r. fold
  r. hemorrhage
  r. imbrication
  r. quadrant neovascularization
  r. scatter photocoagulation
  r. surgery
retinectomy
retinitis
retinoblastoma
retinoblastoma-mental retardation syndrome
retinochoroidectomy
retinocytoma
retinoid therapy
retinoillumination
retinopathy
  r. hemorrhage
retinopexy
  cyanoacrylate r.
  pneumatic r.
retinoscopy
  Copeland r.
  cylinder r.
  fogging r.
  streak r.
retinotomy
retothelioma
retract
retractable stylet
retracted stoma
retractile
  r. testis
retracting suture

retraction
  r. ring
  soft palate r.
  r. space
  wound r.
retractor plication
retrahens aurem
retraining
  computerized diaphragmatic breathing r. (CDBR)
retransplantation
retreatment
  lithotripsy r.
retrenchment
retrieval
  intravascular foreign body r.
  transvaginal ultrasonically guided oocyte r.
retroacetabular lesion
retroadductor space
retroauricular
  r. free flap
  r. lymph nodes
retrobulbar
  r. anesthesia
  r. anesthetic technique
  r. hemorrhage
  r. injection
  r. mass
  r. nerve block
  r. orbital metastasis
  r. space
retrocalcaneal
  r. bursa
retrocardiac
  r. mass
  r. space
retrocaval ureter
retrocecal
  r. abscess
  r. hernia
  r. lymph nodes
  r. recess
retrocervical
retrochiasmal
  r. lesion
  r. optic tract
retroclination
retroclusion
retrocolic
  r. end-to-end pancreatojejunostomy
  r. end-to-side choledochojejunostomy
  r. end-to-side gastrojejunostomy
  r. hernia
retrocollic
retrocorneal membrane
retrocrural space
retrodeviation

retrodiskal
r. pad
r. temporomandibular joint pad inflammation
retrodisplacement
retroduodenal
r. artery
r. fossa
r. perforation
r. recess
retroesophageal
retrofilling method
retroflected
retroflection
retroflexed
retroflexion
endoscopic r.
retrogasserian
r. neurectomy
r. neurotomy
r. procedure
retrogastric space
retrogeniculate lesion
retrograde
r. atrial activation mapping
r. balloon rupture
r. cannulation
r. catheter insertion
r. catheterization
r. duodenogastroscopy
r. endoscopic approach
r. femoral approach
r. hernia
r. incarceration
r. intrarenal surgery
r. nephrostomy puncture
r. obturation
r. root canal filling method
r. sphincterotomy
r. tracheal intubation anesthetic technique
r. transurethral prostatic urethroplasty
r. vascularization of superior mesenteric artery
retrohyoid bursa
retroiliac ureter
retroillumination
retroinguinal space
retrojection
retrojector

retrolabyrinthine
r. presigmoid approach
r. vestibular neurectomy
retrolabyrinthine/retrosigmoid vestibular neurectomy
retrolingual
retrolisthesis
r. positional dyskinesia
retromammary
retromandibular
r. fossa
r. point
r. vein
retromastoid suboccipital craniectomy
retromolar
r. fossa
r. pad
retromylohyoid space
retro-ocular
r.-o. space
retropatellar fat pad
retroperitoneal
r. adenopathy
r. approach
r. cavity
r. cutaneous ureterostomy
r. decompression
r. fetus
r. fistula
r. gas insufflation
r. hematoma
r. hemorrhage
r. hernia
r. infection
r. lymphadenectomy
r. node
r. pelvic lymph node dissection (RPLND)
r. perforation
r. pneumography
r. region
r. soft tissue
r. space
r. viscera
retroperitoneal-iliopsoas abscess
retroperitoneoscopic nephrectomy
retroperitoneoscopy
retroperitoneum
retroperitonitis
retropharyngeal
r. approach
r. hematoma

NOTES

retropharyngeal *(continued)*
  r. hemorrhage
  r. lymph nodes
  r. soft tissue
  r. space
retropharynx
retroplacental hematoma
retroposed
retroposition
retropubic
  r. colpourethrocystopexy
  r. hernia
  r. Lapides-Ball bladder neck
    suspension
  r. space
  r. urethrolysis
  r. urethropexy
  r. urethroscopy
  r. vesiculoprostatectomy
retropulsed bone excision
retropulsion
  r. of posterior fragment
retropyloric
  r. lymph nodes
  r. nodes
retrosacral
  r. fascia
retrosigmoid approach
retrospection
retrosternal
  r. air space
  r. dislocation
  r. hernia
  r. mass
retrotracheal space
retrouterine
retroversioflexion
retroversion
retroverted
retrovesical space
Retrovir injection
retrovirus
  r. infection
retrozygomatic space
retruded
  r. jaw relation
  r. position
retrusive excursion
Retzius
  calcification lines of R.
  R. cavity
  incremental line of R.
  line of R.
  R. space
  space of R.
reunient
reuptake-inhibitor
  monoamine r.-i.

Reuter
  R. bobbin ventilating tube
  R. bobbin ventilation tube
revaccination
revascularization
  brain r.
  cerebral r.
  coronary r.
  r. of graft
  heart laser r.
  lower extremity r.
  myocardial r.
  penile r.
  percutaneous transluminal
    coronary r.
  r. procedure
  renal r.
  repeat r.
  transmyocardial r.
  transmyocardial laser r. (TMLR)
revascularized tissue
reverberation
  echo r.
  r. room
Reverdin
  R. bunionectomy
  R. epidermal free graft
  R. method
  R. osteotomy
Reverdin-Green procedure
Reverdin-Laird
  R.-L. bunionectomy
  R.-L. osteotomy
Reverdin-McBride bunionectomy
reversal
  r. jejunoileal bypass surgery
  JIB r.
  r. line
  narcotic r.
  r. pedicle flap
  pressure r.
  relaxant r.
  sex r.
  vasectomy r.
reverse
  r. augmentation
  r. Barton fracture
  r. bevel incision
  r. Bigelow maneuver
  r. Colles fracture
  r. cross-finger flap
  r. Dillwyn-Evans calcaneal
    osteotomy
  r. Eck fistula
  r. filling procedure
  r. forearm island flap
  r. Hill-Sachs lesion
  r. Mauck procedure

R

r. Monteggia fracture
r. phonation
r. Putti-Platt procedure
r. sigma penoscrotal transposition repair
r. topographic projection
r. Trendelenburg position
r. wedge osteotomy
r. wedge technique
reversed
r. reimplanted appendicocystostomy
r. saphenous vein graft
r. vein graft
reverse-Y incision
reversible
r. decortication
r. shock
Reversol injection
Revex
revision
r. hip arthroplasty
r. procedure
revivification
revulsion
rewarming
Rex-Cantli-Serege line
RF
radiofrequency
RF electrocoagulation
RFB System-I for CDBR
RFCA
radiofrequency catheter ablation
rhabdomyolysis
acute recurrent r.
exertional r.
familial paroxysmal r.
hypoxia-induced r.
idiopathic paroxysmal r.
rhabdomyoma
rhabdomyosarcoma
alveolar r.
rhabdosarcoma
rhabdosphincter
rhachotomy
Capener lateral r.
decompression r.
lateral r.
rhegma
rhegmatogenous
rheologic therapy

Rhese
R. position
R. projection
rheumatoid-related ulceration
rhexis
rhinitis
rhinocanthectomy
rhinocerebral infection
rhinocheiloplasty
rhinocleisis
rhinodymia
rhinokyphectomy
rhinopharyngeal
rhinopharynx
rhinoplasty
English r.
esthetic r.
Indian r.
Italian r.
Joseph r.
rhinoscleroma
rhinoscopy
rhinoseptal approach
rhinotomy
rhizolysis
percutaneous glycerol r.
percutaneous radiofrequency r.
percutaneous retrogasserian glycerol r.
Rhizopus infection
rhizotomy
anterior r.
bilateral ventral r.
cranial nerve r.
Dana posterior r.
dorsal r.
facet r.
Frazier-Spiller r.
glycerol r.
intracranial r.
intradural dorsal spinal root r.
percutaneous radiofrequency r.
posterior r.
radiofrequency r.
selective posterior r.
selective sacral r.
thermal r.
trigeminal r.
rhombic
rhomboatloideus
rhombocele

NOTES

rhomboid
    r. ligament
    r. minor muscle
    r. transposition flap
rhomboidal sinus
rhomboideus
    r. major muscle
rhonchus, pl. rhonchi
    expiratory rhonchi
Rhoton-Merz suction tube
rhoton suction
rhythm
    ectopic r.
    fibrillation r.
    r. method
rhythmic
    r. initiation technique
    r. stabilization
rhytidectomy
rhytidoplasty
rib
    bicipital r.
    bifid r.
    r. cage volume
    cervical r.
    double-exposed r.
    false r.'s
    floating r.'s
    r. fracture
    r. graft
    lumbar r.
    r. notching
    r. removal
    slipping r.
    true r.'s
    vertebral r.'s
    vertebrochondral r.'s
    vertebrosternal r.'s
ribbon
    r. arch technique
    r. gut suture
    r. muscles
Ribes ganglion
Rica mastoid suction tube
rice body
Richard fringe
Richardson procedure
Riche-Cannieu anastomosis
Richet operation
Richter
    R. and Albrich procedure
    R. hernia
    R. suture technique
Richter-Monro line
Ricketts-Abrams technique
rickettsial infection
Rideal-Walker method
Rideau technique

ridge
    bicipital r.'s
    epidermal r.'s
    extension r.
    r. extension
    external oblique r.
    lateral epicondylar r.
    lateral supracondylar r.
    medial epicondylar r.
    medial supracondylar r.
    mesonephric r.
    mylohyoid r.
    oblique r. of trapezium
    osteochondral r.
    pharyngeal r.
    pterygoid r. of sphenoid bone
    r. relation
    sphenoidal r.'s
    supraorbital r.
    temporal r.
    trapezoid r.
    urogenital r.
Ridley sinus
Ridlon procedure
Riedel
    R. frontoethmoidectomy procedure
    R. lobe
Rieger syndrome
Rieux hernia
Rifadin injection
Righini procedure
right
    r. acromiodorsoposterior position
    r. anterior oblique (RAO)
    r. anterior oblique position
    r. anterior oblique projection
    r. anterior occipital (RAO)
    r. anterior pararenal space
    r. antero-oblique position
    r. atrial pressure
    r. border of heart
    r. branch of portal vein
    r. branch of proper hepatic artery
    r. bundle branch block
    r. colic artery
    r. colic flexure
    r. colic lymph nodes
    r. colic vein
    r. crus of diaphragm
    deviation to the r.
    r. duct of caudate lobe
    r. erector spinae musculature
    r. fibrous trigone
    r. frontoanterior position
    r. frontoposterior position
    r. frontotemporal craniotomy
    r. frontotransverse position
    r. gastric artery

r. gastric lymph nodes
r. gastric vein
r. gastroepiploic artery
r. gastroepiploic lymph nodes
r. gastroepiploic vein
r. gastro-omental artery
r. gastro-omental lymph nodes
r. gastro-omental vein
r. heart catheterization
r. hepatic artery
r. hepatic duct
r. hepatic veins
r. inferior pulmonary vein
r. lobe of liver
r. lower extremity
r. lumbar lymph nodes
r. lymphatic duct
r. main bronchus
r. mentoanterior position
r. mentoposterior position
r. mentotransverse position
r. occipitoanterior position
r. occipitoposterior position
r. occipitotransverse position
r. ovarian vein
r. ovarian vein syndrome
r. part of diaphragmatic surface of liver
r. rotation
r. sacroanterior position
r. sacroposterior position
r. sacrotransverse position
r. sagittal fissure
r. scapuloanterior position
r. scapuloposterior position
r. superior intercostal vein
r. superior pulmonary vein
r. suprarenal vein
r. temporoparietal craniotomy
r. testicular vein
r. triangular ligament
r. upper extremity
r. upper quadrant peritonectomy
r. ventricle
r. ventricle-pulmonary artery conduit surgery
r. ventricular end-diastolic pressure
r. ventricular outflow tract (RVOT)
r. ventricular outflow tract tachycardia
r. ventricular systolic pressure

right-angle
    r.-a. chest tube
    r.-a. technique
right-angled end-to-side anastomosis
right-sided
    r.-s. lesion
    r.-s. nail
    r.-s. submandibular transverse incision
    r.-s. thoracotomy
right-side-down position
right-to-left shunt ratio
rigid
    r. body
    r. bronchoscopy
    r. endofluoroscopy
    r. internal fixation
    r. plate fixation
    r. proctoscopy
    r. proctosigmoidoscopy
    r. ureteroscopy
rigidity
    C-D instrumentation r.
    Cotrel pedicle screw r.
    spinal fixation r.
rim
    r. resection
    surgical occlusion r.
rima, pl. **rimae**
    r. pudendi
    r. respiratoria
    r. vestibuli
    r. vocalis
    r. vulvae
rim-enhancing lesion
ring
    A r.
    abdominal r.
    abscess r.
    r. abscess
    amnion r.
    anorectal r.
    anterior limiting r.
    aortic r.
    apex of external r.
    r. apophysis
    arterial r.
    atrial r.
    atrioventricular r.
    B r.
    Balbiani r.
    Bandl r.

R

NOTES

ring *(continued)*
Bickel r.
biofragmentable anastomotic r.
blepharostat r.
Bloomberg SuperNumb anesthetic r.
Bonaccolto-Flieringa scleral r.
Bonaccolto scleral r.
Bores twist fixation r.
Brown-Roberts-Wells base r.
Budde halo r.
Burr corneal r.
Buzard-Thornton fixation r.
Cabot r.
cardiac lymphatic r.
Carpentier r.
Caspar r.
casting r.
cataract mask r.
centering r.
choroidal r.
ciliary r.
Coats white r.
collagenolytic trabecular r.
collagenous trabecular r.
common tendinous r.
congenital r.
conjunctival r.
constriction r.
contractile r.
corneal transplant centering r.
coronary r.
corrin r.
Crawford suture r.
cricoid r.
crural r.
deep inguinal r.
distal esophageal r.
Dollinger tendinous r.
double r.
double-flanged valve sewing r.
doughnut r.
drop-lock r.
dural r.
Duran annuloplasty r.
elastic O r.
enhancing r.
epiphyseal r.
r. epiphysis
esophageal r.
esophageal A, B r.
esophageal contractile r.
esophageal contraction r.
esophageal mucosal r.
esophageal muscular r.
external inguinal r.
extracapsular arterial r.
Falope tubal sterilization r.
femoral r.

fibrous r.
fibrous r. of heart
fibrous r. of intervertebral disk
r. finger
Fischer r.
fixation r.
fixation/anchor r.
Fleischer keratoconus r.
Fleischer-Strumpell r.
Flieringa fixation r.
Flieringa-Kayser copper r.
Flieringa-Kayser fixation r.
Flieringa-LeGrand fixation r.
Flieringa scleral r.
r. fracture
Girard scleral r.
glaucomatous r.
glial r.
gold r.
Graefenberg r.
greater r.
half r.
halo r.
head r.
hymenal r.
ilioinguinal r.
iliopsoas r.
Ilizarov r.
Imlach r.
internal abdominal r.
internal inguinal r.
intrahaustral contraction r.
iris r.
iron Fleischer r.
ischial weightbearing r.
Katena r.
Kayser-Fleischer cornea r.
Klein-Tolentino r.
knitted sewing r.
Lacroix osseous r.
Landolt broken r.
laparotomy sponge r.
lenticular r.
r. lesion
lesser r.
Lower r.
lower esophageal B r.
lower esophageal mucosal r.
Luque r.
lymphatic r. of cardiac part of
  stomach
lymphoid r.
Lyon r.
Martinez corneal transplant
  centering r.
Martinez scleral centering r.
Maxwell r.
Mayo perfusing O r.

R

McKinney fixation r.
McNeill-Goldmann scleral r.
Mertz keratoscopy r.
metal sewing r.
Moran-Karaya r.
mucosal esophageal r.
muscular esophageal r.
Nakayama r.
neonatal r.
Ochsner r.
olive r.
orthosis drop-lock r.
Osbon pressure-point tension r.
osseoligamentous r.
palatopharyngeal r.
pathologic retraction r.
pelvic r.
perfusion O r.
perichondral r.
periureteric venous r.
r. pessary
physiologic retraction r.
placido r.
plastic sewing r.
posterior limiting r.
pressure r.
pressure-point tension r.
prominent Schwalbe r.
prosthetic valve sewing r.
protrusio r.
proximal-to-distal r.
Puig Massana annuloplasty r.
Puig Massana-Shiley annuloplasty r.
pyloric r.
Racestyptine retraction r.
reduction r.
retainer r.
retaining r.
retention r.
retraction r.
rust r.
Saturn r.
Schatzki esophageal r.
Schwalbe anterior border r.
scleral expander r.
scotoma r.
Sculptor annuloplasty r.
sewing r.
Silastic r.
silicone elastomer r.
Smith r.
Soemmerring r.

r. of Soemmerring
sphincter contraction r.
sponge r.
St. Jude annuloplasty r.
r. structure
subcutaneous r.
r. sublimis apponensplasty
superficial inguinal r.
suture r.
symblepharon r.
Tano r.
tantalum O r.
targetoid r.
tentorial r.
Thornton fixating r.
Tolentino r.
tonsillar r.
tracheal r.
trigonal r.
Tru-Arc blood vessel r.
T-shaped constriction r.
tubal r.
tympanic r.
r. ulcer of cornea
umbilical r.
vacuum fixation r.
Valtrac absorbable biofragmentable
   anastomosis r.
vascular r.
Vicussens r.
Vossius lenticular r.
Waldeyer throat r.
Waldeyer tonsillar r.
Walsh pressure r.
Wessely r.
white r.
Wimberger r.
Wolf-Yoon r.
Woronoff r.
Yoon tubal sterilization r.
Zinn r.
zipper r.
ring-disrupting fracture
Ringer
   R. arthroscopy
   R. lactate solution
ring-form congenital cataract
ring-knife
Ring-McLean sump tube
ring-shaped
   r.-s. cataract
ring-wall lesion

NOTES

ringworm of nail
Rinkel serial endpoint titration
Riolan
>anastomosis of R.
>R. anastomosis
>R. arc
>R. arcades
>R. bones
>R. muscle

Riordan
>R. pollicization
>R. tendon transfer technique

Ripstein
>R. anterior sling rectopexy
>R. procedure
>R. rectal prolapse operation

Risdon
>R. approach
>R. incision

Riseborough-Radin classification of intercondylar fracture
risk
>r. of anesthesia
>Goldman classification operative r.
>r. management of anesthesia
>radiation r.
>surgical r.

risorius
>r. muscle

Risser
>R. method
>R. technique

Ritgen maneuver
Ritter-Oleson technique
Ritter suprapubic suction tube
Riva-Rocci method
Rivinus
>R. canals
>R. ducts
>R. gland

Rizzoli operation
RLT
>reduced liver transplant

Roaf syndrome
Robert pelvis
Roberts
>R. approach
>R. syndrome
>R. technique

Robertshaw
>R. bag resuscitator
>R. tube

robertsonian fusion
Robinson
>R. anterior cervical diskectomy
>R. cervical spine fusion
>R. equalizing tube
>R. morcellation

Robinson-Chung-Farahvar
>R.-C.-F. clavicular morcellation
>R.-C.-F. morcellation

Robinson-Southwick fusion technique
Robinul
Robson
>R. point
>R. position

Rochester
>R. method
>R. suction tube
>R. tracheal tube

Rockey-Davis incision
Rockwood
>R. classification of acromioclavicular injury
>R. classification of clavicular fracture
>R. posterior capsulorrhaphy
>R. procedure
>R. resection

Rockwood-Green technique
Rockwood-Matsen capsular shift procedure
rocuronium
>r. bromide

rod
>r. cell of retina
>r. contour preparation
>r. fiber
>r. fracture repair
>r. granule
>r. linkage
>r. migration
>r. placement
>r. rotation prevention
>r. sheath
>r. sleeve fixation
>r. spherule

rod-cone
Rodeck method
rod-hook construct
rodless end-loop stoma
rod-mounted
Rodney Smith biliary stricture repair
rod-shaped
Roeder loop knot
roentgenographic evaluation
Roger-Anderson pin fixation
Rogers cervical fusion technique
Röhrer index
Rokitansky hernia
Rolandic
>R. artery
>R. line

Rolando fracture
role fixation

R

roll
    iliac r.
    r. stitch
    r. tube
rolled shoulder lesion
roller
    r. head perfusion pump
    R. pump suction tube
rollerball
    r. endometrial ablation
    r. technique
Rollet incision
rolling
    r. hiatal hernia
    r. membrane
roll-tube technique
ROM
    range of motion
    ROM therapy
Romazicon
Rood technique
roof fracture
roof-patch graft
room
    operating r. (OR)
    recovery r.
    reverberation r.
    surgical dressing r.
Roos approach
root
    r. amputation
    r. anomaly
    anterior r.
    bifurcation of r.
    r. canal
    r. canal access
    r. canal débridement
    r. canal disinfection
    r. canal electrosterilization
    r. canal filling
    r. canal filling technique obturation
    r. canal ionization
    r. canal orifice
    r. canal point
    r. canal restoration
    r. canal shaping
    r. canal sterilization
    r. canal therapy
    r. canal treatment
    r. compression
    dorsal r.
    r. end resection

    facial r.
    r. formation
    r. fracture
    r. furcation
    r. fusion
    r. infiltration
    r. injection
    lateral r. of median nerve
    r. of lung
    r. of mesentry
    nail r.
    nerve r.
    r.'s of olfactory tract, lateral and
      medial
    r. of penis
    r. perforation
    posterior r.
    spinal r. of accessory nerve
    r. of tongue
    ventral r.
Root-Siegal varus derotational osteotomy
rope flap
ropivacaine
Rorabeck fasciotomy
Rosalki technique
Rosch modification
rose
    r. bengal red solution
    R. position
    R. procedure
rosebud stoma
Rosen
    R. suction
    R. suction tube
**Rosenberg endoscopic anterior cruciate
  ligament reconstruction**
Rosenburg operation
Rosengren operation
Rosenmüller
    R. body
    R. fossa
    R. gland
    R. node
    R. recess
    valve of R.
Rosenthal
    R. classification of nail injuries
    R. fiber
Roser-Nélaton line
Ross
    R. body
    R. procedure

NOTES

Rossetti modification of Nissen fundoplication
Ross-Jones test
rostrad
rostral
    r. cingulotomy
    r. transtentorial herniation
rostralis
rostrate
rostriform
rostrocaudal extent signal abnormality
rostrum
    r. sphenoidale
    r. of the sphenoid bone
rotary
    r. joint
    r. mounted point
    r. shadowing electron microscopy
rotatable coupling head
rotated
    externally r.
rotating
    r. aspiration thromboembolectomy
    r. disk oxygenation
    r. frame imaging
rotating-frame zeugmatography
rotation
    abduction-external r.
    anisotropic r.
    anterior innominate r.
    axial r.
    axis of r.
    Borggreve limb r.
    center of axial r.
    cervical general r.
    clockwise r.
    counterclockwise r.
    r. drawer test
    external r.
    external/internal r.
    eye r.
    r. flap
    flexion in abduction and external r.
    flexion in adduction and internal r.
    flexion, adduction, internal r.
    foot r.
    forceps r.
    r. fracture
    gantry r.
    hip r.
    horizontal external r.
    instantaneous axis of r.
    intentional r.
    internal r.
    internal-external r.
    intersegmental r.
    intestinal r.

    inversion-eversion r.
    inward r.
    r. joint
    knee r.
    left r.
    lumbar r.
    manual r.
    r. mobility
    neutral r.
    optical r.
    organoaxial r.
    outward r.
    pelvic r.
    r. plasty
    polycentric r.
    posterior innominate r.
    pronation-eversion-external r.
    pure r.
    r. recurvatum test
    right r.
    sagittal r.
    short-T2 in anisotropic r.
    shoulder r.
    specific r.
    spine r.
    supination-external r.
    synchronous scapuloclavicular r.
    R. test
    r. testing
    r. therapy
    thoracolumbosacral orthoses - flexion, extension, lateral bending, and transverse r.
    timed intermittent r.
    twin bracket tooth r.
    vertebral r.
    wheel r.
rotational
    r. ablation
    r. burst fracture
    r. contact lithotripsy
    r. coronary atherectomy
    r. correction
    r. deformity
    r. dislocation
    r. flap
    r. osteotomy
    r. thrombectomy
rotationally induced shear-strain lesion
rotation-compression maneuver
rotationplasty
    Kotz-Salzer r.
    Van Ness r.
    Winkelmann r.
rotation-stop washer
rotator
    r. cuff
    r. cuff arthropathy

R

r. cuff lesion
r. cuff muscle
r. cuff repair
r. cuff tear
r. cuff tear arthroplasty
external r.
internal r.
long external r.
medial r.
nucleus r.
short external r.
rotatores
r. cervicis muscles
r. lumborum muscles
r. thoracis muscles
rotatory luxation
rotavirus infection
Rothman Institute total hip program
Roto-Rest bed
rotoscoliotic deformity
Rouget bulb
rouleaux formation
round
r. back deformity
r. body
r. foramen
r. hemorrhage
r. ligament of liver
r. ligament of uterus
r. pelvis
r. shoulder deformity
round-robin classification
round-tip
route
r. of administration
external r.
r. of insertion
Roux-duToit staple capsulorrhaphy
Roux-en-Y
R.-e.-Y. biliary bypass with antrectomy
R.-e.-Y. choledochojejunostomy
R.-e.-Y. distal jejunoileostomy
R.-e.-Y. esophagojejunostomy
R.-e.-Y. gastric bypass
R.-e.-Y. gastroenterostomy
R.-e.-Y. gastrojejunostomy
R.-e.-Y. hepaticojejunal anastomosis
R.-e.-Y. hepaticojejunostomy
R.-e.-Y. limb enteroscopy
R.-e.-Y. loop
R.-e.-Y. loop of jejunum

R.-e.-Y. operation
R.-e.-Y. pancreaticojejunostomy
R.-e.-Y. procedure
R.-e.-Y. procedure with vagotomy
R.-e.-Y. reconstruction
Roux-en-Y-cyst-jejunostomy
Roux-Goldthwait
R.-G. dislocation operation
R.-G. procedure
Roux stasis syndrome
Roveda operation
Rovsing operation
Rowbotham
R. operation
R. orbital decompression
Rowe
R. calcaneal fracture classification
R. and Lowell classification system for fracture-dislocation
R. posterior shoulder approach
Rowe-Lowell hip dislocation classification
Rowe-Zarins shoulder immobilization
Rowinski
R. dacryostomy
R. operation
Rowland pouch
Roxanol SR Oral
Roy-Camille posterior screw plate fixation
Royle-Thompson transfer technique
RPLND
retroperitoneal pelvic lymph node dissection
RPT
rapid pull-through
RPT technique
RSI
rapid sequence induction
RSI orotracheal intubation
rtPA
recombinant tissue-type plasminogen activator
rub
peritoneal friction r.
rubber
r. band ligation
r. band ligation of hemorrhoid
r. suture
r. tissue
rubber-band extraction

NOTES

Rubbrecht
    R. extirpation
    R. operation
Rubens breast flap
Rubin
    R. maneuver
    R. tubal insufflation
rubrobulbar tract
rubroreticular tract
rubrospinal
    r. decussation
    r. tract
Rucker body
rude respiration
Rucdemann
    R. evisceration
    R. operation
Ruedi-Allgower classification
Ruese bone graft
ruffed canal
ruga, pl. rugae
    r. gastrica
    rugae of stomach
    rugae of vagina
    rugae vaginales
rugal columns of vagina
rugation
rugine
rugose
rugosity
rugous
Ruiz
    R. procedure
    R. trapezoidal keratotomy
Ruiz-Mora
    R.-M. correction
    R.-M. procedure
rule
    Fletcher r. of irradiation tolerance
    Steel r. of thirds for spinal cord
      free space
Rungstrom projection
running
    r. locked interdermal suture
    r. stitch
runoff
Runyon classification
rupture
    Achilles tendon r.
    acute hepatic r.
    adductor longus muscle r.
    amnion r.
    aneurysmal r.
    anterior talofibular ligament r.
    aortic r.
    balloon r.
    cardiac r.
    chamber r.

chordae tendineae r.
chordal r.
choroidal r.
collateral ligament r.
crescentic r.
diaphragmatic r.
distal biceps brachii tendon r.
duodenopancreaticocholedochal r.
ERCP-induced splenic r.
esophageal r.
flexor tendon r.
gastric r.
hemidiaphragm r.
hepatic r.
hernia r.
hydatid cyst intrahepatic r.
inflammatory r.
infrapatellar tendon r.
interventricular septal r.
intramural esophageal r.
intraoperative r.
intraperitoneal viscus r.
intrapleural r.
longitudinal ligament r.
Mallory-Weiss mucosal r.
marginal sinus r.
membrane r.
mesenteric r.
myocardial r.
neglected r.
nonpenetrating r.
papillary muscle r.
penetrating r.
penile r.
plaque r.
postmembrane r.
prelabor membrane r.
premature amnion r.
premature membrane r.
premembrane r.
prolonged r.
proximal tendon r.
renal allograft r.
retrograde balloon r.
scleral r.
splenic r.
spontaneous r.
stress r.
tendon r.
testicular r.
total perineal r.
transverse ligament r.
traumatic aortic r.
traumatic choroidal r.
tubal r.
ulnar collateral ligament r.
umbilical hernia r.
urinary bladder r.

uterine r.
valve r.
ventricular septal r.
ruptured
r. abdominal aortic aneurysm
r. disk
r. disk excision
r. episiotomy
r. peliotic lesion
rupture-delivery interval
Rusch
R. endotracheal tube cuff
R. laryngectomy tube
Ruschelit polyvinyl chloride endotracheal tube
Russe
R. bone graft
R. classification
R. technique
Russe-Gerhardt method
Russell
R. fibular head autograft
hooked bundle of R.
R. percutaneous endoscopic gastrostomy

R. suction tube
R. technique
uncinate bundle of R.
Russell-Taylor classification
rust
r. ring
r. ring of cornea
Rüter classification
Rutledge classification of extended hysterectomy
ruyschian membrane
Ruysch membrane
RVOT
right ventricular outflow tract
RWMA
regional wall motion abnormality
Rycroft operation
Rye classification of Hodgkin disease
Ryerson
R. bone graft
R. procedure
R. technique
Ryle duodenal tube

R

NOTES

S-A
    sinoatrial
SA
    septal apical
    spinal anesthesia
    splenic artery
    SA segment
saber-cut
    s.-c. approach
    s.-c. incision
Sabreloc suture
sabre-shin deformity
Sac
    Lap S.
sac
    air s.
    allantoic s.
    alveolar s.
    amniotic s.
    aneurysmal s.
    aortic s.
    bursal s.
    caudal s.
    chorionic s.
    common dural s.
    conjunctival s.
    cupular blind s.
    dental s.
    diverticula of lacrimal s.
    double decidual s.
    drainage of lacrimal s.
    embryonic s.
    empty gestational s.
    enamel s.
    endolymphatic s.
    enterocele s.
    fluid-filled s.
    Föerster lacrimal s.
    s. formation
    gestational s.
    greater peritoneal s.
    heart s.
    hernia s.
    hernial s.
    high ligation of hernia s.
    Hilton s.
    hydrocele s.
    indirect hernial s.
    lacrimal s.
    lateral s.
    lesser s.
    lesser peritoneal s.
    nasolacrimal s.
    omental s.
    pericardial s.

    peritoneal s.
    Pleatman s.
    pleural s.
    preputial s.
    primary yolk s.
    primitive yolk s.
    pseudogestational s.
    pudendal s.
    secondary yolk s.
    tear s.
    thecal s.
    tooth s.
    truncoaortic s.
    vestibular blind s.
    vitelline s.
    wide-mouth s.
    yolk s.
saccadic eccentric target
saccate
sacci (*pl. of* saccus)
sacciform
    s. recess
Saccomanno solution
saccular
    s. aneurysm
    s. collection
    s. spot
sacculated
sacculation
saccule
    s. of larynx
sacculotomy
sacculus, pl. sacculi
    s. communis
    s. endolymphaticus
    s. laryngis
    s. proprius
    s. vestibuli
saccus, pl. sacci
    s. endolymphaticus
    s. reuniens
    s. vaginalis
Sachs
    S. solution
    S. suction tube
Sacks-Vine
    S.-V. feeding gastrostomy tube
    S.-V. PEG tube
saclike cavity
sacrad
sacral
    s. ala
    s. anesthesia
    s. arcuate line
    s. bar technique

S

sacral *(continued)*
    s. bone tumor
    s. brim target point
    s. canal
    s. cornua
    s. crest
    s. flexure of rectum
    s. foramen
    s. fracture
    s. ganglia
    s. hiatus
    s. horizontal plane line
    s. horns
    s. index
    s. lymph nodes
    s. part of spinal cord
    s. pedicle screw fixation
    s. plexus
    s. promontory
    s. region
    s. screw placement
    s. spine fixation
    s. spine fusion
    s. spine stabilization
    s. splanchnic nerve
    s. triangle
    s. venous plexus
    s. vertebrae
sacral-foraminal approach
sacralization
sacrectomy
sacred bone
sacroabdominoperineal pull-through
sacroanterior position
sacrococcygeal
    s. disk
    s. joint
    s. junction
    s. tumor
sacrococcygeus
sacrocolpopexy
sacrodural ligament
sacrofixation operation
sacrogenital folds
sacroiliac (SI)
    s. articulation
    s. buttressing procedure
    s. disarticulation
    s. dislocation
    s. extension fixation
    s. flexion fixation
    s. fracture
sacrolisthesis
sacrolumbalis
sacrolumbar
sacropelvic surface of ilium
sacropexy
    abdominal s.

sacroposterior position
sacrosciatic
sacrospinal
sacrospinous
    s. ligament
    s. ligament suspension
    s. ligament vaginal fixation
sacrotomy
sacrotransverse position
sacrotuberous ligament
sacrouterine fold
sacrovaginal fold
sacrovertebral
sacrovesical fold
sacrum
    assimilation s.
    chordoma of s.
    s. fracture
    s. fusion screw fixation
saddle
    s. block anesthesia
    s. connector base
    s. lesion
    Turkish s.
saddle-nose deformity
Sade modification of Norwood procedure
Saeed technique
Saemisch
    S. operation
    S. section
Saenger
    S. operation
    S. suture technique
Safar operation
Safe-Cuff blood pressure cuff
safe-gastrocutaneous fistulous tract
Safe Response manual resuscitator
SafeTap spinal needle
safe-tract
safety-bolt suture
safety program
Safsite IV therapy system
Saf-T-Flo T-tube connector
Sage-Clark
    S.-C. cheilectomy
    S.-C. technique
Sage Instruments syringe pump
Sage-Salvatore classification of acromioclavicular joint injury
sagitta
sagittal
    s. border of parietal bone
    s. deformity
    s. fontanel
    s. plane
    s. plane instability
    s. projection

s. reconstruction
s. rotation
s. section
s. slice fracture
s. spin-echo image
s. split mandibular osteotomy
s. suture
s. suture line
sagittalis
sagittalization
sagittal-plane imaging
Saha
S. procedure
S. shoulder muscle classification
S. transfer technique
Sahli method
Sakati-Nyhan syndrome
Sakellarides classification of calcaneal fracture
Sakellarides-Deweese technique
Sakoff osteotomy
Salem
S. duodenal sump tube
S. sump action nasogastric tube
saligenin
saline
hypertonic s.
s. injection
s. injection therapy
s. lavage
s. solution
s. technique
saline-epinephrine
hypertonic s.-e. (HSE)
salivary
s. bypass tube
s. duct
s. duct carcinoma
s. fistula
s. gland carcinoma
s. gland infection
s. gland tumor
s. mass
salivation
Salle procedure
salmon
s. patch
s. patch hue
salmon-patch hemorrhage
salpingectomy
salpinges (*pl. of* salpinx)
salpingian

salpingioma
salpingitis
salpingocele
salpingolysis
salpingoneostomy
salpingo-oophorectomy
abdominal s.-o.
bilateral s.-o.
total abdominal hysterectomy and bilateral s.-o.
unilateral s.-o.
salpingo-oophorocele
salpingo-ovariectomy
salpingo-ovariolysis
salpingopalatine membrane
salpingopexy
salpingopharyngeal
s. membrane
s. muscle
salpingopharyngeus
salpingoplasty
salpingorrhaphy
salpingoscopy
salpingostomatomy
salpingostomy
linear s.
salpingotomy
abdominal s.
salpinx, pl. salpinges
s. uterina
Salter
S. epiphyseal fracture classification
S. incremental line
S. innominate osteotomy
S. I-VI fracture
S. pelvic osteotomy
S. technique
Salter-Harris classification of epiphyseal fracture
salting-out procedure
salvage
s. balloon angioplasty
s. cystectomy
limb s.
s. prostatectomy
s. surgery
s. therapy
Salzman method
Samilson
S. crescentic calcaneal osteotomy
S. procedure

S

NOTES

Sammarco-DiRaimondo modification of Elmslie technique
sample
    Bethesda System for cervicovaginal s.
    population s.
sampling
    endocervical s.
    endometrial s.
    fetal tissue s.
    laparoscopic para-aortic lymph node s.
    lymph node s.
    percutaneous fetal tissue s.
    tissue s.
Sampoelesi line
Samson-Davis infant suction tube
sand
    s. body
    urinary s.
Sanders operation
Sandimmune injection
Sandler-Dodge area-length method
Sandoz
    S. Caluso PEG gastrostomy tube
    S. feeding/suction tube
    S. nasogastric feeding tube
    S. suction/feeding tube
    S. suction tube
Sandström bodies
sandwich
    s. patch
    s. staghorn calculus therapy
sandwiched iliac bone graft
Sanger incision
sanguification
sanguineous
    s. exudate
    s. infiltration
    s. inflammation
sanitation
sanitization
Santiani-Stone classification
Santorini
    S. canal
    S. duct
    S. labyrinth
    S. major caruncle
    S. minor caruncle
    S. plexus
    S. vein
SaO$_2$
    arterial oxygen saturation
sap
saphena
saphenectomy

saphenous
    s. branch of descending genicular artery
    s. flap
    s. hiatus
    s. opening
    s. vein bypass
    s. vein bypass graft
    s. vein patch graft
    s. veins
Sappey
    S. fibers
    S. plexus
saprophyte
sarcocele
sarcoid
sarcoidosis
sarcolemmal membrane
sarcology
sarcoma
sarcomatosis
sarcomatosum
    ectropion s.
    fibroma s.
    glioma s.
    lipoma s.
    myxoma s.
sarcophagization
sarcotripsy
Sargenti method
Sarmiento
    S. intertrochanteric osteotomy
    S. trochanteric fracture technique
Sarnes Turbo membrane oxygenator
Sarns
    S. intracardiac suction tube
    S. 7000 MDX pump
sartorial slide procedure
sartorius bursae
Saslow solution
Sassouni classification
satellite
    s. abscess
    s. lesion
    s. metastasis
    s. myofascial trigger point
    S. Plus pulse oximeter
Saticon vacuum chamber pickup tube
Sato
    S. operation
    S. procedure
Satterthwaite method
saturated solution
saturation
    s. analysis
    arterial oxygen s. (SaO$_2$)
    arterial oxyhemoglobin s. (SpO$_2$)
    color s.

s. current
s. index
jugular bulb venous oxygen s.
jugular venous oxygen s. (SjVO$_2$)
mixed venous oxygen s.
s. output
oxygen s.
partial s.
progressive spin s.
receiver s.
s. recovery
secondary s.
selective s.
s. sound pressure level
step-up in oxygen s.
s. time
s. transfer
venous s.
Saturn ring
saucerization
saucerized biopsy
Sauvage
    S. Bionit graft
    S. Dacron graft
    S. filamentous velour graft
Sauve-Kapandji procedure
Savage perineal body
Savin
    S. operation
    S. procedure
Sawyer operation
Saxtorph maneuver
Sayoc
    S. operation
    S. procedure
SB
    septal basal
        SB segment
SBP
    systolic blood pressure
S-BP line
S-B tube
SC
    subtotal colectomy
        SC suspension
SCA-EX 7F graft
Scaglietti
    S. closed reduction technique
    S. procedure scale
scalar classification
scale
    Abbreviated Injury S.

Borg treadmill exertion s.
Bromage s.
Charrière s.
children's coma s.
Cleveland Clinic weighted s. of
    endoscopic procedure
coma s.
ECoG performance status s.
Edinburgh 2 Coma S.
EVM grading of Glasgow
    Coma S.
French s.
Glasgow Coma S.
Karnofsky s.
Lysholm Knee S.
Objective Pain S.
Progressive Ambulation S.
Scaglietti procedure s.
Sessing pressure ulcer
    assessment s.
Shea pressure ulcer assessment s.
sound pressure level s.
visual analog s. (VAS)
Volpicelli functional ambulation s.
scalene
    s. fat pad biopsy
    s. hiatus
    s. lymph node biopsy
    s. maneuver
    s. tubercle
    s. tubercle of Lisfranc
scalenectomy
scalenotomy
    Adson-Coffey s.
scalenus
    s. anterior muscle
    s. medius muscle
    s. minimus muscle
    s. posterior muscle
scaling skin-colored lesion
scalloped closure
scalp
    s. closure
    s. incision
    s. infection
    s. laceration
    s. muscle
    s. sickle flap
scalping
    s. flap
    s. flap of Converse
scalprum

S

NOTES

scan
>biplane s.
>computed tomography s. (CT scan)
>CT s.
>>computed tomography scan
>EMI s.
>iodine-131 whole-body s.
>magnetic resonance imaging s.
>Meckel s.
>omniplane s.
>peritoneovenous shunt patency s.
>s. plane
>pulmonary ventilation s.
>scintillation s.
>sector s.
>stimulation s.
>time position s.
>transesophageal echocardiography s.
>ventilation lung s.
>ventilation/perfusion lung s.

scan-directed biopsy
Scanlon early neonatal neurobehavioral score
scanning
>body s.
>s. electron microscopy
>external s.
>s. force microscopy
>functional activation PET s.
>MEVA Probe for endovaginal s.
>point s.
>real-time sector s.
>scintillation s.
>sector s.
>whole-body s.

Scanzoni maneuver
Scanzoni-Smellie maneuver
Scanz osteotomy
scaphocapitate fusion
scaphohydrocephalus
scaphoid
>s. abdomen
>s. bone
>s. fossa
>s. fossa of sphenoid bone
>s. fracture

scapholunate
>s. dislocation
>s. dissociation

scapi (*pl. of* scapus)
scapula, pl. **scapulae**
>congenital elevation of the s.
>levator scapulae
>swallowtail malformation of s.

scapular
>s. approximation test
>s. elevation
>s. flap

>s. graft
>s. line
>s. notch
>s. peroneal atrophy
>s. region

scapulectomy
>Das Gupta s.
>Phelps s.

scapuloclavicular
>s. articulation

scapulohumeral
scapuloperoneal syndrome
scapulopexy
scapulothoracic
>s. dissociation
>s. fusion

scapus, pl. **scapi**
>s. penis
>s. pili

scar
>s. carcinoma
>chest tube s.
>corneal s.
>episiotomy s.
>facetted corneal s.
>s. formation
>gray-white corneal s.
>iridectomy s.
>osteopetrotic s.
>perineal s.
>sternotomy s.
>thoracotomy s.
>s. tissue
>s. tissue reaction

Scardino
>S. flap
>S. vertical flap pyeloplasty

scarf
>s. maneuver
>s. osteotomy
>s. osteotomy/bunionectomy
>s. Z-osteotomy
>s. Z-osteotomy/bunionectomy
>s. Z-plasty

scarification
>s. test

scarify
Scarpa
>S. fascia
>S. foramina
>S. ganglion
>S. hiatus
>S. liquor
>S. method
>S. sheath
>S. triangle

scarring
>corneal s.

gastrostomy s.
patch test s.
scatoma
scatoscopy
scatter
s. correction
s. photocoagulation
scavenging tube
Schaberg-Harper-Allen technique
Schacher ganglion
Schäfer
S. method
S. method of artificial respiration
Schall laryngectomy tube
Schanz
S. angulation osteotomy
S. femoral osteotomy
Schatzker tibial plateau fracture classification
Schatzki esophageal ring
Schatz maneuver
Schauffler procedure
Schaumann body
Schauta vaginal operation
Schauwecker patellar wiring technique
Schede
S. clot
S. method
S. thoracoplasty
Scheibe malformation
Scheie
S. classification
S. operation
S. syndrome
S. technique
S. thermal sclerostomy
schema
body s.
schematic
Schenk-Eichelter vena cava plastic filter procedure
Schepens
S. operation
S. technique
Schepsis-Leach technique
Scher nail biopsy
scheroma
Schick method
Schiller
S. method
S. solution
Schiller-Duvall body

Schimek operation
schindylesis
Schirmer operation
schistocystis
schistorrhachis
schistosomiasis
ectopic cutaneous s.
schistothorax
Schlatter gastrectomy technique
Schlein elbow arthroplasty
Schlemm
canal of S.
S. canal
Schlesinger solution
Schmalz operation
Schmidel anastomoses
Schmiedt tube
Schneider fixation
schneiderian respiratory membrane
Schnute wedge resection technique
Schober
S. method
S. technique
Schobinger incision
Schoemaker
S. anastomosis
S. gastroenterostomy
S. modification of Billroth I
S. procedure
Schonander
S. procedure
S. technique
Schönbein operation
Schoonmaker-King single-catheter technique
Schreger line
Schreiber maneuver
Schrock procedure
Schroeder operation
Schuchardt
S. operation
S. relaxing incision
Schuind external fixation
Schuknecht
S. classification
S. suction tube
Schuler aspiration/irrigation tube
Schüller
S. ducts
S. method
S. projection

S

NOTES

Schütz
>S. bundle
>tract of S.

Schwalbe
>S. anterior border ring
>S. line
>S. space

schwannoma

Schwartz
>S. dorsiflexory osteotomy
>S. method
>S. tractotomy

Schwarz classification

sciatic
>s. hernia
>s. nerve block
>s. nerve palsy hematoma
>s. plexus
>s. spine

scientific method

Sci-Med-Kolobow membrane lung

Sci-Med Life Systems, Inc., membrane artificial lung

scintillation
>s. scan
>s. scanning
>s. vial

scirrhous lesion

scissor-leg position

scissors dissection

scived incision

sclera, pl. **sclerae**

scleral
>s. buckling operation
>s. buckling procedure
>s. canal
>s. ectasia
>s. exoplant
>s. expander ring
>s. fistula
>s. fistulectomy operation
>s. flap
>s. flap suture
>s. hemorrhage
>s. patch graft
>s. resection
>s. rupture
>s. search coil technique
>s. shortening operation

scleralization

sclerectoiridectomy

sclerectomy
>Holth s.
>Iliff-House s.
>thermal s.

scleriritomy

sclerocorneal
>s. junction
>s. sulcus

sclerodermoid graft-versus-host disease

sclerokeratectomy

scleroma

scleroplasty
>s. operation

sclerosant
>s. solution

sclerosing
>s. adenosis
>s. inflammation
>s. lesion
>s. osteomyelitis of Garré
>s. solution
>s. therapy

sclerosis

sclerostomy
>posterior thermal s.
>Scheie thermal s.

sclerotherapy
>s. complication
>endoscopic injection s.
>endoscopic retrograde s.
>endoscopic variceal s.
>esophageal variceal s.
>fiberoptic injection s.
>injection s.
>intravariceal s.
>paravariceal s.
>variceal s.

sclerotic
>s. calvarial patch
>s. cemental mass
>s. kidney
>s. lesion
>s. line
>s. stomach

scleroticectomy

scleroticochoroidal canal

scleroticotomy

sclerotomy
>anterior s.
>DeWecker anterior s.
>foreign body s.
>Lindner s.
>s. operation
>posterior s.
>s. removal of foreign body
>s. with drainage
>s. with exploration

scoliosis
>s. correction
>s. surgery

scoliotic curve fixation

score
>airway s.

Aldrete s.
Apgar s.
discrimination s.
Dripps-American Surgical
  Association s.
echo s.
Glasgow Coma s.'s
Gleason s.
Injury Severity S.
Lysholm s.
Mangled Extremity Severity S.
Neurologic and Adaptive
  Capacity S. (NACS)
Optimal Observation S.
Scanlon early neonatal
  neurobehavioral s.
Steward Recovery S.
symptom s.
visual analog pain s. (VAPS)
Yale Optimal Observation S.

scotoma
  s. junction
  s. ring
scotomization
scotoscopy
Scott
  S. glenoplasty technique
  S. nasal suction tube
  S. operation
  S. posterior glenoplasty
Scott-Harden tube
scotty-dog
  s.-d. fracture
  s.-d. graft
SCPP
  spinal cord perfusion pressure
scrape
scratch-pad memory
screen
  coagulation s.
  s. filtration pressure
  intravascular coagulation s.
  s. oxygenation
screening
  colonoscopy s.
  endocrine s.
  s. recommendation
  s. test
screw
  s. angulation
  s. epiphysiodesis
  s. fixation

  s. head
  s. implantation
  s. insertion
  s. insertion technique
  s. joint
  s. loosening
  s. position perioperative monitoring
  s. post
  s. stabilization
  s. stripout
screw-and-plate fixation
screw-and-wire fixation
screw-home mechanism
screw-in
screw-plate approach
screw-to-screw compression construct
screw-type abutment
scrobiculus cordis
scrotal
  s. arteries
  s. hematocele
  s. hernia
  s. mass
  s. pouch operation
  s. pouch orchiopexy
  s. raphe
  s. septum
  s. swelling
  s. veins
scrotectomy
  total s.
scrotiform
scrotitis
scrotocele
scrotoplasty
scrotoscopy
scrotum
scrub
  Techni-Care surgical s.
Scudder
  S. method
  S. operation
  S. procedure
  S. technique
Scuderi
  S. procedure
  S. repair
  S. technique
Sculptor annuloplasty ring
Scultetus position
scurvy line
scyphiform

S

NOTES

scyphoid
seal
    cavity s.
    mask s.
SealEasy resuscitation mask
sealed envelope technique
sealer extrusion
sealing perforation
Sealy-Laragh technique
seamless graft
SEA port
searcher
Searcy fixation
seatbelt fracture
Seattle classification
sebaceous adenocarcinoma
Sebileau
    S. hollow
    S. muscle
seborrhea
seborrheica
secobarbital
    s. sodium
Seconal injection
second
    s. cranial nerve
    s. cuneiform bone
    s. degree burn
    s. degree radiation injury
    s. echelon lymph node
    s. gas effect
    s. parallel pelvic plane
    s. tibial muscle
secondary
    s. adhesion
    s. amputation
    s. anesthetic
    s. articulation
    s. closure
    s. expansion
    s. fixation
    s. focal point
    s. fracture
    s. hemorrhage
    s. infection
    s. intention
    s. lesion
    s. membrane
    s. myofascial trigger point
    s. point of ossification
    s. ptosis correction
    s. pulmonary lobule
    s. renal calculus
    s. repair
    s. retroperitoneal organ
    s. saturation
    s. surgery
    s. suture

    s. union
    s. yolk sac
second-echo image
second-generation
second-grade fusion
second-line drug
second-look
    s.-l. laparoscopy
    s.-l. laparotomy
    s.-l. operation
    s.-l. surgery
second-set graft rejection
secretion
secretory
    s. adenocarcinoma
    s. duct
    s. nerve
sectile
sectio, pl. **sectiones**
section
    abdominal s.
    attached cranial s.
    axial s.
    bar s.
    capture cross s.
    cesarean s.
    coronal s.
    cross s.
    cryostat s.
    s. cutting
    detached cranial s.
    diagonal s.
    distal shave s.
    extraperitoneal cesarean s.
    s. freeze substitution technique
    frontal s.
    horizontal s.
    Kerr cesarean s.
    Latzko cesarean s.
    longitudinal s.
    low cervical cesarean s.
    lower uterine segment transverse
        cesarean s.
    low transverse cesarean s.
    median s.
    midfrontal plane coronal s.
    midsagittal s.
    nerve cross s.
    oblique s.
    orbital s.
    parasagittal s.
    perineal s.
    permanent s.
    pituitary stalk s.
    plastic s.
    Porro cesarean s.
    primary cesarean s.
    repeat cesarean s.

Saemisch s.
sagittal s.
tangential s.
thin s.
transperitoneal cesarean s.
transverse s.
vaginal birth after cesarean s.
vertical s.
vestibular nerve s.
sectional
s. root canal filling method
s. technique
sectiones (*pl. of* sectio)
sector
s. cuts
s. iridectomy
s. iridectomy operation
s. scan
s. scanning
sectorial
s. branch
Securat suction tube
sedate
sedation
benzodiazepine conscious s.
conscious s.
ICU s.
intravenous s.
meperidine conscious s.
midazolam conscious s.
sedation-induced hypoventilation
sedative
s. effect
s. therapy
Seddon
S. classification
S. dorsal spine costotransversectomy
S. modification
S. nerve graft
S. technique
sedimentation
s. equilibrium
s. index
Sedlachek program
seeding
instrument-tract s.
needle-tract s.
peritoneal s.
surgical s.
tumor s.
Seessel pouch

SEF
spectral edge frequency
segment
AA s.
AB s.
AM s.
anterior basal s.
anterior inferior s.
anterior superior s.
apical s.
apicoposterior s.
arterial s.'s of kidney
bronchopulmonary s.
cardiac s.
cervical s.'s of spinal cord
coccygeal s.'s of spinal cord
demucosalized augmentation with gastric s.
extramedullary s.
hepatic s.'s
hepatic venous s.'s
IA s.
IB s.
inferior s.
inferior lingular s.
LA s.
lateral basal s.
LB s.
s.'s of liver
lower uterine s. (LUS)
lumbar s.'s of spinal cord
medial basal s.
posterior basal s.
renal s.'s
SA s.
SB s.
SM s.
s.'s of spinal cord
s.'s of spleen
subapical s.
subsuperior s.
superior lingular s.
venous s.'s of the kidney
venous s.'s of liver
segmenta (*pl. of* segmentum)
segmental
s. alveolar osteotomy
s. arteries of kidney
s. bronchus
s. colonic resection
s. compression construct
s. dilatation

NOTES

segmental *(continued)*
    s. epidural anesthesia
    s. explant
    s. fixation
    s. fracture
    s. limb pressure recording
    s. liver graft
    s. lung resection
    s. mandibulectomy
    s. pressure index
    s. pulmonary resection
    s. sphincter
    s. spinal instrumentation (SSI)
    s. surgery
    s. tendon graft
segmentation
    s. anomaly
    k space s.
    s. movement
    s. root canal filling method
    s. sphere
    volume s.
segmentectomy
segmentum, pl. segmenta
    s. apicale
    s. apicoposterius
    s. basale anterius
    s. basale laterale
    s. basale mediale
    s. basale posterius
    s. bronchopulmonale
    s. cardiacum
    segmenta hepatis
    s. inferius
    s. laterale
    segmenta lienis
    s. lingulare inferius
    s. lingulare superius
    segmenta medullae spinalis
    segmenta medullae spinalis
      cervicalia
    segmenta medullae spinalis
      coccygea
    segmenta medullae spinalis
      lumbaria
    segmenta medullae spinalis sacralia
    segmenta medullae spinalis
      thoracica
    segmenta renalia
    s. subapicale
    s. subsuperius
    s. superius
Segond fracture
segregation
Seidelin body
Seiler cartilage
Seinsheimer classification of femoral
  fracture

Seitz metamorphosing respiration
seizure
Selakovich
    S. procedure
    S. procedure for pes valgo planus
Seldinger
    S. cystic duct catheterization
    S. method
    S. percutaneous technique
    S. procedure
    S. retrograde wire/intubation
      technique
selection pressure
selective
    s. anesthesia
    s. bronchial catheterization
      anesthetic technique
    s. catheterization
    s. ductal cannulation
    s. excitation projection
      reconstruction imaging
    s. inguinal node dissection
    s. injection
    s. intracoronary thrombolysis
    s. irradiation
    s. microadenomectomy
    s. photothermolysis
    s. posterior rhizotomy
    s. proximal vagotomy
    s. sacral rhizotomy
    s. saturation
    s. saturation recovery
    s. thoracic spine fusion
selenoid body
self-adhering varus-valgus wedge
self-breast examination
self-catheterization
    clean intermittent s.-c.
self-expandable
self-expanding
self-help
self-infection
self-inflating bulb
self-mutilation
self-obturation
    intermittent s.-o.
self-sealing scleral puncture
self-seal pouch
self-tightening slip knot
Selinger operation
sella
    empty s.
    s. turcica
sellar tumor
Sell-Frank-Johnson extensor shift
  technique
Sellheim incision
Sellick maneuver

Selye
adaptation syndrome of S.
Semb
S. apicolysis
S. nephrectomy technique
semenuria
semicanal
semicanalis
semicartilaginous
semicircular
s. canal
s. ducts
s. line of Douglas
semiclosed
s. anesthesia
s. circle
semicoma
semiconductor
extrinsic s.
semiconstrained total elbow arthroplasty
semi-Fowler position
semihyalinization
semi-impermeable membrane
semilateral position
semilinear canonical correlation
semilunar
s. bone
s. cartilage
s. fibrocartilage
s. flap
s. fold of colon
s. ganglion
s. hiatus
s. line
s. valvular septum
semi-lunate cut
semimembranosus
s. muscle
semimembranous
seminal
s. colliculus
s. duct
s. fluid
s. gland
s. granule
s. hillock
s. tract
s. tract washout
s. vesicle
s. vesicle aspiration
semination
seminiferous

seminoma
seminomatous
seminuria
semioblique position
semiopen
s. anesthesia
s. hemorrhoidectomy
s. sliding tenotomy
semipedunculated lesion
semipermeable membrane
semipronation
semiprone
s. position
semirecumbent position
semispinal
s. muscle
s. muscle of head
s. muscle of neck
s. muscle of thorax
semispinalis
s. capitis muscle
s. cervicis muscle
s. thoracis muscle
semisulcus
semisupination
semisupine
semitendinosus
s. muscle
s. procedure
s. technique
semitendinosus-gracilis graft
semitendinous
semiupright position
Semmes-Weinstein pressure anesthesiometer
Semm Z technique
Sengstaken
S. esophageal tube
S. nasogastric tube
Sengstaken-Blakemore
S.-B. method
S.-B. tube
S.-B. tube insertion
senile
s. ectasia
s. plaque
Senning
S. operation
S. repair
S. transposition procedure
sensate

NOTES

S

sensation
  s. level
  s. time
sense
sensitive
  S. Eyes saline/cleaning solution
  s. plane
  s. plane projection reconstruction
    imaging
  s. point
sensitivity
sensitization
  s. response
sensitizing injection
Sensiv endotracheal tube
sensor
  fiberoptic partial pressure of carbon
    dioxide s.
  fiberoptic PCO_2 s.
  multiparameter s.
  Nellcor Oxsensor II D-25
    disposable adhesive pulse
    oximeter monitor s.'s
  Novametrix combination O_2/CO_2 s.
  s. operation
  Paratrend 7 fiberoptic PCO_2 s.
Sensorcaine-MPF
Sensorcaine with epinephrine
sensorimotor stimulation approach
sensorineural acuity level technique
sensory
  s. block
  s. blockade
  s. examination
  s. extinction
  s. fusion
  s. nerve
  s. nerve fiber bundle
  s. stimulation
  s. tract
sentence classification
sentinel spinous process fracture
SEP
  somatosensory evoked potential
separation
  s. point
  s. of retina
  s. of teeth
Sepracoat coating solution
Seprafilm bioresorbable membrane
sepsis
  Gram-negative s.
  Gram-positive s.
sepsis-induced disseminated intravascular
  coagulation
septa (*pl. of* septum)
septal
  s. apical (SA)

s. basal (SB)
s. hematoma
s. lines
s. midpapillary
s. myectomy
s. myotomy
s. perforation
s. reconstruction
s. resection
s. space
septate
septation
  s. of heart
  s. procedure
septectomy
  atrial s.
  balloon s.
  Blalock-Hanlon atrial s.
  Edwards s.
septic shock
septodermoplasty
septomarginal
  s. tract
septoplasty
  frontal sinus s.
septorhinoplasty
  esthetic s.
septostomy
  atrial s.
  atrial balloon s.
  balloon s.
  balloon atrial s.
  blade atrial s.
septulum, pl. septula
  s. testis
  septula of testis
septum, pl. septa
  s. accessorium
  Bigelow s.
  bridge-like s.
  s. bulbi urethrae
  cartilaginous s.
  s. clitoridis
  Cloquet s.
  comblike s.
  s. corporum cavernosorum clitoridis
  crural s.
  endovenous s.
  femoral s.
  s. femorale
  s. glandis
  s. of glans penis
  interatrial s.
  s. interatriale
  intermuscular s.
  s. intermusculare
  interpulmonary s.
  interradicular septa

septa interradicularia
interventricular s.
s. interventriculare
s. linguae
s. mediastinale
s. membranaceum ventriculorum
membranous s.
s. musculare ventriculorum
pectiniform s.
s. penis
rectovaginal s.
s. rectovaginale
rectovesical s.
s. rectovesicale
scrotal s.
s. scroti
semilunar valvular s.
s. sinuum frontalium
s. sinuum sphenoidalium
s. of sphenoidal sinuses
s. of testis
s. of tongue
urogenital s.
urorectal s.
ventricular s.
Sequeira-Khanuja modification
sequential
s. administration
s. circulator
s. compression stocking
s. line imaging
s. plane imaging
s. point imaging
sequestration
s. bronchopneumonia
sequestrectomy
sequestrotomy
sera (*pl. of* serum)
Serafini hernia
Serafin technique
Seraflo blood line
Sergent white line
serial
s. dilation
s. extraction
s. operation
seriation
series-II humeral head
seriscission
SER-IV fracture
serofibrinous inflammation
serofibrous

serologic examination
seroma
Seroma-Cath
S.-C. drainage tube
S.-C. feeding tube
seromembranous
seromucous gland
seromuscular
s. colocystoplasty
s. enterocystoplasty lined with urothelium
s. intestinal patch graft
s. Lembert suture
seromyotomy
anterior s.
laparoscopic s.
seroprotection
serosa
s. of colon
s. of gallbladder
s. of liver
s. of small intestine
s. of stomach
s. of urinary bladder
s. of uterine tube
s. of uterus
serosanguinous
seroserous
serotonergic tract
serous
s. acute inflammation
s. adenocarcinoma
s. exudate
s. gland
s. layer of peritoneum
s. ligament
s. membrane
serovaccination
serpentine
s. aneurysm
s. incision
serpent infection
serpiginous ulceration
serrated suture
serrate suture
serration
serratus
s. anterior muscle
s. anterior muscle flap
s. posterior inferior muscle
s. posterior superior muscle
serrefine

S

NOTES

serrenocud
Serres angle
Sertoli-cell-only syndrome
serum, pl. sera
    s. bactericidal concentration
    s. bilirubin concentration
    s. calcium concentration
    s. chemistry graft
    s. lithium concentration
    s. neutralization
Services
    Emergency Medical S. (EMS)
Servo
    S. 900 B, C ventilator
    S. ventilator
servocontrolled ventilation pump
sesamoid
    s. bone
    s. cartilage of larynx
sesamoidectomy
    fibular s.
    lateral s.
sessile
    s. adenoma
    s. lesion
Sessing pressure ulcer assessment scale
SET
    signal extraction technology
set
    Catalano intubation s.
    Criticare HN-Isocal tube feeding s.
    Dujovny microsuction dissection s.
    insufflation test s.
    Level One normothermic IV
      fluid s.
    s. point
seton
    s. operation
    s. suture
    S. treatment of high anal fistula
    s. wound
setpoint
setting expansion
seventh cranial nerve
severe deforming osteogenesis imperfecta
Severin classification
Sever-L'Episcopo
    S.-L. repair
    S.-L. repair of shoulder
Sever modification of Fairbank
  technique
sevoflurane
Sewall technique
sewing ring
sex
    s. change operation
    s. reversal
    s. steroid modulation

sextant technique
sexual
    s. aberration
    s. evaluation
    s. gland
sexualization
S-flap incision
S.G.O.
    Surgeon General's Office
shadowing method
Shaffer-Hartmann method
Shaffer operation
Shaffer-Weiss classification
shaft
    s. of femur
    s. of fibula
    s. fracture
    s. of humerus
    s. of radius
    s. of tibia
    s. of ulna
Shaher-Puddu classification
Shah ventilation tube
shallow
    s. inspiration
    s. respiration
sham
    s. injection
    s. surgery
shank
    s. bone
shaping
    root canal s.
sharp
    s. dilaceration
    s. dissection
    s. dissection technique
Sharpoint ophthalmic microsurgical
  suture
Sharrard transfer technique
Sharrard-type kyphectomy
Shauta-Aumreich procedure
shave
    s. biopsy
    s. excision technique
Shea
    S. pressure ulcer assessment scale
    S. procedure
shear fracture
sheath
    anterior layer of rectus
      abdominis s.
    anterior layer of rectus
      abdominis s.
    axillary s.
    carotid s.
    common flexor s.
    crural s.

fascial s.'s of extraocular muscles
femoral s.
fenestrated s.
fibrous tendon s.
giant cell tumor of tendon s.
infundibuliform s.
intertubercular s.
mucous s. of tendon
neurovascular s.
parotid s.
plantar tendon s. of peroneus
longus muscle
s. process of sphenoid bone
prostatic s.
rectus s.
rod s.
Scarpa s.
s. of styloid process
synovial tendon s.
tendon s. of superior oblique
muscle
tendon s. of tibialis anterior
muscle
tendon s. of tibialis posterior
muscle
s. of thyroid gland
vascular s.'s
s.'s of vessels
Waldeyer s.
sheathed artery
Shea-type parasol myringotomy tube
shedding
endometrial s.
Sheehan and Dodge technique
Sheehy
S. collar-button ventilating tube
S. Tytan ventilation tube
Sheen
S. airway reconstruction
S. tip graft
shelf
s. acetabuloplasty
Blumer s.
rectal s.
vocal s.
shell nail
Shelton femoral fracture classification
Shenton line
Shepard
S. drain tube
S. grommet ventilation tube
Shepherd fracture

shepherd's-crook deformity
Sheridan endotracheal tube cuff
Sherk-Probst
S.-P. percutaneous pinning
S.-P. technique
Sherman suction tube
Shigella **infection**
Shiley
S. cuffless fenestrated tube
S. cuffless tracheostomy tube
S. French sump tube
S. laryngectomy tube
S. low-pressure cuffed tracheostomy
tube
S. neonatal tracheostomy tube
S. pediatric tracheostomy tube
S. Tetraflex vascular graft
Shimazaki area-length method
shin bone
Shiner tube
shiny cellophane reflection
ship
Fabricius s.
Shirodkar
S. operation
S. procedure
S. suture technique
shish-kebab technique
shivering
Shoch suture
shock
anesthetic s.
declamping s.
deferred s.
defibrillation s.
endotoxic s.
endotoxin s.
hemorrhagic s.
hyperdynamic s.
hypovolemic s.
irreversible s.
s. lung
s. position
primary s.
reversible s.
septic s.
s. wave lithotripsy
s. wave pressure
shoelace
s. fasciotomy closure
s. stitch
s. suture

NOTES

Shohl solution
Shone anomaly
short
   s. bone
   s. central artery
   s. esophagus type hiatal hernia
   s. external rotator
   s. gastric arteries
   s. gastric veins
   s. head
   s. head of biceps
   s. head of biceps brachii muscle
   s. head of biceps femoris muscle
   s. incubation hepatitis
   s. inversion recovery imaging (STIR)
   s. lever accessory movement technique
   s. lever specific contact procedure
   s. oblique fracture
   s. pulse repetition time/echo time image
   s. saphenous vein
   s. segment spinal fusion
   s. tau inversion recovery (STIR)
   s. TI inversion recovery (STIR)
   s. vinculum
short-acting insulin preparation
short-axis plane
short-bowel syndrome
short-cone technique
short-cuffed endobronchial tube
short-segment lesion
short-T2 in anisotropic rotation
short-wave diathermy
shotgun wound
shotted suture
shoulder
   s. amputation
   s. arthroplasty
   s. blade
   s. disarticulation
   s. dislocation
   s. dislocation bone bank
   s. girdle
   s. reduction
   s. repair
   s. rotation
   Sever-L'Episcopo repair of s.
   s. with bevel preparation
Shouldice
   S. hernia repair
   S. inguinal herniorrhaphy
Shrader fitting
Shrapnell membrane
shrinkage
   tumor s.
shrinker stocking

Shugrue operation
shunt
   s. blockage
   s. cyanosis
   s. index via the inferior mesenteric vein
   s. index via the superior mesenteric vein
   s. infection
   s. to the lung
   s. muscle
   s. pathway
   s. quantification
   s. ratio
   s. surgery
   s. tap
   transjugular intrahepatic portosystemic s. (TIPS)
   s. tubing
shunting
   airway s.
   lumbar-peritoneal s.
   pleuroperitoneal s.
   surgical portosystemic s.
   ventricular peritoneal s.
   ventriculoperitoneal s.
SI
   sacroiliac
   SI joint
sialadenitis
sialoadenectomy
sialoadenotomy
sialocarcinoma
sialocele
sialolithotomy
Sibson
   S. fascia
   S. groove
   S. muscle
Sichi operation
sickle flap
sickle-shaped canal
side
   s. port
   s. posture reduction
side-bending barrier
side-effect
side-entry access
side-lying iliac compression test
SidePort AutoControl airway connector
sideration
sidestream spirometer
sideswipe elbow fracture
side-to-side anastomosis
sidewall
   pelvic s.
   s. structure

SIDS
>sudden infant death syndrome

Siemens
>S. PTCA open-heart suture
>S. Servo 900 B ventilator

Siemens-Elema Servo 900C ventilator

sieve
>s. bone
>s. graft
>molecular s.

Siffert intraepiphyseal osteotomy

Siffert-Storen intraepiphyseal osteotomy

sighing respiration

sigma
>S. method
>s. rectum pouch

sigmoid
>s. arteries
>s. colon
>s. colon carcinoma
>s. cutaneous fistula
>s. cystoplasty
>s. enterocystoplasty
>s. flexure
>s. fossa
>s. kidney
>s. loop reduction
>s. lymph nodes
>s. rectum pouch
>s. sinus
>s. sinus ligation
>s. sulcus
>s. volvulus

sigmoidectomy

sigmoid-end colostomy

sigmoid-loop rod colostomy

sigmoidocystoplasty

sigmoidopexy
>endoscopic s.

sigmoidoproctostomy

sigmoidorectostomy

sigmoidoscopy
>fiberoptic s.
>flexible s.

sigmoidostomy

sigmoidotomy

sigmoidovesical fistula

signal
>s. attenuation
>s. extraction technology (SET)
>s. hemorrhage

signet-ring
>s.-r. adenocarcinoma
>s.-r. carcinoma

sign mechanism for ventilator breathing

SIL/ASCUS lesion

Silastic
>S. collar-reinforced stoma
>S. eustachian tube
>S. graft
>S. intestinal tube
>S. intubation
>S. lunate arthroplasty
>S. ring
>S. sucker suction tube
>S. tracheostomy tube

Silber technique

silence
>electrocerebral s. (ECS)

silent
>s. aspiration
>s. autonephrectomy
>s. gallstones

Silfverskiöld
>S. lengthening technique
>S. procedure

silhouette sign of Felson

silicate restoration

silicone
>s. elastomer ring
>s. elastomer ring vertical
>gastroplasty
>s. implant arthroplasty
>s. implant leakage
>s. injection
>s. intubation
>s. rubber arthroplasty
>s. sponge explant
>s. tube
>s. wrist arthroplasty

silicone-lubricated endotracheal tube

silicone-treated surgical silk suture

siliconoma

siliqua olivae

silk
>s. braided suture
>s. nonabsorbable suture
>s. pop-off suture
>s. stay suture
>surgical s.
>s. traction suture
>virgin s.

silkworm gut suture

NOTES

S

Silky Polydek suture
Sillence type II-IV osteogenesis
  imperfecta
Silovi saphenous vein graft
Siloxane graft
Silva-Costa operation
silver
    s. amalgam restoration
    S. bunionectomy
    s. cone method
    s. dollar technique
    s. nitrate solution
    s. point root canal filling method
    S. procedure
    s. wire suture
silver-fork deformity
Silver-Hildreth operation
silverized catgut suture
Silverstein
    S. permanent aeration tube
    S. tetracaine base powder
    anesthetic
silver-wire
    s.-w. arteriole
    s.-w. reflex
Silvester method
simian line
Simmonds-Menelaus
    S.-M. metatarsal osteotomy
    S.-M. proximal phalangeal
    osteotomy
Simmons
    S. cervical spine fusion
    S. osteotomy
Simon
    S. expansion arch
    S. Nitinol inferior vena cava filter
    S. Nitinol IVC filter
    S. position
    S. suture technique
Simonart bands
Simonton technique
Simplate procedure
simple
    s. cold storage preservation
    s. joint
    s. mastectomy
    s. mastoidectomy
    s. periodontal flap
    s. proximal ligature
    s. skull fracture
    s. sound source
    s. suture
    s. vulvectomy
simplification
Simpson atherectomy
Sims position
simulated-echo

simulation
    Monte Carlo s.
simulator-recorder
    anesthesia s.-r.
simultaneous
    s. bilateral percutaneous
    nephrolithotomy
    s. compression-ventilation CPR
    s. method
    s. pancreas and kidney (SPK)
SIMV
    spontaneous intermittent mandatory
    ventilation
    synchronized intermittent mandatory
    ventilation
Sinarest 12 Hour Nasal solution
sincipital
sinciput
Sinding-Larsen-Johansson lesion
sinew
Singer-Blom endoscopic
    tracheoesophageal puncture technique
Singer-Bloom tube
Singh
    S. osteoporosis classification
    S. osteoporosis index
single
    s. cone root canal filling method
    s. denture construction
    s. fracture
    s. mechanism inhaled anesthetic
    s. midline extraperitoneal incision
    s. onlay cortical bone graft
    s. photon emission computer-aided
    tomography
    s. proximal portal technique
    s. site
    s. site inhaled anesthetic
    s. space technique
    s. strand conformation
    polymorphism analysis
single-balloon
    s.-b. valvotomy
    s.-b. valvuloplasty
single-breath induction of anesthesia
single-channel fiberoptic bronchoscope
single-condylar graft
single-echo
    s.-e. diffusion imaging
single-fraction total body irradiation
single-incision fasciotomy
single-layer closure
single-level spinal fusion
single-pour technique
single-puncture laparoscopy
single-rod construct
single-shot imaging technique
single-slice gradient-echo image

single-stage
    s.-s. tendon graft
    s.-s. tissue transfer
    s.-s. total proctocolectomy
single-stick method
sinistrogyration
sinistrorotation
sinistrorse
sinistrotorsion
sink-trap malformation
sinoaortic denervation
sinoatrial (S-A)
    s. exit block
    s. nodal branch of right coronary artery
    s. nodal function
    s. nodal parasympathectomy
sinonasal
    s. carcinoma
    s. cavity
    s. lesion
    s. tumor
sinoscopy
sinus
    anal s.'s
    s. anales
    s. cavernosus
    cavernous s.
    s. cavity
    cerebral s.'s
    circular s.
    s. circularis
    s. closure
    costomediastinal s.
    cranial s.'s
    s. durae matris
    dural venous s.'s
    s.'s of dura mater
    endodermal s.
    Englisch s.
    s. epididymidis
    s. of epididymis
    s. exit block
    frontal s.
    s. frontalis
    Guérin s.
    Huguier s.
    inferior longitudinal s.
    inferior petrosal s.
    inferior sagittal s.
    s. intercavernosi
    intercavernous s.'s

    s. irrigation
    jugular s.
    s. lactiferi
    lactiferous s.
    laryngeal s.
    s. laryngeus
    lateral s.
    s. line
    longitudinal vertebral venous s.
    Luschka s.
    marginal s.'s of placenta
    Morgagni s.
    s. mucocele
    occipital s.
    s. occipitalis
    osteomyelitic s.
    Palfyn s.
    paranasal s.'s
    s. paranasales
    perineal s.
    petrosal s.
    s. petrosus inferior
    s. petrosus superior
    phrenicocostal s.
    piriform s.
    pleural s.'s
    s. posterior
    prostatic s.
    s. prostaticus
    pulmonary s.'s
    rectal s.'s
    s. rectus
    renal s.
    s. renalis
    rhomboidal s.
    Ridley s.
    s. sagittalis inferior
    s. sagittalis superior
    sigmoid s.
    s. sigmoideus
    sphenoidal s.
    s. sphenoidalis
    sphenoparictal s.
    s. sphenoparietalis
    splenic s.
    straight s.
    superior longitudinal s.
    superior petrosal s.
    superior sagittal s.
    s. surgery
    tentorial s.
    s. tract

S

NOTES

sinus *(continued)*
    transillumination of s.
    transverse pericardial s.
    transverse s. of pericardium
    s. transversus
    s. transversus pericardii
    s. trunci pulmonalis
    urogenital s.
    s. urogenitalis
    venous s.'s
    s. vertebrales longitudinales
sinuscopy
    maxillary s.
sinusitis
sinusoid
sinusoidal
    s. capillary pressure
    s. endothelium
    s. endothelium cornucopia
    s. lesion
    s. relaxation
sinusotomy
    Killian frontal s.
sinuvertebral nerve
siphon
    s. suction tube
siphonage
Sistrunk procedure
site
    angulation at the fracture s.
    arterial entry s.
    carcinoma of uncertain primary s.
    endoscopic biopsy s.
    entry s.
    exit s.
    extranodal s.
    extrapulmonary s.
    fracture s.
    graft s.
    implantation s.
    injection s.
    multiple s.
    nonunion of fracture s.
    patellar tendon graft donor s. (PTGDS)
    pin s.
    single s.
    stoma s.
site-specific surgery
sitting position
situ
    carcinoma in s. (CIS)
    ex s.
    fusion in s.
    in s.
    tumor in s.
situs
    s. inversus

    s. inversus viscerum
    s. perversus
    s. solitus
    s. transversus
Siurala classification
six-portal synovectomy
sixth
    s. cranial nerve
    s. venereal disease
size
    aerodynamic s.
    crosslink plate s.
    lesion s.
    tumor s.
Sjöqvist intramedullary tractotomy
SjVO$_2$
    jugular venous oxygen saturation
skeletal
    s. biopsy
    s. correction
    s. deformity
    s. lesion
    s. metastasis
    s. muscle
    s. tissue
skeletal-extraskeletal angiomatosis
skeletology
skeleton
    appendicular s.
    s. appendiculare
    axial s.
    s. axiale
    cardiac fibrous s.
    fibrous s. of heart
    s. of heart
    s. thoracicus
skeletonization
Skene glands
skewer technique
skew flap
skier fracture
Skillern fracture
skin
    alligator s.
    s. biopsy
    s. bone free graft
    s. closure
    combination s.
    s. conductance
    s. deficit wound
    s. expansion technique
    s. flap
    s. flap necrosis
    s. graft neovagina
    s. grooves
    hidden nail s.
    s. incision
    s. lesion

s. lubrication
s. lubrication therapy
s. measurement
ostomy s.
s. plasty
s. potential response
s. preparation
s. puncture
s. temperature
s. tube
s. window technique
skin-colored lesion
skinned muscle fiber
Skinner classification
skinning
s. colpectomy
s. vulvectomy
skinny-needle biopsy
skin-puncture test
skin-temperature gradient measurement
skin-to-tumor distance
skip
s. areas
s. graft
s. lesion
s. metastasis
ski position
Skoog
S. fasciotomy
S. technique
skull
s. base tumor
s. base tumor resection
s. block
cloverleaf s.
coronal suture line of s.
exophthalmos due to tower s.
s. fracture
maplike s.
steeple s.
skullcap
slack
tissue s.
slant
s. muscle operation
s. of occlusal plane
SLAP
superior labrum anterior position
SLAP lesion
**slaved programmed electrical
stimulation**
Slavianski membrane

sleep
s. dissociation
twilight s.
sleeve
s. fracture
s. graft
s. lobectomy
s. resection
s. technique
slice
s. fracture
s. preparation
sliding
s. abdominal hernia
s. esophageal hiatal hernia
s. flap
s. inlay bone graft
s. nail
s. oblique osteotomy
s. plasty
s. scale method
s. tenotomy
s. tibial bone graft
s. tube
sling
s. and blanket technique
s. immobilization
s. ligation
s. procedure
s. and reef technique
s. suture
s. suture, type I
sling-ring complex
sling/wrapping technique
slipped
s. capital femoral epiphysis
s. hernia
s. Nissen fundoplication
s. Nissen repair
s. vertebral apophysis
slipping rib
slit
s. catheter technique
Cheatle s.
s. hemorrhage
s. illumination
pudendal s.
s. ventricle syndrome
vulvar s.
slit-lamp ophthalmoscopy
Slocum
S. amputation technique

S

NOTES

Slocum *(continued)*
    S. fusion technique
    S. maneuver
· Slo-Flo phosphate topical solution
slope-shouldered lesion
slot
    s. fracture
    s. preparation
slot-blot
    s.-b. hybridization analysis
    s.-b. technique
slot-graft
slotted acetabular augmentation
slot-type preparation
slow
    s. exchange soft tissue
    s. maxillary expansion
    s. respiration
slow-pathway ablation
SLR
    straight leg raising
    SLR with external rotation test
SL technique
Sluder guillotine tonsillectomy
sludging of circulation
SLURPIE procedure
SM-0100
    Bentley Oxi-Sat Meter S.
SMA
    superior mesenteric artery
small
    s. bone enteroscopy
    s. bowel biopsy
    s. bowel enema
    s. bowel enteroscopy
    s. bowel follow-through
      examination
    s. bowel hemorrhage
    s. bowel strangulation
    s. bowel tumor
    s. cardiac vein
    s. fenestra stapedotomy
    s. intestinal membrane
    s. intestine
    s. pancreas
    s. pelvis
    s. polyp removal
    s. saphenous vein
    s. trochanter
small-bowel
    s.-b. resection
    s.-b. tube
smaller
    s. muscle of helix
    s. posterior rectus muscle of head
    s. psoas muscle
smallest
    s. cardiac veins

    s. scalene muscle
    s. splanchnic nerve
small-fragment
Smead-Jones closure
smegma
smegmalith
Smellie method
Smellie-Veit method
smile
    endogenous s.
    exogenous s.
smiley-face knotting technique
smiling incision
Smith
    S. dislocation
    S. eyelid operation
    S. flexor pollicis longus abductor-
      plasty
    S. fracture
    S. Indian technique
    S. modification
    S. modification of Van Lint lid
      block
    S. physical capacities evaluation
    S. ring
    S. trabeculectomy
    S. tube
Smith-Boyce operation
Smith-Indian operation
Smith-Kuhnt-Szymanowski operation
Smith-Lemli-Opitz syndrome
Smith-Petersen
    S.-P. approach
    S.-P. cup arthroplasty
    S.-P. hemiarthroplasty
    S.-P. osteotomy
    S.-P. sacroiliac joint fusion
    S.-P. synovectomy
    S.-P. technique
Smith-Petersen-Cave-Van Gorder
    anterolateral approach
Smith-Robinson
    S.-R. anterior cervical diskectomy
    S.-R. anterior fusion
    S.-R. cervical disk approach
    S.-R. cervical fusion
    S.-R. interbody fusion
    S.-R. operation
    S.-R. procedure
    S.-R. technique
Smithwick sympathectomy
smoker patch
smooth
    s. muscle
    s. muscle relaxant
    s. muscle relaxation
    s. muscular sphincter

s. skin-colored lesion
s. surface cavity

SM segment

SNA
sympathetic nerve activity

snake graft

snap-frozen biopsy

Snaplets-EX

snapshot GRASS technique

snare
s. electrocoagulation
s. excision biopsy
s. loop biopsy
s. technique

Snellen
S. line
S. ptosis operation
S. suture technique

sniffing position

sniff method

S-N line

snout response

Snow procedure

SNP
sodium nitroprusside

snuffbox
anatomical s.

Snyder
S. classification
S. Urevac suction tube

soaking solution

soak therapy

Soave
S. endorectal pull-through
S. operation
S. procedure

socia

social interaction therapy

socket
hard s.
s. joint
s. reconstruction
suspension-type s.
University of California cuff
suspension PTB s.

soda
baking s.
s. lime
s. lime CO_2 absorbent

Sodasorb II CO_2 absorbent

sodium
s. acid carbonate

s. bicarbonate
s. bicitrate
s. bisulfite
Brevital S.
s. bromide
s. butyrate concentration
s. chloride in solution
dantrolene s.
s. fluoride-orthophosphoric acid
    solution
s. fluoride solution
s. hydrogen carbonate
s. hypochlorite solution
indigotin disulfonate s.
methohexital s.
s. morrhuate injection
s. nitroprusside (SNP)
Pentothal S.
primary s. phosphate
secobarbital s.
s. tetradecyl injection
thiamylal s.
thiopental s.
s. thiopental
s. versenate solution

Soemmerring
S. muscle
S. ring
ring of S.
S. ring cataract

Sofield
S. femoral deficiency technique
S. osteotomy
S. pinning

Sofsilk coated and braided suture

soft
s. abdomen
s. callus stage
s. cataract
s. chancre
s. corn
s. event
s. exudate
s. food dysphagia
s. lesion
S. Mate
s. palate
s. palate cancer
s. palate cleft
s. palate paralysis
s. palate retraction
s. parts

NOTES

S

soft *(continued)*
  s. pigment stone
  s. sore
  s. stool
  s. tissue
  s. tissue abnormality
  s. tissue abscess
  s. tissue curettage
  s. tissue dissection
  s. tissue envelope
  s. tissue flap
  s. tissue healing
  s. tissue hinge
  s. tissue injury
  s. tissue integrity
  s. tissue interface
  s. tissue interposition
  s. tissue irritability
  s. tissue lesion
  s. tissue mass
  s. tissue massage
  s. tissue metastasis
  s. tissue mobilization
  s. tissue plication
  s. tissue release
  s. tissue restriction
  s. tissue stranding
  s. tissue stretching
  s. tissue structure
  s. tissue swelling
  s. tissue thickness
  s. tissue undercut
  s. tissue window
  s. tubercle
Softech endotracheal tube
Softgut surgical chromic catgut suture
soft-tissue
  s.-t. damage
  s.-t. necrosis
SOF'WIRE spinal fixation
soilage
  peritoneal s.
Soileau Tytan ventilation tube
soiling
  colostomy s.
solar
  s. ganglia
  s. plexus
Solcia classification
solder
  hard s.
  laser tissue welding s.
soldier patch
sole
  s. laser therapy
soleal line
solid
  s. hidradenoma

  s. phase extraction
  S. Tumor Autologous Marrow
    Transplant Program
solitary
  s. bundle
  s. foramen
  s. glands
  s. pulmonary arteriovenous fistula
  s. pulmonary mass
  s. tract
Solomon-Bloembergen theory of dipole-
  dipole relaxation rate
SoloPass stent/catheter
solubility
solubilization
soluble
  s. gas technique
  s. ligature
Solu-Medrol injection
solute
  total body s.
solution
  10% acetylcysteine 0.05%
    isoproterenol hydrochloride s.
  acid-citrate-dextrose s.
  activating s.
  Adsorbotear Ophthalmic s.
  AIO parenteral s.
  AK-Dilate Ophthalmic s.
  AK-Nefrin Ophthalmic s.
  Akwa Tears s.
  amino acid-based dialysate s.
  Aminofusin L Forte amino acid s.
  Amvisc Plus s.
  antibiotic and saline s.
  Anti-Sept bactericidal scrub s.
  AquaSite Ophthalmic s.
  aqueous s.
  Atrovent Inhalation s.
  azeotropic s.
  bacitracin s.
  BA-EDTA s.
  Balamuth buffer s.
  balanced electrolyte s.
  balanced saline s.
  balanced salt s.
  Balance lavage s.
  Belzer UW liver preservation s.
  Benedict s.
  Betadine Helafoam s.
  Betadine scrub s.
  bile acid-EDTA s.
  Bion Tears s.
  Block-Ace s.
  boric acid s.
  Boston Advance conditioning s.
  Bouin fixative s.
  Bretschneider histidine tryptophan s.

Bretschneider-HTK cardioplegic s.
Brompton s.
buffer s.
buffered saline s.
Bunnell s.
Burow s.
Cajal formol ammonium bromide s.
carbol-fuchsin s.
cardioplegic s.
Chloresium s.
Chlorphed-LA Nasal s.
Cidex activated dialdehyde s.
Cidex Plus s.
cleaning s.
clindamycin phosphate topical s.
cold soak s.
Collins indigo carmine s.
Collins intracellular electrolyte s.
colloid s.
colonic lavage s.
Comfort Tears s.
commercial dialysis s.
s. of contiguity
s. of continuity
CooperVision balanced salt s.
Cornoy s.
Crolom Ophthalmic s.
crystalloid cardioplegic s.
Dakin s.
Dakrina ophthalmic s.
DCI hemolyte s.
Delflex peritoneal dialysis s.
Denhardt s.
developer s.
dexamethasone s.
dextrose s.
Dey-Drop Ophthalmic s.
3,3-diaminobenzidine
  tetrahydrochloride s.
Dianeal dialysis s.
Diaphane s.
diphosphate buffer s.
disclosing s.
disinfecting s.
Domeboro s.
Drabkin s.
Dragendorff s.
Duofilm s.
DuraPrep surgical s.
Duration Nasal s.
Dwelle Ophthalmic s.
Earle s.

ECS cardioplegic s.
electrolyte flush s.
electrolyte-polyethylene glycol
  lavage s.
electrolytic s.
Elliot B s.
Etch-Master electrolyte s.
Euro-Collins s.
extracellular-like, calcium-free s.
  (ECS)
extravasation irrigation s.
eye irrigating s.
Eye-Lube-A s.
Eye-Sed s.
Eye-Sine s.
Eye-Stream s.
Eye Wash s.
Fehling s.
Feldman buffer s.
fixer s.
fluorescein dye and stain s.
fluoride s.
Fonio s.
formaldehyde s.
formol ammonium bromide s.
Fowler s.
FreAmine amino acid s.
Freeman s.
Freezone s.
Fungoid Topical s.
Gallego differentiating s.
Gastrolyte oral s.
gelatin Hank buffered s.
Gey s.
GoLYTELY s.
Gowers s.
graft preservation s.
Hanks balanced salt s.
Hanks buffer s.
hardening s.
Hartman dental s.
Hartmann s.
Hayem s.
Healon s.
heat of s.
heparinized Ringer lactate s.
HepatAmine amino acid s.
HEPES s.
Hibiclens s.
Hollande s.
HSE s.
Hucker-Conn crystal violet s.

NOTES

solution *(continued)*

hydrogen peroxide s.
hydrolysis of s.
hydroxyethyl methacrylate
  polymerizing s.
hydroxyethyl starch s. (HES)
hyperbaric lidocaine spinal s.
hypertonic/hyperoncotic s.
hypertonic saline-epinephrine s.
HypoTears PF s.
hypotonic s.
iced lactated Ringer s.
ICS cardioplegic s.
ideal s.
Indocin ophthalmic s.
Intal Nebulizer s.
intracellular-like, calcium-bearing
  crystalloid s. (ICS)
inulin s.
Iocare balanced salt s.
iodine s.
iodophor s.
Ion Phosphate Fluoride Topical s.
I-Phrine Ophthalmic s.
Iradicav acidulated phosphate
  fluoride s.
irrigating s.
irrigation s.
Isopto Frin ophthalmic s.
Isopto Plain s.
Isopto Tears s.
isotonic sodium chloride s.
Just Tears s.
Krebs s.
Krebs-Henseleit s.
Krebs-Ringer s.
K Sol preservation s.
lacmoid staining s.
Lacril ophthalmic s.
lactated Ringer s.
Lange s.
lavage s.
Liposyn II fat emulsion s.
Liquifilm Forte s.
Liquifilm Tears s.
Locke s.
Locke-Ringer s.
Lotrimin AF s.
LubriTears s.
Lugol iodine s.
Luride topica s.
Lytren electrolyte s.
Massier s.
Mayer-hematoxylin s.
McCarey-Kaufman s.
McKees s.
Mefoxin-saline s.
Melrose s.

Miochol s.
modified Ham F-10 s.
Monsel s.
900 mOsmolar amino acid-
  glucose s.
mucolytic-antifoam s.
Murine s.
Murocel Ophthalmic s.
Mydfrin Ophthalmic s.
NaCl s.
NaFrinse acidulated s.
Nasalcrom Nasal s.
Nature Tears s.
Neosporin ophthalmic s.
Neo-Synephrine Ophthalmic s.
nonideal s.
normal saline s.
NTZ Long Acting Nasal s.
Nu-Tears II s.
OcuCoat PF Ophthalmic s.
ophthalmic s.
oxidation of s.
Pacemaker Nafeen s.
Pacemaker topical fluoride s.
Papanicolaou s.
Pedialyte oral electrolyte
  maintenance s.
Pedialyte RS electrolyte s.
perfusate s.
phosphate buffered saline s.
phosphotope oral s.
physiologic saline s.
physiologic salt s.
pickling s.
Plasmalyte s.
podofilox s.
polyethylene glycol electrolyte s.
polyethylene glycol electrolyte
  lavage s.
povidone-iodine s.
precipitate in s.
Predent disclosing s.
Prefrin ophthalmic s.
preservatives in s.
probenecid-containing s.
pulsatile hypothermic perfusion with
  University of Wisconsin s.
Puralube Tears s.
Rafluor topical s.
Refresh Plus ophthalmic s.
rehydrating s.
relaxing s.
Relief ophthalmic s.
Resectisol Irrigation s.
Resol electrolyte s.
Ringer lactate s.
rose bengal red s.
Saccomanno s.

Sachs s.
saline s.
Saslow s.
saturated s.
Schiller s.
Schlesinger s.
sclerosant s.
sclerosing s.
Sensitive Eyes saline/cleaning s.
Sepracoat coating s.
Shohl s.
silver nitrate s.
Sinarest 12 Hour Nasal s.
Slo-Flo phosphate topical s.
soaking s.
sodium chloride in s.
sodium fluoride s.
sodium fluoride-orthophosphoric
  acid s.
sodium hypochlorite s.
sodium versenate s.
solvent s.
Soyalac fat emulsion s.
Sporicidin cold soak s.
standard s.
sterile Hartmann s.
sterile saline s.
sterility of s.
stroma-free hemoglobin s.
St. Thomas cardioplegic s.
Suby G s.
surgical marking s.
Surgi-Prep s.
Synthamin amino acid s.
taurocholate s.
Tear Drop s.
TearGard Ophthalmic s.
Teargen ophthalmic s.
Tearisol s.
Tears Naturale Free s.
Tears Naturale II s.
Tears Plus s.
Tears Renewed s.
test s.
thrombin s.
Tolerex feeding s.
Transeptic cleansing s.
Trans-Ver-Sal transdermal patch
  Verukan s.
Travamulsion fat emulsion s.
Trump s.
Tyrode s.

Ultra Tears s.
University of Wisconsin s.
UW s.
Vamin amino acid s.
Viscoat s.
Viva-Drops s.
volumetric s.
warm saline s.
Weigert iodine s.
wetting s.
whole-gut lavage s.
Xylocaine viscous s.
Y-type Dianeal peritoneal
  dialysis s.
Zenker s.
zinc sulfate s.
Solvang graft
solvation
solvent
  s. ether
  s. extraction
  s. solution
solvolysis
Soma
soma
somatectomy
  subtotal s.
somatic
  s. nerve
  s. pain
  s. therapy
somaticosplanchnic
somaticovisceral
somatization
Somatome DRG CT technique
somatoprosthetics
somatosensory
  s. evoked potential (SEP, SSEP)
  s. pathway
somatostatin infusion therapy
somatostatinoma
  s. syndrome
somatotropinoma
somatropin injection
Somerville
  S. anterior approach
  S. procedure
  S. technique
somite formation
somnolence
Somogyi method
Sondergaard procedure

NOTES

Sondermann canal
Sones technique
sonication
    s. technique
sonic thrombolysis
sonification
Sonneberg neurectomy
Sonnenberg classification
sonography-guided aspiration
sonoguided biopsy
sonolucent tissue
sonomicrometry
sonomicroscopy
sonorous respiration
Sorbic classification of calcaneal
   fracture
sore
    fungating s.
    hard s.
    pressure s.
    soft s.
    venereal s.
Soren ankle fusion
Soriano operation
Soria operation
Sorondo-Ferré hindquarter amputation
Sorrin operation
Soto-Hall bone graft
Sotradecol injection
sound
    s. analysis
    s. pressure level
    s. pressure level scale
    s. quantity
sound-stimulated fetal movement
source
    endoscopic light s.
    point s.
    s. program
    simple sound s.
Sourdille
    S. keratoplasty
    S. keratoplasty operation
    S. ptosis operation
Southern
    S. blot technique
    S. Eye Bank corneal cutting block
Southey capillary drainage tube
Southwick
    S. biplane trochanteric osteotomy
    S. slide procedure
Southwick-Robinson anterior cervical
   approach
Souttar tube
Soyalac fat emulsion solution
soybean lectin T-lymphocyte-depleted
   marrow graft

space
    abdominal s.
    acromioclavicular s.
    air s.
    alveolar dead s.
    anatomical dead s.
    anatomic dead s.
    anorectal s.
    antecubital s.
    anterior clear s.
    apical s.
    arachnoid s.
    s. available for the cord
    axillary s.
    Berger s.
    s. of body of mandible
    Bogros s.
    Böttcher s.
    Bowman s.
    buccal s.
    buccinator s.
    buccopharyngeal s.
    Burns s.
    s. of Burns
    capsular s.
    carotid s.
    central palmar s.
    Chassaignac s.
    circumlental s.
    Colles s.
    coracoclavicular s.
    costoclavicular s.
    Cotunnius s.
    cranial epidural s.
    craniospinal s.
    danger s.
    dead s.
    deep perineal s.
    deep postanal anorectal s.
    denture s.
    digastric s.
    disk s.
    Disse s.
    s. of Donders
    echo-free s.
    edentulous s.
    embrasure s.
    epidural s.
    episcleral s.
    extracellular s.
    extraction s.
    extradural s.
    extrapleural s.
    extravascular s.
    fascial s.
    fat cell s.
    first web s.
    fixed maintainer s.

s. of Fontana
Fontana s.
freeway s.
geniohyoid s.
gingival s.
H s.
Henke s.
His perivascular s.
Holzknecht s.
incisural s.
increased lateral joint s.
infraglottic s.
inframesocolic s.
infraorbital s.
infratemporal s.
interalveolar s.
intercellular s.
intercondylar s.
intercostal s.
intercristal s.
interdental s.
interfascial s.
interlamellar s.
interocclusal rest s.
interprismatic s.
interproximal s.
interproximate s.
interradicular s.
intersheath s.'s of optic nerve
intersphincteric anorectal s.
interstitial s.
intervaginal s. of optic nerve
intracristal s.
intramembranous s.
s. of iridocorneal angle
ischiorectal anorectal s.
joint s.
k s.
Kiernan s.
lateral central palmar s.
lateral joint s.
lateral midpalmar s.
lateral pharyngeal s.
lattice s.
leeway s.
leptomeningeal s.
Lesgaft s.
life s.
lymph s.
Magendie s.'s
maintainer cast s.
Malacarne s.

mandibular s.
marrow s.
masseteric s.
masseter-mandibulopterygoid s.
masticator s.
masticatory s.
Meckel s.
medial clear s.
medial midpalmar s.
mediastinal s.
medullary s.
middle palmar s.
midpalmar s.
Mohrenheim s.
s. myopia
Nance leeway s.
object s.
obtainer s.
orthodontic maintainer s.
palm s.
paraglottic s.
paralaryngeal s.
parapharyngeal s.
pararenal s.
Parona s.
parotid s.
perforated s.
perianal anorectal s.
perichoroidal s.
peridental s.
peridentinoblastic s.
perihepatic s.
peri-implant s.
perilymphatic s.
perineal s.'s
perinuclear s.
perioptic subarachnoid s.
peripharyngeal s.
perirenal s.
periscleral s.
perisinusoidal s.
peritoneal s.
peritonsillar s.
perivascular s.
perivitelline s.
personal s.
pharyngeal s.
pharyngomaxillary s.
physiological dead s.
plantar s.
pleural s.
pneumatic s.

NOTES

space *(continued)*
    s. of Poirier
    Poiseuille s.
    popliteal s.
    portal s.
    position in s.
    posterior cervical s.
    postpharyngeal s.
    postzygomatic s.
    potassium s.
    predental s.
    preepiglottic s.
    premasseteric s.
    preperitoneal s.
    presacral s.
    preseptal s.
    pretemporal s.
    prevertebral s.
    prezonular s.
    Proust s.
    proximal s.
    proximate s.
    Prussak s.
    pterygomandibular s.
    pterygomaxillary s.
    pterygopalatine s.
    quadrangular s.
    quadrilateral s.
    regainer s.
    Reinke s.
    relief s.
    removable maintainer s.
    retraction s.
    retroadductor s.
    retrobulbar s.
    retrocardiac s.
    retrocrural s.
    retrogastric s.
    retroinguinal s.
    retromylohyoid s.
    retro-ocular s.
    retroperitoneal s.
    retropharyngeal s.
    retropubic s.
    retrosternal air s.
    retrotracheal s.
    retrovesical s.
    retrozygomatic s.
    Retzius s.
    s. of Retzius
    s. of Retzius abscess
    right anterior pararenal s.
    Schwalbe s.
    septal s.
    sphenomaxillary s.
    sphenopalatine s.
    subacromial s.
    subarachnoid s.

    subchorial s.
    subcoracoid s.
    subdural s.
    subgingival s.
    subhepatic s.
    sublingual s.
    submandibular s.
    submasseteric s.
    submaxillary s.
    submental s.
    subperitoneal s.
    subphrenic s.
    subpigment epithelial s.
    subpulmonic pleural s.
    subretinal s.
    subumbilical s.
    superficial perineal s.
    superior joint s.
    supracolic s.
    suprahepatic s.
    suprahepatic s.'s
    suprahyoid s.
    supralevator anorectal s.
    supraomental s.
    suprasternal s.
    supratentorial s.
    Tarin s.
    Tenon s.
    thenar s.
    tibiofibular clear s.
    tissue s.
    Traube semilunar s.
    Trautmann triangular s.
    triangular s.
    vascular s.
    vertebral epidural s.
    vesicocervical s.
    Virchow-Robin s.
    visceral s.
    volume of dead s.
    Waldeyer s.
    web s.
    Westberg s.
    widened retrogastric s.
    yolk s.
    Zang s.
    zygomaticotemporal s.

space-occupying
    s.-o. brain lesion
    s.-o. disease
    s.-o. process

spacing
    excessive s.

Spaeth
    S. cystic bleb operation
    S. ptosis operation

spall

spallation

Spälteholz preparation
span
    levator s.
Spanish blue virgin silk suture
sparganoma
Sparks
    S. mandrel graft
    S. mandrel technique
spasm
spasmolysis
spastic
    s. colon
    s. thumb-in-palm deformity
spatia (*pl. of* spatium)
spatial
    s. localization procedure
Spatial Orientation Memory Test
spatium, pl. spatia
    s. intercostale
    s. interfasciale
    spatia interossea metacarpi
    spatia interossea metatarsi
    s. lateropharyngeum
    s. perilymphaticum
    s. perinei profundum
    s. perinei superficiale
    s. peripharyngeum
    s. retroinguinale
    s. retroperitoneale
    s. retropharyngeum
    s. retropubicum
    s. subdurale
spatulate
spatulated
spatulation
    s. condensation
    graft s.
    ureteral s.
Spaulding classification
speaking tube
Spearman
    S. nonparametric univariate correlation
    S. rank correlation
    S. rank correlation coefficient
    S. rank-order correlation
Speas operation
special
    s. lesion
    s. reference method
specialized nail
species

specific
    s. ionization
    s. modulation
    s. rotation
    s. thrust manipulation
specimen
    catheter s.
spectacle
    s. correction
    s. plane
Spectam injection
spectinomycin hydrochloride
spectometry
    time-of-flight mass s.
spectral
    s. edge
    s. edge frequency (SEF)
    s. edge frequency capnography
    s. line
spectrometer
    Amis 2000 respiratory mass s.
    Centronic 200 MGA respiratory mass s.
    liquid scintillation s.
    mass s.
spectrometry
    gas chromatography-mass s.
    gas isotope ratio mass s.
    isotope dilution-mass s.
    mass s.
spectrophotometry
    endoscopic reflectance s.
    near-infrared s.
spectroscope
    near-infrared s.
    Ohmeda Rascal II Raman s.
    two-wavelength near-infrared s.
spectroscopic
spectroscopy
    clinical s.
    Fourier transform infrared s.
    image-selected in vivo s.
    infrared s.
    magnetic resonance s.
    MR s.
    near-infrared s.
    NMR s.
    Raman s.
    in vivo optical s.
specular
    s. microscopy
    s. reflection

NOTES

speculum examination
speech
    s. correction
    s. detection threshold
Speed
    S. arthroplasty
    S. open reduction
    S. osteotomy graft
    S. radial head fracture classification
    S. sternoclavicular repair
    S. V-Y muscle-plasty
Speed-Boyd
    S.-B. open reduction
    S.-B. radial-ulnar technique
Spemann induction
Spence
    S. and Duckett marsupialization
    S. procedure
Spencer plication of vena cava
Spencer-Watson
    S.-W. Z-plasty
    S.-W. Z-plasty operation
sperm
    s. aspiration
    s. immobilization test
    s. micro-aspiration retrieval
      technique
    s. washing insemination method
spermagglutination
spermatic
    s. cord
    s. duct
    s. fistula
    s. plexus
    s. vein
    s. vein ligation
spermatocele
spermatocelectomy
spermatocyst
spermatogram
spermatolysis
spermatorrhea
spermaturia
spermiduct
spermolith
spermolysis
Spetzler
    S. anterior transoral approach
    S. Microvac suction tube
Spetzler-Martin classification
sphacelation
sphenethmoid
sphenion
sphenobasilar
sphenoccipital
sphenocephaly
sphenoethmoid

sphenoethmoidal
    s. recess
    s. suture
    s. synchondrosis
sphenoethmoidectomy
sphenofrontal
    s. suture
sphenoid
    s. angle
    s. bone
    s. mucocele
    s. process
    s. process of palatine bone
    s. process of septal cartilage
    s. sinus metastasis
sphenoidal
    s. angle of parietal bone
    s. border of temporal bone
    s. conchae
    s. fissure
    s. fontanel
    s. herniation
    s. part of middle cerebral artery
    s. ridges
    s. sinus
    s. spine
    s. turbinated bones
sphenoidale
sphenoidectomy
sphenoidostomy
sphenoidotomy
sphenomalar
sphenomandibular ligament
sphenomaxillary
    s. fissure
    s. fossa
    s. space
    s. suture
spheno-occipital
    s.-o. joint
    s.-o. suture
    s.-o. synchondrosis
spheno-orbital suture
sphenopalatine
    s. canal
    s. foramen
    s. ganglion
    s. ganglionectomy
    s. space
sphenoparietal
    s. sinus
    s. suture
sphenopetrosal
    s. fissure
    s. synchondrosis
sphenorbital
sphenosalpingostaphylinus
sphenosquamosal

sphenosquamous suture
sphenotemporal
sphenotic
    s. foramen
sphenoturbinal
sphenovomerine
    s. suture
sphenozygomatic
    s. suture
sphere
    segmentation s.
spherical lens aberration
spheroid
    s. articulation
    s. joint
spherule
    rod s.
sphincter
    anal ileostomy with preservation
      of s.
    anatomical s.
    s. angularis
    s. ani
    s. ani tertius
    annular s.
    antral s.
    s. antri
    s. of antrum
    artificial s.
    basal s.
    bicanalicular s.
    Boyden s.
    canalicular s.
    choledochal s.
    colic s.
    s. of common bile duct
    s. constrictor cardiae
    s. contraction ring
    duodenal s.
    duodenojejunal s.
    external anal s.
    external rectal s.
    external urethral s.
    extrinsic s.
    first duodenal s.
    functional s.
    s. of gastric antrum
    Glisson s.
    s. of hepatic flexure of colon
    hepatopancreatic s.
    s. of hepatopancreatic ampulla
    Hyrtl s.

    ileal s.
    ileocecocolic s.
    iliopelvic s.
    incompetent s.
    inferior esophageal s.
    s. intermedius
    internal anal s. (IAS)
    internal urethral s.
    intrinsic s.
    lower esophageal s. (LES)
    macroscopic s.
    marginal s.
    mediocolic s.
    microscopic s.
    midgastric transverse s.
    midsigmoid s.
    s. muscle
    s. muscle of common bile duct
    s. muscle of pancreatic duct
    s. muscle of pylorus
    s. muscle of urethra
    s. muscle of urinary bladder
    myovascular s.
    myovenous s.
    Nélaton s.
    O'Beirne s.
    Oddi s.
    s. of Oddi dysfunction
    s. of Oddi pressure
    ostial s.
    palatopharyngeal s.
    pancreatic s.
    s. of pancreatic duct
    pathologic s.
    pelvirectal s.
    s. of the pharyngeal isthmus
    physiological s.
    postpyloric s.
    prepapillary s.
    preprostate urethral s.
    prepyloric s.
    proximal urethral s.
    pyloric s.
    radiological s.
    s. reconstruction
    rectosigmoid s.
    s. repair
    segmental s.
    smooth muscular s.
    striated muscular s.
    superior esophageal s.
    s. of third portion of duodenum

NOTES

sphincter *(continued)*
   unicanalicular s.
   s. urethrae
   s. vaginae
   Varolius s.
   velopharyngeal s.
   s. vesicae
   s. vesicae biliaris
sphincteral
sphincteralgia
sphincterectomy
   endoscopic s.
sphincterial
sphincteric
   s. construction
   s. continence
   s. potency
sphincterismus
sphincteroid
   s. tract of ileum
sphincterolysis
sphincteroplasty
   pancreatic s.
   transduodenal s.
sphincteroscopy
sphincterotomy
   biliary s.
   Doubilet s.
   endoscopic pancreatic duct s.
   Erlangen pull-type s.
   external s.
   Geenen s.
   internal s.
   Mulholland s.
   needle-knife s.
   pancreatic duct s.
   Parks partial s.
   retrograde s.
   transduodenal s.
   transendoscopic s.
   transurethral s.
   urethral s.
sphincter-saving
   s.-s. method
   s.-s. procedure
   s.-s. surgery
   s.-s. technique
sphincter-sparing
   s.-s. method
   s.-s. procedure
   s.-s. resection
   s.-s. technique
sphygmopalpation
sphygmoscopy
spiculated lesion
spider
   s. angioma

   s. pelvis
   s. projection
spigelian
   s. hernia
   s. lobe
   s. vein
Spigelius
   S. hernia
   S. line
   S. lobe
spike burst on electromyogram of colon
spill
   peritoneal s.
spillage
   tumor s.
Spiller-Frazier technique
spiloma
spina, pl. spinae
   s. angularis
   s. bifida
   s. bifida aperta
   s. bifida cystica
   s. bifida manifesta
   s. bifida occulta
   s. dorsalis
   erector spinae
   s. iliaca anterior inferior
   s. iliaca anterior superior
   s. iliaca posterior inferior
   s. iliaca posterior superior
   s. ischiadica
   s. mentalis
   s. ossis sphenoidalis
   s. peronealis
   s. pubis
   s. scapulae
spinal
   s. accessory nerve
   s. accessory nerve-facial nerve
      anastomosis
   s. analgesia
   s. analgesic
   s. anesthesia (SA)
   s. anesthetic
   s. anesthetic technique
   s. angioma
   s. arteries
   s. block
   s. canal
   s. column
   s. column stabilization
   s. compression fracture
   s. concussion
   s. cord compression
   s. cord concussion
   s. cord injury pain
   s. cord perfusion pressure (SCPP)
   s. cord stimulation

s. cord stimulator
s. cord tumor
s. coronal plane deformity
s. decompression
s. deformity/instability
s. delivery
s. dermal sinus tract
s. dural arteriovenous fistula
failed s.
s. fixation
s. fixation rigidity
s. fusion
s. fusion pathomechanics
s. fusion position
s. fusion stimulator
s. fusion technique
s. ganglion
s. gate
s. headache
s. implant load to failure
s. infection
s. infection biopsy
s. inflammation
s. injury operative stabilization
s. instability
s. joint mobilization
s. lesion
s. manipulation
s. marrow
s. metastasis
s. mobilization technique
s. muscle
s. muscle of head
s. muscle of neck
s. muscle of thorax
s. osteotomy
s. osteotomy stabilization
s. part of accessory nerve
s. part of arachnoid
s. point
s. puncture
s. pyramidotomy
s. rod cross-bracing
s. root of accessory nerve
s. tractotomy
s. tract of trigeminal nerve
s. vascular malformation
s. veins
spinalis
s. capitis muscle
s. cervicis muscle
s. thoracis muscle

spinal-locking procedure
spinally administered
spinaloscopy
spinate
spindle
s. cell sarcoma of vagina
Krukenberg corneal s.
spine
alar s.
angular s.
anterior inferior iliac s.
anterior superior iliac s.
Chance fracture thoracolumbar s.
s. deformity
dorsal s.
fixation dysfunction of the
lumbar s.
gibbous deformity of the s.
s. of helix
hemal s.
iliac s.
ischiadic s.
ischial s.
mental s.
neural s.
osteoporotic s.
palpation of anterior superior
iliac s.
palpation of posterior superior
iliac s.
posterior inferior iliac s.
posterior superior iliac s.
pubic s.
s. rotation
s. of scapula
sciatic s.
sphenoidal s.
thoracic s.
tumor metastatic to s.
spin-echo
s.-e. image
s.-e. magnetic resonance imaging
partial saturation s.-e. (PSSE)
Spinelli operation
spinning-top deformity
spinocerebellar tract
spinocostalis
spinogalvanization
spinoglenoid
spinolamellar line
spinolaminar line
spinomuscular

S

NOTES

spinoneural
spino-olivary tract
spinotectal tract
spinothalamic
    s. cordotomy
    s. tract
    s. tractotomy
spinotransversarius
spinous
    s. aspect
    s. interlaminar line
    s. plane
    s. process
    s. process fracture
    s. process of tibia
spiradenoma
spiral
    s. CT technique
    s. dissection
    s. fold of cystic duct
    s. foraminous tract
    s. groove
    s. joint
    s. line
    s. membrane
    s. oblique fracture
    s. suture
spiral-wound endotracheal tube
Spira procedure
spirochetal infection
spirochete infection
spirochetolysis
spirogram
    forced expiratory s.
Spirolyte 201 bedside spirometer
spirometer
    bedside s.
    Capnomac Ultima sidestream s.
    sidestream s.
    Spirolyte 201 bedside s.
Spittler procedure
Spitzka marginal tract
Spivack gastrotomy technique
SPK
    simultaneous pancreas and kidney
    SPK transplant
    SPK transplantation
splanchnapophysial
splanchnapophysis
splanchnectopia
splanchnemphraxis
splanchnic
    s. anesthesia
    s. AV fistula
    s. capillary pressure
    s. ganglion
    s. nerve

    s. oxygenation
    s. wall
splanchnicectomy
    chemical s.
splanchnicotomy
splanchnocele
splanchnocranium
splanchnodiastasis
splanchnolith
splanchnologia
splanchnology
splanchnomicria
splanchnoptosis
splanchnoskelctal
splanchnoskeleton
splanchnosomatic
splanchnotomy
splanchnotribe
S-plasty
SPLATT
    split anterior tibial tendon transfer
        SPLATT procedure
splayfoot deformity
spleen
    accessory s.
    ectopic s.
    floating s.
    s. lesion
    movable s.
    s. tip
splen
    s. accessorius
splenectomy
    greater omentectomy with s.
    incidental s.
splenectopia
spleneolus
splenetic
splenial
splenic
    s. artery (SA)
    s. AV fistula
    s. branches of splenic artery
    s. flexure
    s. flexure carcinoma
    s. flexure colonoscopy
    s. fossa
    s. lesion
    s. lymph nodes
    s. plexus
    s. pulp
    s. recess
    s. rupture
    s. sequestration syndrome
    s. sinus
    s. tissue
    s. vein
spleniculus

spleniform
spleniserrate
splenium
splenius
    s. capitis muscle
    s. cervicis muscle
    s. muscle of head
    s. muscle of neck
splenobronchial fistula
splenocele
splenocleisis
splenocolic
splenogonadal fusion
splenoid
splenolymphatic
splenoma
splenonephric
splenopancreatic
splenopexy
splenophrenic
splenoptosis
splenorenal
    s. ligament
    s. venous anastomosis
splenorrhagia
splenorrhaphy
splenosis
splenotomy
splenule
splenulus
splenunculus
splinted in position of function
splintered fracture
splinter hemorrhage
splinting
    closed reduction/chemical s.
    extracoronal s.
    Strong dorsal extension block s.
splint/stent
    kidney internal s. (KISS)
split
    s. anterior tibial tendon procedure
    s. anterior tibial tendon transfer
    (SPLATT)
    s. calvarial graft
    s. cast method
    s. cuff nipple technique
    s. fixation
    s. fracture
    s. ileostomy
    s. incision
    s. liver

    s. renal function test
    s. skin graft
    s. thin graft
split-and-roll technique
split-bone technique
split-cord malformation
split-course technique
split-hand deformity
split-heel
    s.-h. approach
    s.-h. fracture
    s.-h. incision
split-lung ventilation
split-nail deformity
split-patellar approach
split-shank screw post
split-thickness
    s.-t. periodontal flap
    s.-t. periodontal graft
    s.-t. skin graft
splitting
    s. fracture
    s. lacrimal papilla operation
    s. nail
SpO$_2$
    arterial oxyhemoglobin saturation
spoiled gradient-echo imaging
spondylectomy
spondylitic deformity
spondylodesis
spondylolisthesis
    s. reduction
spondylolysis
spondylophyte
spondylothoracic
spondylotomy
spondylous
sponge
    s. biopsy
    s. explant
    s. graft
    s. ring
    s. tent
spongioblastoma
spongioplasty
spongiosa bone graft
spongiositis
spongy
    s. body of penis
    s. part of the male urethra
    s. urethra
Sponsel oblique osteotomy

NOTES

S

spontaneous
    s. amputation
    s. ascites filtration
    s. breathing
    s. breech extraction
    s. coronary artery dissection
    s. dialytic ultrafiltration
    s. fracture
    s. hyperemic dislocation
    s. intermittent mandatory ventilation (SIMV)
    s. lesion
    s. renal hemorrhage
    s. rupture
    s. ventilation
    s. ventilation anesthetic technique
Sporicidin cold soak solution
spot
    s. compression
    corneal s.
    s. magnification
    milk s.'s
    saccular s.
    utricular s.
S-pouch
    ileal S.-p.
Sprague arthroscopic technique
sprain fracture
Spray
    Fluori-Methane Topical S.
spray-wipe-spray disinfection
spreader graft
spreading fistulation
Sprengel
    S. anomaly
    S. deformity
spring fixation
sprinter fracture
SPT technique
spur
    s. formation
Spurling maneuver
spurring
sputum, pl. **sputa**
    s. induction
    pink frothy s.
SQ
    subcutaneous
squama, pl. **squamae**
    frontal s.
    s. frontalis
    s. occipitalis
    temporal s.
    s. temporalis
squamatization
squamofrontal
squamomastoid
    s. suture

squamo-occipital
squamoparietal
squamopetrosal
squamosa
squamosal
    s. suture
squamotemporal
squamotympanic
    s. fissure
squamous
    s. border
    s. border of parietal bone
    s. border of sphenoid bone
    s. cell carcinoma of eyelid
    s. intraepithelial lesion
    s. margin
    s. part of frontal bone
    s. part of occipital bone
    s. part of temporal bone
    s. suture
squamozygomatic
squared
    kilogram per meter s.
square-shouldered lesion
squarrose
squeak
    bronchopleural leak s.
squeeze
    s. pressure
    s. pressure profile of anal sphincter test
Squibb urostomy pouch
SR
    sustained release
SRCP
    superficial renal cortical perfusion
SRR-5 digital-analogue converter
SS
    SS bobbin myringotomy tube
    SS suture
Ssabanejew-Frank gastrostomy
SSAER
    steady-state auditory evoked response
SSEP
    somatosensory evoked potential
S-shaped
    S-s. body
    S-s. deformity
    S-s. ileal pouch-anal anastomosis
    S-s. incision
    S-s. pouch
SSI
    segmental spinal instrumentation
    anterior-posterior fusion with SSI
St.
    St. Jude annuloplasty ring
    St. Jude composite valve graft

St. Mark polyposis registry
St. Thomas cardioplegic solution
stab
s. incision
s. wound
stability
cardiovascular s.
detrusor s.
s. of fracture
stabilization
anterior internal s.
anterior short-segment s.
s. approach
atlantoaxial s.
atlanto-occipital s.
cervical spine s.
cervicothoracic junction s.
coronoradicular s.
definitive s.
distal radioulnar joint s.
dynamic lumbar s.
flexion compression spine injury s.
fracture s.
Gruca s.
iliac crest bone graft s.
lower cervical spine posterior s.
lumbar spine s.
myoplastic muscle s.
occipitocervical s.
odontoid fracture s.
posterior lower cervical spine s.
prophylactic operative s.
provisional s.
rhythmic s.
sacral spine s.
screw s.
spinal column s.
spinal injury operative s.
spinal osteotomy s.
subluxation s.
thoracolumbar spine s.
s. training
TSRH crosslink s.
wire s.
stabilized
operatively s.
stabilizer
Claussen fragment s.
endodontic s.
stabilizing fulcrum line
stable
s. burst fracture

s. cavitation
s. reduction
stacking
breath s.
Stack shoulder procedure
Stadol
Stafne idiopathic bone cavity
stage
s. B, C carcinoma
Dukes s.
hard callus s.
s. 2, 3 hypoplastic left heart
repair
implant s.
patch s.
rehabilitation s.
soft callus s.
symptom experience s.
tumor s.
staged
s. abdominal repair
s. bilateral stereotactic thalamotomy
s. orchiopexy
s. reconstruction
s. tympanoplasty
staghorn calculus
staging
Ann Arbor classification of
Hodgkin disease s.
Astwood-Coller s. system for
carcinoma
Boden-Gibb tumor s.
FAB s. of carcinoma
FIGO classification s.
Jewett and Strong s.
s. laparotomy
multiple myeloma s.
s. operation
preoperative s.
primary gastric lymphoma s.
surgical s.
surgical-pathologic s.
TNM system for tumor s.
tumor s.
stagnant
s. anoxia
s. hypoxia
s. loop syndrome
stagnation
Staheli
S. shelf procedure
S. technique

NOTES

S

Stähli pigment line
stain
    endocardial s.
    Paget-Eccleston s.
    port-wine s.
staining
    AgNOR s.
    argyrophilic nucleolar organizer
      region s.
    corneal blood s.
    extrinsic environmental s.
    pattern of s.
stainless steel wire suture
stairstep fracture
Stalite root canal post
stalk
    body s.
    s. of epiglottis
Stallard
    S. eyelid operation
    S. flap operation
Stallard-Liegard
    S.-L. operation
    S.-L. suture
staltic
STA-MCA
    superficial temporal artery to middle
      cerebral artery
    STA-MCA anastomosis
Stamey
    S. modification of Pereyra
      procedure
    S. needle suspension
    S. operation
    S. tube
    S. urethropexy
Stamey-Martius procedure
Stamm
    S. gastroplasty
    S. gastrostomy
    S. gastrostomy tube
    S. metatarsal osteotomy
    S. procedure
    S. procedure for intra-articular hip
      fusion
stammering
    s. of the bladder
Stammer method
Stamm-Kader gastrotomy technique
STAMP therapy
Stancel procedure
standard
    s. bone algorithm program
    s. electrode potential
    s. enthalpy of formation
    s. radioenzymatic method
    s. reduction potential
    s. retroperitoneal flank incision

    s. solution
    s. temperature and pressure
    s. therapy
    s. thoracotomy
standardization
Stanford
    S. biopsy method
    S. radical retropubic prostatectomy
Stanford-type aortic dissection
Stanisavljevic technique
Stanley Way procedure
Stanmore shoulder arthroplasty
STANPUMP program
stapedectomy
    House s.
stapedotomy
    small fenestra s.
stapes mobilization
staphylectomy
staphylococcal infection
staphyloma
    s. posticum
staphylopharyngorrhaphy
staphyloplasty
staphylorrhaphy
staphylotomy
staple
    s. capsulorraphy bone bank
    s. capsulorrhaphy
    s. fixation
    s. line dehiscence
    s. suture
stapled
    s. ileal pouch-anal anastomosis
      without proctomucosal proctectomy
    s. ileoanal anastomosis
    s. ileoanal anastomosis without
      mucosectomy
    s. lung reduction
    s. reconstruction
    s. reconstruction method
    s. reconstruction procedure
    s. reconstruction technique
    s. stricturoplasty
Staples
    S. repair
    S. technique
Staples-Black-Broström ligament repair
stapling
    gastric s.
    surgical s.
star
    s. construction test
    s. formation
starch
    alant s.
    hydroxyethyl s. (HES)

Stark
- S. classification
- S. graft

Starkey matrix program
Stark-Moore-Ashworth-Boyes technique
Starlite point
STAR technique
startle technique
Starzl technique
stasis
- s. edema
- s. gallbladder
- s. liver
- s. syndrome
- s. ulceration

state
- central excitatory s.
- S. end-to-end anastomosis
- excited s.
- exhaustion s.
- inotropic s.
- local excitatory s.
- oxidation s.
- thrombin-mediated consumptive s.

static
- s. closure pressure
- s. compliance of the total respiratory system
- s. compression
- s. dilation technique
- s. evaluation
- s. fixation
- s. relation
- s. storage allocation

station
- s. pull-through
- s. pull-through esophageal manometry technique
- s. test

STAT-PACE IIA transesophageal pacing system
status
- acid-base s.
- ASA physical s.
- s. evaluation
- nutritional s.

Stauffer
- S. modification
- S. syndrome

staurion

stay
- length of s. (LOS)
- s. suture

steady-state
- s.-s. auditory evoked response (SSAER)
- s.-s. gradient-echo imaging
- s.-s. ventilatory response

steal
- iliac s.
- s. phenomenon
- renal-splanchnic s.
- subclavian s.

steam autoclave sterilization
steatocystoma
steatoma
Stedman continuous suction tube
steel
- S. correction
- S. maneuver
- s. mesh suture
- S. rule of thirds for spinal cord free space
- S. triple innominate osteotomy

steeple skull
steep Trendelenburg position
steerable cystoscopy
Steffee
- S. instrumentation technique
- S. thumb arthroplasty

Stegemann-Stalder method
stegnosis
Steichen neurovascular free flap
Steinberg infiltration block
Steinbrocker classification
Steindler
- S. flexorplasty
- S. matrixectomy
- S. procedure

Steinert disease
Steinmann
- S. pin fixation
- S. pin with Crowe pilot point

stellate
- s. border breast lesion
- s. ganglion
- s. ganglion block
- s. ganglion block anesthesia
- s. ganglion block anesthetic technique
- s. laceration
- s. ligament

S

NOTES

685

stellate *(continued)*
    s. mass
    s. skull fracture
stellectomy
stem
    s. bronchus
    s. cell gene therapy
    s. cell mobilization
    s. removal
stem-loop structure
Stener-Gunterberg resection
Stener lesion
stenion
stenobregmatic
stenocephalia
stenocephalous
stenocephaly
stenocrotaphy
stenopeic iridectomy
stenosal
stenosed
stenosis, pl. stenoses
    granulation s.
    pulmonary valve s.
    pulmonic valve s.
    subglottic s.
    subglottic tracheal s.
    supracarinal s.
    tracheal s.
stenothorax
stenotic
    s. esophagogastric anastomosis
    s. lesion
    s. stoma
Stensen duct
Stent
stent
    s. apposition
    s. construction
    s. deployment
    s. evaluation
    s. expansion
    S. graft
    s. implantation
    s. incrustation
    S. mass
    s. patency
stent/catheter
    SoloPass s.
stent-graft
    covered s.-g.
stent-induced pneumoperitoneum
stenting
    accessory duct s.
    endoluminal s.
    endoscopic pancreatic s.
    endoscopic papillotomy and s.

    endoscopic retrograde biliary s.
    tumor s.
stent-mounted
stent-through-wire mesh technique
Stenvers projection
step
    corneal graft s.
    s. graft operation
    s. preparation
    s. wedge
step-by-step technique
step-cut
    s.-c. osteotomy
    s.-c. transection
step-down
    s.-d. osteotomy
    s.-d. therapy
stephanial
stephanion
Stephen-Slater valve
stepladder incision technique
step-up in oxygen saturation
stercolith
stercoral
    s. abscess
    s. fistula
    s. ulceration
stercoroma
stereoauscultation
stereochemistry
stereocolpogram
stereoencephalotomy
stereo-identical point
stereomagnification
stereoscopic interrogation
stereoscopy
stereoselective
stereospecific
    s. action
stereotactic
    s. aspiration
    s. automated technique
    s. breast biopsy
    s. catheter drainage
    s. cordotomy
    s. core biopsy
    s. core biopsy method
    s. core biopsy technique
    s. craniotomy
    s. needle core biopsy procedure
    s. operation
    s. percutaneous needle biopsy
    s. puncture
    s. radiation therapy
    s. surgery
    s. surgical ablation
    s. thalamotomy

s. VIM thalamotomy
s. VL thalamotomy
stereotactic-assisted radiation therapy
stereotactic-focused radiation therapy
stereotaxic surgery
stereotaxis
stereotaxy
Steriflex-Braun bacterial filter
sterile
s. abscess
s. field barrier
s. Hartmann solution
s. saline solution
s. technique
s. vaginal examination
sterility
s. of solution
sterilization
autoclave s.
chemical vapor s.
cold s.
defined s.
discontinuous s.
dry heat oven s.
ethylene oxide s.
ETO s.
fractional s.
gas s.
glutaraldehyde s.
intermittent s.
involuntary s.
root canal s.
steam autoclave s.
tubal s.
unsaturated chemical vapor s.
voluntary s.
sterilize
steri-stripped incision
Steri-Strip skin closure
Steritapes closure
sterna (*pl. of* sternum)
Sterna-Band self-locking suture
sternad
sternal
s. angle
s. arteries
s. articular surface of clavicle
s. branches of internal thoracic
artery
s. cartilage
s. extremity of clavicle

s. joints
s. line
s. muscle
s. notch
s. part of diaphragm
s. plane
s. puncture
s. synchondroses
s. wire suture
sternalgia
sternalis
s. muscle
sternal-occipital-mandibular
immobilization
sternal-splitting incision
Sternberger antibody sandwich
technique
sternen
sternochondroscapularis
sternochondroscapular muscle
sternoclavicular
s. angle
s. disk
s. joint
s. joint dislocation
s. joint reconstruction
s. joint reduction
s. ligament
s. muscle
sternoclavicularis
sternocleidal
sternocleidomastoid
s. hemorrhage
s. muscle
s. region
s. vein
sternocleidomastoideus
sternocostal
s. articulations
s. head of pectoralis major muscle
s. joints
s. surface of heart
s. triangle
sternocostalis muscle
sternodynia
sternofascialis
sternoglossal
sternohyoideus
sternohyoid muscle
sternoid
sternomanubrial junction

S

NOTES

687

sternomastoid
    s. artery
    s. muscle
sternopericardial
    s. ligament
sternoschisis
sternothyroid
    s. muscle
    s. muscle flap laryngoplasty
sternothyroideus
sternotomy
    median s.
    s. scar
sternotracheal
sternotrypesis
sternovertebral
sternoxiphoid plane
sternum, pl. sterna
sternum-splitting approach
steroid
    s. concentration
    endogenous s.
    s. injection
stertorous respiration
stethalgia
stetharteritis
stethoscope
    esophageal s.
    pacing esophageal s. (PES)
    Tapscope esophageal pacing s.
Steward Recovery Score
Stewart
    S. distal clavicular excision
    S. styloidectomy
    S. test
Stewart-Hamilton cardiac output
  technique
Steytler-Van Der Walt procedure
Stieda
    S. fracture
    S. process
Stiegmann-Goff technique
stiffening tube
stiffness
    fusion s.
stigma, pl. stigmata
    malpighian stigmas
stigmatization
stigmatoscopy
stilbestrol
Stiles-Bunnell transfer technique
Stilling
    canal of S.
Stillman
    S. method
    S. technique
still radiography technique
stilus

Stimson
    S. anterior shoulder reduction
    technique
    S. gravity method
    gravity method of S.
    S. maneuver
stimulated gracilis neosphincter
  technique
stimulation
    anal electrical s.
    anocutaneous s.
    antidromic s.
    brain s.
    calibrated electrical s.
    cervical carcinoma s.
    direct brain s.
    direct electrical nerve s.
    direct neural s.
    dorsal column s.
    dorsal cord s.
    double burst s.
    double simultaneous s.
    electric s.
    electrical nerve s.
    electrical surface s.
    electrogalvanic s.
    electronic bone s.
    electrophysiological s.
    external-coil electrical s.
    follicle maturation s.
    functional electrical s.
    functional neuromuscular s.
    galvanic s.
    Ganzfeld s.
    gastric electrical s.
    gingival s.
    high-voltage pulsed galvanic s.
    hilum s.
    intracranial s.
    intraoperative cavernous nerve s.
    intravaginal electrical s.
    juxtacrine s.
    lateral electrical surface s.
    magnetic s.
    magnetoelectric s.
    mechanical s.
    microamperage electrical nerve s.
    microamperage neural s.
    Monte Carlo s.
    motor-evoked response to
    transcranial s. (tc-MER)
    neuromuscular electrical s.
    nociceptive s.
    noninvasive programmed s.
    ovulation s.
    paired electrical s.
    pelvic s.
    percutaneous s.

photic s.
programmed electrical s.
repetitive nerve s.
s. scan
sensory s.
slaved programmed electrical s.
spinal cord s.
subthreshold s.
supramaximal tetanic s.
tactile s.
s. test
tetanic s.
thermal s.
s. threshold
train-of-four s.
transcranial s. (TCS)
transcranial electrical s.
transcutaneous cranial electrical s. (TCES)
transcutaneous electric s. (TES)
transcutaneous electrical nerve s.
transcutaneous electrode nerve s.
transesophageal atrial s.
transurethral electrical bladder s.
ultrarapid subthreshold s.
vagal s.
vaginal electrical s.
ventricular-programmed s.
vibroacoustic s.
visual s.

stimulator
ACUTENS transcutaneous nerve s.
Anustim electronic neuromuscular s.
Atrostim phrenic nerve s.
Axostim nerve s.
Bard Neurostim peripheral nerve s.
Concept nerve s.
dorsal column s.
electric nerve s.
Electro-Acuscope s.
electrogalvanic s.
Gatron nerve s.
implantable neural s.
Myotest train-of-four nerve s.
nerve s.
OrthoGen implantable s. for nonunion of fracture
spinal cord s.
spinal fusion s.
surgical nerve s.
Theratouch 4.7 s.

transcutaneous electrical neuromuscular s.
transcutaneous nerve s.
Ultratone electrical transcutaneous neuromuscular s.
URYS 800 nerve s.
WR surgical nerve s.

stimulus, pl. stimuli
double extra s.
external s.
flicker-fusion s.
noxious stimuli
summation of stimuli
train-of-four s.
transcutaneous tetanic s.

stippled epiphysis
STIR
short inversion recovery imaging
short tau inversion recovery
short TI inversion recovery
STIR technique

stitch
s. abscess
Allgöwer s.
baseball s.
bow-tie s.
Bunnell s.
Connell s.
cuticular s.
figure-eight s.
Fothergill s.
Frost s.
funnel s.
intersymphyseal s.
intracuticular s.
marker s.
mattress s.
McCall s.
Pulvertaft fish-mouth s.
roll s.
running s.
shoelace s.
tagging s.
tilt s.
tracheal safety s.
triple-throw square knot s.
Tyrrell-Gray s.
s. with twists
zipper s.
Stocker
S. line
S. operation

S

NOTES

Stockholm technique for radium therapy
stockinette tube
stocking
    s. anesthesia
    compression s.
    graduated compression s.
    leg-compression s.
    pneumatic compression s.
    sequential compression s.
    shrinker s.
    venous pressure gradient support s.
stocking-seam incision
Stock operation
Stoffel operation
Stoll dilution egg count technique
stoma, pl. **stomata**
    abdominal s.
    anastomotic s.
    Benchekroun s.
    bowel s.
    concealed umbilical s.
    diverting s.
    dusky s.
    end s.
    end-loop s.
    gastroenterostomy s.
    gastrointestinal s.
    Gomez horizontal gastroplasty with reinforced s.
    ileostomy s.
    Laws gastroplasty with Silastic collar-reinforced s.
    loop s.
    maturing the s.
    Mitrofanoff s.
    nippled s.
    permanent s.
    prolapsed s.
    retracted s.
    rodless end-loop s.
    rosebud s.
    Silastic collar-reinforced s.
    s. site
    stenotic s.
    tracheostomy s.
    ureteral s.
    ureteric s.
    Wang pleural s.
stomach
    s. adenocarcinoma
    bilocular s.
    s. cancer metastasis
    Dieulafoy vascular malformation of the s.
    drain-trap s.
    hourglass s.
    insufflation of s.

    leather-bottle s.
    s. reefing
    sclerotic s.
    thoracic s.
    trifid s.
    s. tube
    wallet s.
    water-trap s.
stomachal
stomachic
stomal
    s. invagination
    s. ulceration
stomata (*pl. of* stoma)
stomatal
Stomate extension tube
stomatic
stomatomy
stomatonoma
stomatoplastic
stomatoplasty
stomatoscopy
    diagnostic fiberoptic s.
stomatotomy
stomocephalus
stone
    biliary tract s.
    bladder s.
    endoscopic extraction pancreatic duct s.
    s. extraction
    extraction bile duct s.
    extraction pancreatic s.
    extrahepatic s.
    s. fragmentation
    s. granuloma formation
    mounted point s.
    S. procedure
    soft pigment s.
    s. surgery
    vein s.
stone-tissue
stony-hard eye
Stookey-Scarff operation
stool
    s. evacuation
    hard s.
    s. impaction
    soft s.
stopcock
    ACCEL s.
    Burron Discofix s.
    Discofix s.
stop-valve airway obstruction
storage allocation
storm
    thyroid s.
Storz suction tube

Stovall-Black method
strabismus
    s. surgery
strabotomy
straddle fracture
straight
    s. canal
    s. catheter test
    s. leg raising (SLR)
    s. part of cricothyroid muscle
    s. seminiferous tubule
    s. sinus
    s. tube
    s. tube stylet
    s. venules of kidney
straightening maneuver
straight-in ventriculostomy
straight-pin teeth
strain
    compression s.
    lysogenic s.
strain/counterstrain technique
straining
    excessive s.
Straith eyelid operation
Strampelli-Valvo operation
stranding
    soft tissue s.
strangulated
    s. hernia
strangulation
    s. necrosis
    small bowel s.
strangury
strap
    external elastic s.
    s. muscles
    S. operation
strapping
    adhesive s.
Strassman
    S. metroplasty
    S. technique
    transverse fundal incision of S.
stratiform fibrocartilage
stratum, pl. strata
    s. circulare tunicae
    s. circulare tunicae muscularis coli
    s. circulare tunicae muscularis
     gastricae
    s. circulare tunicae muscularis recti

    s. circulare tunicae muscularis
     ventriculi
    s. fibrosum
    s. longitudinale tunicae muscularis
    s. longitudinale tunicae muscularis
     coli
    s. longitudinale tunicae muscularis
     gastricae
    s. longitudinale tunicae muscularis
     recti
    s. nucleare externum et internum
     retinae
    s. nucleare externum retinae
    s. plexiforme externum et internum
     retinae
    s. subcutaneum
    s. synoviale
Straub technique
Strauss method
straw
    filter s.
strawberry angioma
Strayer
    S. procedure
    S. tendon technique
streak retinoscopy
Streatfield-Fox operation
Streatfield operation
Streatfield-Snellen operation
strength
    bone-screw interface s.
    C-D instrumentation fixation s.
    cervical extension s.
    Cotrel pedicle screw fixation s.
    extensor hallucis longus s.
    extrinsic muscle s.
    graft s.
    isometric cervical extension s.
    pedicle screw pull-out s.
strength-duration curve
Stren intraepiphyseal osteotomy
streptococcal infection
Streptococcus **infection**
streptozotocin
stress
    s. dorsiflexion projection
    s. fracture
    s. lesion
    operative s.
    s. reaction in exenteration
    s. relaxation
    s. response

S

NOTES

stress *(continued)*
    s. rupture
    surgical s.
    s. ulceration
    s. ulcer hemorrhage
    s. urethral pressure profile
    s. urinary incontinence
stress-induced gastric ulceration
stress-redistribution-reinjection thallium-201 imaging
stretcher
stretching
    soft tissue s.
stretch injury
stria, pl. **striae**
    corneal s.
    striae of Zahn
striate body
striated
    s. duct
    s. muscle
    s. muscle innervation
    s. muscular sphincter
striation
    tabby-cat s.
    tigroid s.
Strickland
    S. modification
    S. technique
    S. tendon repair
stricture
    s. prophylaxis
stricturoplasty
    Finney s.
    stapled s.
    Thal s.
stricturotomy
    endoscopic s.
stridor
    nonorganic s.
stridulous respiration
string
    s. method for treatment of penile incarceration
    s. test
strip
    s. biopsy
    s. biopsy resection technique
    s. perforation
    s. procedure
    s. resection
stripe
    paratracheal tissue s.
    properitoneal flank s.
stripout
    screw s.

stripping
    s. membrane
    s. program
Stroganoff method
stroke
    s. ejection rate
    exploratory s.
stroma
    s. ovarii
    s. plexus
    s. vitreum
stroma-free hemoglobin solution
stromal
    s. line
    s. neovascularization
stromatolysis
stromatosis
Strombeck nipple transposition
Strong dorsal extension block splinting
strongyloma
strophocephaly
Stroud pectinated area
structural
    s. anomaly
    s. lesion
structure
    cord s.'s
    echodense s.
    extra-articular s.
    graft s.
    helix-loop-helix s.
    implant s.
    ossification of cartilaginous s.
    ring s.
    sidewall s.
    soft tissue s.
    stem-loop s.
strumectomy
    median s.
strumiform
strut
    s. fracture
    s. fusion technique
    s. graft
    s. plate fixation
struvite
    s. calculus
    s. crystal formation
ST segment elevation
studding
    peritoneal s.
Studebaker technique
Student-Newman-Keuls test
Studer
    S. pouch procedure
    S. reservoir urinary diversion
study
    acoustic stimulation s.

altitude simulation s.
bead chain s.
bulb tip retrograde s.
coronary artery surgery s. (CASS)
electrophysiology s.
exercise s.
injection s.
postirradiation s.
pressure s.
pressure-flow electromyography s.
prospective s.
tissue s.
T-tube s.
Veterans Administration
  Cooperative s.

stump
s. embolization syndrome
s. invagination
s. ligation
s. pressure

stunned myocardium
stupe
Sturmdorf
S. hemostatic suture
S. operation

stuttering
exteriorized s.
urinary s.

style
stylet
articulating s.
Cooper endotracheal s.
endotracheal s.
illuminating s.
jet s.
lighted s.
retractable s.
straight tube s.
surgical s.
The Hockey Stick articulating s.
tourniquet-eyed ratchet s.
Trachlight lighted intubating s.
Tubestat lighted s.
Universal curved-tube s.
Universal straight-tube s.

styliform
styloauricularis
styloauricular muscle
styloglossus
s. muscle

stylohyal

stylohyoid
s. branch of facial nerve
s. ligament
s. muscle

styloid
s. cornu
s. process of temporal bone
s. prominence

styloidectomy
Stewart s.

stylolaryngeus
stylomandibular
s. ligament
s. membrane

stylomastoid
s. artery
s. foramen
s. vein

stylomaxillary
s. ligament

stylopharyngeal muscle
stylopharyngeus
s. muscle

stylostaphyline
stylosteophyte
Stylus cardiovascular suture
stype
styptic
s. collodion
s. colloid

Suarez-Villafranca operation
Suave-Kapanje arthroplasty
subabdominal
subabdominoperitoneal
subacromial
s. bursa
s. space

subacute
s. combined degeneration of the
  spinal cord
s. inflammation

subanal
subanesthetic
s. concentration

subannular mattress suture
subaortic lymph nodes
subapical
s. segment

subaponeurotic
subarachnoid
s. anesthesia
s. block

S

NOTES

693

subarachnoid *(continued)*
   s. cavity
   s. cistern
   s. hemorrhage
   s. injection
   s. space
subarcuate fossa
subareolar
subastragalar
   s. dislocation
subaural
subauricular
subaxial
subaxillary
subcapital
   s. fracture
   s. osteotomy
subcapsular
   s. hemorrhage
   s. renal hematoma
subcartilaginous
subcaudate tractotomy
subcecal
   s. fossa
subchondral
subchorial
   s. hemorrhage
   s. space
subchorionic
   s. hematoma
   s. hemorrhage
subchoroidal approach
subclavian
   s. arteriovenous fistula
   s. artery
   s. artery bypass graft
   s. central venous catheter insertion
   s. duct
   s. groove
   s. line
   s. loop
   s. lymphatic trunk
   s. muscle
   s. nerve
   s. periarterial plexus
   s. perivascular block
   s. plexus
   s. steal
   s. steal syndrome
   s. sulcus
   s. triangle
   s. vein
   s. vein catheterization
   s. vein patch angioplasty
subclavicular
   s. approach

subclavius
   s. muscle
   s. tendon graft
subcoma
   s. therapy
subcondylar
   s. deformity
   s. oblique osteotomy
subconjunctival
   s. hemorrhage
   s. injection
subcoracoid
   s. bursa
   s. shoulder dislocation
   s. space
subcorneal
   s. blister
subcortical hemorrhage
subcostal
   s. artery
   s. flank incision
   s. groove
   s. line
   s. muscle
   s. nerve
   s. plane
   s. port
   s. transperitoneal incision
subcostosternal
subcranial
subcruralis
subcrureus
subcutaneous (SQ)
   s. acromial bursa
   s. arterial bypass graft
   s. bursa of the laryngeal
     prominence
   s. bursa of lateral malleolus
   s. bursa of medial malleolus
   s. bursa of tibial tuberosity
   s. calcaneal bursa
   s. defibrillator patch
   s. emphysema
   s. fasciotomy
   s. flap
   s. fungal infection
   s. implantation
   s. implanted injection port
   s. infrapatellar bursa
   s. injection
   s. mastectomy
   s. necrotizing infection
   s. olecranon bursa
   s. operation
   s. part of external anal sphincter
   s. portion of external anal
     sphincter
   s. ring

s. suture
s. tibialis posterior tenotomy
s. tissue
s. transfusion
s. veins of abdomen
subcuticular suture
subdeltoid
s. bursa
s. fat plane obliteration
subdiaphragmatic
s. abscess
subdigastric node
subdorsal
subduce
subdural
s. block
s. cavity
s. cleft
s. grid implantation
s. hematorrhachis
s. hemorrhage
s. interhemispheric hematoma
s. puncture
s. space
subendocardial
subependymal
s. extension
s. hemorrhage
subependymoma
subepithelial
s. connective tissue graft
s. hemorrhage
s. membrane
subepithelium
subfalcial herniation
subfascial
s. hematoma
s. prepatellar bursa
subfrontal approach
subfrontal-transbasal approach
subgaleal
s. emphysema
s. hematoma
s. hemorrhage
subgingival space
subglenoid
s. shoulder dislocation
subglottic
s. lesion
s. pressure
s. stenosis
s. tracheal stenosis

subgluteal hematoma
subgrundation
subhepatic
s. abscess
s. recess
s. space
subhyaloid
s. hemorrhage
subhyoid
s. bursa
subiculum
subiliac
subilium
subimplant membrane
subinfection
subinguinal
s. fossa
s. microsurgical varicocelectomy
s. triangle
s. varicocelectomy
subintimal hemorrhage
subjacent tissue
subjugal
subjunctival hemorrhage
sublabial
s. incision
s. midline rhinoseptal approach
s. perforation
sublaminar fixation
sublation
sublesional ulceration
sublethal x-ray damage repair
subligamentous dissection
sublimation
heat of s.
Sublimaze injection
sublingual
s. bursa
s. caruncula
s. crescent
s. fossa
s. ganglion
s. gland
s. hematoma
s. pit
s. space
s. space abscess
s. vein
sublumbar
subluxation
s. of lens
s. stabilization

S

NOTES

submammary
submandibular
  s. duct
  s. fossa
  s. lymph nodes
  s. space
  s. space abscess
submandibulectomy
submasseteric
  s. space
  s. space abscess
submaxillary
  s. duct
  s. fossa
  s. space
submembranous placental hematoma
submental
  s. artery
  s. fistula
  s. hematoma
  s. lymph nodes
  s. space
  s. space abscess
  s. triangle
  s. vein
  s. vertex projection
submentovertical projection
submucosal
  s. dissection
  s. gastric hemorrhage
  s. mass
  s. plexus
  s. Teflon injection
  s. upper gastrointestinal tract lesion
  s. urethral augmentation
  s. vascular dilation
submucous
  s. membrane
  s. resection
submuscular implantation
subnarcotic
subnasal
subneural
suboccipital
  s. decompression
  s. muscles
  s. nerve
  s. part of vertebral artery
  s. region
  s. triangle
  s. venous plexus
suboccipital-subtemporal approach
suboccipital-transmeatal approach
suboccluding ligature
suboptimal
  s. examination
  s. surgery
subparalyzing dose

subparietal
subpatellar
subpectoral
  s. implantation
  s. implantation technique
  s. plane
  s. pocket
subpelviperitoneal
subpericardial
subperiosteal
  s. dissection
  s. exposure
  s. fracture
  s. hematoma
  s. hemorrhage
  s. implant abutment
  s. implant one-phase technique
  s. infection
subperitoneal
  s. fascia
  s. space
subperitoneoabdominal
subperitoneopelvic
subpetrosal
subpharyngeal
subphrenic
  s. abscess
  s. recesses
  s. space
subpigment epithelial space
subpleural
subplexal
subpopliteal recess
subpopulation
subpreputial
subpubic
  s. angle
subpulmonary
subpulmonic pleural space
subpyloric
  s. lymph nodes
  s. node
subretinal
  s. hemorrhage
  s. neovascularization
  s. neovascular membrane
  s. space
subsarcolemma cisterna
subsartorial
  s. canal
subscapular
  s. artery
  s. branches of axillary artery
  s. bursa
  s. fossa
  s. group of axillary lymph nodes
  s. muscle
  s. nerve

subscapularis
    s. muscle
subsector
subsegmentectomy
    hepatic s.
subspinale
    s. point A
subspinous
substance
    cement s.
    compact s.
    s. concentration
    corneal s.
    cortical s.
    exogenous s.
    exophthalmos-producing s.
    extracellular ground s.
    glandular s. of prostate
    medullary s.
    müllerian inhibiting s.
    muscular s. of prostate
    s. P
    tumor polysaccharide s.
    vasoactive s.
substantia
    s. compacta
    s. compacta ossium
    s. corticalis
    s. glandularis prostatae
    s. medullaris
    s. muscularis prostatae
substernal
    s. angle
substernomastoid
substitute
    Biobrane/HF experimental skin s.
    blood s.
    hypo-oncotic plasma s.
    low pressure bladder s.
substitutional cardiac surgery
substitution transfusion
substructure
subsuperior segment
subtalar
    s. articulation
    s. dislocation
subtemporal
    s. decompression
    s. dissection
subtemporal-intradural approach
subtendinous
    s. bursa of gastrocnemius muscle

    s. bursa of the tibialis anterior muscle
    s. iliac bursa
    s. prepatellar bursa
subtentorial lesion
subthreshold stimulation
subthyroideus
subtotal
    s. colectomy (SC)
    s. distal pancreatectomy
    s. esophagectomy
    s. gastrectomy
    s. gastric exclusion
    s. gastric resection
    s. glossectomy
    s. lateral meniscectomy
    s. maxillectomy
    s. proctocolectomy
    s. somatectomy
    s. supraglottic laryngectomy
    s. thyroidectomy
subtraction technique
subtrochanteric
    s. femoral fracture
    s. osteotomy
subtrochlear
subumbilical
    s. space
subungual hematoma
suburethral
    s. rectus fascial sling procedure
subvaginal
subvertebral
subvitrinal
subvolution
subxiphoid limited pericardiotomy
Suby G solution
subzonal
    s. insemination
subzygomatic
succenturiate
successive approximation
succinylcholine
    s. chloride
succinyldicholine
succinylsulfathiazole
sucker
    Yankauer s.
sucking wound
Sucostrin injection

S

NOTES

Sucquet
  S. anastomosis
  S. canal
Sucquet-Hoyer
  S.-H. anastomosis
  S.-H. canal
suction
  Adson s.
  airway s.
  s. aspiration
  Barton s.
  s. biopsy
  Bowen s.
  bulb s.
  continuous NG s.
  s. curettage
  s. cylinder
  diastolic s.
  s. dissection
  s. drainage
  Ferguson s.
  Frazier s.
  Gomco s.
  s. injury
  lavage and s.
  low intermittent s.
  s. method
  nasogastric s.
  nasopharyngeal s.
  nasotracheal s.
  NG s.
  perilimbal s.
  Pleur-evac s.
  s. pump
  s. Regugauge regulator
  rhoton s.
  Rosen s.
  s. suspension
  s. tube
  s. tubing
  Vabra s.
  Vactro perilimbal s.
  Wangensteen s.
  Yankauer s.
suctioning
  endotracheal s.
suction-irrigation technique
sudation
Suda type I, II, III classification of papilla
sudden infant death syndrome (SIDS)
Sudeck critical point
sudomotor
sudoriferous
  s. duct
  s. glands
Sufenta injection

sufentanil
  s. citrate
sufentanil/enflurane technique
sufentanil/midazolam technique
suffocate
suffocation
Sugarbaker operation
sugar-icing liver
suggillation
  postmortem s.
Sugioka transtrochanteric rotational osteotomy
Sugiura
  S. esophageal variceal transection
  S. procedure
suit
  body-exhaust s.
suite
  endoscopy s.
sulcal
  s. artery
sulcate
sulci (*pl. of* sulcus)
sulciform
sulcomarginal tract
sulculus
sulcus, pl. sulci
  s. ampullaris
  ampullary s.
  s. angularis
  s. arteriae occipitalis
  s. arteriae temporalis mediae
  s. arteriae vertebralis
  sulci arteriosi
  atrioventricular s.
  s. auriculae anterior
  s. auriculae posterior
  s. bicipitalis lateralis
  s. bicipitalis medialis
  calcaneal s.
  s. calcanei
  s. caroticus
  carotid s.
  s. carpi
  s. coronarius
  coronary s.
  s. costae
  s. costae arteriae subclaviae
  s. fixated position
  s. fixation
  implant gingival s.
  inferior petrosal s.
  s. infraorbitalis
  internal spiral s.
  intertubercular s.
  s. intertubercularis
  mentolabial s.
  s. mentolabialis

s. for middle temporal artery
s. musculi subclavii
s. mylohyoideus
s. nervi petrosi majoris
s. nervi petrosi minoris
s. nervi radialis
s. nervi spinalis
s. nervi ulnaris
nymphocaruncular s.
s. nymphocaruncularis
nymphohymenal s.
s. obturatorius
s. of occipital artery
s. olfactorius cavum nasi
olfactory s. of nasal cavity
sulci paracolici
s. popliteus
preauricular s.
s. pulmonalis
pulmonary s.
sclerocorneal s.
sigmoid s.
s. sinus petrosi inferioris
s. sinus petrosi superioris
s. sinus sagittalis superioris
s. sinus sigmoidei
s. sinus transversi
s. spinosus
s. spiralis externus
s. spiralis internus
subclavian s.
s. subclavianus
s. subclavius
superior petrosal s.
supra-acetabular s.
s. supra-acetabularis
talar s.
s. tali
s. tendinis musculi peronei longi
s. for transverse sinus
s. of umbilical vein
s. venae subclaviae
sulci venosi
s. for vertebral artery
sulfacytine
sulfate
butacaine s.
mephentermine s.
morphine s.
sulfation
sulfonation
sulfuric ether

sulfur and silver point
Sullivan III nasal continuous positive air pressure device
sulmazole
summation of stimuli
Summerskill operation
sump
s. nasogastric tube
s. syndrome
sun
s. and chemical combination damage
s. exposure
Sunderland classification of nerve injury
superacromial
superanal
superciliary arch
supercilii
musculus corrugator s.
supercilium
superduct
superexcitation
superfecundation
superfetation
superficial
s. angioma
s. back muscles
s. brachial artery
s. branch of the lateral plantar nerve
s. branch of the medial plantar artery
s. branch of the radial nerve
s. branch of the superior gluteal artery
s. branch of the ulnar nerve
s. burn
s. cardiac plexus
s. cervical artery
s. cervical nerve
s. circumflex iliac artery
s. corneal line
s. dorsal sacrococcygeal ligament
s. dorsal veins of clitoris
s. dorsal veins of penis
s. epigastric artery
s. epigastric vein
s. external pudendal artery
s. fascia
s. fascia of penis
s. fascia of perineum

NOTES

superficial *(continued)*
- s. head of flexor pollicis brevis muscle
- s. implantation
- s. infection
- s. inguinal lymph nodes
- s. inguinal pouch
- s. inguinal ring
- s. keratectomy
- s. lamellar keratoplasty
- s. layer of deep cervical fascia
- s. layer of temporalis fascia
- s. line of cornea
- s. lingual muscle
- s. lymphatic vessel
- s. palmar artery
- s. palmar branch of radial artery
- s. parotidectomy
- s. parotid lymph nodes
- s. part of external anal sphincter
- s. part of masseter muscle
- s. perineal pouch
- s. perineal space
- s. peroneal nerve
- s. posterior sacrococcygeal ligament
- s. radiation
- s. renal cortical perfusion (SRCP)
- s. temporal artery
- s. temporal artery to middle cerebral artery (STA-MCA)
- s. temporal plexus
- s. temporal veins
- s. transverse muscle of perineum
- s. transverse perineal muscle
- s. volar artery

superficialis
- s. volae

superfine fiberscope
supergenual
superimpregnation
superinfection
superior
- s. aberrant ductule
- s. anastomotic vein
- s. angle of scapula
- s. arcuate bundle
- s. articular facet of atlas
- s. articular process of sacrum
- s. azygoesophageal recess
- s. basal vein
- s. border of pancreas
- s. border of petrous part of temporal bone
- s. border of scapula
- s. border of spleen
- s. border of suprarenal gland
- s. branch of the pubic bone
- s. branch of the superior gluteal artery
- s. branch of the transverse cervical nerve
- s. bursa of biceps femoris
- s. carotid triangle
- s. cerebellar artery
- s. cerebral veins
- s. cervical cardiac branches of vagus nerve
- s. cervical cardiac nerve
- s. cervical ganglion
- s. cervical ganglionectomy
- s. constrictor muscle of pharynx
- s. costal facet
- s. costal pit
- s. costotransverse ligament
- s. dislocation
- s. duodenal fold
- s. duodenal fossa
- s. duodenal recess
- s. epigastric artery
- s. epigastric veins
- s. esophageal sphincter
- s. fascia of pelvic diaphragm
- s. fascia of urogenital diaphragm
- s. flexure of duodenum
- s. ganglion of glossopharyngeal nerve
- s. ganglion of vagus nerve
- s. gastric lymph nodes
- s. gluteal artery
- s. gluteal nerve
- s. gluteal neurovascular bundle
- s. hemorrhoidal artery
- s. hemorrhoidal plexus
- s. hemorrhoidal vein
- s. horn of thyroid cartilage
- s. hypogastric plexus
- s. hypophysial artery
- s. ileocecal recess
- s. intercostal artery
- s. intercostal vein
- s. internal parietal artery
- s. joint space
- s. labial artery
- s. labial branches of infraorbital nerve
- s. labial vein
- s. labrum anterior position (SLAP)
- s. labrum anterior and posterior lesion
- s. laryngeal cavity
- s. laryngeal nerve
- s. laryngeal nerve external branch
- s. laryngeal vein
- s. lateral genicular artery
- s. ligament of epididymis

s. lingular segment
s. longitudinal muscle of tongue
s. longitudinal sinus
s. maxillary nerve
s. medial genicular artery
s. mediastinum
s. mesenteric artery (SMA)
s. mesenteric ganglion
s. mesenteric lymph nodes
s. mesenteric plexus
s. mesenteric vein
s. mesenterorenal bypass technique
s. nuchal line
s. oblique extraocular muscle
s. oblique muscle of head
s. omental recess
s. orbital fissure
s. pancreaticoduodenal artery
s. part of diaphragmatic surface of liver
s. part of duodenum
s. part of vestibular ganglion
s. pelvic aperture
s. peroneal retinaculum
s. petrosal sinus
s. petrosal sulcus
s. phrenic artery
s. phrenic lymph nodes
s. phrenic veins
s. pole
s. pole of kidney
s. pole of testis
s. posterior serratus muscle
s. pubic ligament
s. pubic ramotomy
s. pubic ramus
s. rectal artery
s. rectal lymph nodes
s. rectal plexus
s. rectal vein
s. rectus extraocular muscle
s. root of cervical loop
s. sagittal sinus
s. sector iridectomy
s. segmental artery of kidney
s. suprarenal arteries
s. surface of horizontal plate of palatine bone
s. tarsus
s. temporal line
s. temporal venule of retina
s. thoracic aperture

s. thoracic artery
s. thyroid artery
s. thyroid notch
s. thyroid plexus
s. thyroid tubercle
s. thyroid vein
s. tibial articulation
s. tracheobronchial lymph nodes
s. transverse scapular ligament
s. trunk of brachial plexus
s. ulnar collateral artery
s. vena cava
s. vena cava filter
s. vesical artery

superior-intradural approach
superioris
cisterna s.
levator palpebrae s.
musculus levator palpebrae s.
superiosus
levator palpebrae s.
superius
incision s.
superlactation
superligamen
supernumerary
s. breast
s. organs
superovulation
s. induction
superpetrosal
superpigmentation
superselective vagotomy
supersensitivity
superstructure
supinate
supination
s. deformity
s. injury
s. reflex
supination-adduction
s.-a. fracture
supination-eversion
s.-e. fracture
s.-e. injury
supination-external
s.-e. rotation
s.-e. rotation injury
s.-e. rotation IV fracture
supination-inversion
s.-i. rotation injury
supination-plantar flexion injury

NOTES

S

supinator
    s. crest
    s. longus reflex
    s. muscle
supine
    s. hypotensive syndrome
    s. position
supine-oblique approach
Supolene suture
supplementary
    s. canal
    s. oxygen
    s. respiration
supply
    tumor blood s.
support
    advanced trauma life s. (ATLS)
    Dale ventilator tubing s.
    excessive lip s.
    external s.
    extracorporeal life s. (ECLS)
    inspiratory pressure s.
    Thompson chin s.
    ventilator s.
    volume-assured pressure s.
supporting tissue
suppository
    Itinerol B$_6$ s.
suppressed respiration
suppression
    failure of fixation s.
    twitch s.
suppressor
    tumor s.
suppurant
suppurate
suppuration
    alveodental s.
    pulmonary s.
suppurative
    s. acute inflammation
    s. chronic inflammation
    s. exudate
    s. granulomatous inflammation
supra-acetabular
    s.-a. groove
    s.-a. sulcus
supra-acromial
supra-anal
supra-annular mitral valve replacement
supra-arytenoid cartilage
supra-auricular
    s.-a. point
supra-axillary
suprabuccal
supracarinal stenosis
supracerebellar approach
supracervical hysterectomy

suprachoroid
    s. layer
suprachoroidal hemorrhage
suprachoroidea
supraciliary
    s. canal
supraclavicular
    s. approach
    s. block
    s. brachial block anesthesia
    s. examination
    s. lymph node biopsy
    s. lymph nodes
    s. muscle
    s. part of brachial plexus
    s. triangle
supraclavicularis
supraclinoid aneurysm
supracolic space
supracondylar
    s. amputation
    s. humeral fracture
    s. process
    s. suspension
    s. varus osteotomy
    s. Y-shaped fracture
supracondyloid
supracostal
supracotyloid
supracrestal
    s. line
    s. plane
supracristal
    s. plane
supradiaphragmatic
supraduodenal
    s. approach
    s. artery
supraepicondylar
    s. process
supraglottic laryngectomy
supraglottoplasty
suprahepatic
    s. inferior vena cava
    s. space
    s. spaces
suprahyoid
    s. branch of lingual artery
    s. gland
    s. muscles
    s. neck dissection
    s. space
suprailiac aortic mesenteric graft
suprainguinal
suprainterparietal bone
supraintestinal
supralevator
    s. anorectal space

s. pelvic exenteration
s. perirectal abscess
supralumbar
supramalleolar
s. flap
s. varus derotation osteotomy
supramammary
supramandibular
supramastoid
s. fossa
supramaxillary
supramaximal tetanic stimulation
suprameatal
s. pit
s. triangle
supramental
supramentale
point B, s.
Supramid
S. bridle collagen suture
S. Extra suture
S. graft
S. lens implant suture
supranasal
Suprane
supraneural
supranormal hemodynamic therapy
supranuclear lesion
supraomental space
supraomohyoid neck dissection
supraoptic canal
supraopticohypophysial tract
supraorbital
s. arch
s. artery
s. canal
s. foramen
s. margin
s. nerve
s. notch
s. pericranial flap
s. point
s. ridge
s. vein
supraorbital-pterional approach
supraorbitomeatal
suprapapillary Roux-en-Y
    duodenojejunostomy
suprapatellar
s. bursa
s. pouch
suprapelvic

supraperiosteal flap
suprapineal recess
suprapleural membrane
supraprostatectomy
suprapubic
s. cystotomy
s. cystotomy tract urethral atresia
s. lithotomy
s. needle aspiration
s. port
s. prostatectomy
s. puncture
s. urethrovesical suspension
    operation
suprapyloric
s. lymph node
s. node
suprarenal
s. body
s. capsule
s. cortex
s. gland
s. impression
s. medulla
s. plexus
s. veins
suprarenalectomy
suprascapular
s. artery
s. ligament
s. nerve
s. nerve compression
s. notch
s. vein
suprasellar
s. low-density lesion
s. mass
s. subarachnoid cistern
suprasphincteric fistula
supraspinal
supraspinalis
s. muscle
supraspinatus
s. muscle
supraspinous
s. fossa
s. ligament
s. muscle
suprasternal
s. bone
s. examination
s. notch

S

NOTES

suprasternal *(continued)*
   s. plane
   s. space
suprasymphysary
supratemporal
supratentorial
   s. approach
   s. arteriovenous malformation
   s. craniotomy
   s. lesion
   s. space
suprathoracic
Suprathreshold Adaptation Test
supratonsillar
   s. recess
supratragic tubercle
supratrochlear veins
supraumbilical incision
supravaginal
   s. portion of cervix
supravalvar
supravalvular
supraventricular crest
supraversion
supravesical fossa
supreme
   s. intercostal artery
   s. intercostal vein
sural
   s. artery
   s. nerve bridge graft
   s. nerve cable graft
   s. region
Sureclosure closure
SureGrip manual resuscitator
surface
   acromial articular s. of clavicle
   anterior articular s. of dens
   anterior s. of cornea
   anterior s. of eyelids
   anterior s. of kidney
   anterior s. of maxilla
   anterior s. of pancreas
   anterior s. of prostate
   anterior s. of suprarenal gland
   anterior s. of ulna
   articular s. of acromion
   articular s. of head of rib
   articular s. of tubercle of rib
   arytenoidal articular s. of cricoid
   auricular s. of ilium
   auricular s. of sacrum
   buccal s.
   colic s. of spleen
   s. cooling technique
   costal s.
   costal s. of scapula
   denture foundation s.

   s. disinfection
dorsal s. of scapula
endosteal s.
s. epithelium
extensor s.
external s.
external s. of frontal bone
external s. of parietal bone
foundation s.
glenoid s.
implant-bearing s.
inferior s. of petrous part of
   temporal bone
inferior s. of tongue
inferolateral s. of prostate
infratemporal s. of maxilla
interlobar s.'s of lung
internal s.
internal s. of frontal bone
internal s. of parietal bone
intestinal s. of uterus
s. irradiation
s. landmark
lateral s. of testis
lateral s. of zygomatic bone
maxillary s. of greater wing of
   sphenoid bone
maxillary s. of palatine bone
medial s. of ovary
medial s. of testis
s. membrane
nasal s. of maxilla
nasal s. of palatine bone
orbital s.
posterior s. of arytenoid cartilage
posterior s. of cornea
posterior s. of eyelids
posterior s. of kidney
posterior s. of pancreas
posterior s. of petrous part of
   temporal bone
posterior s. of prostate
posterior s. of suprarenal gland
posterior talar articular s. of
   calcaneus
s. projection
pulmonary s. of heart
renal s. of spleen
renal s. of suprarenal gland
renal s. of the suprarenal gland
s. replacement hip arthroplasty
sacropelvic s. of ilium
sternal articular s. of clavicle
sternocostal s. of heart
symphysial s. of pubis
temporal s.
thyroidal articular s. of cricoid
urethral s. of penis

vesical s. of uterus
visceral s. of liver
visceral s. of the spleen
surface-projection rendering image
surfactant
    bovine lavage extract s.
    hydrolysis of s.
Sur-Fit
    S.-F. Mini pouch
    S.-F. urostomy pouch
Surgaloy metallic suture
Surgeon General's Office (S.G.O.)
surgeon's knot
surgery
    ablative s.
    ablative cardiac s.
    access flap in osseous s.
    acne s.
    adult scoliosis s.
    ambulatory s.
    anorectal s.
    anterior cervical spine s.
    anterior cervicothoracic junction s.
    anterior lower cervical spine s.
    antiglaucoma s.
    antireflux s.
    apically repositioned flap in
      mucogingival s.
    arthroscopic laser s.
    aseptic s.
    asymmetric s.
    bariatric s.
    bat ear s.
    bench s.
    breast-conserving s.
    bypass s.
    cardiac s.
    cardiothoracic s.
    cataract s.
    cervical decompression s.
    cervical disk s.
    cervicothoracic junction s.
    ciliodestructive s.
    closed s.
    closed-eye s.
    colon and rectal s.
    colorectal s.
    combination s.
    computer-assisted stereotactic s.
    concomitant antireflux s.
    conservation s.
    conservative s.

corneal s.
coronary artery bypass grafting s.
cosmetic s.
craniofacial s.
cranio-orbital s.
cytoreductive s.
debulking s.
decompressive s.
dental s.
dentofacial s.
dialysis access s.
double jaw s.
DREZ s.
ear s.
ECA-PCA bypass s.
elective cosmetic s. (ECS)
endodontic s.
endoscopic sinus s.
epilepsy s.
esthetic s.
excisional cardiac s.
extracorporeal s.
extracranial-intracranial bypass s.
eyelid s.
eye muscle s.
failed s.
featural s.
fetal s.
filtration s.
first ray s.
fistulizing s.
full flap in mucogingival s.
functional endoscopic sinus s.
gastric bypass s.
gastric reduction s.
glaucoma s.
hypotensive s.
hysteroscopic s.
ileal pouch s.
inadequate s.
intestinal s.
intra-abdominal s.
intradural tumor s.
intraorbital s.
jejunoileal bypass s.
keyhole s.
knee replacement s.
lacrimal s.
laparoscopic s.
laparoscopically assisted s.
laryngeal framework s.
laser s.

S

NOTES

surgery *(continued)*
　　laser-filtering s.
　　left ventricle-aorta conduit s.
　　limb-salvage s.
　　limb-sparing s.
　　local s.
　　lower extremity s.
　　lower posterior lumbar spine and
　　　sacrum s.
　　lung volume reduction s.
　　major s.
　　mandibular s.
　　maxillary s.
　　maxillofacial s.
　　microscopically controlled s.
　　minimal access general s.
　　minimally invasive s.
　　minor s.
　　Mohs micrographic s.
　　mucogingival s.
　　nasal s.
　　nephron-sparing s.
　　neurologic s.
　　nonbench s.
　　noncardiac s.
　　oblique flap in mucogingival s.
　　open disk s.
　　open heart s. (OHS)
　　oral and maxillofacial s.
　　orbital s.
　　orthognathic s.
　　orthopaedic s.
　　orthopedic s.
　　osseous s.
　　palliative s.
　　parenchymal sparing s.
　　pediatric s.
　　pedicle flap in mucogingival s.
　　pelvic colonic s.
　　pelvic-floor s.
　　penile venous ligation s.
　　periapical s.
　　peripheral vascular s.
　　plastic s.
　　portal-systemic shunt s.
　　posterior lower cervical spine s.
　　posterior lumbar interbody fusion s.
　　posterior lumbar spine and
　　　sacrum s.
　　posterior upper cervical spine s.
　　preprosthetic s.
　　primary perineal hypospadias s.
　　radical s.
　　radioimmunoguided s.
　　reconstructive preprosthetic s.
　　rectovaginal s.
　　reoperative aesthetic s.
　　reoperative bariatric s.

　　reparative cardiac s.
　　resective s.
　　retinal s.
　　retrograde intrarenal s.
　　reversal jejunoileal bypass s.
　　right ventricle-pulmonary artery
　　　conduit s.
　　salvage s.
　　scoliosis s.
　　secondary s.
　　second-look s.
　　segmental s.
　　sham s.
　　shunt s.
　　sinus s.
　　site-specific s.
　　sphincter-saving s.
　　stereotactic s.
　　stereotaxic s.
　　stone s.
　　strabismus s.
　　suboptimal s.
　　substitutional cardiac s.
　　symmetric s.
　　telepresence s.
　　telerobotic-assisted laparoscopic s.
　　thoracic and thoracolumbar spine s.
　　thyroglossal cyst s.
　　transsexual s.
　　transsphenoidal s.
　　transsphincteric s.
　　trauma s.
　　tubal reconstruction s.
　　urologic s.
　　vaginal s.
　　vascular s.
　　video-assisted thoracic s. (VATS)
　　video-assisted thoracoscopic s.
　　visco s.
　　vitreous s.
　　weight reduction s.
surgical
　　s. abdomen
　　s. ablation
　　s. anatomy
　　s. anesthesia
　　s. approach
　　s. autoimmunization
　　s. bone impression
　　s. cholecystectomy
　　s. cholecystostomy
　　s. chromic suture
　　s. correction
　　s. crown lengthening
　　s. cystgastrostomy
　　s. decompression
　　s. defect
　　s. diathermy

s. dressing room
s. emergency
s. emphysema
s. endarterectomy
s. endodontics
s. enucleation
s. enucleation method
s. enucleation procedure
s. enucleation technique
s. eruption
s. erysipelas
s. excision biopsy
s. extirpation
s. flap
s. gut suture
s. incision
s. infection
s. instrument post
s. intervention
s. keratometry
s. ligation
s. linen suture
s. maggot
s. management
s. margin
s. marking solution
s. mask
s. neck
s. neck fracture
s. nerve stimulator
s. neurangiographic technique
s. occlusion rim
s. oncology
s. orthodontia
s. orthodontics
s. patch grafting
s. pathology
s. perspective
s. portosystemic shunting
s. positioning
s. preparation
s. pulp exposure
s. reduction
s. repair
s. resection
s. retention
s. risk
s. seeding
s. silk
s. silk suture
s. staging
s. stapling

s. steel suture
s. stress
s. stylet
s. therapy
s. treatment objective
s. tuberculosis
s. vagotomy
s. weight loss
s. wound
surgical-pathologic staging
surgical-radiologic minicholecystostomy
Surgicel implantation
Surgicraft suture
Surgidac suture
Surgidev suture
Surgigut suture
Surgilar suture
Surgilene blue monofilament
  polypropylene suture
Surgiloid suture
Surgilon
    S. braided nylon suture
    S. monofilament polypropylene
    suture
Surgilope suture
SurgiMed suture
Surgi-Prep solution
Surgipro suture
Surgiset suture
Surgitek One-Step percutaneous
  endoscopic gastrostomy
Surgiwip suture ligature
surrenal
Survector
surveillance
    endoscopic s.
    s. technique
survey
    s. line
    s. program
    radiation s.
survival
    graft s.
survivor
suspended inspiration
suspension
    Aldridge-Studdefort urethral s.
    Alexander-Adams uterine s.
    Baldy-Webster uterine s.
    bladder neck s.
    Burch bladder s.
    Coffey s.

NOTES

S

suspension *(continued)*
    corset s.
    cuff s.
    endoscopic bladder neck s.
    extraperitoneal laparoscopic bladder
      neck s.
    fingertrap s.
    flexible hinge s.
    Gilliam-Doleris uterine s.
    Gittes-Loughlin bladder neck s.
    s. laryngoscopy
    minimal-incision pubovaginal s.
    Olshausen s.
    Pereyra bladder neck s.
    Pereyra needle s.
    Raz bladder neck s.
    Raz four-quadrant s.
    Raz needle s.
    Raz urethral s.
    retropubic Lapides-Ball bladder
      neck s.
    sacrospinous ligament s.
    SC s.
    Stamey needle s.
    suction s.
    supracondylar s.
    urethral s.
    uterine s.
suspension-type socket
suspensory
    s. ligament of axilla
    s. ligament of clitoris
    s. ligament of penis
    s. ligaments of breast
    s. ligaments of Cooper
    s. ligament of testis
    s. ligament of thyroid gland
    s. muscle of duodenum
    s. sling operation
Sustagen nasogastric tube
sustained
    s. pressure technique
    s. release (SR)
sustentacular
    s. tissue
sustentaculum
    s. lienis
    s. tali
Sutherland-Greenfield osteotomy
Sutherland-Rowe incision
Sutupak suture
sutura, pl. **suturae**
    s. coronalis
    suturae cranii
    s. ethmoidolacrimalis
    s. ethmoidomaxillaris
    s. frontalis
    s. frontoethmoidalis

    s. frontolacrimalis
    s. frontomaxillaris
    s. frontonasalis
    s. frontozygomatica
    s. incisiva
    s. infraorbitalis
    s. intermaxillaris
    s. internasalis
    s. interparietalis
    s. lacrimoconchalis
    s. lacrimomaxillaris
    s. lambdoidea
    s. metopica
    s. nasofrontalis
    s. nasomaxillaris
    s. notha
    s. occipitomastoidea
    s. palatina mediana
    s. palatina transversa
    s. palatoethmoidalis
    s. palatomaxillaris
    s. parietomastoidea
    s. plana
    s. sagittalis
    s. serrata
    s. sphenoethmoidalis
    s. sphenofrontalis
    s. sphenomaxillaris
    s. spheno-orbitalis
    s. sphenoparietalis
    s. sphenosquamosa
    s. sphenovomeriana
    s. sphenozygomatica
    s. squamosa
    s. squamosomastoidea
    s. temporozygomatica
    s. zygomaticofrontalis
    s. zygomaticomaxillaris
    s. zygomaticotemporalis
sutural
    s. bones
    s. diastasis
    s. ligament
suture
    absorbable surgical s.
    Acutrol s.
    adjustable s.
    Albert s.
    Alcon s.
    already-threaded s.
    aluminum-bronze wire s.
    American silk s.
    anastomotic s.
    Ancap braided silk s.
    anchoring s.
    s. anchor technique
    Appolito s.
    apposition of skull s.

approximation s.
Arroyo encircling s.
arterial silk s.
Atraloc s.
atraumatic braided silk s.
atraumatic chromic s.
Aureomycin s.
Barraquer silk s.
bastard s.
Bell s.
16-bite nylon s.
black braided nylon s.
black braided silk s.
black silk sling s.
black twisted s.
blanket s.
blue-black monofilament s.
blue cotton s.
blue twisted cotton s.
bolster s.
bone wax s.
Bozeman s.
braided Ethibond s.
braided Mersilene s.
braided Nurolon s.
braided nylon s.
braided polyamide s.
braided silk s.
braided Vicryl s.
braided wire s.
Bralon s.
bridge s.
s. bridge
bridle s.
bronze wire s.
Brown-Sharp gauge s.
B&S gauge s.
bulb s.
Bunnell crisscross s.
Bunnell figure-eight s.
buried lock s.
button s.
cable wire s.
canaliculus rod and s.
capitonnage s.
Caprolactam s.
cardinal s.
Cardioflon s.
cardiovascular Prolene s.
cardiovascular silk s.
catgut s.
celluloid linen s.

cervical s.
chain s.
Chinese fingertrap s.
Chinese twisted silk s.
chloramine catgut s.
chopstick retention s.
chromated catgut s.
chromic blue-dyed s.
chromic catgut s.
chromic collagen s.
chromic gut s.
chromicized catgut s.
circular s.
circumcisional s.
coaptation s.
coated polyester s.
coated Vicryl s.
cobbler s.
cocoon thread s.
collagen s.
compound s.
compression s.
Connell s.
continuous running horizontal
  mattress s.
continuous running monofilament s.
continuous sling s.
control release s.
core s.
s. of cornea operation
corner s.
coronal s.
cotton Duknatel s.
cotton nonabsorbable s.
Cottony Dacron s.
cranial s.
Cushing s.
Czerny s.
Czerny-Lembert s.
Dacron bolstered s.
Dacron traction s.
20-day chromic catgut s.
40-day chromic catgut s.
Degnon s.
dekalon s.
Deklene polypropylene s.
Deknatel silk s.
delayed s.
dentate s.
dermal s.
Dermalene polyethylene s.
Dermalon cuticular s.

NOTES

suture *(continued)*

Dexon absorbable synthetic polyglycolic acid s.
Dexon II s.
Dexon Plus s.
D&G s.
DG Softgut s.
Docktor s.
Donati s.
double right-angle s.
doubly armed s.
Dulox s.
Dupuytren s.
dynamic supporting s.
Edinburgh s.
elastic s.
Endoknot s.
Endoloop s.
end-on mattress s.
end-to-end s.
end-to-side s.
epitenon s.
EPTFE vascular s.
Equisetene s.
Ethibond polyester s.
Ethicon-Atraloc s.
Ethicon micropoint s.
Ethicon Sabreloc s.
Ethicon silk s.
Ethiflex retention s.
Ethilon nylon s.
Ethi-pack s.
ethmoidomaxillary s.
everting mattress s.
external lock s.
extrachromic s.
s. of eyeball operation
Faden s.
false s.
far-and-near s.
fascial s.
s. fatigue
figure-of-eight s.
filament s.
fine chromic s.
fine silk s.
fingertrap s.
fish-mouth end-to-end s.
s. fixation
Flaxedil s.
Flexitone s.
Flexon steel s.
formaldehyde catgut s.
Foster s.
Frater s.
frontal s.
frontoethmoidal s.
frontolacrimal s.
frontomaxillary s.
frontonasal s.
frontozygomatic s.
Frost s.
furrier s.
Gailliard-Arlt s.
Gambee s.
gastrointestinal surgical gut s.
gastrointestinal surgical linen s.
gastrointestinal surgical silk s.
Gély s.
general closure s.
Gillis s.
GI pop-off silk s.
glover s.
glue-in s.
Gore-Tex nonabsorbable s.
gossamer silk s.
Gould s.
grasping s.
green braided s.
green monofilament polyglyconate s.
groove s.
Gussenbauer s.
gut s.
guy steading s.
Halsted s.
harmonic s.
heavy-gauge s.
heavy monofilament s.
heavy retention s.
heavy silk retention s.
heavy wire s.
helical s.
hemostatic s.
Herculon s.
horizontal mattress s.
Horsley s.
IKI catgut s.
implanted s.
incisive s.
India rubber s.
infraorbital s.
interendognathic s.
intermaxillary s.
internasal s.
interparietal s.
interrupted pledgeted s.
intracameral s.
intracuticular s.
intradermal s.
inverting s.
iodine catgut s.
iodized surgical gut s.
iodochromic catgut s.
iris s.
s. of iris operation

Ivalon s.
Jobert de Lamballe s.
s. joint
Kal-Dermic s.
kangaroo tendon s.
Kessler grasping s.
Kessler-Kleinert s.
Kessler-Tajima s.
lacidem s.
lacrimoconchal s.
lacrimomaxillary s.
lambdoid s.
lambdoidal s.
lancet s.
Lapra-Ty s.
lateral trap s.
lead s.
lead-shot tie s.
Lembert inverting seromuscular s.
lens s.'s
s. of lens
Ligapak s.
s. ligated
s. ligature
s. line
s. line cancer
s. line dehiscence
linen s.
lock s.
locking horizontal mattress s.
lock-stitch s.
Look s.
loop s.
Lukens catgut s.
Mannis s.
Marlex s.
Mason-Allen s.
mattress s.
Maxam s.
Maxon absorbable s.
Mayo linen s.
McLaughlin modification of
  Bunnell pull-out s.
McLean s.
Measuroll s.
median palatine s.
Medrafil wire s.
Mersilene braided nonabsorbable s.
mesh s.
metal band s.
metallic s.
metopic s.

micropoint s.
middle palatine s.
mild chromic s.
Millipore s.
modified Kessler s.
modified Kessler-Tajima s.
Monocryl poliglecaprone s.
monofilament absorbable s.
monofilament clear s.
monofilament green s.
monofilament nylon s.
monofilament polypropylene s.
monofilament skin s.
monofilament steel s.
monofilament wire s.
Monosof s.
multifilament steel s.
multistrand s.
s. of muscle operation
nail s.
nasomaxillary s.
natural s.
nerve s.
neurocentral s.
neurosurgical s.
Nicoladoni s.
nonabsorbable surgical s.
nonresorbable s.
Novofil s.
Nurolon s.
nylon 66 s.
nylon monofilament s.
nylon retention s.
occipitomastoid s.
oiled silk s.
Ophthalon s.
over-and-over s.
Oyloidin s.
Pagenstecher linen thread s.
palatine s.
palatoethmoidal s.
palatomaxillary s.
Pancoast s.
Paré s.
parietomastoid s.
Parker-Kerr s.
PDS Vicryl s.
Pearsall Chinese twisted s.
Pearsall silk s.
pericostal s.
Perlon s.
Perma-Hand braided silk s.

NOTES

S

suture *(continued)*

petrosquamous s.
petrotympanic s.
pickup spatula s.
pin s.
pink twisted cotton s.
plain catgut s.
plain collagen s.
plain gut s.
plane s.
plastic s.
pledget s.
pledgeted Ethibond s.
pledgeted mattress s.
plication s.
s. plication
polyamide s.
polybutester s.
Polydek s.
polydioxanone s.
polyester fiber s.
polyethylene s.
polyfilament s.
polygalactic acid s.
polygalactide s.
polygalactin 910 s.
polyglecaprone 25 s.
polyglycol s.
polyglycolic acid s.
polyglyconate s.
polypropylene button s.
Polysorb s.
pop-off s.
posterior fixation s.
premaxillary s.
primary s.
Prolene polypropylene s.
Proxi-Strip s.
pull-out wire s.
Pulvertaft end-to-end s.
Pulvertaft interweave s.
Purlon s.
pursestring s.
PVB s.
pyoktanin catgut s.
pyroglycolic acid s.
Quickert s.
quilted s.
Ramsey County pyoktanin catgut s.
reabsorbable s.
reinforcing s.
relaxation s.
Reo Macrodex s.
s. repair
retention s.
retracting s.
ribbon gut s.
s. ring

rubber s.
running locked interdermal s.
Sabreloc s.
safety-bolt s.
sagittal s.
scleral flap s.
s. of sclera operation
secondary s.
seromuscular Lembert s.
serrate s.
serrated s.
seton s.
Sharpoint ophthalmic microsurgical s.
Shoch s.
shoelace s.
shotted s.
Siemens PTCA open-heart s.
silicone-treated surgical silk s.
silk braided s.
silk nonabsorbable s.
silk pop-off s.
silk stay s.
silk traction s.
silkworm gut s.
Silky Polydek s.
silverized catgut s.
silver wire s.
simple s.
sling s.
Sofsilk coated and braided s.
Softgut surgical chromic catgut s.
Spanish blue virgin silk s.
sphenoethmoidal s.
sphenofrontal s.
sphenomaxillary s.
spheno-occipital s.
spheno-orbital s.
sphenoparietal s.
sphenosquamous s.
sphenovomerine s.
sphenozygomatic s.
spiral s.
squamomastoid s.
squamosal s.
squamous s.
SS s.
stainless steel wire s.
Stallard-Liegard s.
staple s.
stay s.
steel mesh s.
Sterna-Band self-locking s.
sternal wire s.
Sturmdorf hemostatic s.
Stylus cardiovascular s.
subannular mattress s.
subcutaneous s.

subcuticular s.
Supolene s.
Supramid bridle collagen s.
Supramid Extra s.
Supramid lens implant s.
Surgaloy metallic s.
surgical chromic s.
surgical gut s.
surgical linen s.
surgical silk s.
surgical steel s.
Surgicraft s.
Surgidac s.
Surgidev s.
Surgigut s.
Surgilar s.
Surgilene blue monofilament
   polypropylene s.
Surgiloid s.
Surgilon braided nylon s.
Surgilon monofilament
   polypropylene s.
Surgilope s.
SurgiMed s.
Surgipro s.
Surgiset s.
Sutupak s.
swaged s.
swaged-on s.
Swedgeon s.
Swiss blue virgin silk s.
synthetic absorbable s.
Tajima modified Kessler s.
tantalum wire monofilament s.
Tapercut s.
Teflon-coated Dacron s.
Teflon-pledgeted s.
temporozygomatic s.
tendon s.
tension s.
tension-free s.
Tevdek pledgeted s.
Thermo-Flex s.
thread s.
through-the-wall mattress s.
Ti-Cron s.
tiger gut s.
Tom Jones s.
traction s.
transfixion s.
transition s.
transosseus s.

transparenchymal s.
transverse palatine s.
twisted cotton s.
twisted dermal s.
twisted linen s.
twisted virgin silk s.
Tycron s.
tympanomastoid s.
tympanosquamosal s.
Tyrrell-Gray s.
umbilical tape s.
unabsorbable s.
undyed s.
uninterrupted s.
vascular silk s.
vertical mattress s.
Vicryl pop-off s.
Vicryl Rapide s.
Vicryl SH s.
Vienna wire s.
virgin silk s.
Viro-Tec s.
wedge-and-groove s.
whipstitch s.
white braided silk s.
white nylon s.
white twisted s.
wide s.
wing s.
wire Zytor s.
Worst s.
Z s.
zygomaticofrontal s.
zygomaticomaxillary s.
zygomaticotemporal s.
suturectomy
sutured
   doubly s.
sutureless
   s. bowel anastomosis
   s. colostomy closure
suture-ligation
suture-ligature
SutureStrip Plus wound closure
suturing
   direct s.
   intracorporeal s.
suxamethonium
swab
swage
swaged-on suture
swaged suture

S

NOTES

swallow method
swallowtail malformation of scapula
Swan-Ganz tube
Swan incision
Swank high-flow arterial blood filter
swan-neck
    s.-n. deformity reduction
    s.-n. finger deformity
Swanson
    S. classification
    S. Convex condylar arthroplasty
    S. radial head implant arthroplasty
    S. reconstruction
    S. silicone wrist arthroplasty
    S. technique
sweat
    s. duct
    s. gland adenocarcinoma
    s. gland adenoma
    s. glands
Swedgeon suture
Swedish approach
Sweet method
swelling
    external s.
    genital s.'s
    levator s.
    lysosomal s.
    scrotal s.
    soft tissue s.
Swenson pull-through procedure
Swiss
    S. blue virgin silk suture
    S. roll embedding technique
    S. Therapy eye mask
switch
    compression s.
    s. operation
    s. procedure
switched B-gradient technique
swivel dislocation
sword-fighting
sycoma
sycosiform fungous infection
Sydney
    S. line
    S. system gastritis classification
sylvian
    s. approach
    s. cistern
    s. dissection
    s. fistula
    s. hematoma
    s. line
    s. point
Sylvius
    valve of S.
symblepharon ring

Syme
    S. ankle disarticulation amputation
    S. external urethrotomy
    S. procedure
Symington anococcygeal body
symmetric
    s. surgery
    s. thumb duplication
    s. vertebral fusion
symmetry
    s. operation
    s. plane
sympathectomy
    cervical perivascular s.
    cervicothoracic s.
    chemical s.
    Leriche s.
    lumbar s.
    periarterial s.
    preganglionic s.
    presacral s.
    Smithwick s.
    visceral s.
sympathetic
    s. block
    s. blockade
    s. blockade anesthetic technique
    s. branch to submandibular ganglion
    s. ganglion block anesthetic technique
    s. microneurography
    s. nerve
    s. nerve activity (SNA)
    s. nerve block
    s. part
    s. projection
    s. trunk
sympathetically
    s. maintained pain
    s. mediated pain
sympathetoblastoma
sympathic
sympathicectomy
sympathicoblastoma
sympathicogonioma
sympathicotripsy
sympathoadrenal
    s. response
sympathoblastoma
sympathoexcitation
    reflex s.
    s. reflex
sympathoexcitatory response
sympathogonioma
sympatholysis
sympatholytic agent

sympathomimetic
    s. agent
    s. drug
β-sympathomimetic agent
symperitoneal
symphyseotomy
symphyses (*pl. of* symphysis)
symphysial
    s. surface of pubis
symphysic
symphysion
symphysiotomy
symphysis, pl. **symphyses**
    cardiac s.
    intervertebral s.
    s. intervertebralis
    s. mandibulae
    mandibular s.
    manubriosternal s.
    s. manubriosternalis
    mental s.
    s. mentalis
    s. menti
    pleural s.
    pubic s.
    s. pubica
    s. pubis
    s. pubis diastasis
    s. sacrococcygea
symptom
    s. experience stage
    s. formation
    s. magnification syndrome
    s. score
symptomatic infection
symptothermal method
synadelphus
synanastomosis
synandrogenic
synapse
    excitatory s.
synaptosome
synarthrodia
synarthrodial
    s. joint
synarthrosis
syncephalus
synchondrodial joint
synchondroseotomy
synchondrosis, pl. **synchondroses**
    anterior intraoccipital s.
    s. arycorniculata

    arycorniculate s.
    cranial synchondroses
    synchondroses cranii
    s. epiphyseos
    s. intraoccipitalis anterior
    s. intraoccipitalis posterior
    s. manubriosternalis
    s. petro-occipitalis
    posterior intraoccipital s.
    sphenoethmoidal s.
    spheno-occipital s.
    s. spheno-occipitalis
    s. sphenopetrosa
    sphenopetrosal s.
    sternal synchondroses
    synchondroses sternales
    s. xiphosternalis
synchondrotomy
synchrocyclotron operation
synchronization
synchronized
    s. fibrillation
    s. intermittent mandatory ventilation (SIMV)
    s. intermittent mechanical ventilation
synchronous
    s. bladder reconstruction
    s. intermittent mandatory ventilation
    s. lesion
    s. scapuloclavicular rotation
    s. urinary tract infection
syncope
syncretio
syncytial knot
syncytiovascular membrane
syndactyl
syndactylia
syndactylization
syndactylous
syndactyly
    Diamond-Gould reduction s.
    Kelikian-Clayton-Loseff surgical s.
    reduction s.
syndectomy
syndesmectomy
syndesmectopia
syndesmodial joint
syndesmopexy
syndesmophyte
    bridging s.
syndesmoplasty

S

NOTES

syndesmorrhaphy
syndesmotic
syndesmotomy
syndrome
    abdominal compartment s.
    abdominal muscle deficiency s.
    acrofacial s.
    acute disconnection s.
    acute respiratory distress s.
    (ARDS)
    adhesive s.
    adrenal feminization s.
    adult respiratory distress s. (ARDS)
    afferent loop s.
    aglossia-adactylia s.
    Alport s.
    amniotic infection s.
    angio-osteohypertrophy s.
    ankyloglossia superior s.
    anomalous innominate artery
    compression s.
    anterior spinal artery s.
    Apert s.
    Arnold-Chiari s.
    Ascher s.
    Behçet s.
    bent-nail s.
    bile-plug s.
    billowing mitral valve s.
    black patch s.
    blind loop s.
    blind pouch s.
    Bloodgood s.
    body cast s.
    Boerhaave s.
    bowel bypass s.
    brittle nail s.
    Burnett s.
    calcaneal spur s.
    callosal disconnection s.
    camptomelic s.
    capsular exfoliation s.
    Caroli s.
    cauda equina s.
    central anticholinergic s.
    central cord s.
    central heel pad s.
    cerebellomedullary malformation s.
    cerebellopontine angle s.
    cervical acceleration-deceleration s.
    cervical compression s.
    cervical fusion s.
    Cheatle s.
    Chiari II s.
    chronic hyperventilation s.
    cloverleaf skull s.
    coarctation s.
    common peroneal nerve s.

    compartment s.
    compartment compression s.
    compression s.
    congenital central hypoventilation s.
    congenital ring s.
    Cooper s.
    cord traction s.
    Crouzon s.
    crush s.
    cutaneomucouveal s.
    Dandy-Walker s.
    D chromosome ring s.
    deafferentation pain s.
    Dejerine-Roussy s.
    de Quervain s.
    dialysis disequilibrium s.
    dialysis encephalopathy s.
    disconnection s.
    dumping s.
    dural shunt s.
    Eagle-Barrett s.
    ectopic ACTH s.
    embryonic fixation s.
    euthyroid sick s.
    excited skin s.
    exertional anterior compartment s.
    exertional compartment s.
    exertional deep posterior
    compartment s.
    exfoliation s.
    extra-articular pain s.
    extrapyramidal s.
    failed back surgery s.
    familial aortic ectasia s.
    familial atypical multiple mole
    melanoma s.
    familial cardiac myxoma s.
    familial cholestasis s.
    female urethral s.
    feminization s.
    fetal aspiration s.
    fibrofascial compartment s.
    first arch s.
    flapping valve s.
    floppy valve s.
    Fraley s.
    Franceschetti s.
    Fraser s.
    functional prepubertal castration s.
    G s.
    gastrojejunal loop obstruction s.
    glomangiomatous osseous
    malformation s.
    glucagonoma s.
    Gorlin-Chaudhry-Moss s.
    Hadju-Cheney acro-osteolysis s.
    Hallermann-Streiff s.
    Hallermann-Streiff-François s.

Hanhart s.
head-bobbing doll s.
hemangioma-thrombocytopenia s.
hemispheric disconnection s.
hemolytic uremic s.
hepatorenal s.
hereditary flat adenoma s.
Hinman s.
Hutchison s.
hyaline membrane s.
hypersensitive xiphoid s.
hyperventilation s.
immotile cilia s.
impaired regeneration s.
infantile choriocarcinoma s.
innominate artery compression s.
intersection s.
iridocorneal endothelial s.
iridocorneal epithelial s.
Jeune s.
jugular foramen s.
Klippel-Trenaunay-Weber s.
Larsen s.
lateral patellar compression s.
levator ani s.
levator scapulae s.
loculation s.
lower nephron s.
Luys body s.
malignant external otitis s.
Mallory-Weiss s.
mandibulofacial dysotosis s.
mandibulo-oculofacial s.
mangled extremity s.
Marfan s.
MASS s.
massive bowel resection s.
maternal deprivation s.
meconium aspiration s.
meconium plug s.
megacystic s.
megacystitis-megaureter s.
megacystitis-microcolon-intestinal
  hypoperistalsis s.
Mendelson s.
minimal-change nephrotic s.
minimal-lesion nephrotic s.
Mirizzi s.
mitral valve prolapse s.
Mohr s.
monofixation s.
mucocutaneous lymph node s.

mucocutaneous pigmentation of
  Peutz-Jeghers s.
mucosal neuroma s.
mucous plug s.
müllerian duct derivation s.
multiple endocrine neoplasia s.
multiple hamartoma s.
multiple mucosal neuroma s.
multiple neuroma s.
multiple pterygium s.
myofascial pain s.
nail-patella s.
nail-patella-elbow s.
naviculocapitate fracture s.
nephritic s.
nerve compression-degeneration s.
neuroleptic malignant s. (NMS)
nevoid basal cell carcinoma s.
OAV s.
obesity-hypoventilation s.
ocular-mucous membrane s.
oculobuccogenital s.
oculomandibulofacial s.
oculovertebral s.
OFD s.
Ogilvie s.
optic tract s.
orofaciodigital s.
osteogenesis imperfecta congenita s.
osteomyelofibrotic s.
osteopathia striata s.
osteoporosis pseudoglioma s.
Ostrum-Furst s.
otomandibular s.
ovarian hyperstimulation s.
ovarian overstimulation s.
ovarian vein s.
pacemaker s.
Paget-von Schrötter s.
Papillon-Léage and Psaume s.
pericardiotomy s.
pericolic membrane s.
peroneal compartment s.
persistent müllerian duct s.
pharyngeal pouch s.
Phocas s.
placental hemangioma s.
popliteal web s.
postadrenalectomy s.
postcardiotomy s.
postcholecystectomy s.
postcolonoscopy distention s.

S

NOTES

717

syndrome *(continued)*
postcommissurotomy s.
postembolization s.
posterior interosseous nerve compression s.
postfundoplication s.
postgastrectomy s.
postirradiation s.
postlaminectomy s.
postpericardiotomy s.
postphlebitic s.
postpolypectomy coagulation s.
posttubal ligation s.
postvagotomy s.
preexcitation s.
prolapsed mitral valve s.
pronator teres s.
proximal loop s.
prune-belly s.
pseudo-blind loop s.
pseudoexfoliation s.
pseudolymphoma s.
pseudoxanthoma elasticum s.
pulmonary acid aspiration s.
quadrilateral space s.
rapid tumor lysis s.
Reclus I s.
red-eyed shunt s.
Reifenstein s.
Reiter s.
renal crush s.
respiratory distress s. (RDS)
retinoblastoma-mental retardation s.
Rieger s.
right ovarian vein s.
Roaf s.
Roberts s.
Roux stasis s.
Sakati-Nyhan s.
scapuloperoneal s.
Scheie s.
Sertoli-cell-only s.
short-bowel s.
slit ventricle s.
Smith-Lemli-Opitz s.
somatostatinoma s.
splenic sequestration s.
stagnant loop s.
stasis s.
Stauffer s.
stump embolization s.
subclavian steal s.
sudden infant death s. (SIDS)
sump s.
supine hypotensive s.
symptom magnification s.
Takayasu s.
terminal reservoir s.
testicular feminization s.
tethered cord s.
third and fourth pharyngeal pouch s.
thoracic compression s.
thoracic endometriosis s.
thoracic outlet s.
Thorn s.
Tillaux-Phocas s.
tooth-and-nail s.
transient compartment s.
translocation Down s.
transplant lung s.
transurethral resection s.
Treacher Collins s.
trisomy 8 s.
trisomy C s.
tumor lysis s.
TUR s.
Turcot s.
urethral s.
uterine hernia s.
uveo-encephalitic s.
valgus extension overload s.
vanished testis s.
vascular ring s.
VATER association s.
vertebral subluxation s.
vibration s.
vibrator hand s.
visual deprivation s.
vitreoretinal traction s.
Wartenberg s.
Weyers-Thier s.
yellow nail s.
synechia, pl. **synechiae**
synechiotomy
Paufique s.
synechotomy
synectenterotomy
synencephalocele
synergism
synergistic
s. interaction
s. muscles
synergy
drug s.
syngeneic
s. graft
s. tissue
s. transplantation
syngenesioplastic transplantation
syngenesioplasty
syngenesiotransplantation
syngnathia
syngraft
synonychia
synorchidism

synoscheos
synostectomy
synosteology
synostosis
synotia
synovectomy
    Albright s.
    arthroscopic s.
    carpal s.
    dorsal s.
    Inglis-Ranawat-Straub elbow s.
    palmar s.
    Porter-Richardson-Vainio s.
    six-portal s.
    Smith-Petersen s.
    volar s.
    Wilkinson s.
synovia (*pl. of* synovium)
synovial
    s. biopsy
    s. bursa
    s. cavity
    s. fistula
    s. fluid
    s. fluid examination
    s. fold
    s. frena
    s. frenula
    s. fringe
    s. glands
    s. herniation
    s. joint
    s. ligament
    s. membrane
    s. tendon sheath
    s. tissue
    s. villi
synovioma
    benign giant cell s.
    malignant s.
synoviparous
synovitis
synovium, pl. synovia
synpolydactyly
Synthamin amino acid solution
synthesis
    s. of continuity
synthetic
    s. absorbable suture
    s. augmentation
    s. bone graft

    s. lysine analog antifibrinolytic
      drug
    s. method
    s. vascular bypass graft
syphilid
syphilis
syphilitic fever
syphiloma
    s. of Fournier
syringadenoma
syringe
    S. Avitene
    s. cap
syringeal
syringectomy
syringe-type infusion pump
syringoadenoma
syringocarcinoma
syringocele
syringocisternostomy
syringocystadenoma
syringocystoma
syringohydromyelic cavity
syringoma
syringomeningocele
syringomyelia
syringomyelic
    s. dissociation
    s. hemorrhage
syringomyelocele
syringomyelomeningocele
syringomyelus
syringotome
syringotomy
syrinx
syssarcosic
syssarcosis
syssarcotic
system
    Acorn II nebulizer s.
    Acoustic Pharyngometer two-
      microphone imaging s.
    Advanced Catheter S.'s
    anesthetic s.
    Baxter-PCA-on-demand s.
    Bioject injector s.
    cell salvage s.
    circle s.
    closed anesthesia s.
    Comfort and sedation scoring s.
    compliance of the total
      respiratory s.

S

NOTES

system *(continued)*
- Datex As/3 anesthesia s.
- Escort II patient monitoring s.
- forced-air patient warming s.
- Mallinckrodt sensory s.
- M1156A monitoring s.
- Mcginnis balloon s.
- MERA F breathing s.
- needle-free s.
- needleless intravenous administration s.
- Neuroguard TCD Monitoring S.
- Neuropack Four mini evoked potential measuring s.
- neurotransmitter s.'s
- Omni-Trak 3100 MRI vital Signs Monitoring S.
- open anesthesia s.
- Pain Relief Scoring S.
- pediatric anesthesia s.
- peripheral access s. (PAS)
- pin-index safety s.
- pneumotachograph/pressure transducer s.
- Safsite IV therapy s.
- static compliance of the total respiratory s.
- STAT-PACE IIA transesophageal pacing s.
- Tapscope transesophageal pacing s.
- Trach Care closed suctioning s.
- vaporizer exclusion s.
- Venflon needless injection port s.

systema
- s. alimentarium
- s. digestorium
- s. lymphaticum
- s. nervosum
- s. nervosum autonomicum
- s. respiratorium
- s. skeletale
- s. urogenitale

systematic
- s. method
- s. sextant biopsy

systematization

systemic
- s. absorption
- s. arteriovenous fistula
- s. dissection
- s. endotoxemia
- s. fungal infection
- s. lesion
- s. mean arterial pressure
- s. to pulmonary artery anastomosis
- s. radioimmunoglobulin therapy
- s. venodilation
- s. venous circulation

systolic
- s. blood pressure (SBP)
- s. ejection murmur
- s. ejection rate
- s. left ventricular pressure
- s. pressure time index

Szymanowski-Kuhnt operation

Szymanowski operation

T

   T fracture
   T incision
   T myelotomy
   T tube
T1
   first twitch height
t
   t test
T1, T2 relaxation
T1-weighted spin-echo image
T2 relaxation rate
T2-weighted spin-echo image
tabatière anatomique
tabby-cat striation
tabetic dissociation
tablature
table
   inner t. of skull
   outer t. of skull
   vitreous t.
tabulation
TACC
   thoracic aortic cross-clamping
Tachdjian
   T. classification
   T. procedure
tachycardia
   atrial ectopic t.
   automatic ectopic t.
   bundle-branch reentrant t.
   ectopic atrial t.
   endless-loop t.
   endocardial mapping of
      ventricular t.
   exercise-induced ventricular t.
   junctional ectopic t.
   pacemaker-mediated t.
   right ventricular outflow tract t.
   torsade de pointes ventricular t.
      (TdPVT)
   t. traumosa exophthalmica
tachyphylaxis
tacrine
Tactilaze angioplasty
tactile
   t. anesthesia
   t. stimulation
taenia strip of soft tissue
TAER
   transient auditory evoked response
tag
tagging stitch
tagliacotian operation

tail
   t. bone
   t. of epididymis
   t. of helix
   t. of pancreas
   t. vertebrae
tailor bunionectomy
Tajima
   T. method
   T. modified Kessler suture
   T. suture technique
Takayasu
   T. disease
   T. syndrome
takedown
   bilateral ureterostomy t.
   colostomy t.
   t. of colostomy
   t. of pelvic sling procedure
talar
   t. avulsion fracture
   t. canal
   t. dislocation
   t. neck fracture
   t. osteochondral fracture
   t. sulcus
talc
   t. insufflation
   t. operation
   t. pleurodesis
talectomy
   Trumble t.
Talesnick scapholunate repair
talipes cavus deformity
talocalcaneal
   t. angle
   t. articulation
   t. fusion
talocalcaneonavicular articulation
talonavicular
   t. fusion
taloscaphoid
talotibial
talus
   beaking of head of t.
   truncated-wedge tarsometatarsal
      arthrodesis vertical t.
Talwin NX
tamed iodine
tamp
   interbody graft t.
   tension band wire t.
tampon
   Corner t.
   t. tube

T

tamponade
  balloon tube t.
  low-pressure t.
  t. needle tract
  tract t.
tamponage
tamponing
Tanagho
  T. bladder flap urethroplasty
  T. bladder neck reconstruction
tandem
  t. clipping technique
  t. colonoscopy
  t. construction
  t. lesion
tangential
  t. biopsy
  t. colonic submucosal injection
  t. projection
  t. section
  t. wound
tangent screen examination
tank
  oxygen t.
Tanne corneal cutting block
Tanner operation
Tano ring
Tansley operation
tantalum
  t. cranioplasty
  t. O ring
  t. wire monofilament suture
tap
  peritoneal t.
  shunt t.
tape mark
Tapercut suture
tapered-tip
taper-point
tapetum
tapinocephalic
tapinocephaly
tapping
  glabellar t.
Tapscope
  T. esophageal pacing stethoscope
  T. transesophageal pacing system
target
  fixation t.
  t. gland
  t. lesion
  saccadic eccentric t.
target-controlled infusion (TCI)
targeting
  magnetite in tumor t.
targetoid ring
Tarin space
Tarkowski method

tar preparation
tarsal
  t. amputation
  t. bone fracture
  t. canal
  t. dislocation
  t. fold
  t. joint infection
  t. laceration
  t. medullostomy
  t. membrane
  t. strip procedure
  t. wedge osteotomy
tarsectomy
  Blaskovics t.
  Kuhnt t.
tarsen
tarsi (*pl. of* tarsus)
tarsocheiloplasty
tarsoconjunctival flap
tarsometatarsal
  t. amputation
  t. articulation
  t. dislocation
  t. fracture-dislocation
  t. truncated-wedge arthrodesis
tarsophalangeal
tarsoplasty
tarsorrhaphy
  bilateral temporary t.
  lateral t.
tarsotomy
  transverse t.
tarsus, pl. tarsi
  t. inferior
  inferior t.
  t. superior
  superior t.
tartrate
  butorphanol t.
  dihydrocodeine t.
  levorphanol t.
  vinorelbine t.
Tasia operation
tattoo of cornea operation
taurocholate solution
Taussig-Bing anomaly
Taussig-Morton node dissection
Tawara node
taxis
Taylor
  T. approach
  T. procedure
  T. technique
Taylor-Daniel-Weiland technique
Taylor-Townsend-Corlett iliac crest bone graft

TBW
    total body weight
TC
    total colectomy
TCD
    transcranial Doppler
      TCD recanalization
T-cell line
TCES
    transcutaneous cranial electrical
      stimulation
TCI
    target-controlled infusion
tc-MER
    motor-evoked response to transcranial
      stimulation
T-condylar fracture
T-configuration
TCS
    transcranial stimulation
TD
    thermodilution
TDCO
    thermodilution cardiac output
TdPVT
    torsade de pointes ventricular tachycardia
TE
    thromboembolic
      TE fistula
teacup fracture
Teale-Knapp operation
TEAP
    transesophageal atrial pacing
      TEAP threshold
tear
    bucket-handle t.
    T. Drop solution
    t. duct tube
    flap meniscal t.
    Mallory-Weiss t.
    T.'s Naturale Free solution
    T.'s Naturale II solution
    Neer acromioplasty for rotator
      cuff t.
    T.'s Plus solution
    T.'s Renewed solution
    rotator cuff t.
    t. sac
teardrop
    t. fracture
    t. line
TearGard Ophthalmic solution

Teargen ophthalmic solution
tearing
    excessive t.
Tearisol solution
teat
technic
Techni-Care surgical scrub
technique
    abdominal pressure t.
    abduction traction t.
    ablative t.
    Ace-Colles frame t.
    acid etch bonding t.
    adduction traction t.
    afterloading t.
    agglutination t.
    airbrasive t.
    air-gap t.
    airway occlusion t.
    Albert suture t.
    Alexander t.
    American laryngectomy t.
    Amplatz t.
    Amspacher-Messenbaugh t.
    Anderson-Hutchins t.
    Andrews t.
    anesthetic t.
    angiographic road-mapping t.
    angle bisection t.
    antegrade double balloon/double
      wire t.
    antegrade/retrograde cardioplegia t.
    anterior quadriceps
      musculocutaneous flap t.
    anterior sandwich patch t.
    anterograde transseptal t.
    antireflux ureteral implantation t.
    AO t.
    APAAP t.
    Araki-Sako t.
    Argyll-Robertson suture t.
    Armaly-Drance t.
    Armistead t.
    Aronson-Prager t.
    arterial cannulation anesthetic t.
    arthrographic capsular distension
      and rupture t.
    ascending t.
    aseptic t.
    ASIF screw fixation t.
    Asnis t.
    assay t.

NOTES

723

technique *(continued)*
assisted reproductive t.
Atasoy V-Y t.
Atkinson t.
atrial-well t.
autosuture t.
Avila t.
avulsion t.
Axenfeld suture t.
axillary block anesthetic t.
axillary perivascular t.
Ayre spatula-Zelsmyr cytobrush t.
Badgley t.
bag-of-bones t.
Bailey-Badgley t.
Bailey-Dubow t.
Baker t.
Balacescu-Golden t.
balanced anesthetic t.
balloon catheter t.
balloon-catheter and basket-
retrieval t.
Bandi t.
Banks-Laufman t.
Barbour t.
Barcat t.
bare scleral t.
Barkan t.
barrier t.
Barsky t.
baseball suture t.
basic t.
basket fragmentation t.
basketing t.
Bass t.
Bassini t.
Batch-Spittler-McFaddin t.
Bauer-Tondra-Trusler t.
Baumgard-Schwartz tennis elbow t.
Beall-Webel-Bailey t.
Beckenbaugh t.
Becker t.
Béclard suture t.
Becton t.
Begg light wire differential
force t.
Bellemore-Barrett-Middleton-Scougall-
Whiteway t.
Bell-Tawse open reduction t.
Belsey fundoplication t.
Belt t.
bench surgical t.
Bentall inclusion t.
Bertrandi suture t.
Beverly-Douglas lip-tongue
adhesion t.
Bevin-Aurglass t.
bilateral inguinal hernia repair t.

Billroth I, II t.
bioprogressive t.
Bircher-Weber t.
bisecting angle t.
bisecting-the-angle t.
bitewing t.
Black t.
Black-Broström staple t.
Blackburn t.
bladder neck preserving t.
Blair t.
Blair-Byars hypospadias t.
blanket suture t.
Bleck recession t.
Blenderm patch t.
blind nasal intubation anesthetic t.
blind nasotracheal intubation
anesthetic t.
blind-spot projection t.
Bloom-Raney modification of
Smith-Robinson t.
Blount tracing t.
Blundell-Jones t.
Bohlman cervical fusion t.
Bohlman triple-wire t.
bolster suture t.
bolus intravenous anesthetic t.
bone t.
Bonfiglio-Bardenstein t.
Bonfiglio modification of
Phemister t.
Bonola t.
boost t.
bootstrap two-vessel t.
Bora t.
Borggreve-Hall t.
bougienage t.
Bowers t.
Bowles t.
Box t.
Boyd-Anderson t.
Boyden chamber t.
Boyd-McLeod tennis elbow t.
Boyes brachioradialis transfer t.
Bozeman suture t.
Braasch bulb t.
brachial plexus block anesthetic t.
Brackett-Osgood-Putti-Abbott t.
Brackin t.
Brady-Jewett t.
Brand tendon transfer t.
Brannon-Wickström t.
breast-conserving t.
Brecher-Cronkite t.
Brecher new methylene blue t.
Brenner gastrojejunostomy t.
Brockenbrough t.
Brockhurst t.

bronchoscopy anesthetic t.
Brooks t.
Brooks-Jenkins atlantoaxial fusion t.
Brooks-Seddon transfer t.
Broström injection t.
Brown t.
Brown-Beard t.
Brown-Brenn t.
Brown-Wickham t.
Bruhat t.
Bruser t.
Bryan-Morrey t.
Buck-Gramcko t.
Bugg-Boyd t.
bulk pack t.
Buncke t.
Bunnell atraumatic t.
Bunnell tendon transfer t.
Burch bladder suspension t.
Burgess t.
buried mass far-and-near suture t.
Burkhalter modification of Stiles-Bunnell t.
Burkhalter transfer t.
Burrows t.
button t.
Buxton bolus suture t.
bypass t.
Caldwell-Coleman flatfoot t.
Callahan fusion t.
Camino catheter t.
Camitz t.
Campbell t.
Canale t.
canal-wall-up t.
Capello t.
Cape Town t.
capping t.
capsule flap t.
capsule forceps t.
cardiovascular imaging t.
Carey Ranvier t.
Carnesale t.
carotid preservation t.
Carrell fibular substitution t.
catheterization t.
catheter-securing t.
caudal epidural anesthetic t.
cavernosal alpha blockade t.
Cave-Rowe shoulder dislocation t.
celiac plexus block anesthetic t.
cell separation t.

cement t.
cementless t.
central anesthetic t.
central slip sparing t.
central venous cannulation anesthetic t.
cephalotrigonal t.
cervical plexus block anesthetic t.
cervical screw insertion t.
cervical spondylotic myelopathy fusion t.
chain suture t.
channel shoulder pin t.
Charters t.
Chaves-Rapp muscle transfer t.
Cherney suture t.
chevron t.
chew-in t.
Chiari t.
Childress ankle fixation t.
chloramine-T t.
Cho tendon t.
Chow t.
Chrisman-Snook ankle t.
Cierny-Mader t.
Cincinnati t.
circulatory arrest anesthetic t.
clamshell t.
Clancy ligament t.
Clark transfer t.
Class V Multiple Step Build-up t.
Clayton-Fowler t.
clearance t.
Cleveland-Bosworth-Thompson t.
clip t.
closed-circuit anesthetic t.
closed tubule fixation t.
Cloward t.
cobalt-60 moving strip t.
Cobb scoliosis measuring t.
Codivilla tendon lengthening t.
Coffey t.
Coffey-Witzel jejunostomy t.
Cofield t.
Cohen cross-trigonal t.
cold saline-induced paresthesia t.
Cole t.
Coleman flatfoot t.
Collis broken femoral stem t.
Collis-Nissen fundoplication t.
Coltart fracture t.
combination of isotonics t.

NOTES

technique *(continued)*

combined spinal/epidural anesthetic t.
compensation t.
composite addition t.
composite pelvic resection t.
compression t.
computer-assisted continuous infusion anesthetic t.
computer-controlled drug administration anesthetic t.
computer-controlled infusion anesthetic t.
Connolly t.
continuous anesthetic t.
continuous gum t.
continuous infusion anesthetic t.
continuous pull-through t.
continuous spinal anesthetic t.
continuous suture t.
continuous-wave t.
contoured anterior spinal plate t.
contraceptive t.
contract relax t.
controlled release anesthetic t.
controlled water added t.
conventional t.
Conyers t.
Coomassie brilliant blue t.
Coonse-Adams t.
Cope t.
Copeland t.
coracoclavicular t.
Corbin t.
coronary flow reserve t.
costotransversectomy t.
cough CPR t.
Counsellor-Flor modification of McIndoe t.
Cozen-Brockway t.
crash t.
Crawford graft inclusion t.
Crawford-Marxen-Osterfeld t.
Creech t.
Crego tendon transfer t.
cricoid pressure anesthetic t.
cross-facial t.
cross-section t.
Crown suture t.
Crutchfield reduction t.
cryosurgical t.
Cubbins shoulder dislocation t.
Culcher-Sussman t.
culturing t.
cup-patch t.
Cupper suture t.
Curtis t.
Curtis-Fisher knee t.

cutdown t.
Darrach-McLaughlin shoulder t.
Davey-Rorabeck-Fowler decompression t.
Davis drainage t.
Debeyre-Patte-Elmelik rotator cuff t.
decompression t.
decortication t.
DEFT t.
Deisting prostatic dilation t.
deliberate hypotension anesthetic t.
demand-adapted administration anesthetic t.
Denis Browne urethroplasty t.
Dennis t.
de novo needle knife t.
DePalma modified patellar t.
depth pulse t.
descending t.
destructive interference t.
Devonshire t.
Dewar-Barrington clavicular dislocation t.
Dewar-Harris shoulder t.
Dewar posterior cervical fusion t.
Deyerle femoral fracture t.
Dias-Giegerich fracture t.
Dickinson calcaneal bursitis t.
Dickson transplant t.
Dieffenbach-Duplay hypospadias t.
differential force t.
differential spinal block anesthetic t.
digital subtraction t.
dilator and sheath t.
dilution-filtration t.
Dimon-Hughston t.
Diprivan t.
direct/indirect t.
direct insertion t.
distraction t.
Dixon t.
DOC exchange t.
Dolenc t.
Doll trochanteric reattachment t.
Doppler auto-correlation t.
Dor fundoplication t.
dot-blot t.
Dotter t.
Dotter-Judkins t.
double-balloon t.
double-dummy t.
double-folded cup-patch t.
double-freeze t.
double-looped semitendinosus t.
double-rod t.
double-sealant t.
double-staple t.

double-stapled ileoanal reservoir t.
double-stick t.
double-tube t.
double-wire t.
Douglas bag t.
dowel t.
doweling spondylolisthesis t.
Drake tandem clipping t.
DREZ modification of Eriksson t.
drilling t.
driven equilibrium Fourier
 transform t.
Drummond spinous wiring t.
Drummond wire t.
dry field t.
dual impression t.
Dufourmentel t.
Dunn t.
Dunn-Brittain foot stabilization t.
Duplay I, II t.
DuVries deltoid ligament
 reconstruction t.
Dyban t.
dye dilution t.
dynamic bolus tracking t.
Eames t.
Eastwood t.
Eaton-Littler t.
Eaton-Malerich fracture-dislocation t.
Eberle contracture release t.
ECG signal-averaging t.
Ecker-Lotke-Glazer tendon
 reconstruction t.
edgewise t.
Eftekhar broken femoral stem t.
Eggers tendon transfer t.
Eisenberger t.
Eklund t.
elliptical excision t.
Ellis t. for Barton fracture
Ellis-Jones peroneal tendon t.
Ellison t.
Ellis skin traction t.
Emmet suture t.
en bloc, no-touch t.
Ender femoral fracture t.
endobronchial intubation
 anesthetic t.
endodontic t.
endofluoroscopic t.
endorectal ileoanal pull-through t.
endoscopic mucosal resection t.

endovascular t.
end-to-end reconstruction t.
end-to-side vasoepididymostomy t.
entangling t.
enucleation t.
epiaortic imaging t.
epidural anesthetic t.
epidural blood patch anesthetic t.
epithelialization t.
Erickson-Leider-Brown t.
Eriksson brachial block t.
Eriksson ligament t.
erysiphake t.
esophageal banding t.
Essex-Lopresti axial fixation t.
Essex-Lopresti calcaneal fracture t.
Evans ankle reconstruction t.
evoked potential t.
exchange t.
excisional biopsy t.
excision-curettage t.
Exorcist t.
extra-anatomical renal
 revascularization t.
extra-anatomic bypass t.
extra-articular t.
extracorporeal t.
extraction balloon t.
extradural anesthetic t.
extravesical ureteral
 reimplantation t.
extremity mobilization t.
extubation anesthetic t.
ex vivo t.
FA t.
facet excision t.
Fahey t.
Fahey-O'Brien t.
Fairbanks t.
Falk vesicovaginal fistula t.
Farmer t.
fast exposure t.
fat-suppression t.
feeder-frond t.
femoral 3-in-1 t.
Ferkel torticollis t.
ferning t.
fiberoptic bronchoscopy anesthetic t.
fiberoptic endoscopy anesthetic t.
fiberoptic intubation anesthetic t.
fiberoptic tracheal intubation
 anesthetic t.

T

NOTES

technique *(continued)*

Fick t.
Ficoll-Hypaque t.
Fielding modification of Gallie t.
filling first t.
finger fracture t.
Finochietto-Billroth I gastrectomy t.
first-line screening t.
first-pass t.
first rib resection via subclavicular
    approach t.
Fish cuneiform osteotomy t.
fixation t.
FLAK t.
Flamm t.
flap t.
Flatt t.
flicker-fusion frequency t.
Flick-Gould t.
flip-flap t.
floppy Nissen fundoplication t.
flow detection t.
flow interruption t.
flow mapping t.
fluid loading anesthetic t.
fluoroscopic pushing t.
flush and bathe t.
flushing t.
Flynn t.
Fones t.
Forbes modification of Phemister
    graft t.
Ford triangulation t.
Forest-Hastings t.
forward triangle t.
four-maximal breath
    preoxygenation t.
four-port t.
Fowler t.
Fowles dislocation t.
Frank permanent gastrotomy t.
Fraunfelder t.
Fraunfelder "no touch" t.
Freebody-Bendall-Taylor fusion t.
free-hand suturing t.
French fracture t.
Fried-Hendel tendon t.
FRODO t.
Froimson t.
frontalis sling t.
functional t.
Furnas-Haq-Somers t.
fusion t.
Gaenslen split-heel t.
Gallie atlantoaxial fusion t.
Gallie wiring t.
Galveston t.
Ganley t.

Garceau tendon t.
gaseous laparoscopy t.
gasless laparoscopy t.
gastric valve tightening t.
gated t.
Gaur balloon distension t.
Gelman t.
general anesthetic t.
George Lewis t.
Ger t.
Getty decompression t.
Giannestras modification of
    Lapidus t.
Gilbert-Tamai-Weiland t.
Gillies-Millard cocked-hat t.
Gill-Manning-White
    spondylolisthesis t.
Gill sliding graft t.
Gil-Vernet t.
Gittes t.
Gledhill t.
Glen Anderson t.
gliding-hole-first t.
gloved-fist t.
Glover suture t.
Glynn-Neibauer t.
Goebell-Frangenheim-Stoeckel t.
Goldberg t.
Goldmann kinetic t.
Goldmann static t.
Goldner-Clippinger t.
gold plate t.
gold seed implantation t.
Goldstein spinal fusion t.
Gomco t.
Goodwin t.
Goodwin-Hohenfellner t.
Goodwin-Scott t.
Gordon-Broström t.
Gordon joint injection t.
Gordon-Taylor t.
Gould suture t.
grabbing t.
gracilis flap t.
grasping t.
Graves t.
gravimetric t.
Green-Banks t.
Greulich-Pyle t.
Grice-Green t.
Grimelius t.
Gritti-Stokes knee amputation t.
Grosse-Kempf tibial t.
Groves-Goldner t.
Grüntzig t.
Guhl t.
guidewire exchange t.
guidewire and mini-snare t.

Guttmann t.
Guyon ankle amputation t.
Hackethal stacked nailing t.
Håkanson t.
half-mouth t.
Hall t.
Halsted suture t.
Hamas t.
Hamou t.
Hardinge t.
Hark t.
Harmon transfer t.
Harriluque t.
Harris suture t.
Hartel t.
Hartmann reconstruction t.
Hassmann-Brunn-Neer elbow t.
Hauri t.
Hauser patellar realignment t.
Hawkins inside-out nephrostomy t.
Hawkins single-stick t.
head turn t.
Heaney t.
Heller myotomy with Dor
  fundoplication t.
hemostat t.
Hendler unitunnel t.
Henning inside-to-outside t.
Henry acromioclavicular t.
Hermodsson internal rotation t.
Hey-Groves fascia lata t.
Hey-Groves-Kirk t.
Hey-Groves ligament
  reconstruction t.
Heyman-Herndon-Strong t.
Higgins t.
high-amplitude sucking t.
high-heat casting t.
high-kV t.
high-tension suturing t.
Hill-Nahai-Vasconez-Mathes t.
Hitchcock tendon t.
Hodgson t.
Hofmeister t.
Hohl-Moore t.
Hokc-Kite t.
hold-relax t.
hole-in-one t.
Hood t.
Hoppenfeld-Deboer t.
Hori t.
hot biopsy t.

Hotchkiss-McManus PAS t.
hot dog t.
Houghton-Akroyd fracture t.
House t.
Hovanian transfer t.
Howard t.
Hughes modification of Burch t.
Hughston-Jacobson t.
Hungerford t.
Hunt-Early t.
Huntington tibial t.
hybridization-subtraction t.
hybridoma t.
hydroflow t.
hydrogen inhalation t.
hygroscopic t.
hypogastric plexus block
  anesthetic t.
hypothermia anesthetic t.
Ilizarov limb-lengthening t.
immediate extension t.
immersion t.
impression t.
indicator dilution t.
indirect t.
indocyanine green indicator
  dilution t.
induced hypotension anesthetic t.
induction anesthetic t.
infiltration anesthetic t.
Inglis-Cooper t.
Inglis-Ranawat-Straub t.
inhalation anesthetic t.
injection t.
Insall ligament reconstruction t.
insemination swim-up t.
inside-out t.
inside-to-outside t.
insufflation anesthetic t.
intercostal nerve block anesthetic t.
interference screw t.
internal jugular vein cannulation
  anesthetic t.
internal jugular vein catheterization
  anesthetic t.
internal jugular vein puncture
  anesthetic t.
interpleural anesthetic t.
interscalene block anesthetic t.
interspinous segmental spinal
  instrumentation t.
intra-articular anesthetic t.

NOTES

technique *(continued)*
    intracorporeal knotting t.
    intradermal tattooing t.
    intramuscular preanesthetic
      medication anesthetic t.
    intraperitoneal t.
    intrathecal cannulation anesthetic t.
    intrathecal morphine anesthetic t.
    intravenous cannulation anesthetic t.
    intravenous oxygen-15 water
      bolus t.
    intubation anesthetic t.
    invagination t.
    inverting knot t.
    ischemic-tourniquet t.
    isometric t.
    Jaboulay-Doyen-Winkleman t.
    Jacobs locking-hook spinal rod t.
    Jansey t.
    Jeffery t.
    jejunoileal bypass reversal t.
    Jerne t.
    jet ventilation anesthetic t.
    J loop t.
    Johnson pelvic fracture t.
    Johnson staple t.
    Johnston pursestring suture t.
    Jones-Brackett t.
    Jones and Jones wedge t.
    Jones-Politano t.
    Jorgensen t.
    Judd pyloroplasty t.
    Judkins t.
    Judkins-Sones t.
    jugular t.
    Kader-Senn gastrotomy t.
    Kapandji t.
    Kapel elbow dislocation t.
    Kaplan t.
    Kashiwagi t.
    Kates-Kessel-Kay t.
    Kato thick smear t.
    Kaufer tendon t.
    Kaufmann t.
    Kehr t.
    Kelikian-Clayton-Loseff t.
    Kelikian-Riashi-Gleason t.
    Kellogg-Speed fusion t.
    Kelly suture t.
    Kendrick t.
    Kendrick-Sharma-Hassler-Herndon t.
    Kennedy ligament t.
    Kern t.
    Kessler suture t.
    Kety-Schmidt inert gas saturation t.
    keyhole tenodesis t.
    Keystone t.
    Kidde cannula t.

King t.
King-Richards dislocation t.
King-Steelquist t.
Kirk thigh amputation t.
kissing balloon t.
Kjolbe t.
Klein t.
Klisic-Jankovic t.
Knoll refraction t.
Knott t.
Kock t.
Krawkow-Cohn t.
Krawkow-Thomas-Jones t.
Krempen-Craig-Sotelo tibial
  nonunion t.
Krönig t.
Kumar-Cowell-Ramsey t.
Kumar spica cast t.
Küntscher t.
Kutler finger amputation t.
Labbé gastrotomy t.
labiolingual t.
Lamaze t.
Lamb-Marks-Bayne t.
Lambrinudi t.
laparoscopic colposuspension t.
laparoscopic lymph node
  dissection t.
laparoscopic Nissen
  fundoplication t.
laparoscopic para-aortic lymph node
  sampling t.
Lapides t.
Lapidus hammertoe t.
large-core t.
Larson t.
laryngeal mask insertion
  anesthetic t.
laryngoscopy anesthetic t.
laser welding t.
lateral bending t.
lateral window t.
Laurell t.
Lazarus-Nelson t.
Leach t.
Leadbetter modification t.
Leboyer t.
Le Dentu suture t.
Le Dran suture t.
LeDuc t.
Lee t.
Lefèvre gastrectomy t.
Le Fort suture t.
Lehman t.
Leibolt t.
Leksell t.
Lenart-Kullman t.
letterbox t.

Lewit stretch t.
Lich extravesical t.
Lich-Gregoire t.
Lichtman t.
lid-loading t.
Liebolt radioulnar t.
light-around-wire t.
Limberg t.
limb-saving t.
Lindholm t.
lingual split-bone t.
Lipscomb t.
Lister t.
Little t.
Littler t.
Littler-Cooley t.
Littre suture t.
Lloyd-Roberts fracture t.
localization t.
local standby anesthesia t.
Löffler suture t.
long cone t.
long posterior flap t.
3-loop t.
loop gastric bypass t.
Losee modification of MacIntosh t.
Losee sling and reef t.
loss-of-resistance t.
lost wax pattern t.
LowDye taping t.
low-flow anesthetic t.
Lown t.
Ludloff t.
lumbar accessory movement t.
lumbar anesthetic t.
Luque instrumentation concave t.
Luque instrumentation convex t.
Luque sublaminar wiring t.
Lyden t.
Lyden-Lehman t.
Lynn t.
MacIntosh t.
macroelectrode t.
Madden t.
Magerl translaminar facet screw fixation t.
Magilligan measuring t.
Magnuson t.
Ma-Griffith t.
Maitland t.
Majestro-Ruda-Frost tendon t.
Malawer excision t.

Mallory t.
Mancini t.
mandibular swing t.
Mankin t.
Manske t.
manual t.
manual push-pull t.
Maquet t.
Marbach-Weil t.
March t.
Marcus-Balourdas-Heiple ankle fusion t.
Marks-Bayne t. for thumb duplication
Marlex plug t.
Marshall ligament repair t.
Marshall-McIntosh t.
marsupialization t.
Martin patellar wiring t.
Martin reduction t.
masking t.
masquerade t.
MAST t.
Mathieu t.
Matti-Russe t.
Mazet t.
McCauley t.
McConnell t.
McElfresh-Dobyns-O'Brien t.
McElvenny t.
McFarland-Osborne t.
McFarlane t.
McGoon t.
McKeever-Buck elbow t.
McLaughlin-Hay t.
McLean t.
McMaster t.
McReynolds open reduction t.
McVay t.
Meares-Stamey t.
mechanical ventilation anesthetic t.
medial cortical overlap t.
medial heel skive t.
Mehn-Quigley t.
membrane catheter t.
Menghini biopsy t.
Mensor-Scheck t.
Merendino t.
Messerklinger t.
Meyerding-Van Demark t.
Michal II t.
microsurgery t.

NOTES

technique *(continued)*

microtransducer t.
micro-tubulotomy t.
microvascular t.
midface degloving t.
Milch cuff resection of ulna t.
Milch elbow t.
Milford mallet finger t.
Millen t.
mille pattes t.
Millesi modified t.
minimal-access t.
minimal leak t.
minimally invasive surgical t.
Mital elbow release t.
miter t.
Mitrofanoff continent urinary diversion t.
Mizuno t.
Mizuno-Hirohata-Kashiwagi t.
modified Belsey fundoplication t.
modified brachial t.
modified Cantwell t.
modified Hassan open t.
modified Pomeroy t.
modified Sacks-Vine push-pull t.
modified Seldinger t.
modified Toupe t.
Moe scoliosis t.
Mohs fresh-tissue t.
Mohs fresh tissue chemosurgery t.
Mohs microsurgery t.
monitored anesthesia care anesthetic t.
monitoring t.
Monticelli-Spinelli distraction t.
Moore t.
morcellation t.
Morgan-Casscells meniscus suturing t.
Morrison t.
Mose t.
motor point block anesthetic t.
MPGR t.
MP-RAGE t.
Mubarak-Hargens decompression t.
mucosal relaxing incision t.
Mueller t.
Mullins blade t.
multiple inert gas elimination t. (MIGET)
multiple-port incisions t.
muscle energy t.
muscle-splitting t.
Nalebuff-Millender lateral band mobilization t.
nasotracheal intubation anesthetic t.
nasovesicular catheter t.

Nealon t.
needle-knife t.
needle thoracentesis t.
needle-through-needle single interspace t.
nerve stimulator anesthetic t.
neural arch resection t.
neuroablative t.
neuroleptanalgesia anesthetic t.
Neviaser acromioclavicular t.
Neviaser-Wilson-Gardner t.
Nicholas five-in-one reconstruction t.
Nicholas ligament t.
Niebauer-King t.
Nikaidoh-Bex t.
Nirschl t.
Nissen fundoplication t.
Nissen-Rosseti fundoplication t.
nitrous oxide/opioid/barbiturate anesthetic t.
nitrous oxide-oxygen-opioid anesthetic t. (N_2O/O_2/opioid anesthetic technique)
no-leak t.
noninvasive t.
non-rib-spreading thoracotomy incision t.
N_2O/O_2/opioid anesthetic t. nitrous oxide-oxygen-opioid anesthetic technique
Norfolk t.
Northern blot t.
no-touch t.
N2-Sargenti t.
Oakley-Fulthorpe t.
Ober-Barr transfer t.
Ober tendon t.
O'Brien akinesia t.
Obtura injectable t.
Ochterlony gel diffusion t.
off-center isoperistaltic t.
Ogata t.
Okamura t.
Ollier t.
Omer-Capen t.
one-lung ventilation anesthetic t.
one-phase subperiosteal implant t.
one-pour t.
onlay t.
onlay-tube-onlay urethroplasty t.
open drop t.
open flap t.
open palm t.
open-sky t.
operative t.
O'Phelan t.
oral anesthetic t.

Orandi t.
orbital exenteration gastroscopic access t.
Orticochea scalping t.
Osborne-Cotterill elbow t.
Osgood modified t.
Osmond-Clarke t.
Ostrup harvesting t.
Ouchterlony t.
outside-to-outside arthroscopy t.
Overhauser t.
over-the-wire t.
Oxford t.
Pacey t.
Pack t.
Pagenstecher suture t.
Palfyn suture t.
Palmer t.
Palmer-Widen shoulder t.
Palomo t.
pants-over-vest t.
Papineau t.
Paquin t.
paradoxical t.
parallel t.
paralleling t.
paresthesia anesthetic t.
Parrish-Mann hammertoe t.
Parvin gravity t.
PAS t.
passive gliding t.
patch t.
Paterson t.
patient-controlled analgesia anesthetic t.
Paulos ligament t.
Pauwels t.
Peacock transposing t.
peg and socket t.
pelviscopic clip ligation t.
Percoll t.
percutaneous t.
perfusion hypothermia t.
perfusion measurement t.
peribulbar anesthetic t.
peripheral nerve block anesthetic t.
Perry t.
Perry-Nickel t.
Perry-O'Brien-Hodgson t.
Perry-Robinson cervical t.
Pheasant elbow t.
Phemister-Bonfiglio t.

Phemister onlay bone graft t.
phrenic nerve block anesthetic t.
Pichlmayer t.
Pierrot-Murphy tendon t.
plaque t.
plastic matrix t.
PNF t.
Pólya t.
Ponsky pull or guidewire insertion t.
porcelain cervical contact and single bake t.
porcelain cervical ditching t.
Porstmann t.
Porter-Richardson-Vainio t.
posterior flap t.
posterolateral costotransversectomy t.
postresection filling t.
Pratt t.
presaturation t.
preservation t.
pressure half-time t.
Pringle vascular control t.
Proetz displacement t.
prograde t.
projection-reconstruction t.
projective t.
pseudobiopsy t.
PSSE t.
Puddu tendon t.
pull-through t.
pulmonary artery catheterization anesthetic t.
Pulvertaft weave t.
push-back t.
push plus retraction t.
push-pull T t.
quadrant sampling t.
Quartey t.
Quénu nail plate removal t.
quick angulation t.
Quickert three-suture t.
radiographic t.
radionuclide t.
Rainville t.
Ralston-Thompson pseudoarthrosis t.
Ranawat DeFiore-Straub t.
rapid pull-through esophageal manometry t.
rapid scan t.
rapid-sequence induction anesthetic t.

T

NOTES

733

technique *(continued)*
    Rashkind balloon t.
    Ray-Clancy-Lemon t.
    Rayhack t.
    reattribution t.
    rebreathing t.
    Rebuck skin window t.
    recanalization t.
    recombinant DNA t.
    reconstruction t.
    rectal anesthetic t.
    reduction t.
    regional anesthetic t.
    Reichel-Pólya t.
    Reichenheim t.
    relaxation t.
    rescue t.
    retained papilla t.
    retrobulbar anesthetic t.
    retrograde tracheal intubation anesthetic t.
    reverse wedge t.
    rhythmic initiation t.
    ribbon arch t.
    Richter suture t.
    Ricketts-Abrams t.
    Rideau t.
    right-angle t.
    Riordan tendon transfer t.
    Risser t.
    Ritter-Oleson t.
    Roberts t.
    Robinson-Southwick fusion t.
    Rockwood-Green t.
    Rogers cervical fusion t.
    rollerball t.
    roll-tube t.
    Rood t.
    Rosalki t.
    Royle-Thompson transfer t.
    RPT t.
    Russe t.
    Russell t.
    Ryerson t.
    sacral bar t.
    Saeed t.
    Saenger suture t.
    Sage-Clark t.
    Saha transfer t.
    Sakellarides-Deweese t.
    saline t.
    Salter t.
    Sammarco-DiRaimondo modification of Elmslie t.
    Sarmiento trochanteric fracture t.
    Scaglietti closed reduction t.
    Schaberg-Harper-Allen t.
    Schauwecker patellar wiring t.
    Scheie t.
    Schepens t.
    Schepsis-Leach t.
    Schlatter gastrectomy t.
    Schnute wedge resection t.
    Schober t.
    Schonander t.
    Schoonmaker-King single-catheter t.
    scleral search coil t.
    Scott glenoplasty t.
    screw insertion t.
    Scudder t.
    Scuderi t.
    sealed envelope t.
    Sealy-Laragh t.
    sectional t.
    section freeze substitution t.
    Seddon t.
    Seldinger percutaneous t.
    Seldinger retrograde wire/intubation t.
    selective bronchial catheterization anesthetic t.
    Sell-Frank-Johnson extensor shift t.
    Semb nephrectomy t.
    semitendinosus t.
    Semm Z t.
    sensorineural acuity level t.
    Serafin t.
    Sever modification of Fairbank t.
    Sewall t.
    sextant t.
    sharp dissection t.
    Sharrard transfer t.
    shave excision t.
    Sheehan and Dodge t.
    Sherk-Probst t.
    Shirodkar suture t.
    shish-kebab t.
    short-cone t.
    short lever accessory movement t.
    Silber t.
    Silfverskiöld lengthening t.
    silver dollar t.
    Simon suture t.
    Simonton t.
    Singer-Blom endoscopic tracheoesophageal puncture t.
    single-pour t.
    single proximal portal t.
    single-shot imaging t.
    single space t.
    skewer t.
    skin expansion t.
    skin window t.
    Skoog t.
    SL t.
    sleeve t.

sling and blanket t.
sling and reef t.
sling/wrapping t.
slit catheter t.
Slocum amputation t.
Slocum fusion t.
slot-blot t.
smiley-face knotting t.
Smith Indian t.
Smith-Petersen t.
Smith-Robinson t.
snapshot GRASS t.
snare t.
Snellen suture t.
Sofield femoral deficiency t.
soluble gas t.
Somatome DRG CT t.
Somerville t.
Sones t.
sonication t.
Southern blot t.
Sparks mandrel t.
Speed-Boyd radial-ulnar t.
sperm micro-aspiration retrieval t.
sphincter-saving t.
sphincter-sparing t.
Spiller-Frazier t.
spinal anesthetic t.
spinal fusion t.
spinal mobilization t.
spiral CT t.
Spivack gastrotomy t.
split-and-roll t.
split-bone t.
split-course t.
split cuff nipple t.
spontaneous ventilation anesthetic t.
Sprague arthroscopic t.
SPT t.
Staheli t.
Stamm-Kader gastrotomy t.
Stanisavljevic t.
stapled reconstruction t.
Staples t.
STAR t.
Stark-Moore-Ashworth-Boyes t.
startle t.
Starzl t.
static dilation t.
station pull-through esophageal
  manometry t.
Steffee instrumentation t.

stellate ganglion block anesthetic t.
stent-through-wire mesh t.
step-by-step t.
stepladder incision t.
stereotactic automated t.
stereotactic core biopsy t.
sterile t.
Sternberger antibody sandwich t.
Stewart-Hamilton cardiac output t.
Stiegmann-Goff t.
Stiles-Bunnell transfer t.
Stillman t.
still radiography t.
Stimson anterior shoulder
  reduction t.
stimulated gracilis neosphincter t.
STIR t.
Stoll dilution egg count t.
strain/counterstrain t.
Strassman t.
Straub t.
Strayer tendon t.
Strickland t.
strip biopsy resection t.
strut fusion t.
Studebaker t.
subpectoral implantation t.
subperiosteal implant one-phase t.
subtraction t.
suction-irrigation t.
sufentanil/enflurane t.
sufentanil/midazolam t.
superior mesenterorenal bypass t.
surface cooling t.
surgical enucleation t.
surgical neurangiographic t.
surveillance t.
sustained pressure t.
suture anchor t.
Swanson t.
Swiss roll embedding t.
switched B-gradient t.
sympathetic blockade anesthetic t.
sympathetic ganglion block
  anesthetic t.
Tajima suture t.
tandem clipping t.
Taylor t.
Taylor-Daniel-Weiland t.
telescoping suture t.
tension band wiring t.
Terzis t.

NOTES

technique *(continued)*

test dose anesthetic t.
Teuffer t.
Thal fundoplication t.
thermal expansion t.
thermocatalytic t.
thermodilution t.
thermo-photocatalytic t.
thiopental/sufentanil/desflurane/nitrous oxide anesthetic t.
Thomas t.
Thomas-Thompson-Straub transfer t.
Thompson t.
Thompson-Henry t.
Thompson-Loomer t.
thoracic epidural anesthetic t.
thoracolumbar spondylosis surgical t.
threaded-hole-first t.
three-portal t.
tissue-sparing t.
titration t.
Todd-Evans stepladder tracheal dilatation t.
Tohen tendon t.
Tompkins median bivalving t.
tongue-and-groove suture t.
topical anesthetic t.
Torg t.
Torgerson-Leach modified t.
total etch t.
total fundoplication t.
total intravenous anesthetic t.
Toupe t.
tracheal extubation anesthetic t.
tracheal intubation anesthetic t.
tracheal suction anesthetic t.
transarterial anesthetic t.
transcranial electrical stimulation anesthetic t.
transdermal anesthetic t.
transiliac bar t.
translaryngeal guided intubation anesthetic t.
transmucosal drug administration anesthetic t.
transtracheal jet ventilation anesthetic t.
trapezius stimulation anesthetic t.
Trethowan-Stamm-Simmonds-Menelaus-Haddad t.
triangulation t.
triangulation t. for arthroscope
triple-wire t.
trocar t.
trocar-cannula t.
Trusler aortic valve t.
tubal ligation band t.

tube-shift t.
tube-within-tube t.
Tuffier morcellement t.
Tullos t.
tumbling t.
Turco clubfoot release t.
turn-and-suction t.
turn-and-suction biopsy t.
Turnbull t.
twist-off t.
two-layer open t.
two-needle t.
two-patch t.
two-portal t.
two-pour t.
two-sleeve t.
two-stage tendon grafting t.
two-step t.
ultrasound anesthetic t.
uncut Collis-Nissen fundoplication t.
underlay fascia t.
unilateral inguinal hernia repair t.
unitunnel t.
unlocking spiral t.
upgated t.
Ussing chamber t.
Van Lint modified t.
Van Milligen eyelid repair t.
Vastamäki t.
Veleanu-Rosianu-Ionescu t.
velocity catheter t.
venous access t.
ventral bending t.
Verdan t.
vertical-cut t.
Vidal-Ardrey fracture t.
video-assisted t.
videofluoroscopic t.
video transurethral resection t.
Vim-Silverman t.
volumetric t.
Volz-Turner reattachment t.
von Haberer-Finney gastrectomy t.
Vulpius-Compere tendon t.
Wadsworth t.
Wagner open reduction t.
Wagoner cervical t.
Waldhausen subclavian flap t.
Wallace t.
Wanger reduction t.
Warner-Farber ankle fixation t.
Warwick and Ashken t.
wash t.
washed field t.
water-suppression t.
Watkins fusion t.
Watson t.
Watson-Cheyne t.

wax-matrix t.
wax pattern thermal expansion t.
Weaver-Dunn acromioclavicular t.
Weber-Brunner-Freuler-Boitzy t.
Weber-Vasey traction-absorption
  wiring t.
Weckesser t.
Weinstein-Ponseti t.
Wertheim-Bohlman t.
West-Soto-Hall patellar t.
Whitesides t.
Whitesides-Kelly cervical t.
whole blood lysis t.
Wick catheter t.
Wickham t.
Williams-Haddad t.
Willi glass crown t.
Wilson t.
Wilson-Jacobs tibial fracture
  fixation t.
Wilson-McKeever shoulder t.
window t.
Windson-Insall-Vince grafting t.
Winograd t.
Winter spondylolisthesis t.
wire removal t.
Wirth-Jager tendon t.
Wölfler suture t.
Woodward t.
^{133}Xe intravenous injection t.
xenon-washout t.
Young t.
Young-Dees t.
Zancolli rerouting t.
Zariczny t.
Zarins-Rowe ligament t.
Zavala t.
Zazepen-Gamidov t.
Zeier transfer t.
Zielke t.
Zoeller-Clancy t.
Zuker and Manktelow t.
technocausis
technology
endoscopic t.
fluorescent optode t.
signal extraction t. (SET)
tectobulbar tract
tectocephalic
tectocephaly
tectology

tectonic
t. epikeratoplasty
t. keratoplasty
tectopontine tract
tectora
membrane t.
tectorial membrane
tectospinal
t. decussation
t. tract
TEE
transesophageal echocardiography
teeth
extruded t.
full-surface micro mesh t.
t. ligation
Logan traction bow with t.
separation of t.
straight-pin t.
tube t.
TEF
tracheoesophageal fistula
Teflon
T. nasobiliary tube
T. periurethral injection
T. sling rectopexy
T. tube graft
Teflon-coated Dacron suture
Teflon-pledgeted suture
teflurane
TEG
thromboelastograph
thromboelastography
tegmentotomy
tela, pl. **telae**
t. subcutanea
t. submucosa
t. submucosa pharyngis
t. subserosa
t. vasculosa
telangiectasia
telangioma
telecobalt therapy
Telectronic electrical stimulation device
telelectrocardiogram
telencephalic malformation
telencephalization
telepresence surgery
telerobotic-assisted laparoscopic surgery
telescoping
t. nail
t. suture technique

T

NOTES

televised radiofluoroscopy
TeLinde operation
TEM
    transanal endoscopic microsurgery
temperature
    ambient t.
    axilla t.
    basal body t.
    bladder t.
    body t.
    brain t.
    esophagus t.
    flash-point t.
    t. gradient
    heat production t.
    intraoperative core body t.
    normal body t.
    t., pulse, and respiration
    skin t.
    t. threshold
temperature-compensated vaporizer
Temp-Kuff blood pressure cuff
temple
tempora (*pl. of* tempus)
temporal
    t. aponeurosis
    t. apophysis
    t. artery biopsy
    t. bone
    t. bone fracture
    t. bone tumor
    t. branch of facial nerve
    t. canal
    t. fascia
    t. fossa
    t. line
    t. lobectomy
    t. lobe radiation
    t. muscle
    t. orientation
    t. plane
    t. process
    t. region of head
    t. ridge
    t. space infection
    t. squama
    t. surface
    t. veins
    t. venules of retina
    t. wedge
temporal-cerebral arterial anastomosis
temporalis
    t. fascia flap
    t. muscle
    t. muscle flap
temporary
    t. cavity phenomenon
    t. diverting colostomy

    t. end colostomy
    t. loop ileostomy
    t. pacemaker placement
    t. restoration
temporization
temporoauricular
temporofrontal tract
temporohyoid
temporomalar
temporomandibular
    t. articular disk
    t. joint
    t. joint articulation
    t. joint dislocation
    t. ligament
    t. luxation
    t. nerve
temporomaxillary
    t. vein
temporo-occipital
temporoparietal
    t. muscle
temporoparietalis muscle
temporopontine tract
temporosphenoid
temporozygomatic
    t. suture
tempus, pl. tempora
Tena pouch
tender
    t. line
    t. point
tenderness
tendines (*pl. of* tendo)
tendinitis
tendinomyoplastic amputation
tendinoplasty
tendinosuture
tendinous
    t. arch
    t. arch of levator ani muscle
    t. arch of pelvic fascia
    t. chiasm of the digital tendons
    t. cords
    t. inscription
    t. insertion
    t. opening
tendo, pl. tendines
    t. Achillis
    t. calcaneus
    t. conjunctivus
tendolysis
tendon
    Achilles t.
    attenuation of t.
    calcaneal t.
    calcanean t.
    central t. of diaphragm

t. centralization
central t. of perineum
common extensor t.
conjoined t.
conjoint t.
digital extensor t.
elbow extensor t.
t. excursion
extensor carpi radialis brevis t.
extensor carpi radialis longus t.
extensor carpi ulnaris t.
extensor digiti minimi t.
extensor digiti quinti t.
extensor digitorum brevis t.
extensor digitorum communis t.
extensor digitorum longus t.
extensor hallucis longus t.
extensor indicis proprius t.
extensor pollicis brevis t.
extensor pollicis longus t.
extensor quinti t.
t. graft
hamstring t.
heel t.
t. interposition arthroplasty
long head biceps t.
obturator internus t.
peroneal t.
peroneal brevis t.
peroneal longus t.
pronator teres t.
t. repair
t. rupture
t. sheath of superior oblique
   muscle
t. sheath of tibialis anterior muscle
t. sheath of tibialis posterior
   muscle
t. suture
tenotomy of ocular t.
thumb extensor t.
toe extensor t.
t. transplantation
trefoil t.
wrist extensor t.
tendoplasty
tendotomy
tendovaginal
tenectomy
tenesmus
tenia, pl. **teniae**
   teniae coli

colic teniae
free t.
t. libera
mesocolic t.
t. mesocolica
omental t.
t. omentalis
t. terminalis
teniae of Valsalva
tenial
teniamyotomy
tenodesis
   calcaneal t.
   extensor t.
   MacIntosh extra-articular t.
tenolysis
tenomyoplasty
tenomyotomy
Tenon
   T. membrane
   T. space
tenonectomy
tenontology
tenontomyoplasty
tenontomyotomy
tenontoplastic
tenontoplasty
tenontotomy
tenophyte
tenoplastic
   t. reconstruction
tenoplasty
tenorrhaphy
tenosuture
tenosynovectomy
   dorsal t.
   flexor t.
tenosynovitis
tenotomy
   adductor t.
   Arroyo t.
   Arruga t.
   Braun shoulder t.
   curb t.
   extensor t.
   Fowler central slip t.
   free t.
   graduated t.
   intrasheath t.
   t. of metatarsophalangeal joint
   t. of ocular tendon
   t. operation

NOTES

tenotomy *(continued)*
    percutaneous t.
    semiopen sliding t.
    sliding t.
    subcutaneous tibialis posterior t.
    transverse t.
    Veleanu-Rosianu-Ionescu adductor t.
    Z marginal t.
    Z-plasty t.
tensile
Tensilon injection
tension
    t. by applanation
    t. band fixation
    t. band wire tamp
    t. band wiring technique
    t. endothorax
    extrapolated end-tidal carbon
      dioxide t. (PETCO$_2$)
    t. fracture
    isometric venous t.
    t. suture
    twitch t.
tension-free
    t.-f. anastomosis
    t.-f. Millesi nerve graft
    t.-f. suture
tension-length relation
tensor
    t. fascia femoris flap
    t. fascia lata muscle
    t. fascia lata muscle flap
    t. insertion
    t. muscle of fascia lata
    t. muscle of soft palate
    t. tarsi muscle
    t. veli palati muscle
tent
    oxygen t.
    sponge t.
tenth cranial nerve
tentorial
    t. herniation
    t. laceration
    t. notch
    t. pressure
    t. ring
    t. sinus
tentorium
    t. cerebelli
    t. of hypophysis
Tenzel rotational cheek flap
teratoblastoma
teratocarcinoma
    pineal t.
teratogenic medication
teratogen-induced malformation
teratologic dislocation

teratomatous
teratoneuroma
teratospermia
terebration
teres
    anterior pronator t.
    t. major muscle
    pronator t.
tergal
tergum
terminad
terminal
    t. bronchiole
    t. cisterna
    t. colostomy
    t. crest
    t. duct carcinoma
    t. filum
    t. ganglion
    t. head
    t. hinge position
    t. ileal pouch
    t. ileal resection
    t. ileostomy
    t. ileum intubation
    t. jaw relation record
    t. line
    t. neosalpingostomy
    nociceptor afferent peripheral t.
    t. part
    t. plane
    t. reservoir syndrome
    t. Syme procedure
    t. ventriculostomy
    t. web
terminalization
termino-terminal anastomosis
terminus, pl. termini
    termini generales
    incision t.
terrace
Terramycin I.M. injection
Terson operation
tertiary amputation
Terzis technique
TES
    transcutaneous electric stimulation
tessellation
Tessier
    T. classification
    T. craniofacial operation
    T. osteotomy
test
    abduction external rotation t.
    acoustic stimulation t.
    Adson t.
    air t.
    Allen t.

T

Apley compression t.
articulation t.
artificial erection t.
axial compression t.
balloon expulsion t.
baroreceptor t.
Behçet skin puncture t.
Bielschowsky-Parks head-tilt, three-step t.
Bielschowsky three-step head-tilt t.
bladder neck elevation t.
Bonney t.
breast stimulation contraction t.
breath excretion t.
Brodie-Trendelenburg tourniquet t.
bronchial inhalation challenge t.
bronchoprovocation t.
caffeine and halothane contracture t. (CHCT)
carpal compression t.
cavity t.
chlormerodrin accumulation t.
CLO t.
closed patch t.
CO_2 inhalation t.
cold pressor t. (CPT)
compression t.
concentration performance t.
confrontation visual field t.
corneal staining t.
Cortrosyn stimulation t.
Crampton t.
deep articulation t.
diagnostic articulation t.
differential ureteral catheterization t.
Digit Symbol Substitution T.
disk space saline acceptance t.
t. dose anesthetic technique
double Maddox rod t.
DR-70 tumor marker t.
Dunnett t.
Dupuy-Dutemps dacryocystorhinostomy dye t.
Durkan carpal compression t.
dye exclusion t.
dye reduction spot t.
ergonovine provocation t.
excitability t.
external rotation-abduction stress t.
external rotation-recurvatum t.
extrastimulus t.
extrinsic entrapment t.

fast-flush t.
Feagin shoulder dislocation t.
femoral nerve traction t.
fetal acoustic stimulation t.
Finger Oscillation T.
fistula t.
flexion-rotation-drawer knee instability t.
fluctuation t.
fluorescein instillation t.
fluorescein string t.
foramen compression t.
foraminal compression t.
forced generation t.
forearm ischemic exercise t.
forearm supination t.
forward traction t.
Friberg microsurgical agglutination t.
gastric accommodation t.
germ tube t.
hair bulb incubation t.
head compression t.
head distraction t.
head-down tilt t.
head-dropping t.
head-tilt t.
head-up tilt t.
head-up tilt-table t.
high-altitude simulation t.
Hollander t.
Howard t.
Hughston external rotation recurvatum t.
human ovum fertilization t.
hyperventilation t.
iliac compression t.
implantation t.
Ingram-Withers-Speltz motor t.
t. injection
Korotkoff t.
Kruskal-Wallis t.
labyrinthine fistula t.
lacrimal irrigation t.
lidocaine t.
line t.
lumbar extension t.
lumbar rotation t.
Luria-Delbruck fluctuation t.
Maddox rod t.
Maddox wing t.
Mann-Whitney t.

NOTES

test *(continued)*
   Marshall t.
   Marshall-Marchetti t.
   Maudsley Mentation T.
   maximum stimulation t.
   MHA-TP t.
   mobilization t.
   MUGA exercise stress t.
   Multistage Maximal Effort exercise stress t.
   nasal provocation t.
   nerve excitability t.
   neutralization t.
   nipple stimulation t.
   nonparametric t.
   Noyes flexion rotation drawer t.
   Object Classification T.
   obturator t.
   occlusive patch t.
   one-hour office pad t.
   one-minute endoscopy room t.
   open application t.
   open patch t.
   Pachon t.
   parametric t.
   Parks-Bielschowsky three-step head-tilt t.
   penetration t.
   Peptavlon stimulation t.
   percutaneous pressure ureteral perfusion t.
   perimeter corneal reflex t.
   perineal nerve terminal motor latency t.
   peritoneal equilibration t.
   Perthes t.
   prick puncture t.
   prism adaptation t.
   promontory stimulation t.
   prone extension t.
   protection t.
   provocation t.
   provocative chelation t.
   Q-tip t.
   Rapoport t.
   regurgitation t.
   Ross-Jones t.
   Rotation t.
   rotation drawer t.
   rotation recurvatum t.
   scapular approximation t.
   scarification t.
   screening t.
   side-lying iliac compression t.
   skin-puncture t.
   SLR with external rotation t.
   t. solution
   Spatial Orientation Memory T.
   sperm immobilization t.
   split renal function t.
   squeeze pressure profile of anal sphincter t.
   star construction t.
   station t.
   Stewart t.
   stimulation t.
   straight catheter t.
   string t.
   Student-Newman-Keuls t.
   Suprathreshold Adaptation T.
   t t.
   Thompson t.
   tissue compression t.
   tourniquet t.
   traction t.
   transillumination t.
   Trieger t.
   trunk incurvation t.
   t. tube
   tube dilution t.
   tube precipitin t.
   tumor skin t.
   twitch height t.
   two-point discrimination t.
   University of Pennsylvania Smell Identification T.
   vaginal cornification t.
   vaginal mucification t.
   Valpar Whole Body Range of Motion T.
   vertical compression t.
   vibration threshold t.
   Visual-Motor Integration T.
   in vitro contracture t.
   Von Frey t.
   walking ventilation t.
   washout t.
   Whitaker pressure-perfusion t.
   Wilcoxon signed-rank t.
   wire loop t.
testalgia
Tes-Tape
testectomy
tester
   Neurometer CPT/C quantitative sensory nerve function t.
testes *(pl. of* testis)
testicle
testicular
   t. adrenal-like tissue
   t. appendage
   t. artery
   t. biopsy
   t. carcinoma
   t. cord
   t. duct

t. ectopia
t. feminization syndrome
t. mass
t. metastasis
t. plexus
t. rupture
t. tumor
t. veins
testiculus
testing
compression t.
confrontation t.
Disk-Criminator sensory t.
Doppler ultrasound segmental blood
pressure t.
Model 810 axial closed-loop
hydraulic mechanical t.
palpation t.
patch t.
penile injection t.
rotation t.
tilt-table t.
testis, pl. **testes**
t. cords
cryptorchid t.
dystopia transversa externa t.
ectopia t.
ectopic t.
t. fracture
interstitial cell tumor of t.
movable t.
occult primary tumor of t.
retractile t.
undescended t.
yolk sac tumor of t.
testitis
testoid
tetanic
t. fade
t. stimulation
t. stimulation method
tetanization
tetanus
cephalic t.
extensor t.
head t.
traumatic t.
tetany
duration t.
hyperventilation t.
postoperative t.
tethered cord syndrome

tetracaine
t. hydrochloride
hyperbaric t.
liposome-encapsulated t. (LET)
t. with dextrose
tetraethylammonium
tetragonus
tetralogy of Fallot
Teuffer
T. technique
T. tendo calcaneus repair
Teutleben ligament
Tevdek pledgeted suture
TEVP
transesophageal ventricular pacing
Texas Scottish Rite Hospital (TSRH)
texture
echo t.
TFD
transdermal fentanyl device
T-fracture
T-grommet ventilation tube
Thal
T. esophageal stricture repair
T. esophagogastroscopy
T. esophagogastrostomy
T. fundic patch operation
T. fundoplasty
T. fundoplication
T. fundoplication method
T. fundoplication procedure
T. fundoplication technique
T. stricturoplasty
thalamectomy
thalamencephalic
thalamencephalon
thalamic
t. circulation
t. pain
t. plane
thalamic-subthalamic hemorrhage
**thalamocaudate arteriovenous
malformation**
thalamostriate veins
thalamotomy
gamma t.
staged bilateral stereotactic t.
stereotactic t.
stereotactic VIM t.
stereotactic VL t.
Vim t.
VL t.

T

NOTES

THAM
　　tris(hydroxymethyl)-aminomethane
thanatopsy
Thane method
theater
thebesian
　　t. circulation
　　t. veins
thecal
　　t. sac
　　t. sac compression
thecoma
　　luteinized t.
　　ovarian t.
Theden method
The Hockey Stick articulating stylet
Theile muscle
Theirsch-Duplay repair
thele
theleplasty
thenad
thenal
thenar
　　t. eminence
　　t. flap
　　t. prominence
　　t. space
thenen
thenyldiamine hydrochloride
theory
　　Burnet-Talmadge-Lederberg t. of
　　　antibody formation
　　Ehrlich t. of antibody formation
　　Jerne t. of antibody formation
　　Pauling t. of antibody formation
TheraPEP pre-respiratory therapy
　treatment
therapeutic
　　t. anesthesia
　　t. approach
　　t. colonoscopy
　　t. dissection
　　t. insemination
　　t. iridectomy
　　t. irradiation
　　t. laparoscopy
　　t. nerve block
　　t. phlebotomy
　　t. upper endoscopy
TheraPulse bed
therapy
　　ablation t.
　　ablative laser t.
　　active appliance t.
　　active assistive motion t.
　　adjuvant chemoradiation t.
　　adjuvant drug t.
　　adjuvant whole-brain radiation t.

aerosol t.
alternate-day t.
amplitude-summation interferential
　current t.
anaclitic t.
angina-guided t.
antiarrhythmic t.
antiemetic t.
antihormonal t.
antireflux t.
antithrombotic t.
apotreptic t.
argon laser t.
around-the-clock oral maintenance
　bronchodilator t.
augmentation t.
balloon photodynamic t.
belly bath t.
biomagnetic t.
bite plane t.
boron neutron-capture t.
Bragg peak proton-beam t.
brisement t.
buprenorphine narcotic analgesic t.
Cancell t.
cerebral protective t.
chest physical t.
Clinitron air-fluidized t.
coagulative laser t.
combined chemoradiation t.
compartmental
　radioimmunoglobulin t.
concomitant t.
conditioning t.
conformal radiation t.
conservative t.
contact dissolution t.
continuous renal replacement t.
convulsive t.
corrective t.
Crozat t.
deep chest t.
device t.
diagnostic surgical t.
diathermic t.
diclofenac analgesic t.
dilation t.
dressing t.
electrical stimulation t.
electric aversion t.
electric differential t.
electroconvulsive t.
electrotherapeutic sleep t.
endocavitary radiation t.
endoscopic hemostatic t.
endoscopic injection t.
endoscopic laser t.
endoscopic pancreatic t.

endourological t.
endovascular t.
enterostomal t.
esophageal photodynamic t.
ethanol injection t.
expansion and activator t.
extended field irradiation t.
external beam radiation t.
external vacuum t.
external x-ray t.
ex vivo gene t.
factor replacement t.
fast neutron radiation t.
fetal drug t.
focused radiation t.
fractionated radiation t.
frappage t.
frequency-difference interferential current t.
functional orthodontic t.
gastrointestinal complication of radiation t.
gene replacement t.
gene-transfer t.
grenz ray t.
HDR intracavitary radiation t.
hemofiltration t.
hepatic arterial t.
high-dose t.
high-voltage t.
hyperbaric oxygen t.
hyperthermia t.
ImmTher t.
immunocompetent tissue t.
implosive t.
incremental t.
indirect pulpal t.
Indoklon t.
InFerno moist heat t.
infrared t.
inhalation t.
injection t.
innovative t.
instillation t.
insulin coma t.
insulin shock t.
interlesional t.
internal radiation t.
interstitial photodynamic t.
interstitial radiation t.
intra-arterial t.
intracavernous injection t.

intracavitary radiation boost t.
intracorporeal injection t.
intralesional t.
intraperitoneal radiation t.
intrathecal t.
intravascular fluid t.
intravenous ozone t.
intraventricular t.
invasive t.
ischemia-guided medical t.
isolation perfusion t.
I.V. fluid t.
Kelsey unloading exercise t.
ketoprofen analgesic t.
laser t.
LDR intracavitary radiation t.
Livingstone t.
long-term oxygen t.
Lymphapress compression t.
Manchester system for radium t.
manipulative t.
microcurrent t.
microwave t.
morphine narcotic analgesic t.
MTBE t.
multimodal adjuvant t.
multimodality t.
multiple t.
myoablative t.
myofunctional t.
Nd:YAG laser t.
neoadjuvant t.
neodymium:YAG laser t.
neutron beam t.
neutron capture t.
nonspecific t.
occlusal t.
occlusion t.
occlusive t.
occupational t.
ocular radiation t.
orthodontic t.
outpatient physical t.
oxygen t.
palliative t.
pancreatic intraluminal radiation t.
parenteral t.
Paris method for radium t.
particle beam radiation t.
PEI t.
PEMF t.
penile injection t.

NOTES

therapy *(continued)*
 penile vein occlusion t.
 percussion t.
 percutaneous embolization t.
 percutaneous ethanol injection t.
 percutaneous microwave
  coagulation t.
 percutaneous transcatheter t.
 perfusion t.
 periodontal t.
 perioperative antibiotic t.
 photoradiation t.
 physical t.
 placebo t.
 Polar wrap t.
 pool t.
 positional release t.
 postnatal t.
 postoperative anticoagulation t.
 postradiation t.
 posttransplant immunosuppression t.
 prenatal t.
 preventive intravesical t.
 primary healing after radiation t.
 progestational t.
 progestogen support t.
 programmed t.
 prophylactic antibiotic t.
 protein shock t.
 proton pump inhibition t.
 pulp canal t.
 pyretic t.
 quadrangular t.
 quadrantectomy, axillary dissection,
  radiation t.
 quadruple t.
 quatro t.
 radiation t.
 radioimmunoglobulin t.
 radiopharmaceutical t.
 range of motion t.
 red-filter t.
 reflex t.
 rehydration t.
 renal infusion t.
 renal replacement t.
 rescue t.
 retinoid t.
 rheologic t.
 ROM t.
 root canal t.
 rotation t.
 saline injection t.
 salvage t.
 sandwich staghorn calculus t.
 sclerosing t.
 sedative t.
 skin lubrication t.

 soak t.
 social interaction t.
 sole laser t.
 somatic t.
 somatostatin infusion t.
 STAMP t.
 standard t.
 stem cell gene t.
 step-down t.
 stereotactic-assisted radiation t.
 stereotactic-focused radiation t.
 stereotactic radiation t.
 Stockholm technique for radium t.
 subcoma t.
 supranormal hemodynamic t.
 surgical t.
 systemic radioimmunoglobulin t.
 telecobalt t.
 thermal t.
 three-cornered t.
 three-dimensional conformal
  radiation t.
 timed-sequential t.
 tocolytic t.
 tongue thrust t.
 total push t.
 transcatheter arterial embolization t.
 transfusion t.
 transurethral collagen injection t.
 transvenous t.
 triadic t.
 trial of conservative t.
 trimodality t.
 triple intrathecal t.
 tumor t.
 ultrasonic t.
 ultrasound t.
 ultrasound-guided shock wave t.
 voice t.
 volume t.
 whole-brain radiation t.
 wide-field radiation t.
 wide-range radiation t.
 will t.
 xenogenic cell t.
 x-ray t.

Theratouch 4.7 stimulator
therencephalous
thermal
 t. anesthesia
 t. balance
 t. coefficient expansion
 t. death point
 t. disinfection
 t. expansion technique
 t. keratoplasty
 t. rhizotomy
 t. sclerectomy

t. stimulation
t. therapy
thermally active method
thermal/perfusion balloon angioplasty
thermic anesthesia
thermistor
t. rectal thermometer
Yellow Springs Instruments t.
thermocatalytic technique
thermocauterectomy
thermocautery
thermochemotherapy
thermocoagulation
thermocouple
21-G needle t.
22-G needle t.
Mon-a-Therm t.
needle t.
thermodilution (TD)
t. cardiac output (TDCO)
t. method
t. technique
Thermo-Flex suture
thermogenesis
nonshivering t.
thermogram
thermographic examination
thermokeratoplasty
thermolysis
thermometer
basal body t.
Coretemp deep tissue t.
FirstTemp t.
Iso-Thermex 16-channel
electronic t.
Mon-a-Therm 6510 two-channel t.
thermistor rectal t.
thermometry
tympanic t.
thermopenetration
thermo-photocatalytic technique
thermoregulation
perianesthetic t.
thermoregulatory vasoconstriction
thermorhizotomy
thermosclerectomy
thermosclerostomy
thermosclerotomy
thermosector
ThermoVent heat and moisture
exchanger
thialbarbital

thiamylal sodium
thickened
t. nail
t. synovial membrane
thickening
endocardial t.
heel pad t.
postlumpectomy skin t.
thickness
Breslow t.
endometrial t.
end-systolic wall t. (ESWT)
soft tissue t.
Thiersch
T. anal incontinence operation
T. graft operation
T. medium split free graft
T. method
T. procedure
T. thin split free graft
T. tube
Thiersch-Duplay
T.-D. proximal tube procedure
T.-D. tube graft
T.-D. urethral construction
T.-D. urethroplasty
thiethylperazine maleate
thigh
t. bone
t. graft arteriovenous fistula
t. joint
thimble valvotomy
thin
t. basement membrane
t. basement membrane disease
t. section
thin-needle biopsy
thinning
corneal t.
thin-section axial image
thiol
t. augmentation
t. modification
thiolysis
thiopental
sodium t.
t. sodium
thiopental/sufentanil/desflurane/nitrous
oxide
t./s./d./n.o. anesthesia
t./s./d./n.o. anesthetic technique
Thioplex

T

NOTES

thiotepa
thiourea-resorcinol method
third
    t. cranial nerve
    t. degree burn
    t. degree radiation injury
    t. and fourth pharyngeal pouch syndrome
    t. occipital nerve
    t. parallel pelvic plane
    t. trochanter
    t. ventriculostomy
third-grade fusion
Thiry fistula
Thiry-Vella fistula
Thoma
    T. ampulla
Thomas
    T. classification
    T. extrapolated bar graft
    T. operation
    T. procedure
    T. technique
Thomas-Thompson-Straub transfer technique
Thom flap laryngeal reconstruction method
Thompson
    T. anterolateral approach
    T. anteromedial approach
    T. capsule flap pyeloplasty
    T. chin support
    T. excision
    T. ligament
    T. line
    T. posterior radial approach
    T. procedure
    T. quadricepsplasty
    T. resection
    T. technique
    T. telescoping V osteotomy
    T. test
Thompson-Epstein classification of femoral fracture
Thompson-Hatina method
Thompson-Henry technique
Thompson-Loomer technique
Thoms method
thoracal
thoracentesis
    needle t.
thoraces (*pl. of* thorax)
thoracic
    t. anesthesia
    t. aorta
    t. aortic cross-clamping (TACC)
    t. aortic dissection
    t. aortic plexus

    t. approach
    t. axis
    t. cage
    t. cardiac branches of vagus nerve
    t. cardiac nerve
    t. cavity
    t. compression syndrome
    t. diskectomy
    t. disk herniation
    t. duct
    t. duct fistula
    t. endometriosis syndrome
    t. epidural analgesia
    t. epidural anesthetic technique
    t. epidural catheterization
    t. facet fusion
    t. ganglia
    t. girdle
    t. great vessel
    t. index
    t. inlet soft tissue
    t. interspinales muscles
    t. interspinal muscle
    t. intertransversarii muscles
    t. intertransverse muscles
    t. kidney
    t. limb
    t. longissimus muscle
    t. outlet syndrome
    t. part of aorta
    t. part of esophagus
    t. part of spinal cord
    t. part of thoracic duct
    t. plane
    t. respiration
    t. rotator muscles
    t. spinal fusion
    t. spinal nerve
    t. spine
    t. spine biopsy
    t. spine fracture
    t. spine kyphotic deformity
    t. spine scoliotic deformity
    t. spine vertebral osteosynthesis
    t. splanchnic nerve
    t. stomach
    t. and thoracolumbar spine surgery
    t. veins
    t. vertebrae
    t. vertebral body
    t. wall
thoracicoabdominal
thoracicoacromial
thoracicohumeral
thoracis
    compages t.
thoracoabdominal
    t. esophagogastrectomy

t. extrapleural approach
t. incision
t. intrapleural approach
t. nerve
t. retroperitoneal lymphadenectomy
thoracoacromial
t. artery
t. flap
t. trunk
t. vein
thoracoceloschisis
thoracocentesis
thoracocyllosis
thoracocyrtosis
thoracodorsal
t. artery
t. nerve
thoracoepigastric
t. flap
t. vein
thoracograph
thoracolaparotomy
thoracolumbar
t. aponeurosis
t. burst fracture
t. fascia
t. junction surgical exposure
t. retroperitoneal approach
t. spine anterior exposure
t. spine fracture
t. spine fracture-dislocation
t. spine stabilization
t. spine vertebral osteosynthesis
t. spondylosis surgical technique
thoracolumbosacral orthoses - flexion, extension, lateral bending, and transverse rotation
thoracolysis
thoracomelus
thoracophrenolaparotomy
thoracoplasty
conventional t.
costoversion t.
Delorme t.
Fowler t.
Schede t.
Wilms t.
thoracopneumoplasty
thoracoschisis
thoracoscopic
t. pericardiectomy
t. talc insufflation

thoracoscopy
thoracostenosis
thoracosternotomy
thoracostomy
closed chest t.
tube t.
t. tube
thoracotomy
t. approach
axillary t.
esophagectomy with t.
t. incision
left-sided t.
Lewis t.
muscle-sparing t.
open t.
resuscitative t.
right-sided t.
t. scar
standard t.
Thora-Drain III chest drainage
Thora-Klex chest tube
Thora-Port port
thorascopic
t. apical pleurectomy
t. drainage
thorax, pl. thoraces
Peyrot t.
Thorel bundle
Thorn
T. maneuver
T. syndrome
Thornell microlaryngoscopy
Thornton fixating ring
thoroscopy
thread
t. suture
threaded-hole-first technique
three-body wear
three-bottle tidal suction tube
Three Color Concept of wound classification
three-cornered
t.-c. bone
t.-c. therapy
three-dimensional
t.-d. conformal radiation therapy
t.-d. Fourier transform gradient-echo imaging
t.-d. projection reconstruction imaging
t.-d. reconstruction

T

NOTES

three-dimensional-FATS method
three-loop ileal pouch
three-part fracture
three-pin Mayfield head fixation
three-plane deformity
three-point
    t.-p. bending moment
    t.-p. touch
three-portal technique
three-snip punctum operation
threshold
    apneic t.
    atrial defibrillation t.
    current perception t. (CPT)
    defibrillation t.
    detection t.
    displacement t.
    double-point t.
    experimental t.
    fibrillation t.
    flicker-fusion t.
    median detection t.
    noise detection t.
    pacemaker t.
    pressure pain t. (PPT)
    t. shift method
    speech detection t.
    stimulation t.
    TEAP t.
    temperature t.
    ventilation t.
throat
    t. anesthesia
Throat-E-Vac suction device
thrombase
thrombasthenia
thrombectomy
    chemical t.
    mechanical t.
    percutaneous rotational t.
    rotational t.
thrombi (pl. of thrombus)
thrombin
    human t.
    t. solution
thrombin-mediated consumptive state
thromboasthenia
thromboelastogram
thromboelastograph (TEG)
thromboelastographer
thromboelastography (TEG)
thromboembolectomy
    percutaneous aspiration t.
    rotating aspiration t.
thromboembolic (TE)
    t. fistula
thromboembolism

thromboendarterectomy
    pulmonary t. (PTE)
    renal t.
thrombolysis
    coronary t.
    T. in Myocardial Infarction (TIMI)
    selective intracoronary t.
    sonic t.
thrombopathy
thrombophlebitis
thromboplastin
    tissue t.
thrombosed internal and external hemorrhoid
thrombosin
thrombostasis
thrombotic
Thrombo-Wellcotest method
thrombus, pl. thrombi
    t. extension
through-and-through
    t.-a.-t. fracture
    t.-a.-t. laceration
    t.-a.-t. V-shaped horizontal osteotomy
through drainage
through-knee amputation
through-the-scope
    t.-t.-s. balloon dilation
    t.-t.-s. balloon removal
through-the-wall mattress suture
thrower fracture
thrust manipulation
thulium:YAG laser angioplasty
thumb
    t. deformity
    t. duplication
    t. extensor tendon
    t. metacarpophalangeal joint approach
    t. reconstruction
    t. web
thumb-in-palm deformity
thumbprinting
thymectomy
    neonatal t.
    video-assisted thoracoscopic t.
thymic
    t. arteries
    t. branches of internal thoracic artery
    t. carcinoma
    t. mass
    t. veins
thymicolymphatic
thymocyte NA+/H+ exchanger
thymol flocculation
thymolipoma

thymoma
thymus
    t. gland
thymusectomy
thyration indicator
thyroarytenoid
    t. muscle
thyrocele
thyrocervical
    t. trunk
thyrochondrotomy
thyroepiglottic
    t. ligament
    t. muscle
thyroglossal
    t. cyst surgery
    t. duct
    t. fistula
thyrohyal
thyrohyoid
    t. membrane
    t. muscle
thyroid
    t. adenoma
    t. axis
    t. body
    t. carcinoma
    t. cartilage
    t. eminence
    t. endocrine disorder
    t. gland
    t. hormone serum concentration
    t. ima artery
    t. lobectomy
    t. lymph nodes
    t. needle biopsy
    t. nodule ablation
    t. storm
    t. tissue
    t. tumor
    t. veins
thyroidal articular surface of cricoid
thyroidea
    t. accessoria
thyroidectomy
    completion t.
    near-total t.
    provocative food t.
    subtotal t.
thyrointoxication
thyrolaryngeal
thyrolingual duct

thyromental distance
thyropalatine
thyroparathyroidectomy
thyropharyngeal
thyroplasty
thyroptosis
thyrotomy
thyrotoxic coma
thyroxine
Ti
    inspiratory time
tibia, pl. tibiae
    corticotomy of proximal t.
    lateral condyle of t.
    medial condyle of t.
    Phemister medial approach to t.
tibiad
tibial
    t. acceleration
    t. augmentation block
    t. bending fracture
    t. bone defect regeneration
    t. bone graft
    t. condyle fracture
    t. crest
    t. diaphyseal fracture
    t. epiphysis
    t. intertendinous bursa
    t. metaphysis
    t. open fracture
    t. plafond fracture
    t. plateau fracture
    t. plateau fracture-dislocation
    t. shaft fracture
    t. triplane fracture
    t. tuberosity fracture
    t. tuberosity osteotomy
tibiale posticum
tibialis
    t. posterior dislocation
tibiocalcaneal
    t. arthrodesis
    t. medullary nailing
    t. part of deltoid ligament
tibiocalcanean
tibiofascialis
tibiofemoral
    t. articulation
tibiofibular
    t. articulation
    t. clear space
    t. diastasis

NOTES

T

tibiofibular *(continued)*
    t. fusion
    t. joint dislocation
    t. line
tibionavicular
    t. part of deltoid ligament
tibioperoneal
    t. trunk angioplasty
    t. vessel angioplasty
tibioscaphoid
tibiotalar fusion
tibiotalocalcaneal
    t. arthrodesis
    t. fusion
Tibone posterior capsulorrhaphy
Ti-Cron suture
tidal
    t. drainage
    t. volume
tie
    circumferential suture t.
ties-over-stent
tiger gut suture
tightening
    gastric valve t.
tight Nissen repair
tight-to-shaft (TTS)
    t.-t.-s. Aire-Cuf tracheostomy tube
tigroid striation
tigrolysis
Tikhoff-Linberg
    T.-L. procedure
    T.-L. shoulder girdle resection
Tilden method
tile
    T. classification
    t. plate facet replacement
Tillaux
    extraocular muscles of T.
Tillaux-Chaput fracture
Tillaux-Kleiger fracture
Tillaux-Phocas syndrome
Tillett operation
tilt
    base-ring t.
    head-up t.
    t. stitch
tilt-table testing
time
    acceleration t.
    activated clotting t. (ACT)
    association t.
    blood-brain equilibration t.
    carotid ejection t.
    celite-activated clotting t. (CACT)
    cerebral circulation t.
    circulation t.
    concentration times t.

    correlation t.
    deceleration t.
    decimal reduction t.
    duration t.
    ejection t.
    electrode response t.
    execution t.
    explosive doubling t.
    forced expiratory t.
    helium equilibration t.
    inspiration t.
    inspiratory t. (Ti)
    interhemispheric propagation t.
    isovolumic relaxation t.
    Ivy method of bleeding t.
    kaolin-activated clotting t. (KACT)
    left ventricular ejection t.
    t. of maximum concentration
    mean circulation t.
    nucleation t.
    t. position scan
    preservation t.
    t. pressure
    procedure t.
    recalcification t.
    t. to recovery
    relaxation t.
    saturation t.
    sensation t.
    total respiratory t. (Ttot)
    total tourniquet t.
    tourniquet t.
    tumor doubling t.
    ventilator t.
    ventricular activation t.
    voice termination t.
    warm ischemic t.
time/concentration curve
time-cycled ventilation
timed
    t. forced expiratory volume
    t. intermittent rotation
timed-sequential therapy
time-of-flight mass spectometry
TIMI
    Thrombolysis in Myocardial Infarction
    TIMI classification
Tim knot
T-incision
Tiny-Tef ventilation tube
Tiny Tytan ventilation tube
tip
    t. angle
    t. of auricle
    t. of medial malleolus
    nasal t.
    t. of nose
    overprojecting nasal t.

papillary t.
papillary muscle t.
t. of posterior horn
pyramidal t.
rectal t.
spleen t.
t. of tongue
tip-deflecting
tip-of-the-tongue phenomenon
TIPS
transjugular intrahepatic portosystemic shunt
TIPS procedure
Tissomat
tissue
abdominal adipose t.
aberrant t.
t. ablation
acellular pannus t.
acinar t.
adipose t.
ampullary granulation t.
anechoic t.
angiomatous neoplastic t.
anisotropic t.
t. approximation
t. architecture
areolar connective t.
atrioventricular conduction t.
attenuating t.
t. bank
bile pigment demonstration in t.
t. blocking
border t.
breast biopsy t.
bronchial-associated lymphoid t.
brown adipose t.
bursa-equivalent t.
bursal t.
cancellous t.
capsular support t.
cartilaginous t.
caseated t.
cementoid t.
cervical soft t.
chromaffin t.
cicatricial t.
t. coagulation
collagenous t.
t. compression
t. compression test
t. conductivity

t. confirmation
conjunctiva-associated lymphoid t.
connective t.
coronal pulp t.
crushed t.
cryostat t.
cutaneous t.
denuded connective t.
t. detritus
devitalized t.
diffuse lymphatic t.
donor t.
t. Doppler imaging
earlobe adipose t.
echogenic t.
ectopic endometrial t.
elastic t.
episcleral t.
t. expansion
extra-articular t.
extracapsular t.
extraperitoneal t.
exuberant granulation t.
fatty prostatic t.
fetal lymphoid t.
fibroadipose t.
fibroblastic t.
fibroelastic t.
fibrofatty breast t.
fibrous connective t.
fibrous scar t.
t. fluke
t. fusion
Gamgee t.
gastrointestinal-associated lymphoid t.
gingival t.
glandular t.
t. glue
granulation t.
granulomatous t.
gut-associated lymphoid t. (GALT)
hard and soft t.
hemangiomatous t.
hematopoietic t.
hilar structure scar t.
His-Purkinje t.
histiocytic t.
t. homogeneity
hyperplastic t.
hypertrophic granulation t.
t. imprint

T

NOTES

tissue *(continued)*
    inflammation of connective t.
    interdental t.
    interfascicular fibrous t.
    t. interposition
    interstitial t.
    intervening connective t.
    intralobular connective t.
    isotropic t.
    keratinized t.
    ligamentous support t.
    t. ligand
    lipoma-like t.
    lipomatous t.
    t. lymph
    lymphoid t.
    mammary t.
    maternal t.
    mesenchymal t.
    mesothelial t.
    mineralized t.
    t. molding
    mucosa-associated lymphoid t.
    muscular t.
    myeloid t.
    myocardial t.
    nasion soft t.
    t. necrosis
    necrotic hyalinized t.
    neoplastic t.
    nephrogenic t.
    neural t.
    nodal t.
    nonviable t.
    normal t.
    nuclear t.
    t. nutrition
    oral t.
    orbital adipose t.
    orbitonasal t.
    osseous t.
    t. oxygenation
    paracancerous t.
    paraoral t.
    paratransplantal t.
    paravaginal soft t.
    parenchymal t.
    penoid t.
    t. perfusion
    periadvential t.
    periapical t.
    periarticular t.
    pericanalicular connective t.
    peri-implant t.
    perilobular connective t.
    perinephric t.
    perineural t.
    perinodal t.

periosteal t.
peripheral t.
peripheral lymphoid t.
periprostatic t.
pharyngeal t.
t. pH monitoring
placental t.
preepiglottic soft t.
t. preservation
t. pressure
t. pressure measurement
pressure-sensitive t.
pressure-tolerant t.
prevertebral soft t.
pterygial t.
redundant sac t.
t. regencration
t. remodeling
t. renewal
t. repair
residual ductal t.
t. resistance
t. respiration
retroperitoneal soft t.
retropharyngeal soft t.
revascularized t.
rubber t.
t. sampling
scar t.
skeletal t.
t. slack
slow exchange soft t.
soft t.
sonolucent t.
t. space
splenic t.
t. study
subcutaneous t.
subjacent t.
supporting t.
sustentacular t.
syngeneic t.
synovial t.
taenia strip of soft t.
testicular adrenal-like t.
t. texture abnormality
thoracic inlet soft t.
t. thromboplastin
thyroid t.
t. tolerance
t. tolerance dose
t. transfer
t. transplant
t. transplantation
t. trimming
trophoblastic t.
tuberculosis granulation t.
t. typing

vascular t.
viable t.
viscoelastic t.
t. water content
t. welding
xenogeneic t.
tissue-base relationship
tissue-bearing area
tissue-borne
tissue-equivalent
tissue-sparing technique
tissue-supported base
tissue-tissue-supported base
titanium Greenfield vena cava filter
titratable
titration
coulometric t.
Dean and Webb t.
heparin-protamine t.
potentiometric t.
Rinkel serial endpoint t.
t. technique
titubation
head t.
TIVA
total intravenous anesthesia
TKR
total knee arthroscopy
T-lesion
TME
total mesorectal excision
TMLR
transmyocardial laser revascularization
T-myelotomy
T-nail
TNM
tumor, node, metastasis
TNM carcinoma classification
TNM classification of carcinoma
TNM system for tumor staging
to-and-fro anesthesia
tocolysis
tocolytic therapy
Todd-Evans stepladder tracheal dilatation technique
toddler fracture
Tod muscle
toe
t. block anesthesia
Butler procedure to correct overlapping t.'s
catheter t.

t. extensor
t. extensor muscle
t. extensor tendon
extra t.
great t.
toe-phalanx transplantation
TOF
train-of-four
Tohen tendon technique
toilet
cavity t.
t. of cavity
peritoneal t.
pulmonary t.
tolazoline
Toldt
T. fascia
line of T.
T. membrane
white line of T.
Tolentino ring
tolerance
anesthetic t.
pressure t.
tissue t.
Tolerex feeding solution
Tom
T. Jones closure
T. Jones suture
tome
tomentum
tomography
computed t.
expiratory computed t.
positron emission t. (PET)
single photon emission computer-aided t.
ultrafast CT electron beam t.
Tompkins median bivalving technique
tongue
t. bone
crenation of t.
extrinsic muscles of the t.
t. fasciculation
t. flap
t. fracture
mandibular t.
mucous membrane of t.
t. plication
t. pressure
t. thrust classification
t. thrust therapy

NOTES

755

tongue-and-groove suture technique
tongue-in-groove operation
tongue-jaw-neck dissection
tonometer
    hollow visceral t.
    indentation t.
    TRIP nasogastric t.
tonometry
    applanation t.
    gastric t.
    indentation t.
    nasogastric t.
tonsil
tonsilla, pl. tonsillae
    t. adenoidea
    t. intestinalis
    t. lingualis
    t. palatina
    t. pharyngealis
    t. tubaria
tonsillar
    t. branch of the facial artery
    t. branch of glossopharyngeal nerve
    t. crypt
    t. herniation
    t. ring
    t. suction tube
tonsillectomy
    t. and adenoidectomy
    Sluder guillotine t.
tonsilloadenoidectomy
tooth
    t. extraction
    t. fracture
    t. hemisection
    t. immobilization
    t. mass
    t. migration
    t. perforation
    t. plane
    t. position
    t. sac
    t. transplantation
    t. tube
tooth-and-nail syndrome
tooth-to-tooth position
topectomy
Topel knot
tophus
topical
    t. anesthetic
    t. anesthetic technique
    EMLA T.
    Exelderm t.
    t. iodine application
    t. oropharyngeal anesthesia
    Pontocaine T.
    t. Xylocaine

topicalization
Topinard facial angle
topistic
topographic projection
Toposar injection
top-up
    epidural t.-u.
Toradol
    T. injection
    T. Oral
Torek
    T. operation
    T. orchiopexy
    T. resection of thoracic esophagus
Torg
    T. classification
    T. knee reconstruction
    T. technique
Torgerson-Leach modified technique
tori (pl. of torus)
toric ablation
Torkildsen ventriculocisternostomy
Torode-Zieg classification
Toronto pelvic fracture classification
TORP
    total ossicular replacement prosthesis
Torpin cul-de-sac resection
torque
    light wire t.
    translation of t.
    unwanted screw t.
torr
    t. pressure
torrential hemorrhage
torsade de pointes ventricular
  tachycardia (TdPVT)
torsion
    t. of appendage
    biliary tract t.
    extravaginal testicular t.
    intravaginal t.
    perinatal t.
    t. testis
    t. of testis
torsional fracture
torso
torsoclusion
tortipelvis
toruloma
torulopsis infection
torus, pl. tori
    t. fracture
total
    t. abdominal colectomy
    t. abdominal evisceration
    t. abdominal hysterectomy
    t. abdominal hysterectomy and
      bilateral salpingo-oophorectomy

t. ankle arthroplasty
t. articular replacement arthroplasty
t. articular resurfacing arthroplasty
t. axial node irradiation
t. bilateral vagotomy
t. biopsy
t. body fat
t. body hypothermia
t. body irradiation
t. body solute
t. body water
t. body weight (TBW)
t. breech extraction
t. colectomy (TC)
t. colonoscopy
t. cystectomy
t. ear obliteration
t. elbow arthroplasty
t. etch technique
t. ethmoidectomy
t. exchangeable potassium
  measurement
t. excisional operation
t. fundoplication
t. fundoplication method
t. fundoplication procedure
t. fundoplication technique
t. gastrectomy
t. gastric wrap
t. glossectomy
t. graft area rejection
t. hip arthroplasty
t. hip replacement
t. hypophysectomy
t. internal reflection
t. intravenous anesthesia (TIVA)
t. intravenous anesthetic technique
t. keratoplasty
t. knee arthroplasty
t. knee arthroscopy (TKR)
t. laryngectomy
t. laryngopharyngectomy
t. L-chain concentration
t. lymphoid irradiation
t. mastectomy
t. meniscectomy
t. mesorectal excision (TME)
t. nodal irradiation
t. ossicular replacement prosthesis
  (TORP)
t. pancreatectomy
t. parenteral alimentation

t. parenteral nutrition (TPN)
t. patellectomy
t. patellofemoral joint arthroplasty
t. pelvic exenteration
t. perineal prostatectomy
t. perineal rupture
t. proctocolectomy
t. proctocolectomy with ileoanal
  anastomosis and J pouch
t. prostatoseminal vesiculectomy
t. protein concentration
t. pulpotomy
t. push therapy
t. respiratory time (Ttot)
t. retrocolic end-to-side
  gastrojejunostomy
t. scrotectomy
t. shoulder arthroplasty
t. space analysis
t. spinal anesthesia
t. time to intubation (TTI)
t. tourniquet time
t. transfusion
t. transurethral resection of prostate
t. vascular isolation (TVI)
t. wrist arthroplasty

totally stapled restorative
proctocolectomy
Toti
  T. operation
  T. procedure
Toti-Mosher operation
touch
  three-point t.
touch-up procedure
Touma T-type grommet ventilation tube
Toupe
  T. method
  T. procedure
  T. technique
Toupet
  T. fundoplication
  T. hemifundoplication
tourniquet
  t. control
  t. ischemia
  t. ischemic pain
  t. occlusion
  t. paralysis
  t. pressure
  t. test
  t. time

T

NOTES

tourniquet-eyed
>   t.-e. ratchet stylet
tourniquet-induced pain
Tourtual
>   T. canal
>   T. membrane
Tovell tube
Towako method
tower
>   Concept traction t.
Towne projection
Townley-Paton operation
toxemia
toxic
>   t. dilation of colon
>   t. epidermal necrolysis
>   t. granulation
toxicity
>   endocrine t.
>   extramedullary t.
>   neostigmine t.
>   oxygen t.
>   radiation-induced pulmonary t.
toxin
>   botulinum A t.
>   t. exposure
>   extracellular t.
Toynbee
>   T. diagnostic tube
>   T. muscle
T-piece
>   Ayre T.-p.
TPN
>   total parenteral nutrition
TPR
>   transsphenoidal pituitary resection
trabecula, pl. **trabeculae**
>   trabeculae corporis spongiosi penis
>   trabeculae lienis
>   trabeculae of spleen
>   trabeculae splenicae
>   t. testis
trabecular
>   t. bone fracture
>   t. membrane
>   t. network
trabeculated
>   t. bladder
>   t. bone lesion
trabeculation
trabeculectomy
>   Cairns t.
>   t. operation
>   Smith t.
trabeculopexy
>   argon laser t.

trabeculoplasty
>   argon laser t.
>   laser t.
trabeculotomy
trace anesthetic
tracer dilution
Trach Care closed suctioning system
trachea
tracheal
>   t. adenoma
>   t. agenesis
>   t. aspiration
>   t. bifurcation angle
>   t. block
>   t. branches
>   t. cartilages
>   t. compression
>   t. extubation anesthetic technique
>   t. fenestration
>   t. fracture
>   t. glands
>   t. intubation
>   t. intubation anesthetic technique
>   t. lymph nodes
>   t. reconstruction
>   t. ring
>   t. safety stitch
>   t. stenosis
>   t. suction anesthetic technique
>   t. topical analgesia
>   t. triangle
>   t. tube
>   t. tube changer
>   t. tube cuff
>   t. tug
>   t. tumor
>   t. ulceration
>   t. web
trachealis
>   t. muscle
trachelalis
trachelectomy
trachelematoma
trachelian
tracheloclavicular muscle
trachelomastoid
trachelo-occipitalis
trachelopexy
tracheloplasty
trachelorrhaphy
trachelos
tracheloschisis
trachelotomy
tracheoaerocele
tracheobiliary
>   t. fistula

tracheobronchial
    t. anomaly
    t. foreign body
tracheobronchoesophageal fistula
tracheobronchoscopy
tracheocele
tracheocutaneous fistula
tracheoesophageal
    t. fistula (TEF)
    t. puncture
tracheolaryngeal
tracheopharyngeal
tracheoplasty
tracheostomy
    t. cuff
    elective dilatational t.
    flap t.
    Great Ormond Street t.
    Montgomery t.
    percutaneous dilational t.
    t. stoma
    t. tube
tracheotomy
    t. tube
Trachlight lighted intubating stylet
trachoma
    t. gland
track
    pin t.
    radial suture t.
Tracoe tracheostomy tube
Tracrium
tract
    abnormal fetal urogenital t.
    aerodigestive t.
    alimentary t.
    anterior corticospinal t.
    anterior pyramidal t.
    anterior spinocerebellar t.
    anterior spinothalamic t.
    Arnold t.
    association t.
    atriodextrofascicular t.
    atriofascicular t.
    atrio-Hisian bypass t.
    atrionodal bypass t.
    auditory t.
    benign mesothelioma of genital t.
    biliary t.
    bronchial t.
    Burdach t.
    bypass t.

    central tegmental t.
    cerebellorubral t.
    cerebellothalamic t.
    cholinergic t.
    Collier t.
    concealed bypass t.
    corticobulbar t.
    corticopontine t.
    corticospinal t.
    crossed pyramidal t.
    cuneocerebellar t.
    dead t.
    deiterospinal t.
    dental sinus t.
    dentatothalamic t.
    dermal sinus t.
    digestive t.
    t. dilation
    direct pyramidal t.
    dopaminergic t.
    dorsal spinocerebellar t.
    dorsolateral t.
    extrapyramidal t.
    fastigiobulbar t.
    fetal urogenital t.
    fistulous t.
    Flechsig t.
    frontopontine t.
    frontotemporal t.
    gastrointestinal t.
    geniculocalcarine t.
    geniculotemporal t.
    genital t.
    genitourinary t.
    GI t.
    Gowers t.
    habenulointerpeduncular t.
    hepatic outflow t.
    Hoche t.
    hypothalamohypophysial t.
    ileal inflow t.
    ileal outflow t.
    iliopubic t.
    iliotibial t.
    infected t.
    inflammatory sinus t.
    inflow t.
    intestinal t.
    intramural fistulous t.
    lateral corticospinal t.
    lateral lemniscus t.
    lateral pyramidal t.

NOTES

tract *(continued)*
    lateral root of optic t.
    lateral spinothalamic t.
    left ventricular outflow t. (LVOT)
    leiomyoma of uveal t.
    Lissauer t.
    Loewenthal t.
    mamillothalamic t.
    Marchi t.
    medial root of optic t.
    mesolimbic-mesocortical t.
    Monakow t.
    t. of Münzer and Wiener
    nasal t.
    needle t.
    nerve t.
    nigrostriatal t.
    nodo-Hisian bypass t.
    nodoventricular t.
    nucleus of solitary t.
    occipitocollicular t.
    occipitopontine t.
    occipitotectal t.
    olfactory t.
    olivocerebellar t.
    olivospinal t.
    optic t.
    oro-respiratory t.
    outflow t.
    pancreaticobiliary t.
    parietopontine t.
    perineal sinus t.
    portal t.
    posterior spinocerebellar t.
    prepyramidal t.
    pulmonary outflow t.
    pyramidal t.
    reproductive t.
    respiratory t.
    reticulospinal t.
    retrochiasmal optic t.
    right ventricular outflow t. (RVOT)
    rubrobulbar t.
    rubroreticular t.
    rubrospinal t.
    safe-gastrocutaneous fistulous t.
    t. of Schütz
    seminal t.
    sensory t.
    septomarginal t.
    serotonergic t.
    sinus t.
    solitary t.
    sphincteroid t. of ileum
    spinal dermal sinus t.
    spinocerebellar t.
    spino-olivary t.
    spinotectal t.

    spinothalamic t.
    spiral foraminous t.
    Spitzka marginal t.
    sulcomarginal t.
    supraopticohypophysial t.
    t. tamponade
    tamponade needle t.
    tectobulbar t.
    tectopontine t.
    tectospinal t.
    temporofrontal t.
    temporopontine t.
    tree-barking urinary t.
    T-tube t.
    tuberoinfundibular t.
    Türck t.
    UGI t.
    upper aerodigestive t.
    upper gastrointestinal t.
    upper respiratory t.
    urinary t.
    urogenital t.
    uveal t.
    ventral spinocerebellar t.
    ventral spinothalamic t.
    ventricular outflow t.
    vestibulospinal t.
    vocal t.
    Waldeyer t.
    Wolff-Parkinson-White bypass t.

traction
    t. alopecia
    t. aneurysm
    t. application
    t. atrophy
    t. band
    t. detachment
    t. epiphysis
    t. fracture
    t. headache
    t. suture
    t. test

tractotomy
    anterolateral t.
    bulbar t.
    bulbar cephalic pain t.
    intramedullary t.
    mesencephalic t.
    pontine t.
    pyramidal t.
    Schwartz t.
    Sjöqvist intramedullary t.
    spinal t.
    spinothalamic t.
    subcaudate t.
    trigeminal t.
    Walker t.

tractus
  t. iliotibialis
trafficking
  membrane t.
tragicus muscle
training
  joint protection t.
  stabilization t.
train-of-four (TOF)
  t.-o.-f. stimulation
  t.-o.-f. stimulus
  t.-o.-f. transmission
Trainor-Nida operation
Trainor operation
trajector
Trake-Fit endotracheal tube
TRALI
  transfusion-related lung injury
TRAM
  transverse rectus abdominis muscle
  TRAM flap
tramadol
tram lines
trampoline fracture
Tramscope 12
trance coma
Trandate injection
tranquilization
tranquilizer
transabdominal
  t. mucosectomy
  t. preperitoneal repair
transacromial approach
transactivation
transanal
  t. endoscopic microsurgery (TEM)
  t. endoscopic microsurgical resection
  t. excision
  t. mucosectomy
  t. mucosectomy with hand-sewn anastomosis
transanimation
transantral
  t. ethmoidal approach
  t. ethmoidectomy
transaortic valve gradient
transarterial anesthetic technique
transarticular wire fixation
transaxial scan plane

transaxillary
  t. apical bullectomy
  t. approach
transbrachioradialis approach
transbronchial
  t. lung biopsy
  t. needle aspiration
transcallosal transventricular approach
transcanine approach
transcaphoid fracture
transcapillary hydrostatic pressure gradient
transcapitate
  t. fracture
  t. fracture-dislocation
transcapitellar wire fixation
transcarpal amputation
transcatheter
  t. ablation
  t. arterial embolization therapy
  t. closure
transcavernous transpetrous apex approach
transcerebellar hemispheric approach
transcervical
  t. approach
  t. balloon tuboplasty
  t. femoral fracture
  t. intrafallopian tube transfer
  t. resection
transchondral fracture
transclavicular approach
transcochlear
  t. approach
  t. cochleovestibular neurectomy
  t. vestibular neurectomy
transcondylar fracture
transcortical
  t. transventricular approach
transcranial
  t. Doppler (TCD)
  t. electrical stimulation
  t. electrical stimulation anesthetic technique
  t. frontal-temporal-orbital approach
  t. stimulation (TCS)
transcranial-supraorbital approach
transcubital approach
transcutaneous
  t. biopsy
  t. cranial electrical stimulation (TCES)

NOTES

transcutaneous *(continued)*
t. electrical nerve stimulation
t. electrical neuromuscular
  stimulator
t. electric stimulation (TES)
t. electrode nerve stimulation
t. nerve stimulator
t. oxygen monitoring
t. oxygen pressure measurement
t. partial pressure of oxygen
t. tetanic stimulus
transdermal
t. administration
t. analgesic
t. anesthesia
t. anesthetic technique
Duragesic T.
t. fentanyl device (TFD)
t. medication patch
transduodenal
t. approach
t. endoscopic decompression
t. sphincteroplasty
t. sphincterotomy
transect
transection
aortic t.
t. and devascularization operation
esophageal t.
step-cut t.
Sugiura esophageal variceal t.
traumatic aortic t.
transendoscopic
t. electrocoagulation
t. laser photocoagulation
t. procedure
t. sphincterotomy
transepiphyseal fracture
Transeptic cleansing solution
transesophageal
t. atrial pacing (TEAP)
t. atrial stimulation
t. echocardiography (TEE)
t. echocardiography scan
t. echocardiography with pacing
t. endoscopy
t. ligation of varix
t. varix ligation
t. ventricular pacing (TEVP)
transethmoidal
transfemoral venous catheterization
transfer
barber pole stripe t.
composite free tissue t.
composite tissue t.
dermal fat-free tissue t.
free flap t.

free tissue t.
microvascular free flap t.
Ober-Barr procedure for
  brachioradialis t.
placental t.
pronuclear stage t. (PROST)
saturation t.
single-stage tissue t.
split anterior tibial tendon t.
  (SPLATT)
tissue t.
transcervical intrafallopian tube t.
in vitro fertilization-embryo t.
wraparound neurovascular composite
  free tissue t.
transfibular approach
transfixation
transfixion
t. of iris operation
t. suture
transforaminal passage
transform
driven equilibrium Fourier t.
  (DEFT)
transformary mass
transformation zone
transfrontal approach
transfuse
transfusion
allogeneic blood t.
arterial t.
coagulation factor t.
direct t.
double-volume exchange t.
drip t.
exchange t.
exsanguination t.
immediate t.
indirect t.
intraperitoneal blood t.
intraperitoneal fetal t.
intrauterine intraperitoneal fetal t.
mediate t.
peritoneal t.
subcutaneous t.
substitution t.
t. therapy
total t.
transfusion-related lung injury (TRALI)
transgastric
t. fine-needle-aspiration biopsy
t. ligation
t. plication
transgastrostomic enteroscopy
transglomerular hydrostatic filtration
  pressure
transgluteal approach

transhamate
 t. fracture
 t. fracture-dislocation
transhepatic antegrade biliary drainage procedure
transhiatal
 t. approach
 t. blunt esophagectomy
transhyoid pharyngotomy
transient
 t. auditory evoked response (TAER)
 t. cavitation
 t. compartment syndrome
 t. hiatal hernia
 t. lesion
 t. osteoporosis of hip
 t. visual obscuration
transiliac
 t. amputation
 t. bar technique
 t. fracture
 t. rod fixation
transillumination
 t. of head
 t. of sinus
 t. test
transischiac
transition
 cervicothoracic t.
 t. suture
transitional
 t. epithelium
 t. respiration
 t. zone biopsy
transjugular
 t. hepatic biopsy
 t. intrahepatic portosystemic shunt (TIPS)
 t. liver biopsy
translabyrinthine and suboccipital approach
translaryngeal
 t. endotracheal tube
 t. guided intubation anesthetic technique
 t. tracheal intubation
translation
 anterior t.
 anteroposterior t.
 caudal t.
 cephalad t.

coronal plane deformity sagittal t.
 dorsal t.
 force t. (FTR)
 t. injury
 t. mobility
 t. motion
 posterior t.
 pure t.
 t. of torque
 ulnar t.
 vertical t.
translational
 t. fracture
 t. position
translocation Down syndrome
translucent
 t. drain tube
 t. myringotomy tube
transluminal
 t. coronary angioplasty
 t. extraction atherectomy
transmandibular-glossopharyngeal approach
transmandibular projection
transmastoid approach
transmeatal
 t. approach
 t. tympanoplasty incision
transmembrane hydraulic pressure
transmesenteric
 t. hernia
 t. plication
transmetatarsal amputation
transmigration
 ovular t.
transmission
 double burst t.
 t. electron microscopy
 iatrogenic t.
 neuromuscular t.
 pressure t.
 train-of-four t.
transmucosal
 t. delivery
 t. drug administration anesthetic technique
transmural
 t. approach
 t. hydrostatic pressure gradient
 t. pressure
transmutation

T

NOTES

transmyocardial
   t. laser revascularization (TMLR)
   t. perfusion pressure
   t. revascularization
transnasal
   t. administration
   t. bile duct catheterization
   t. endoscopy
transocular
transolecranon approach
transoral
   t. approach
   t. odontoid resection
transorbital
   t. leukotomy
   t. lobotomy
   t. projection
transosseus suture
transpalatal approach
transpapillary
   t. approach
   t. biopsy
   t. cannulation
   t. catheterization
   t. endoscopic cholecystotomy
transparenchymal suture
transparietal
transpedicular
   t. approach
   t. screw-rod fixation
transpelvic amputation
transperineal palladium 103
transperineurial passage
transperitoneal
   t. approach
   t. cesarean section
   t. exposure
   t. laparoscopic adrenalectomy
   t. laparoscopic nephrectomy
   t. laparoscopic nephroureterectomy
transplacental hemorrhage
transplant
   acute rejection of liver t.
   corneal t.
   fetal tissue t.
   Gallie t.
   lamellar corneal t.
   t. lung syndrome
   t. nephrectomy
   orthotopic liver t. (OLT)
   penetrating corneal t.
   placental tissue t.
   reduced liver t. (RLT)
   t. rejection
   rejection cardiomyopathy t.
   SPK t.
   tissue t.
transplantar

transplantation
   adrenal medulla t.
   allogeneic t.
   allograft t.
   anhepatic stage of liver t.
   autogenous tooth t.
   autologous blood stem cell t.
   bone marrow t.
   Bosworth femoroischial t.
   brain t.
   t. of cornea
   corneal t.
   Cowen-Loftus toe-phalanx t.
   femoroischial t.
   fetal liver t.
   fetal thymus t.
   heart t.
   hepatocyte t.
   heterotopic t.
   homogenous tooth t.
   homotopic t.
   kidney t.
   liver t.
   living-related donor t. (LRLT)
   t. of muscle operation
   muscle-tendon t.
   neonatal pulmonary t.
   organ t.
   orthoptic t.
   orthotopic t.
   orthotopic liver t. (OLT)
   osteoarticular allograft t.
   pancreaticoduodenal t.
   piggyback liver t.
   pigment cell t.
   pituitary gland t.
   renal t.
   SPK t.
   syngeneic t.
   syngenesioplastic t.
   tendon t.
   tissue t.
   toe-phalanx t.
   tooth t.
   xenograft t.
transplantectomy
transpleural
transposition
   t. flap
   penoscrotal t.
   Strombeck nipple t.
   Z-plasty t.
transpubic incision
transpupillary cyclophotocoagulation
transpyloric
   t. feeding tube
   t. plane
transradial approach

transrectal
t. approach
t. surgical treatment
t. ultrasound-guided-sextant biopsy
transsacral fracture
transscaphoid
t. dislocation fracture
t. perilunate dislocation
transsection
transseptal
t. approach
t. left heart catheterization
t. orchiopexy
t. puncture
transsexual
t. surgery
transsexualism
transsinus approach
transsphenoidal
t. approach
t. evacuation
t. hypophysectomy
t. microsurgical resection
t. operation
t. pituitary resection (TPR)
t. removal
t. surgery
transsphincteric
t. anal fistula
t. surgery
transstenotic pressure gradient measurement
transsternal approach
transsylvian approach
transtentorial
t. approach
t. herniation
transthermia
transthoracic
t. approach
t. diskectomy
t. dissection
t. esophagectomy
t. needle aspiration
t. needle aspiration biopsy
t. percutaneous fine-needle aspiration biopsy
t. vertebral body resection
transthoracotomy
transtorcular approach
transtracheal
t. aspirate

t. aspiration
t. jet
t. jet ventilation
t. jet ventilation anesthetic technique
transtriquetral
t. fracture
t. fracture-dislocation
transtrochanteric
t. approach
t. rotational osteotomy
transtubercular plane
transtympanic neurectomy
transubstantiation
transudation
transudative inflammation
transureteroureteral anastomosis
transureteroureterostomy (TUU)
transurethral
t. ablative prostatectomy
t. balloon dilatation
t. balloon dilation
t. collagen injection therapy
t. electrical bladder stimulation
t. evaporation of prostate
t. laser incision of the prostate
t. marsupialization
t. needle ablation
t. resection
t. resection of bladder
t. resection of bladder tumor
t. resection of prostate
t. resection of prostate ulceration
t. resection syndrome
t. sphincterotomy
t. ultrasound-guided laser-induced prostatectomy
t. ureterorenoscopy
t. vaporization of prostate
transvaginal
t. approach
t. Burch procedure
t. fallopian tube catheterization
t. tubal catheterization
t. ultrasonically guided oocyte retrieval
t. urethrolysis
transvector
transvenous
t. approach
t. liver biopsy
t. therapy

NOTES

transventricular mitral valve
  commissurotomy
transversalis fascia
Trans-Ver-Sal transdermal patch
  Verukan solution
transverse
  t. abdominal incision
  t. anthelicine groove
  apical t. (AP-T)
  t. approach
  t. artery of neck
  t. arytenoid muscle
  t. atlantal ligament
  t. cervical artery
  t. cervical nerve
  t. cervical veins
  t. colectomy
  t. colon
  t. comminuted fracture
  t. costal facet
  deep-gastric t. (DG-T)
  t. diaphyseal osteotomy
  t. ductules of epoöphoron
  t. duodenotomy
  t. facial artery
  t. facial fracture
  t. facial vein
  t. fissure of the lung
  five-chamber t. (5C-T)
  t. fixation
  t. fixator application
  t. foramen
  four-chamber t. (4C-T)
  t. fundal incision of Strassman
  t. head
  t. ligament of the atlas
  t. ligament of pelvis
  t. ligament of perineum
  t. ligament rupture
  t. lines of sacrum
  lower uterine segment t. (LUST)
  t. magnetization phase
  t. maxillary fracture
  t. metatarsal osteotomy
  midpapillary t. (MP-T)
  mitral valve-t. (MV-T)
  t. muscle of abdomen
  t. muscle of auricle
  t. muscle of chin
  t. muscle of nape
  t. muscle of thorax
  t. muscle of tongue
  t. nerve of neck
  t. oval pelvis
  t. palatine fold
  t. palatine suture
  t. pancreatic artery

  t. part of left branch of portal
    vein
  t. pericardial sinus
  t. perineal ligament
  t. plane
  t. plane motion insufficiency
  t. process
  t. process fracture
  t. projection
  t. rectal folds
  t. rectus abdominis muscle
    (TRAM)
  t. rectus abdominis muscle flap
  t. relaxation
  t. relaxation rate
  t. resection
  t. scapular artery
  t. section
  t. section of heart
  t. section imaging
  t. semilunar skin incision
  t. sinus of pericardium
  t. supracondylar osteotomy
  t. suture of Krause
  t. tarsotomy
  t. tenotomy
  t. umbilical line
  t. vein of face
  t. vein of scapula
  t. veins of neck
  t. vesical fold
transversectomy
transverse-loop rod colostomy
transversely oriented endplate
  compression fracture
transversocostal
transversospinalis muscle
transversospinal muscle
transversostomy
transversourethralis
transversovertical index
transversus
  t. abdominis muscle
  t. menti muscle
  t. nuchae muscle
  t. thoracis muscle
transxiphoid approach
Trantas operation
tranylcypromine
trap-door
  t.-d. approach
  t.-d. fragment
  t.-d. scleral buckle operation
trapezial
trapeziform
trapeziometacarpal fusion
trapezium
  t. fracture

trapezius
t. flap
t. stimulation anesthetic technique
trapezoid
t. body
t. incision
t. line
t. method
t. ridge
trapezoidal
t. incision
t. keratotomy
t. osteotomy
trap incision
Trasylol
Traube-Hering curves
Traube semilunar space
trauma, pl. **traumas, traumata**
blunt t.
corneal t.
external t.
foreign body t.
genital tract t.
head t.
intraoral t.
penetrating t.
perineal impact t.
t. surgery
traumasthenia
traumatic
t. amputation
t. anesthesia
t. aortic rupture
t. aortic transection
t. cardiac arrest
t. cervical disk herniation
t. choroidal rupture
T. Coma Data Bank
t. corneal abrasion
t. diaphragmatic hernia
t. dislocation
t. false aneurysm
t. fistula
t. fracture
t. inflammation
t. intracranial hematoma
t. lesion
t. progressive encephalopathy
t. pseudomeningocele
t. renal mass
t. rupture of the diaphragm
t. tetanus

traumatism
traumatize
traumatology
traumatonesis
traumatopathy
traumatopnea
traumatosepsis
traumatotherapy
Trautmann triangular space
Travamulsion fat emulsion solution
Treacher Collins syndrome
treatment
acidification t.
allocation of t.
anoplasty t.
Boyd-Ingram-Bourkhard t.
Carrel t.
cholecystectomy t.
chronic anoplasty t.
compression rod t.
Dakin-Carrel t.
distraction/compression scoliosis t.
dual compression scoliosis t.
duration of t.
endoscopic t.
endovascular t.
esophageal dilation t.
experimental t.
ex vivo marrow t.
ferromagnetic microembolization t.
Gelfoam particles transarterial embolization t.
insulin coma t.
intracavernosal injection t.
lipiodol transarterial embolization t.
mitomycin transarterial embolization t.
photocoagulation t.
P32 intraperitoneal t.
rectovaginal surgical t.
root canal t.
Seton t. of high anal fistula
TheraPEP pre-respiratory therapy t.
transrectal surgical t.
ureteral surgical t.
Trecator-SC
tree
cannulation of the biliary t.
endobronchial t.
iliac arterial t.
tree-barking urinary tract

NOTES

trefoil
>> t. deformity
>> t. tendon

Treitz
>> T. arch
>> T. fascia
>> T. fossa
>> T. hernia
>> T. ligament
>> T. muscle

trellis formation

trema

trematode infection

Trendelenburg
>> T. operation
>> T. position

trepanation
>> t. of cornea
>> corneal t.
>> dental t.

trephination
>> dental t.
>> open-sky t.

trephine needle biopsy

Treponema pallidum
>> *T. p.* immobilization
>> microhemagglutination *T. p.* (MHA-TP)

Trethowan metatarsal osteotomy

Trethowan-Stamm-Simmonds-Menelaus-Haddad technique

Treves fold

triad
>> acute compression t.
>> Beck t.
>> Charcot t.
>> hepatic t.
>> t. knee repair
>> portal t.
>> wall-echo shadow t.

triadic therapy

trial
>> t. cementation
>> t. of conservative therapy
>> European Carotid Surgery T. (ECST)
>> t. point
>> t. reduction

triangle
>> anal t.
>> anterior t. of neck
>> Assézat t.
>> auricular t.
>> t. of auscultation
>> axillary t.
>> Béclard t.
>> Burow t.
>> Calot t.
>> carotid t.
>> cephalic t.
>> cervical t.
>> digastric t.
>> Elaut t.
>> facial t.
>> Farabeuf t.
>> femoral t.
>> frontal t.
>> Grynfcltt t.
>> Hesselbach t.
>> inferior carotid t.
>> inferior occipital t.
>> infraclavicular t.
>> inguinal t.
>> interscalene t.
>> Labbé t.
>> Langenbeck t.
>> Lesser t.
>> Lesshaft t.
>> Lieutaud t.
>> lumbar t.
>> lumbocostoabdominal t.
>> Macewen t.
>> Malgaigne t.
>> Marcille t.
>> muscular t.
>> occipital t.
>> omoclavicular t.
>> omotracheal t.
>> Petit lumbar t.
>> Pirogoff t.
>> posterior t. of neck
>> pubourethral t.
>> sacral t.
>> t. of safety
>> Scarpa t.
>> sternocostal t.
>> subclavian t.
>> subinguinal t.
>> submental t.
>> suboccipital t.
>> superior carotid t.
>> supraclavicular t.
>> suprameatal t.
>> tracheal t.
>> umbilicomammillary t.
>> urogenital t.
>> t. of vertebral artery
>> vesical t.
>> Weber t.

triangular
>> t. advancement flap
>> t. bone
>> t. capsulotomy
>> t. cartilage
>> t. fascia
>> t. ligaments of liver

t. muscle
t. space
triangularis
triangulation
indirect t.
t. stapling method
t. technique
t. technique for arthroscope
triaxial total elbow arthroplasty
tribromoethanol
triceps
t. bursa
tricepsplasty
trichangion
trichiasis repair
trichilemmoma
desmoplastic t.
trichion
trichloride
ethinyl t.
trichloroacetic acid
trichloroethane
trichloroethanol
trichloroethene
trichloroethyl alcohol
trichloroethylene
trichlorofluoromethane
trichloromethane
trichloromonofluoromethane
dichlorodifluoromethane and t.
trichodiscoma
tricholemmoma
trichoma
Trichomonas infection
trichoscopy
tricipital
triclofos
tricorn
tricornute
tricorrectional bunionectomy
tricortical iliac crest bone graft
tricuspid
t. position
t. valve annuloplasty
t. valve annulus
t. valve area
t. valve disease
t. valve flow
t. valve repair
t. valvuloplasty
tridermoma
Tridil injection

Trieger test
triethiodide
gallamine t.
trifacial
t. nerve
trifid stomach
2,2,2-trifluoroethyl vinyl
trifurcation
t. injury
t. involvement
popliteal artery t.
trigastric
trigeminal
t. cave
t. cavity
t. decompression
t. dermatome
t. ganglion
t. impression
t. nerve
t. rhizotomy
t. tractotomy
trigeminus
trigger
t. point
t. point injection
triggered ventilation
trigona (*pl. of* trigonum)
trigonal ring
trigone
t. of bladder
fibrous t.'s of heart
inguinal t.
left fibrous t.
Lieutaud t.
right fibrous t.
vertebrocostal t.
trigonitis
trigonocephaly
trigonum, pl. trigona
t. caroticum
t. cervicale
t. cervicale anterius
t. cervicale posterius
t. colli
t. femorale
trigona fibrosa cordis
t. fibrosum dextrum
t. fibrosum sinistrum
t. inguinale
t. lumbale
t. lumbocostale

NOTES

769

trigonum *(continued)*
    t. musculare
    t. omoclaviculare
    t. omotracheale
    t. sternocostale
    t. submentale
    t. vesicae
Trilene
Trillat procedure
trilobate
trimalleolar ankle fracture
Trimar
trimetaphan camsylate
trimethaphan
    t. camsylate
trimethylene
trimethylethylene
trimming
    tissue t.
trimodality therapy
triophthalmos
triotus
triphalangeal thumb deformity
triphenyltetrazolium staining method
triphosphate
    adenosine t.
Tripier
    T. operation
    T. operation throw square knot
triplane
    t. osteotomy
    t. tibial fracture
triple
    t. buccal tube
    t. hemisection
    t. innominate osteotomy
    t. intrathecal therapy
    t. ligamentous repair
    t. lobe hepatectomy
    t. loop pouch
    t. point
triple-balloon valvuloplasty
triple-lumen Sengstaken-Blakemore tube
triple-throw square knot stitch
triple-wire
    t.-w. procedure
    t.-w. technique
triplication
TRIP nasogastric tonometer
tripod
    t. fracture
    Haller t.
tripodia
tri-point
tripsinization
triquetral
    t. bone
    t. fracture

triquetrolunate dislocation
triquetropisiform articulation
triquetrous cartilage
triquetrum
triradial
triradiate
    t. acetabular extensile approach
    t. line
    t. transtrochanteric approach
triradius
triscaphe fusion
trisection
    pulse t.
trisegmentectomy
tris(hydroxymethyl)-aminomethane (THAM)
trisomy
    t. C syndrome
    t. 8 syndrome
trisplanchnic
tristichia
triticeal cartilage
triticeum
trituration
trivalve
Trobicin injection
trocar
    t. cystostomy
    t. drainage method
    t. technique
    t. wound
trocar-cannula technique
trocar-related injury
trochanter
    greater t.
    lesser t.
    t. major
    t. minor
    small t.
    t. tertius
    third t.
trochanterian
trochanteric
    t. bursa
    t. crest
    t. migration
    t. osteotomy
trochanterplasty
trochantin
trochantinian
trochlea, pl. trochleae
    t. femoris
    t. humeri
    t. of humerus
    t. muscularis
    t. phalangis
    t. tali
    t. of the talus

trochlear
- t. fossa
- t. fovea
- t. process
- t. synovial bursa

trochleariform
trochlearis
trochleiform
trochoid
- t. articulation
- t. joint

Trolard vein
tromethamine
- ketorolac t.

Tronzo classification of intertrochanteric fracture
trophectoderm biopsy
trophic
- t. fracture
- t. lesion

trophoblastic tissue
troponin C
trough line
trousers
- anti-shock military t.

Trousseau point
Troutman operation
Tru-Arc blood vessel ring
Truc
- T. flap
- T. operation

true
- t. aneurysm
- t. exfoliation
- t. knot
- t. muscles of back
- t. pelvis
- t. ribs
- t. vertebra
- t. vocal cord

Trumble talectomy
trumpet
- nasal t.

Trump solution
truncal
- t. vagotomy
- t. vagotomy and gastroenterostomy
- t. vagotomy and pyloroplasty

truncated tarsometatarsal wedge arthrodesis
truncated-wedge
- t.-w. arthrodesis

- t.-w. tarsometatarsal arthrodesis
- vertical talus

truncation phenomenon
truncoaortic sac
truncus, pl. trunci
- t. arteriosus communis
- t. brachiocephalicus
- t. bronchiomediastinalis
- t. celiacus
- t. costocervicalis
- t. fascicularis atrioventricularis
- t. inferior plexus brachialis
- trunci intestinales
- t. jugularis
- t. linguofacialis
- trunci lumbales
- t. lumbosacralis
- t. medius plexus brachialis
- trunci plexus brachialis
- t. pulmonalis
- t. subclavius
- t. superior plexus brachialis
- t. sympathicus
- t. thyrocervicalis
- t. vagalis

trunk
- accessory nerve t.
- t. of atrioventricular bundle
- bifurcation of pulmonary t.
- t.'s of brachial plexus
- brachiocephalic t.
- bronchomediastinal t.
- celiac t.
- costocervical t.
- t. duplication
- t. incurvation test
- inferior t. of brachial plexus
- intestinal t.'s
- jugular lymphatic t.
- linguofacial t.
- lumbar t.'s
- lumbosacral t.
- middle t. of brachial plexus
- nerve t.
- pulmonary t.
- subclavian lymphatic t.
- superior t. of brachial plexus
- sympathetic t.
- thoracoacromial t.
- thyrocervical t.
- vagal t.

T

NOTES

Trusler
> T. aortic valve technique
> T. technique of aortic valvuloplasty

truss

trypsin
> crystallized t.

trypsinization

Tsai-Stillwell procedure

Tscherne classification

**Tscherne-Gotzen tibial fracture
  classification**

T-shaped
> T.-s. capsulotomy
> T.-s. constriction ring
> T.-s. incision

T-sign

TSRH
> Texas Scottish Rite Hospital
> TSRH crosslink stabilization
> TSRH double-rod construct
> TSRH pedicle screw-laminar claw
> construct
> TSRH rod fixation

Tsuji laminaplasty

TTI
> total time to intubation

Ttot
> total respiratory time

TTS
> tight-to-shaft
> TTS Aire-Cuf endotracheal tube
> TTS Aire-Cuf tracheostomy tube
> TTS balloon dilation

T7, T9, T11 dermatome

T-tube
> T.-t. drainage
> T.-t. round suction tube
> T.-t. study
> T.-t. tract
> T.-t. tract choledochofiberoscopy
> T.-t. tract choledochoscopy

T-type myringotomy tube

tuba, pl. tubae
> t. fallopiana
> t. uterina

tubage

tubal
> t. branch of the uterine artery
> t. insufflation
> t. ligation
> t. ligation band technique
> t. reconstruction surgery
> t. ring
> t. rupture
> t. sterilization

tubatorsion

tube
> Abbott t.

Abbott-Miller t.
Abbott-Rawson t.
Abbott-Rawson double-lumen
  gastrointestinal t.
AccuMark calibrated infant
  feeding t.
Activent-Sheehy tympanotomy t.
Adson suction t.
AF t.
air t.
Aire-Cuf endotracheal t.
Aire-Cuf tracheostomy t.
Air-Lon laryngectomy t.
Air-Lon tracheal t.
alar lamina of neural t.
alar plate of neural t.
Alesen t.
American circle nephrostomy t.
American tracheotomy t.
Anderson flexible suction t.
Anderson gastric t.
Andrews-Pynchon t.
Andrews-Pynchon suction t.
angled pleural t.
angled suction t.
angulated buccal t.
anterior chamber t.
Anthony suction t.
antifog t.
aortic sump t.
Argyle chest t.
Argyle-Dennis t.
Argyle endotracheal t.
Argyle feeding t.
Argyle-Salem sump t.
Argyle Sentinel Seal chest t.
Arm-a-Med endotracheal t.
armored endotracheal t.
Armstrong grommet ventilation t.
Armstrong V-Vent t.
Arrow t.
ascites drainage t.
Asepto suction t.
Aspisafe nasogastric t.
Atkins-Cannard tracheal t.
Atkins-Cannard tracheotomy t.
Atkinson silicone rubber t.
auditory t.
Axiom double sump t.
Ayre t.
Babcock t.
Baerveldt glaucoma implant t.
Baker jejunostomy t.
Baker self-sumping t.
Baldwin butterfly ventilation t.
Bard gastrostomy feeding t.
Bardic t.
Bard PEG t.

Barnes suction t.
Baron ear t.
Baron-Frazier suction t.
basal lamina of neural t.
basal plate of neural t.
Baylor cardiovascular sump t.
Baylor intracardiac sump t.
Beall-Feldman-Cooley sump t.
Beardsley empyema t.
Bellocq t.
Bellucci suction t.
Bel-O-Pak suction t.
Bettman empyema t.
Billroth t.
Binova Medical Technologies
  customized tracheostomy t.
Biolite ventilation t.
Biosystems feeding t.
Bivona Fome-Cuff t.
Bivona sleep apnea tracheostomy t.
Bivona TTS tracheostomy t.
Blakemore esophageal t.
Blakemore nasogastric t.
Blakemore-Sengstaken t.
Blue Line cuffed endotracheal t.
blunt suction t.
bobbin myringotomy t.
Bouchut laryngeal t.
Bourdon t.
Bower PEG t.
Bowman t.
Boyce modification of Sengstaken-
  Blakemore t.
Brawley nasal suction t.
bronchial t.'s
Broncho-Cath double-lumen
  endotracheal t.
Broncho-Cath endobronchial t.
bronchoscopy disposable suction t.
Bruecke t.
buccal t.
Bucy-Frazier suction t.
Bucy suction t.
Buie rectal suction t.
bulboventricular t.
Butler tonsillar suction t.
Buyes air-vent suction t.
Caluso PEG t.
Caluso PEG gastrostomy t.
Cantor t.
Cantor intestinal t.
Carabelli endobronchial t.

Carden bronchoscopy t.
Carlens double-lumen
  endotracheal t.
Carl Zeiss myringotomy t.
Carrel t.
Casselberry sphenoid t.
cast buccal t.
Castelli-Paparella collar button t.
cast-like t.
Cattell forked-type T t.
t. cecostomy
Celestin endoesophageal t.
Celestin esophageal t.
Celestin latex rubber t.
t. changer
Charnley drain t.
Chauffen-Pratt t.
Chaussier t.
chest t.
Chevalier Jackson tracheal t.
Clerf laryngectomy t.
closed suction t.
closed water-seal suction t.
Coakley wash t.
Cole endotracheal t.
Cole orotracheal t.
Cole pediatric t.
Cole uncuffed endotracheal t.
collar button t.
Colton empyema t.
Combitube endotracheal t.
Combitube esophageal tracheal t.
Comfit endotracheal t.
Compat feeding t.
Cone-Bucy suction t.
Cone suction t.
Contigen t.
continuous suction t.
Cook County tracheal suction t.
Cooley-Anthony suction t.
Cooley aortic sump t.
Cooley graft suction t.
Cooley intracardiac suction t.
Cooley sump suction t.
Cooley vascular suction t.
Coolidge t.
Cope loop nephrostomy t.
corneal t.
Corpak feeding t.
Corpak weighted-tip, self-
  lubricating t.
Costen suction t.

NOTES

tube *(continued)*
Cottle suction t.
Coupland nasal suction t.
Crawford t.
cricothyrotomy trocar t.
Crookes-Hittorf t.
cuffed endotracheal t.
cuffed tracheostomy t.
CUI myringotomy t.
cystostomy t.
Dandy suction t.
David pharyngolaryngectomy t.
Davol t.
Dawson-Yuhl suction t.
Deane t.
Dean wash t.
Deaver t.
DeBakey-Adson suction t.
DeBakey suction t.
Debove t.
decompression t.
t. decompression
Denker t.
Dennis t.
Dennis intestinal t.
DePaul t.
DeVilbiss suction t.
Devine-Millard-Frazier fiberoptic suction t.
diagnostic t.
DIC tracheostomy t.
digestive t.
t. dilution test
disposable Yankauer suction t.
Dobbhoff feeding t.
Dobbhoff gastric decompression t.
Dobbhoff PEG t.
Doesel-Huzly bronchoscopic t.
Donaldson t.
Donaldson eustachian t.
Donaldson ventilation t.
dorsal plate of neural t.
double-cannula tracheostomy t.
double-focus t.
double-lumen endobronchial t.
double-lumen suction irrigation t.
double setup endotracheal t.
Dow Corning t.
drainage t.
drain-to-wall suction t.
Dreiling t.
Dr. Twiss duodenal t.
dual-lumen sump nasogastric t.
dual percutaneous gastrostomy t.
Duke t.
Dundas-Grant t.
Duralite t.
Durham tracheostomy t.

Eastman suction t.
E. Benson Hood Laboratories esophageal t.
E. Benson Hood Laboratories salivary bypass t.
edgewise buccal t.
Edlich gastric lavage t.
Einhorn t.
embryonic neural t.
empyema t.
encircling polyethylene t.
end t.
endobrachial double-lumen t.
endobronchial t.
endocardial t.
endoesophageal t.
endoneural t.
endoneurial t.
endoscopic t.
endoscopic gastrostomy t.
Endosoft reinforced cuffed t.
endothelial t.
endotracheal t. (ETT)
Endotrol endotracheal t.
Endotrol tracheal t.
ENDO-Tube nasal jejunal feeding t.
enteral feeding t.
enteroclysis t.
EntriStar feeding t.
EntriStar polyethylene PEG t.
EntriStar polyurethane PEG t.
Eppendorf t.
ESKA-Buess esophageal t.
Esmarch t.
esophageal t.
ET t.
eustachian t.
Ewald t.
extension t.
t. extrusion
fallopian t.
Fay suction t.
t. feeding
feeding gastrostomy t.
fenestrated t.
fenestrated tracheostomy t.
Ferguson-Frazier suction t.
Feuerstein drainage t.
Feuerstein split ventilation t.
fiberoptic suction t.
fil d'Arion silicone t.
fimbriated end of fallopian t.
Finsterer myringotomy split t.
Finsterer suction t.
Fitzpatrick suction t.
flanged Teflon t.
t. flap graft

Flexiflo enteral feeding t.
Flexiflo gastrostomy t.
Flexiflo Inverta-Peg t.
Flexiflo Sacks-Vine t.
Flexiflo stoma creator t.
Flexiflo Stomate gastrostomy t.
Flexiflo suction feeding t.
Flexiflo tap-fill enteral t.
Flexiflo Taptainer t.
Flexiflo tungsten-weighted
  feeding t.
Flexiflo Versa-PEG t.
flow regulated suction t.
fluffy-cuffed t.
Fome-Cuf endotracheal t.
Fome-Cuf tracheostomy t.
four-lumen t.
Franco triflange ventilation t.
Frazier aspirating t.
Frazier Britetrac nasal suction t.
Frazier nasal suction t.
Frazier-Paparella mastoid suction t.
Frederick-Miller t.
Fuller bivalve trach t.
fusion t.
Gabriel Tucker t.
gastric augment and single
  pedicle t.
gastrointestinal t.
gastrostomy feeding t.
Gavriliu gastric t.
GBH bypass t.
germ t.
Gillquist-Stille arthroplasty
  suction t.
Gillquist suction t.
Glasser gastrostomy t.
Glover suction t.
glow modulator t.
glutaraldehyde-tanned bovine
  collagen t.
Gomco suction t.
Goode Trim t.
Goode T-tube ventilating t.
Gore-Tex t.
Gott t.
Grafco Martin laryngectomy t.
graft suction t.
Great Ormond Street pediatric
  tracheostomy t.
Great Ormond Street
  tracheostomy t.

Greiling gastroduodenal t.
grommet drain t.
grommet ventilating t.
Guibor t.
Guibor duct t.
Guibor Silastic t.
Guilford-Wright suction t.
Guisez t.
guttered T t.
Gwathmey suction t.
Haering t.
Hagan surface suction t.
Haldane-Priestley t.
Hardy suction t.
Har-el pharyngeal t.
Harris t.
Heimlich t.
Heimlich-Gavrilu gastric t.
Helsper tracheostomy vent t.
Hemagard collection t.
Hemovac suction t.
heparin-bonded Bott-type t.
Herring t.
Hi-Lo Jet tracheal t.
Holter t.
horizontal t.
Hossli suction t.
Hough-Cadogan suction t.
House-Baron suction t.
House endolymphatic shunt t.
House-Radpour suction t.
House-Stevenson suction t.
House suction t.
House-Urban t.
Hubbard airplane vent t.
Humphrey coronary sinus-sucker
  suction t.
Hymlek portable chest t.
Hyperflex tracheostomy t.
Immergut suction t.
Inconel t.
indicator t.
infusion t.
insertion t.
intestinal t.
intracardiac suction t.
intracardiac sump t.
intratracheal t.
irrigation t.
Israel suction t.
Jackson cane-shaped tracheal t.
Jackson cone-shaped tracheal t.

NOTES

tube *(continued)*
Jackson laryngectomy t.
Jackson open-end aspirating t.
Jackson-Pratt suction t.
Jackson-Rees endotracheal t.
Jackson silver tracheostomy t.
Jackson tracheal t.
Jackson velvet-eye aspirating t.
Jacques gastric t.
Jako laryngeal suction t.
Jako suction t.
Jarit-Poole abdominal suction t.
Jarit-Yankauer suction t.
Javid bypass t.
jejunal feeding t.
jejunostomy t.
Jergesen t.
Jiffy t.
Johnson intestinal t.
Jones Pyrex t.
Jones tear duct t.
J-shaped t.
Jutte t.
Kangaroo gastrostomy feeding t.
Kangaroo silicone gastrostomy feeding t.
Kaslow gastrointestinal t.
Kaslow intestinal t.
Kay-Cross suction tip suction t.
Kelly t.
Keofeed feeding t.
KeyMed esophageal t.
Killian suction t.
Kistner plastic tracheostomy t.
Klein ventilation t.
Knoche t.
knuckle of t.
Kozlowski t.
Kritter irrigation t.
Kuhn endotracheal t.
Kurze suction t.
Lacor t.
Lahey Y-tube t.
Lanz low-pressure cuff endotracheal t.
Lar-A-Jext laryngectomy t.
large-bore gastric lavage t.
LaRocca nasolacrimal t.
laryngeal suction t.
laryngectomy t.
Laryngoflex reinforced endotracheal t.
laser laryngeal suction t.
Laser-Trach endotracheal t.
t. leakage
Leiter t.
Lell tracheal t.
Lennarson t.
Lepley-Ernst tracheal t.
Levin-Davol t.
Levin duodenal t.
Lewis laryngectomy t.
Lezius suction t.
life-saving t.
Lindeman-Silverstein Arrow t.
Lindeman-Silverstein ventilation t.
Lindholm tracheal t.
Linton esophageal t.
Linton-Nachlas t.
long intestinal t.
Lonnecken t.
Lo-Por tracheal t.
Lord-Blakemore t.
Lore-Lawrence trachea t.
Lore-Lawrence tracheotomy t.
Lore suction t.
L.T. Jones tear duct t.
Luer speaking t.
Luer tracheal t.
Lyon t.
MacKenty laryngectomy t.
Mackler intraluminal t.
Mackray short-cuffed endobronchial t.
Madoff suction t.
Magill Safety Clear Plus endotracheal t.
Malecot gastrostomy t.
Malecot nephrostomy t.
Malis-Frazier suction t.
malleable multipore suction t.
Mallinckrodt endotracheal t.
Mallinckrodt Laser-Flex t.
marked t.
Martin laryngectomy t.
Martin tracheostomy t.
Mason suction t.
McGowan-Keeley t.
McMurtry-Schlesinger shunt t.
Medena t.
mediastinal t.
Medina t.
Medoc-Celestin pulsion t.
medullary t.
mesh myringotomy t.
metal-weighted Silastic feeding t.
Methodist vascular suction t.
MIC gastrostomy t.
MIC jejunal t.
MIC jejunostomy t.
Mic-Key gastrostomy t.
Microfuge t.
microlaryngeal endotracheal t.
Micron bobbin ventilation t.
t. migration
Mik gastrostomy t.

Miller t.
Miller-Abbott double-lumen
 intestinal t.
Miller-Abbott intestinal t.
Miller endotracheal t.
Millin suction t.
Mill-Rose t.
Milroy-Piper suction t.
Minnesota t.
Mixter t.
modified Minnesota t.
modified suction t.
molar t.
Momberg t.
Montando t.
Montefiore tracheal t.
Montgomery esophageal t.
Montgomery salivary bypass t.
Montgomery tracheal t.
Morch swivel tracheostomy t.
Moretz Tiny Tytan ventilation t.
Morse-Andrews suction t.
Morse-Ferguson suction t.
Morse suction t.
Mosher intubation t.
Mosher life-saving suction t.
Mosher life-saving tracheal t.
Moss gastrostomy t.
Moss Mark IV t.
Moss Suction Buster t.
Moulton lacrimal duct t.
Mousseau-Barbin esophageal t.
Mousseau-Barbin prosthetic t.
Mueller-Frazier suction t.
Mueller-Pool suction t.
Mueller-Pynchon suction t.
Mueller suction t.
Mueller-Yankauer suction t.
Muldoon t.
Myerson wash t.
myringotomy drain t.
Nachlas gastrointestinal t.
Nachlas-Linton t.
nasal Rae t.
nasal suction t.
nasobiliary t.
nasocystic drainage t.
nasoduodenal feeding t.
nasoenteric feeding t.
nasogastric feeding t.
nasoileal t.
nasojejunal feeding t.

nasotracheal t.
NCC Hi-Lo Jet endotracheal t.
negative pressure t.
negative pressure-controlled t.
nephrostomy t.
nephrotomy t.
Neuber bone t.
neural t.
New Luer-type speaking t.
NG t.
Nilsson suction t.
Nishizaki-Wakabayashi suction t.
NIXIE t.
NJ feeding t.
Norton endotracheal t.
Nunez ventricular ventilation t.
Nuport PEG t.
Nyhus-Nelson gastric decompression
 and jejunal feeding t.
Nystroem abdominal suction t.
O'Beirne sphincter t.
Ochsner gallbladder t.
O'Dwyer t.
O'Hanlon-Poole suction t.
Olympus One-Step Button
 gastrostomy t.
Ommaya ventricular t.
opaque myringotomy t.
oroendotracheal t.
orogastric Ewald t.
oropharyngeal t.
orotracheal t.
Ossoff-Karlan laser suction t.
otopharyngeal t.
Oxford nonkinking cuffed t.
Panda gastrostomy t.
Panda nasoenteric feeding t.
Panje t.
Paparella-Frazier suction t.
Paparella myringotomy t.
Paparella ventilation t.
Parker t.
Paul intestinal drainage t.
Paul-Mixter t.
pediatric feeding t.
pediatric nasogastric t.
Pedi PEG t.
Pee Wee low-profile gastrostomy t.
PEG t.
PEG-400 t.
PEJ t.

T

NOTES

tube *(continued)*

percutaneous endoscopic gastrostomy t.
percutaneous endoscopic placement of jejunal t.
Per-Lee equalizing t.
Per-Lee myringotomy t.
Per-Lee ventilation t.
Pertrach percutaneous tracheostomy t.
pharyngotympanic t.
Pierce antrum wash t.
pigtail nephrostomy t.
Pilling duralite t.
Pitt talking tracheostomy t.
t. placement
plastic-cuffed tracheostomy t.
pleural t.
Pleur-evac suction t.
Polisar-Lyons adapted tracheal t.
polyethylene t.
polyvinyl chloride t.
Ponsky-Gauderer PEG t.
Ponsky PEG t.
Poole abdominal suction t.
Poole suction t.
Poppen suction t.
Portex Per-Fit tracheostomy t.
Portex preformed blue line tracheal t.
Porto-Vac suction t.
postpyloric feeding t.
t. precipitin test
preformed polyvinyl chloride endotracheal t.
Pribram suction t.
primordial catheter t.
Procter-Livingstone t.
Proctor suction t.
proctosigmoid disposable suction t.
Puestow-Olander gastrointestinal t.
pus t.
Pynchon suction t.
Pyrex t.
Questek laser t.
Quickert-Dryden t.
Quinton t.
Radpour-House suction t.
RAE endotracheal t.
RAE-Flex tracheal t.
Rand-House suction t.
Rand-Radpour suction t.
rectal t.
rectifier t.
Redivac suction t.
Rehfuss duodenal t.
Rehfuss stomach t.
Reinecke-Carroll lacrimal t.

reinforced tracheostomy t.
t. removal
t. replacement
Replogle t.
Reuter bobbin ventilating t.
Reuter bobbin ventilation t.
Rhoton-Merz suction t.
Rica mastoid suction t.
right-angle chest t.
Ring-McLean sump t.
Ritter suprapubic suction t.
Robertshaw t.
Robinson equalizing t.
Rochester suction t.
Rochester tracheal t.
roll t.
Roller pump suction t.
Rosen suction t.
Ruschelit polyvinyl chloride endotracheal t.
Rusch laryngectomy t.
Russell suction t.
Ryle duodenal t.
Sachs suction t.
Sacks-Vine feeding gastrostomy t.
Sacks-Vine PEG t.
Salem duodenal sump t.
Salem sump action nasogastric t.
salivary bypass t.
Samson-Davis infant suction t.
Sandoz Caluso PEG gastrostomy t.
Sandoz feeding/suction t.
Sandoz nasogastric feeding t.
Sandoz suction t.
Sandoz suction/feeding t.
Sarns intracardiac suction t.
Saticon vacuum chamber pickup t.
S-B t.
scavenging t.
Schall laryngectomy t.
Schmiedt t.
Schuknecht suction t.
Schuler aspiration/irrigation t.
Scott-Harden t.
Scott nasal suction t.
Securat suction t.
Sengstaken-Blakemore t.
Sengstaken esophageal t.
Sengstaken nasogastric t.
Sensiv endotracheal t.
Seroma-Cath drainage t.
Seroma-Cath feeding t.
Shah ventilation t.
Shea-type parasol myringotomy t.
Sheehy collar-button ventilating t.
Sheehy Tytan ventilation t.
Shepard drain t.
Shepard grommet ventilation t.

Sherman suction t.
Shiley cuffless fenestrated t.
Shiley cuffless tracheostomy t.
Shiley French sump t.
Shiley laryngectomy t.
Shiley low-pressure cuffed
 tracheostomy t.
Shiley neonatal tracheostomy t.
Shiley pediatric tracheostomy t.
Shiner t.
short-cuffed endobronchial t.
Silastic eustachian t.
Silastic intestinal t.
Silastic sucker suction t.
Silastic tracheostomy t.
silicone t.
silicone-lubricated endotracheal t.
Silverstein permanent aeration t.
Singer-Bloom t.
siphon suction t.
skin t.
sliding t.
small-bowel t.
Smith t.
Snyder Urevac suction t.
Softech endotracheal t.
Soileau Tytan ventilation t.
Southey capillary drainage t.
Souttar t.
speaking t.
Spetzler Microvac suction t.
spiral-wound endotracheal t.
SS bobbin myringotomy t.
Stamey t.
Stamm gastrostomy t.
Stedman continuous suction t.
stiffening t.
stockinette t.
stomach t.
Stomate extension t.
Storz suction t.
straight t.
suction t.
sump nasogastric t.
Sustagen nasogastric t.
Swan-Ganz t.
T t.
tampon t.
tear duct t.
t. teeth
Teflon nasobiliary t.
test t.

T-grommet ventilation t.
Thiersch t.
thoracostomy t.
t. thoracostomy
Thora-Klex chest t.
three-bottle tidal suction t.
tight-to-shaft Aire-Cuf
 tracheostomy t.
Tiny-Tef ventilation t.
Tiny Tytan ventilation t.
tonsillar suction t.
tooth t.
Touma T-type grommet
 ventilation t.
Tovell t.
Toynbee diagnostic t.
tracheal t.
tracheostomy t.
tracheotomy t.
Tracoe tracheostomy t.
Trake-Fit endotracheal t.
translaryngeal endotracheal t.
translucent drain t.
translucent myringotomy t.
transpyloric feeding t.
triple buccal t.
triple-lumen Sengstaken-
 Blakemore t.
TTS Aire-Cuf endotracheal t.
TTS Aire-Cuf tracheostomy t.
T-tube round suction t.
T-type myringotomy t.
Tucker aspirating t.
Tucker flexible tip t.
Tucker tracheal t.
Turkel t.
twist-in drain t.
twist-in myringotomy t.
tympanostomy t.
tympanotomy t.
Tytan grommet ventilation t.
uncuffed endotracheal t.
underwater-seal suction t.
Univent Inoue t.
Univent single-lumen
 endotracheal t.
urinary drainage t.
uterine t.
UTTS endotracheal t.
U-tube t.
Vacutainer t.
vacuum t.

NOTES

tube *(continued)*
    Valentine irrigation t.
    Van Alyea antral wash t.
    vascular suction t.
    vent t.
    ventilation t.
    ventral plate of neural t.
    Venturi bobbin myringotomy t.
    Venturi collar-button
      myringotomy t.
    Venturi grommet myringotomy t.
    Venturi pediatric myringotomy t.
    Vernon antral wash t.
    vertical t.
    vinyl t.
    Vinyon-N cloth t.
    Vivonex gastrostomy t.
    Vivonex Moss t.
    V. Mueller-Frazier suction t.
    V. Mueller-Poole suction t.
    Voltolini ear t.
    Von Eichen antral wash t.
    Vortex tracheotomy t.
    Wangensteen suction t.
    Wannagat suction t.
    wash t.
    water-seal chest t.
    Webster infusion t.
    Weck suction t.
    Welch Allyn suction t.
    Wendl t.
    Wepsic suction t.
    White t.
    Williams esophageal t.
    Willscher t.
    Wilson-Cook nasobiliary t.
    Wilson-Cook NJFT-series feeding t.
    Winsburg-White bladder t.
    wire-wound endotracheal t.
    Wolf suction t.
    Woodbridge t.
    Wookey skin t.
    woven dacron t.
    Wullstein microsuction t.
    Wurbs-type nasobiliary t.
    Xomed endotracheal t.
    Xomed straight-shank t.
    Xomed-Treace ventilation t.
    Yankauer aspirating t.
    Yankauer suction t.
    Yankauer-type suction t.
    Yasargil microsuction t.
    Yasargil suction t.
    Yeder suction t.
    Zollner suction t.
    Zyler t.
tube-carina distance
tubectomy

tubed
    t. free skin graft
    t. groin flap
    t. pedicle flap
    t. urethroplasty
tube-fed patient
tube-occluding
tube-patient distance
tuber, pl. **tubera**
    calcaneal t.
    t. calcanei
    t. calcis
    frontal t.
    t. frontale
    t. ischiadicum
    t. of ischium
    omental t.
    t. omentale
    parietal t.
    t. parietale
    t. radii
    t. zygomaticum
tubercle
    accessory t.
    anterior t. of atlas
    anterior t. of cervical vertebrae
    t. of anterior scalene muscle
    articular t. of temporal bone
    auricular t.
    calcaneal t.
    carotid t.
    Chassaignac t.
    conoid t.
    corniculate t.
    cuneiform t.
    dissection t.
    dorsal t. of radius
    genital t.
    Gerdy t.
    greater t. of humerus
    hard t.
    iliac t.
    t. of iliac crest
    inferior thyroid t.
    infraglenoid t.
    jugular t.
    labial t.
    lateral t. of posterior process of
      talus
    Lisfranc t.
    Lister t.
    mamillary t.
    marginal t.
    marginal t. of zygomatic bone
    medial t. of posterior process of
      talus
    mental t.
    Morgagni t.

obturator t.
orbital t. of zygomatic bone
t. osteotomy
pharyngeal t.
posterior t. of atlas
posterior t. of cervical vertebrae
Princeteau t.
prosector t.
pterygoid t.
pubic t.
t. of rib
t. of root of zygoma
t. of saddle
scalene t.
scalene t. of Lisfranc
t. of scaphoid bone
soft t.
superior thyroid t.
supratragic t.
t. of trapezium
t. of upper lip
wedge-shaped t.
Whitnall t.
Wrisberg t.
tubercula (*pl. of* tuberculum)
tuberculation
tuberculization
tuberculocele
tuberculoma
tuberculosis
central nervous system t.
endobronchial t.
endometrial t.
extra-articular t.
extrapulmonary t.
extrathoracic t.
exudative t.
t. granulation tissue
inhalation t.
peritoneal t.
reactivation t.
reinfection t.
surgical t.
tuberculous
t. abscess
t. caseation
t. infiltration
t. lesion
tuberculum, pl. tubercula
t. anterius atlantis
t. anterius vertebrarum cervicalium
t. articulare ossis temporalis

t. auriculae
t. calcanei
t. caroticum
t. costae
t. cuneiforme
t. dorsale
t. iliacum
t. intercondylare
t. jugulare
t. labii superioris
t. laterale processus posterioris tali
t. majus humeri
t. marginale ossis zygomatici
t. mediale processus posterioris tali
t. mentale
t. minus humeri
t. musculi scaleni anterioris
t. obturatorium
t. ossis scaphoidei
t. ossis trapezii
t. pharyngeum
t. posterius atlantis
t. posterius vertebrarum cervicalium
t. pubicum
t. sellae
t. superius
t. supratragicum
t. thyroideum inferius
t. thyroideum superius
tuberoinfundibular tract
tuberositas
t. costalis
t. pterygoidea
t. sacralis
tuberosity
costal t.
t. fragment
pterygoid t.
reduction t.
t. reduction
t. for serratus anterior muscle
tube-shift technique
Tubestat lighted stylet
tube-to-film distance
tube-within-tube technique
tubi (*pl. of* tubus)
tubing
evacuator t.
Ott insufflator filter t.
polyethylene t.
pressure-separator t.

T

NOTES

tubing *(continued)*
    shunt t.
    suction t.
tuboabdominal
***d*-tubocurarine**
    dimethyl *d*-tubocurarine
tubocurarine chloride
tuboligamentous
tubo-ovarian
tubo-ovariectomy
tuboperitoneal
tuboplasty
    balloon t.
    transcervical balloon t.
    ultrasound transcervical t.
tubotorsion
tubouterine
    t. implantation
tubovaginal
tubular
    t. aneurysm
    t. basement membrane
    t. colonic duplication
    t. excretory mass
    t. reconstruction
    t. regeneration
    t. respiration
    t. vertical gastroplasty
tubularized
    t. bladder neck reconstruction
    t. cecal flap
tubulation
tubule
    Albarran y Dominguez t.'s
    convoluted seminiferous t.
    Henle t.'s
    mesonephric t.
    paragenital t.'s
    straight seminiferous t.
    uriniferous t.
tubuli *(pl. of* tubulus)
tubulization
tubulovillar lesion
tubulus, pl. **tubuli**
    tubuli biliferi
    tubuli epoöphori
    tubuli galactophori
    tubuli lactiferi
tubus, pl. **tubi**
    t. digestorius
    t. medullaris
    t. vertebralis
tuck
    t. position
    t. procedure
Tucker
    T. aspirating tube

    T. flexible tip tube
    T. tracheal tube
Tudor-Thomas
    T.-T. graft
    T.-T. operation
Tuffier morcellement technique
tuft
    t. fracture
tug
    tracheal t.
Tukey post-hoc correction
tulle gras
Tullos technique
tumbling
    t. procedure
    t. technique
    t. technique operation
tumor
    t. ablation
    adenoid t.
    ampullary t.
    aortic body t.
    t. ascites
    t. bed
    biliary tract t.
    bleeding t.
    blood t.
    t. blood supply
    blood vessel t.
    t. blush
    bone t.
    brain t.
    brown fat t.
    t. bulk
    t. burden
    t. capsule
    cardiac t.
    carotid body t.
    celiac t.
    t. cell-host bone relationship
    t. cell purging
    cervical t.
    colon t.
    colorectal t.
    debulking of t.
    deep t.
    t. defect
    t. doubling time
    dumbbell t.
    duodenal t.
    t. embolism
    t. encapsulation
    endocrine t.
    t. erosion
    esophageal t.
    eye t.
    eyelid t.
    t. of eyelid

focal t.
foci of t.
fungating t.
genital tract t.
gritty t.
t. growth
hepatic t.
t. hypoxia
t. imaging
t. infiltration
t. of interior of eye
invasive t.
lacrimal gland t.
liver t.
lumbar t.
lung t.
t. lysis syndrome
t. mass
mediastinal t.
t. metastatic to spine
musculoskeletal t.
t. necrosis
t. neovasculature
t., node, metastasis (TNM)
t., node, metastasis classification
ocular t.
optic nerve t.
t. of optic nerve
oral cavity t.
orbital t.
ovarian t.
t. oxygenation
pituitary t.
t. ploidy
t. plop
t. polysaccharide substance
potato t. of neck
primary t.
t. progression
t. promoter
pulmonary t.
t. receptor protein negative
recurrent t.
t. registry
t. regression
renal t.
t. resection
sacral bone t.
sacrococcygeal t.
salivary gland t.
t. seeding
sellar t.

t. shrinkage
sinonasal t.
t. in situ
t. size
t. skin test
skull base t.
small bowel t.
t. spillage
spinal cord t.
t. stage
t. stage grouping
t. staging
t. stenting
t. suppressor
temporal bone t.
testicular t.
t. therapy
thyroid t.
tracheal t.
transurethral resection of bladder t.
t. vascularity
t. vessel
t. volume
tumor-associated
tumor-cell product
tumor:cerebellum ratio
tumor-free margin
tumorigenesis
    foreign body t.
tumor-like bone condition
tumor-specific
tumor-targeting ability
tunable dye laser lithotripsy
tunic
    fibrous t. of corpus spongiosum
    mucosal t.'s
    muscular t.'s
    muscular t. of gallbladder
tunica, pl. **tunicae**
    t. adventitia
    t. albuginea of corpora cavernosa
    t. albuginea corporis spongiosi
    t. albuginea corporum cavernosorum
    t. albuginea of corpus spongiosum
    t. albuginea testis
    t. albuginea of testis
    t. carnea
    t. dartos
    t. elastica
    t. fibrosa
    t. fibrosa hepatis
    t. fibrosa lienis

NOTES

tunica *(continued)*
    t. fibrosa renis
    t. fibrosa splenis
tunicae funiculi spermatici
    t. intima
    t. media
    t. mucosa
    t. mucosa bronchiorum
    t. mucosa cavitatis tympani
    t. mucosa coli
    t. mucosa ductus deferentis
    t. mucosa esophagi
    t. mucosa gastrica [ventriculi]
    t. mucosa intestini tenuis
    t. mucosa laryngis
    t. mucosa linguae
    t. mucosa pharyngis
    t. mucosa tracheae
    t. mucosa tubae uterinae
    t. mucosa ureteris
    t. mucosa urethrae femininae
    t. mucosa uteri
    t. mucosa vaginae
    t. mucosa vesicae biliaris
    t. mucosa vesicae felleae
    t. mucosa vesicae urinariae
    t. mucosa vesiculae seminalis
    t. muscularis
    t. muscularis bronchiorum
    t. muscularis coli
    t. muscularis ductus deferentis
    t. muscularis esophagi
    t. muscularis gastrica
    t. muscularis intestini tenuis
    t. muscularis pharyngis
    t. muscularis recti
    t. muscularis tracheae
    t. muscularis tubae uterinae
    t. muscularis ureteris
    t. muscularis urethrae femininae
    t. muscularis uteri
    t. muscularis vaginae
    t. muscularis ventriculi
    t. muscularis vesicae biliaris
    t. muscularis vesicae felleae
    t. muscularis vesicae urinariae
    t. propria lienis
    t. reflexa
    t. serosa coli
    t. serosa gastrica
    t. serosa hepatis
    t. serosa intestini tenuis
    t. serosa peritonei
    t. serosa tubae uterinae
    t. serosa uteri
    t. serosa ventriculi
    t. serosa vesicae biliaris
    t. serosa vesicae felleae

    t. serosa vesicae urinariae
    t. submucosa
    t. vaginalis blanket wrap
    t. vaginalis communis
    t. vaginalis testis
    t. vasculosa testis
tunnel
    catheter t.
    t. creation
    t. graft
    t. infection
    t. and sling fixation
tunneled ventriculostomy
Tupper arthroplasty
turbid peritoneal fluid
turbinal
turbinate
turbinated
turbinectomy
turbinoplasty
Türck
    T. bundle
    T. tract
Turco clubfoot release technique
Turco-Spinella tendo calcaneus repair
Turcot syndrome
Turkel tube
Turkish saddle
Turk line
turn-and-suction
    t.-a.-s. biopsy technique
    t.-a.-s. technique
Turnbull
    T. colostomy
    T. end-loop ileostomy
    T. multiple ostomy operation
    T. technique
turned-up pulp deformity
turnover flap
TUR syndrome
turunda
tutamen, pl. **tutamina**
    tutamina cerebri
TUU
    transureteroureterostomy
TVI
    total vascular isolation
Tweed
    T. method
    T. method of dentofacial analysis
twelfth cranial nerve
twilight sleep
twin
    t. bracket tooth rotation
    t. formation
    t. method
Twining line
twirling method

twisted
  t. cotton suture
  t. dermal suture
  t. linen suture
  t. virgin silk suture
twist-in
  t.-i. drain tube
  t.-i. myringotomy tube
twist-off technique
twists
  stitch with t.
twitch
  t. depression
  evoked t.
  t. height
  t. height test
  t. response
  t. suppression
  t. tension
two-bellied muscle
two-chamber longitudinal (2C-L)
two-dimensional
  t.-d. Fourier transformation imaging
  t.-d. Fourier transform gradient-echo
    imaging
  t.-d. monitoring
two-dye method
two-flight exertional dyspnea
two-inclinometer method
two-layer
  t.-l. anastomosis
  t.-l. enteroenterostomy
  t.-l. open technique
two-loop J-shaped ileal pouch
**two-microphone acoustic reflection
  method**
two-needle technique
two-part fracture
two-patch technique
two-piece ostomy pouch
two-plane
  t.-p. deformity
  t.-p. fluoroscopy
  t.-p. occlusion
two-point
  t.-p. discrimination test
  t.-p. nerve block
two-portal technique
two-pour technique
two-sleeve technique
two-stage
  t.-s. hip fusion

  t.-s. procedure
  t.-s. repair
  t.-s. Syme amputation
  t.-s. tendon grafting technique
  t.-s. tendon graft reconstruction
two-step
  t.-s. orchiopexy
  t.-s. procedure
  t.-s. technique
two-team dissection
**two-wavelength near-infrared
  spectroscope**
Tycos pressure infusion line
Tycron suture
tylectomy
tylion
tyloma
tympanic
  t. bone
  t. canal
  t. cavity
  t. membrane
  t. membrane measurement
  t. neurectomy
  t. part of temporal bone
  t. ring
  t. thermometry
tympanohyal bone
tympanomastoid
  t. fissure
  t. suture
tympanomastoidectomy
tympanomeatal flap
tympanoplasty
  t. mastoidectomy
  t. ossiculoplasty
  staged t.
  type I–V t.
tympanosquamosal
  t. suture
tympanosquamous fissure
tympanostomy
  t. tube
tympanotemporal
tympanotomy
  t. tube
tyndallization
type
  t. C pelvic ring fracture
  t. I, II, III, IIIA, IIIB, IIIC open
    fracture

NOTES

785

type *(continued)*
    t. I–IV canal
    t. I–V tympanoplasty
typhlectasis
typhlectomy
typhlodicliditis
typhloempyema
typhlolithiasis
typhlon
typhlopexy
typhlorrhaphy
typhlostomy

typhlotomy
typhloureterostomy
typing
    tissue t.
Tyrode solution
tyroma
Tyrrell fascia
Tyrrell-Gray
    T.-G. stitch
    T.-G. suture
Tyson glands
Tytan grommet ventilation tube

U
- U pouch
- U pouch construction

UA
- umbilical arterial
- UA blood

UGI
- UGI endoscopy
- UGI tract

Uhl
- U. anomaly
- U. malformation

UICC
- International Union Against Cancer
- Union Internationale Contre le Cancer
- UICC tumor classification

UICC-RO resection

ulcer
- u. lesion

ulceration
- acute hemorrhagic u.
- anal u.
- anastomotic u.
- aphthous u.
- A.S.A.-induced gastric u.
- catarrhal marginal u.
- CMV-associated u.
- CMV-induced esophageal u.
- collar-button u.
- u. of cornea
- corneal u.
- diffuse u.
- duodenal u.
- esophageal u.
- gastric u.
- gastrointestinal u.
- genital u.
- herpes epithelial tropic u.
- intertrigo with u.
- intestinal u.
- labial u.
- marginal u.
- mucosal u.
- mucous membrane u.
- nasal mucosal u.
- necrotic u.
- oral u.
- u. of oral mucosa
- patchy colonic u.
- postbulbar u.
- radiation-induced u.
- rectal u.
- rheumatoid-related u.
- serpiginous u.
- stasis u.

stercoral u.
- stomal u.
- stress u.
- stress-induced gastric u.
- sublesional u.
- tracheal u.
- transurethral resection of prostate u.

ulcerative
- u. colitis
- u. inflammation

ulcerogenic fistula

ulcerogranuloma

ulectomy

ulegyria

uletomy

Ullmann line

Ulloa operation

ulna, pl. **ulnae**

ulnar
- u. artery
- u. branch of medial antebrachial cutaneous nerve
- u. bursa
- u. collateral ligament rupture
- u. communicating branch of superficial radial nerve
- u. deviation deformity
- u. drift deformity
- u. eminence of wrist
- u. fracture
- u. head
- u. head excision
- u. hemiresection interposition arthroplasty
- u. motor neurectomy
- u. translation

ulnaris
- extensor carpi u. (ECU)

ulocarcinoma

uloid

ulotomy

Ultane

Ultiva

ultra
- u. high-magnification endoscopy
- U. Tears solution

ultrabrachycephalic

Ultracaine

ultrafast CT electron beam tomography

ultrafiltration
- continuous arteriovenous u.
- dialytic u.
- extracorporeal u.

ultrafiltration *(continued)*
    glomerular u.
    spontaneous dialytic u.
ultrahigh frequency ventilation
ultrahigh-frequency ventilation
ultraligation
ultrarapid subthreshold stimulation
ultrasonic
    u. aspiration
    u. attenuation
    u. endovaginal finding
    u. fragmentation
    u. lithotresis
    u. lithotripsy
    u. therapy
ultrasonication
ultrasonographically-guided injection
ultrasonosurgery
ultrasound
    u. anesthetic technique
    u. therapy
    u. transcervical tuboplasty
ultrasound-assisted percutaneous
  endoscopic gastrostomy
ultrasound-guided
    u.-g. automated large-core breast
      biopsy
    u.-g. bronchoscopy
    u.-g. core breast biopsy
    u.-g. fine-needle aspiration
    u.-g. nephrostomy puncture
    u.-g. shock wave therapy
ultraterminal excementosis
Ultratone electrical transcutaneous
  neuromuscular stimulator
ultraviolet (UV)
    u. blood irradiation
    psoralens, u. A (PUVA)
Ultravist injection
ultropaque method
ULT-Svi calibrated end-tidal gas
  analyzer
umbilical
    u. arterial (UA)
    u. artery
    u. artery catheterization
    u. artery line
    u. circulation
    u. cord
    u. cord anomaly
    u. cord hematoma
    u. fissure
    u. fistula
    u. fossa
    u. hernia
    u. hernia rupture
    u. herniorrhaphy
    u. mass

    u. notch
    u. part of left branch of portal
      vein
    u. port
    u. prevesical fascia
    u. region
    u. ring
    u. tape suture
    u. vein (UV)
    u. vein catheterization
    u. vein to maternal vein (UV/MV)
    u. vein recanalization
    u. venous
umbilicate
umbilication
umbilicomammillary triangle
umbilicovesical fascia
umbilicus
umbrella
    u. closure
unabsorbable suture
unattended laboratory operation
unavoidable hemorrhage
unbanded gastroplasty
uncal
    u. herniation
unci (*pl. of* uncus)
unciform
    u. bone
unciforme
uncinate
    u. bundle of Russell
    u. pancreas
    u. procedure
    u. process fracture
    u. process mass
    u. process of pancreas
uncinatum
uncinectomy
uncipressure
uncommitted metaphyseal lesion
unconstrained shoulder arthroplasty
uncovertebral
    u. joints
uncuffed endotracheal tube
uncus, pl. **unci**
uncut
    u. Collis-Nissen fundoplication
    u. Collis-Nissen fundoplication
      method
    u. Collis-Nissen fundoplication
      procedure
    u. Collis-Nissen fundoplication
      technique
underangulation
undercorrection
undercut
    soft tissue u.

underlay fascia technique
underresuscitation
undersensing
    pacemaker u.
underventilation
underwater-seal suction tube
undescended testis
undifferentiated
    u. adenocarcinoma
    u. connective tissue disease
    u. embryonal sarcoma of liver
undifferentiation
undisplaced fracture
undiversion
Undritz anomaly
undulating membrane
undyed suture
uniaxial joint
unicaliceal kidney
unicanalicular sphincter
unicompartmental knee arthroplasty
unicondylar fracture
unification
unifocal optic nerve lesion
unilateral
    u. anesthesia
    u. diaphragmatic elevation
    u. hemidysplasia cornification disorder
    u. hemilaminectomy
    u. hypophysectomy
    u. inguinal hernia repair
    u. inguinal hernia repair method
    u. inguinal hernia repair procedure
    u. inguinal hernia repair technique
    u. interfacetal dislocation
    u. intrafacetal dislocation
    u. nephrectomy
    u. pedicle cannulation
    u. pneumoretroperitoneum
    u. sacroiliac approach
    u. salpingo-oophorectomy
    u. subcostal incision
unilocular
    u. cystic lesion
    u. joint
unimalleolar fracture
Unimar J-needle
uninhibited neurogenic bladder
unintegration
uninterrupted suture

union
    delayed fracture u.
    fibrous u.
    U. Internationale Contre le Cancer (UICC)
    osteonal bone u.
    primary u.
    secondary u.
    vicious u.
unipedicled flap
Unipen injection
unipennate
    u. muscle
unipolar cauterization
uniportal arthroscopic microdiskectomy
Uni-Shunt
unit
    Bair Hugger patient heating u.
    day care surgical u. (DCSU)
    Deltatrac metabolic u.
    Flowtron DVT prophylactic deep venous thrombosis u.
    Hounsfield u. (HU)
    intensive care u. (ICU)
    Kreiselman resuscitation u.
    low-grade suction u.
    u. of mass
    u. membrane
    neurosurgical intensive care u. (NICU)
    Ohmeda intermittent suction u.
    postanesthesia care u. (PACU)
United
    U. Bongort Life-style pouch
    U. Max-E drainable pouch
    U. Surgical Bongort Life-style pouch
    U. Surgical Convex insert
    U. Surgical Featherlite ileostomy pouch
    U. Surgical Shear Plus drainable pouch
    U. Surgical Soft & Secure pouch
uniting
    u. canal
    u. cartilage
    u. duct
unitunnel technique
Univent
    U. Inoue tube
    U. single-lumen endotracheal tube

U

NOTES

Universal
U. curved-tube stylet
U. distal radius fracture classification
U. straight-tube stylet
University
U. of California cuff suspension PTB socket
U. of Pennsylvania Smell Identification Test
U. of Wisconsin preservation fluid
U. of Wisconsin solution
unlocking spiral technique
unplanned valgus osteotomy
unreduced dislocation
unrepositioned flap
unresectable
u. metastasis
unsaturated chemical vapor sterilization
unsex
unstable
u. bladder
u. fracture
u. fracture-dislocation
unstrained jaw relation
unstriated muscle
untethering procedure
ununited fracture
unusual opportunistic infection
unwanted screw torque
up-and-down staircases procedure
upgated technique
UPJ
ureteropelvic junction
upper
u. aerodigestive tract
u. airway obstruction
u. alimentary endoscopy
u. cervical spine anterior exposure
u. cervical spine fusion
u. cervical spine procedure
u. endoscopy and colonoscopy
u. esophageal sphincter relaxation
u. extremity
u. extremity nerve block
u. eyelid
u. gastrointestinal endoscopy
u. gastrointestinal panendoscopy
u. gastrointestinal tract
u. genital tract infection
u. GI hemorrhage
u. GI tract foreign body
u. incisor angulation
u. jaw
u. jaw bone
u. lid
u. lip
u. midclavicular line

u. motor neuron lesion
u. respiratory tract
u. respiratory tract infection
u. respiratory tract mucosa
u. subscapular nerve
u. thoracic splanchnic nerve
u. tract disease
u. trapezius flap
up-regulation
u.-r. of the receptor
upright position
upright-Y incision
upsiloid
uptake
placental u.
urachal
u. carcinoma
u. fistula
u. fold
u. ligament
uraniscoplasty
uraniscorrhaphy
uranoplasty
Wardill-Kilner four-flap u.
uranorrhaphy
uranostaphyloplasty
uranostaphylorrhaphy
uraroma
urate-associated inflammation
urates
uratoma
Urbaniak
U. neurovascular free flap
U. scapular flap
Urban operation
urea hydrolysis
urea-impermeable membrane
Ureaphil injection
urecchysis
uredema
urelcosis
uremic
u. coma
u. gastrointestinal lesion
u. inflammation
ureter
constrictions of u.
curlicue u.
ectopic u.
extravesical infrasphincteric ectopic u.
u. implantation
postcaval u.
retrocaval u.
retroiliac u.
ureteral
u. bladder augmentation
u. branches

u. carcinoma
u. catheterization
u. colic
u. duplication
u. ectopia
u. fistula
u. meatotomy
u. meatus
u. patch procedure
u. perforation
u. pressure
u. reimplantation
u. spatulation
u. stent placement
u. stoma
u. stoma removal
u. surgical treatment

ureteralgia
ureterectasia
ureterectomy
distal u.
ureteric
u. branches
u. branches of the ovarian artery
u. branches of the renal artery
u. branches of the testicular artery
u. fold
u. orifice
u. pelvis
u. plexus
u. stoma
ureteritis
ureterocalicostomy
ureterocele
ectopic u.
orthotopic u.
pyoureter ectopic u.
ureterocelorraphy
ureterocolic
u. fistula
ureterocolonic anastomosis
ureterocolostomy
ureterocutaneous fistula
ureterocystoplasty
ureterocystostomy
ureteroendoscopy
ureteroenteric
ureteroenterostomy
ureterohydronephrosis
ureteroileal anastomosis
ureteroileocecoproctostomy
ureteroileoneocystostomy

ureteroileostomy
Bricker u.
ureterolithiasis
ureterolithotomy
laparoscopic u.
ureterolysis
combined u.
extravesical u.
intravesical u.
Lich-Gregoire u.
Pacquin u.
Politano-Leadbetter u.
ureteroneocystostomy
Glen Anderson u.
u. herniation
Politano-Leadbetter u.
reoperative u.
ureteroneopyelostomy
ureteronephrectomy
ureteropelvic
u. junction (UPJ)
u. obstruction
ureteroperitoneal fistula
ureteroplasty
ileal patch u.
ureteroproctostomy
ureteropyelitis
ureteropyeloneostomy
ureteropyelonephrostomy
uretcropyeloplasty
ureteropyeloscopy
flexible u.
ureteropyelostomy
ureteropyosis
ureterorcctostomy
ureterorenoscopy
transurethral u.
ureterorrhagia
ureterorrhaphy
ureteroscopy
rigid u.
ureterosigmoid
u. anastomosis
ureterosigmoidostomy
ileocecal u.
Maydl u.
ureterostenoma
ureterostenosis
ureterostoma
ureterostomy
cutaneous loop u.
Davis intubated u.

U

NOTES

ureterostomy *(continued)*
    high-loop cutaneous u.
    low-loop cutaneous u.
    retroperitoneal cutaneous u.
ureterotomy
    Davis intubated u.
    intubated u.
ureterotrigonoenterostomy
ureterotubal anastomosis
ureteroureteral
    u. anastomosis
ureteroureterostomy
ureterouterine fistula
ureterovaginal fistula
ureterovesical
    u. obstruction
ureterovesicostomy
urethan
urethra
    anterior u.
    external opening of u.
    female u.
    u. feminina
    fixed drain pipe u.
    male u.
    u. masculina
    membranous u.
    u. muliebris
    penile u.
    posterior u.
    prostatic u.
    spongy u.
    u. virilis
urethral
    u. artery
    u. calculus
    u. carcinoma
    u. carina of vagina
    u. caruncle
    u. closure mechanism
    u. closure pressure profile
    u. coaptation
    u. crest of female
    u. crest of male
    u. dilation
    u. diverticulectomy
    u. glands
    u. groove
    u. lacuna
    u. openings
    u. papilla
    u. pressure
    u. pressure measurement
    u. sphincterotomy
    u. surface of penis
    u. suspension
    u. syndrome
    u. vesicle suspension procedure

urethralgia
urethrectomy
urethremorrhagia
urethrism
urethritis
urethrobalanoplasty
urethrobulbar
urethrocavernous fistula
urethrocecal anastomosis
urethrocele
urethrocystometry
urethrocystopexy
urethrocystoplasty
urethrocystoscopy
urethrodynia
urethrohymenal fusion
urethrolysis
    retropubic u.
    transvaginal u.
urethropenile
urethroperineal
urethroperineoscrotal
urethropexy
    Gittes u.
    Lapides-Ball u.
    Marshall-Marchetti-Krantz u.
    retropubic u.
    Stamey u.
urethroplasty
    Badenoch u.
    Cantwell-Ransley u.
    Cecil u.
    modified Young u.
    onlay island flap u.
    pedicle flap u.
    prostatic u.
    retrograde transurethral prostatic u.
    Tanagho bladder flap u.
    Thiersch-Duplay u.
    tubed u.
urethroprostatic
urethrorectal
    u. fistula
urethrorrhagia
urethrorrhaphy
urethrorrhea
urethroscopic
urethroscopy
    retropubic u.
urethrospasm
urethrostaxis
urethrostenosis
urethrostomy
    perineal u.
    Poncet perineal u.
urethrotomy
    direct vision internal u.
    endoscopic optical u.

external u.
internal u.
perineal u.
Syme external u.
urethrovaginal
u. fistula
urethrovesical
urethrovesicopexy
urge incontinence
urinary
u. apparatus
u. bladder
u. bladder rupture
u. calculus
u. catheterization
u. conduit
u. drainage tube
u. exertional incontinence
u. extraversion
u. fistula
u. organs
u. sand
u. stuttering
u. tract
u. tract abnormality
u. tract anomaly
u. tract disease
u. tract disorder
u. tract infection
u. tract obstruction
urinary-umbilical fistula
urinary-vaginal fistula
urinate
urination
urine
u. specimen collection
uriniferous
u. tubule
urinogenital
urinogenous
urinoma
urinoscopy
urinosexual
urocele
urocheras
urochesia
urocyst
urocystic
urocystis
urodynamics
urodynia

urogenital
u. anomaly
u. apparatus
u. canal
u. cleft
u. diaphragm
u. fistula
u. membrane
u. region
u. ridge
u. septum
u. sinus
u. tract
u. triangle
urogenous
urolith
urolithiasis
urolithic
urolithology
urologic
u. anesthesia
u. complication
u. surgery
u. system cancer
urological evaluation
urologist
urology
Uromat dilation
uroncus
uronephrosis
uronoscopy
uropathy
obstructive u.
uropoiesis
uropoietic
uropsammus
urorectal
u. membrane
u. septum
uroscheocele
uroschesis
uroscopy
urosepsin
urosepsis
urostomy
urothelial
u. basement membrane
u. carcinoma
urothelium
seromuscular enterocystoplasty lined
with u.
urothorax

U

NOTES

urticaria
urtication
URYS 800 nerve stimulator
u-score method
use
> off-label u.

use-dependent sodium channel blocker
U-shaped
> U.-s. incision
> U.-s. scalp flap

Ussing chamber technique
uterectomy
uterine
> u. anomaly
> u. artery
> u. aspiration
> u. cavity
> u. compression
> u. evaluation
> u. fibromyoma
> u. glands
> u. hematoma
> u. hernia syndrome
> u. incision
> u. infection
> u. lysosome level
> u. mass
> u. opening of uterine tubes
> u. ostium of uterine tubes
> u. papillary serous carcinoma
> u. part of uterine tube
> u. perforation
> u. relaxation
> u. rupture
> u. sarcoma metastasis
> u. suspension
> u. tube
> u. veins
> u. venous plexus

uteroabdominal
uterocervical
uterocystostomy
uterofixation
uterolysis
> laparoscopic u.

utero-ovarian
uteroparietal
uteropelvic
uteroperitoneal fistula
uteropexy
uteroplacental
> u. circulation

uteroplasty
uterosacral
> u. block
> u. ligament

uteroscopy

uterotomy
uterotubal
uterovaginal
> u. canal
> u. plexus

uteroventral
uterovesical
> u. fold
> u. ligament
> u. pouch

uterus
> Dührssen vaginofixation of u.
> masculine u.
> opening of u.

utricle
> prostatic u.

utricular spot
utriculitis
utriculocele
utriculosaccular
> u. duct

utriculus
> u. prostaticus

UTTS endotracheal tube
U-tube tube
U-turn maneuver
UV
> ultraviolet
> umbilical vein
>> UV blood
>> UV irradiation

uveal
> u. metastasis
> u. tract

uveitis
> endogenous u.

uveo-encephalitic syndrome
uveoplasty
uviofast
uvioresistant
uviosensitive
UV/MV
> umbilical vein to maternal vein
>> UV/MV ratio

uvula
> u. of bladder
> Lieutaud u.
> u. vesicae

uvular muscle
uvulectomy
uvulopalatopharyngoplasty
uvulopalatoplasty
> laser-assisted u.

uvulotomy
UW solution
Uyemura operation

V.
>V. Mueller-Frazier suction tube
>V. Mueller-Poole suction tube

V$_E$
>minute ventilation

V$_A$
Vabra suction
vaccinia infection
vaccinization
VACTERL anomaly
Vactro perilimbal suction
vacuolation
vacuole
vacuolization
>basket-weave v.
>isometric tubular v.

Vacutainer tube
Vacutron suction regulator
vacuum
>v. aspiration
>v. extraction
>v. extractor delivery
>v. fixation ring
>v. tube

VAE
>venous air embolism

vagal
>v. arrest
>v. body
>v. part of accessory nerve
>v. stimulation
>v. trunk

vagectomy
vagina, pl. vaginae
>v. carotica
>vaginae fibrosae digitorum manus
>vaginae fibrosae digitorum pedis
>v. fibrosa tendinis
>v. intertubercularis
>v. masculina
>v. musculi recti abdominis
>v. processus styloidei
>in situ carcinoma of v.
>spindle cell sarcoma of v.
>vaginae synoviales digitorum manus
>vaginae synoviales digitorum pedis
>v. synovialis tendinis
>v. synovialis trochleae
>vaginae vasorum

vaginal
>v. adenocarcinoma
>v. anomaly
>v. artery
>v. birth after cesarean section
>v. carcinoma

>v. celiotomy
>v. columns
>v. cone biopsy
>v. construction
>v. cornification test
>v. cystourethropexy
>v. ectopic anus
>v. electrical stimulation
>v. examination
>v. fistula
>v. foreign body
>v. gland
>v. hematoma
>v. hysterectomy
>v. hysterotomy
>v. infection
>v. inflammation
>v. laceration
>v. lithotomy
>v. mass
>v. mucification test
>v. myomectomy
>v. needle suspension procedure
>v. nerve
>v. opening
>v. orifice
>v. perineorrhaphy
>v. portion of cervix
>v. process
>v. process of peritoneum
>v. process of sphenoid bone
>v. process of testis
>v. surgery
>v. venous plexus
>v. vesicostomy
>v. wall approach
>v. wall repair
>v. wall sling procedure

vaginalis
>patent processus v.

vaginapexy
vaginate
vaginectomy
vaginitis
vaginoabdominal
vaginocele
vaginofixation
vaginohysterectomy
vaginolabial
vaginoperineal
vaginoperineoplasty
vaginoperineorrhaphy
vaginoperineotomy
vaginoperitoneal

vaginopexy
    Norman Miller v.
vaginoplasty
    cutback-type v.
    Fenton v.
    posterior flap v.
vaginoscopy
    pediatric v.
vaginotomy
vaginourethroplasty
vaginovesical
vaginovulvar
vagoaccessorius
vagoglossopharyngeal
vagolysis
vagotomy
    v. and antrectomy with
      gastroduodenostomy
    bilateral v.
    highly selective v.
    laparoscopic v.
    laser laparoscopic v.
    medical v.
    parietal cell v.
    posterior truncal v.
    proximal gastric v.
    v. and pyloroplasty
    Roux-en-Y procedure with v.
    selective proximal v.
    superselective v.
    surgical v.
    total bilateral v.
    truncal v.
vagovagal reflex
vagus
    v. nerve
Vaino MP arthroplasty
Valentine
    V. irrigation tube
    V. position
valgus
    v. angulation
    v. deformity
    v. extension osteotomy
    v. extension overload syndrome
    v. high tibial osteotomy
    v. intertrochanteric-wedge osteotomy
    v. subtrochanteric osteotomy
    v. wedge-prop osteotomy
    v. Y-shaped prop osteotomy
valgus-external rotation injury
Valium
    V. injection
    V. Oral
vallecula, pl. valleculae
    epiglottic v.
    v. epiglottica
Valleix point

Valls-Ottolenghim-Schajowicz needle biopsy
Valmid
Valpar Whole Body Range of Motion Test
Valpius-Compere procedure
Valrelease Oral
Valsalva
    V. maneuver
    V. muscle
Valtrac absorbable biofragmentable anastomosis ring
value
    acid-base v.
valva, pl. valvae
    v. atrioventricularis dextra
    v. atrioventricularis sinistra
    v. ileocecalis
    v. mitralis
    v. trunci pulmonalis
valve
    v. ablation
    v. of Bauhin
    v. bladder
    v. cinefluoroscopy
    v. cusps
    v. debris
    expiratory v.
    Fink v.
    Frumin v.
    Georgia v.
    v. of Guérin
    v. of Hasner
    v. of Heister
    high-pressure relief v.
    v. of Houston
    Lanz pressure regulating v.
    v. leaflet
    Lewis-Leigh v.
    nonrebreathing v.
    v. orifice area
    v. patency
    pop-off v.
    v. replacement
    v. of Rosenmüller
    v. rupture
    Stephen-Slater v.
    v. of Sylvius
    v. of Vieussens
    v. wrapping
valvectomy
valvoplasty
valvotomy
    aortic v.
    balloon aortic v.
    balloon mitral v.
    balloon pulmonary v.
    balloon tricuspid v.

double-balloon v.
Inoue balloon mitral v.
Longmire v.
mitral balloon v.
mitral valve v.
percutaneous mitral balloon v.
rectal v.
repeat balloon mitral v.
single-balloon v.
thimble v.

valvula, pl. **valvulae**
Amussat v.
valvulae anales
v. foraminis ovalis
v. fossae navicularis
Gerlach v.
v. lymphatica
v. processus vermiformis
v. pylori
valvulae pylori
v. semilunaris
v. semilunaris dextra valvae aortae
v. semilunaris dextra valvae trunci
  pulmonalis
v. semilunaris posterior valvae
  aortae
v. semilunaris sinistra valvae aortae
v. sinus coronarii
v. spiralis
v. venae cavae inferioris

valvule
lymphatic v.

valvulectomy
valvuloplasty
aortic v.
bailout v.
balloon aortic v.
balloon dilation v.
balloon mitral v.
balloon pulmonary v.
Carpentier tricuspid v.
double-balloon v.
intracoronary thrombolysis
  balloon v.
mitral v.
multiple-balloon v.
percutaneous balloon aortic v.
percutaneous balloon mitral v.
percutaneous balloon pulmonic v.
percutaneous transluminal balloon v.
pulmonary v.
single-balloon v.

tricuspid v.
triple-balloon v.
Trusler technique of aortic v.

valvulotomy
balloon v.
v. procedure

Vamin amino acid solution

VAMP
venous/arterial management protection
Baxter VAMP
VAMP device

van
V. Alyea antral wash tube
v. Buren disease
V. de Kramer fecal fat procedure
V. Herick modification
V. Hoorne canal
V. Hoorn maneuver
V. Lint anesthesia
V. Lint flap
V. Lint injection
V. Lint modified technique
V. Milligen eyelid repair technique
V. Milligen operation
V. Ness procedure
V. Ness rotationplasty

Vancocin injection
Vancoled injection
vanished testis syndrome
Vannas capsulotomy
vapocauterization

vapor
anesthetic v.
partial pressure of water v.
v. pressure
V. 19 vaporizer

vaporization
Contact Laser v.
heat of v.
laser v.

vaporize
vaporizer
draw-over v.
v. exclusion system
flow-over v.
Goldman v.
Muraco v.
Ohmeda Sevotec 5 v.
Penlon v.
temperature-compensated v.
Vapor 19 v.

NOTES

VAPS
  visual analog pain score
variability
    heart rate v. (HRV)
    interpretation v.
variable
    v. positive airway pressure
    v. release compression
    v. screw placement
variable-dose patient-controlled
  anesthesia (VDPCA)
varication
variceal
    v. band ligation
    v. bleeding
    v. column
    v. decompression
    v. hemorrhage
    v. pressure
    v. sclerotherapy
    v. sclerotherapy in esophagus
    v. wall
varicella infection
varicella-zoster virus infection
varicelliform lesion
varices (*pl. of* varix)
varicocele
varicocelectomy
    laparoscopic v.
    microsurgical inguinal v.
    subinguinal v.
    subinguinal microsurgical v.
varicose
    v. aneurysm
    v. vein stripping and ligation
varicotomy
variocele
variolation
variolization
Varivas R denatured homologous vein
  graft
varix, pl. varices
    v. anastomoticus
    aneurysmal v.
    ectopic varices
    endoscopic band ligation of varices
    v. ligation
    Okuda transhepatic obliteration
      of v.
    percutaneous transhepatic
      obliteration of esophageal v.
    transesophageal ligation of v.
Varolius sphincter
varus
    v. hindfoot deformity
    v. rotational osteotomy
    v. rotation shortening osteotomy
    v. supramalleolar osteotomy

varus-valgus plane
VAS
  visual analog scale
vas, pl. vasa
    v. aberrans hepatis
    v. aberrans of Roth
    vasa aberrantes
    v. afferens
    v. anastomoticum
    vasa brevia
    vasa chylifera
    v. deferens
    vasa nervorum
vascular
    v. anastomosis
    v. anomaly
    v. bundle
    v. bypass graft
    v. cannulation
    v. circle
    v. complication
    v. ectasia
    v. endothelium
    v. exclusion
    v. fold of the cecum
    v. laceration
    v. laceration repair
    v. lesion
    v. loop
    v. malformation
    v. metastasis
    v. nerve
    v. patch graft
    v. pedicle
    v. perforation
    v. plexus
    v. pressure
    v. rejection
    v. renal mass
    v. ring
    v. ring division
    v. ring syndrome
    v. sheaths
    v. silk suture
    v. space
    v. suction tube
    v. surgery
    v. tissue
    v. zone
vascularity
    tumor v.
vascularization
vascularize
vascularized
    v. bone graft
    v. fibular graft
    v. free flap
    v. rib graft

vasculature
    extracranial v.
    extracranial cerebral v.
vasculitic lesion
vasculitis
vasculocardiac
vasculomyelinopathy
vasculopathy
    graft v.
Vascutek
    V. gelseal vascular graft
    V. knitted vascular graft
    V. woven vascular graft
vasectomy
    no-scalpel v.
    v. reversal
vasoactive
    v. medication
    v. substance
vasocillator
vasoconstriction
    hypoxic pulmonary v. (HPV)
    isoflurane-induced v.
    thermoregulatory v.
vasocutaneous fistula
vasodilatation
vasodilation
vasodilator
    v. administration
    v. agent
    arterial-selective intravenous v.
vasodilator-stimulated rCBF single photon emission computed tomographic measurement
vasoepididymostomy
vasoganglion
vasoligation
vasomotor nerve
vasoneuropathy
vasoneurosis
vaso-orchidostomy
vasopressor
vasoproliferation
vasopuncture
vasoreflex
vasorelaxation
vasosection
vasostimulant
vasostomy
vasotomy
vasovagal
vasovasostomy

vasovesiculectomy
Vastamäki technique
vastus
VATER
    V. association
    V. association syndrome
Vater
    ampulla of V.
    V. ampulla
    V. fold
VATS
    video-assisted thoracic surgery
    VATS procedure
Vaughan Williams antiarrhythmic drug classification
vault
    cranial v.
VBG
    vertical banded gastroplasty
    VBG pouch
VDPCA
    variable-dose patient-controlled anesthesia
Veau classification
Vecchietti
    V. method
    V. operation
VECO$_2$
    carbon dioxide elimination
vection
vector
    v. phase
    v. product
    v. profile
    v. quantity
vecuronium
    v. bromide
    v. neuromuscular blocking
vegetative lesion
vehicle
veil
    aqueduct v.
    Jackson v.
vein
    aberrant obturator v.
    accessory cephalic v.
    accessory hemiazygos v.
    accessory saphenous v.
    accessory vertebral v.
    anastomotic v.'s
    anterior auricular v.
    anterior cardiac v.'s

V

NOTES

799

vein *(continued)*
anterior cerebral v.
anterior facial v.
anterior intercostal v.'s
anterior jugular v.
anterior scrotal v.'s
anterior vertebral v.
appendicular v.
aqueous v.
arciform v.'s of kidney
arcuate v.'s of kidney
arterial v.
ascending lumbar v.
auricular v.'s
autogenous v.
axillary v.
azygos v.
basal v.'s
basilic v.
basivertebral v.
brachiocephalic v.'s
bronchial v.'s
Browning v.
v. of bulb of penis
Burow v.
capillary v.
cardiac v.'s
cavernous v.'s of penis
cavernous transformation of the
  portal v.
central v.'s of liver
central v. of suprarenal gland
cephalic v.
cerebellar v.'s
cerebral v.'s
cervical v.
choroid v.
circumflex v.'s
colic v.'s
common basal v.
common facial v.
condylar emissary v.
coronary v.
costoaxillary v.
v. decompression
deep cervical v.
deep v.'s of clitoris
deep dorsal v. of clitoris
deep dorsal v. of penis
deep epigastric v.
deep facial v.
deep lingual v.
deep v. of penis
deep temporal v.'s
digital v.'s
dorsal v.'s of clitoris
dorsal digital v.'s of toes
dorsal v.'s of penis

dorsal scapular v.
dorsispinal v.'s
emissary v.
endophlebitis of retinal v.
epigastric v.'s
esophageal v.'s
ethmoidal v.'s
external jugular v.
external pudendal v.'s
external spermatic v.
extrahepatic portal v.
v.'s of eyelids
facial v.
frontal v.'s
v. of Galen malformation
gastric v.'s
gastroepiploic v.'s
v. graft
great cardiac v.
great cerebral v.
great v. of Galen
great saphenous v.
hemiazygos v.
hemorrhoidal v.'s
hepatic portal v.
highest intercostal v.
human umbilical v. (HUV)
hypogastric v.
ileal v.'s
ileocolic v.
inferior anastomotic v.
inferior basal v.
inferior cardiac v.
inferior cerebral v.'s
inferior epigastric v.
v.'s of inferior eyelid
inferior hemorrhoidal v.'s
inferior labial v.
inferior laryngeal v.
inferior mesenteric v.
inferior phrenic v.
inferior rectal v.'s
inferior thyroid v.
innominate cardiac v.'s
intercapitular v.'s
intercostal v.'s
interlobar v.'s of kidney
interlobular v.'s of kidney
interlobular v.'s of liver
intermediate basilic v.
intermediate cephalic v.
internal jugular v.
internal pudendal v.
internal thoracic v.
intervertebral v.
jejunal and ileal v.'s
jugular v.'s
v.'s of kidney

Labbé v.
labial v.'s
labyrinthine v.'s
large saphenous v.
laryngeal v.'s
lateral thoracic v.
left colic v.
left coronary v.
left gastric v.
left gastroepiploic v.
left gastroomental v.
left hepatic v.'s
left inferior pulmonary v.
left ovarian v.
left superior intercostal v.
left superior pulmonary v.
left suprarenal v.
left testicular v.
left umbilical v.
lingual v.
long saphenous v.
long thoracic v.
lumbar v.'s
Marshall oblique v.
median basilic v.
median cephalic v.
median v. of neck
median sacral v.
mediastinal v.'s
meningeal v.'s
mesenteric v.'s
middle cardiac v.
middle colic v.
middle hemorrhoidal v.'s
middle hepatic v.'s
middle meningeal v.'s
middle rectal v.'s
middle temporal v.
middle thyroid v.
musculophrenic v.'s
nasofrontal v.
oblique v. of left atrium
occipital cerebral v.'s
occipital emissary v.
ovarian v.'s
pancreatic v.'s
pancreaticoduodenal v.'s
paraumbilical v.'s
parietal emissary v.
parotid v.'s
v. patch
v. patch angioplasty

patent v.
pericardiacophrenic v.'s
pericardial v.'s
peritoneal v.
peroneal v.
petrosal v.
pharyngeal v.'s
phrenic v.'s
portal v.
posterior anterior jugular v.
posterior auricular v.
posterior facial v.
posterior intercostal v.'s
posterior labial v.'s
posterior v. of left ventricle
posterior parotid v.'s
posterior scrotal v.'s
prepyloric v.
v. of pterygoid canal
pudendal v.'s
pulmonary v.'s
pyloric v.
renal v.'s
retromandibular v.
right colic v.
right gastric v.
right gastroepiploic v.
right gastro-omental v.
right hepatic v.'s
right inferior pulmonary v.
right ovarian v.
right superior intercostal v.
right superior pulmonary v.
right suprarenal v.
right testicular v.
Santorini v.
saphenous v.'s
scrotal v.'s
v. of septum pellucidum
short gastric v.'s
short saphenous v.
shunt index via the inferior mesenteric v.
shunt index via the superior mesenteric v.
small cardiac v.
smallest cardiac v.'s
small saphenous v.
spermatic v.
spigelian v.
spinal v.'s
splenic v.

NOTES

vein *(continued)*
    sternocleidomastoid v.
    v. stone
    stylomastoid v.
    subclavian v.
    subcutaneous v.'s of abdomen
    sublingual v.
    submental v.
    superficial dorsal v.'s of clitoris
    superficial dorsal v.'s of penis
    superficial epigastric v.
    superficial temporal v.'s
    superior anastomotic v.
    superior basal v.
    superior cerebral v.'s
    superior epigastric v.'s
    v.'s of superior eyelid
    superior hemorrhoidal v.
    superior intercostal v.
    superior labial v.
    superior laryngeal v.
    superior mesenteric v.
    superior phrenic v.'s
    superior rectal v.
    superior thyroid v.
    supraorbital v.
    suprarenal v.'s
    suprascapular v.
    supratrochlear v.'s
    supreme intercostal v.
    temporal v.'s
    v.'s of temporomandibular joint
    temporomaxillary v.
    testicular v.'s
    thalamostriate v.'s
    thebesian v.'s
    thoracic v.'s
    thoracoacromial v.
    thoracoepigastric v.
    thymic v.'s
    thyroid v.'s
    transverse cervical v.'s
    transverse v. of face
    transverse facial v.
    transverse v.'s of neck
    transverse v. of scapula
    Trolard v.
    umbilical v. (UV)
    umbilical vein to maternal v. (UV/MV)
    uterine v.'s
    v. valve wrapping
    vertebral v.
    v.'s of vertebral column
    Vesalius v.
    vesical v.'s
    vestibular v.'s
    v. of vestibular aqueduct
    v. of vestibular bulb
    vidian v.
    Vieussens v.'s
Veirs canaliculus repair
vela (*pl. of* velum)
velamen, pl. velamina
velamentous
    v. insertion
    v. insertion of cord
velamentum
velamina (*pl. of* velamen)
velar
Velcro closure
Veleanu-Rosianu-Ionescu
    V.-R.-I. adductor tenotomy
    V.-R.-I. technique
Velex woven Dacron vascular graft
veliform
Vella fistula
vellication
vellus
velocity catheter technique
velopharyngeal
    v. closure
    v. port
    v. sphincter
veloplasty
    functional v.
velour collar graft
Velpeau
    V. canal
    V. deformity
    V. fossa
    V. hernia
velum, pl. vela
    corneal v.
    v. palatinum
    v. pendulum palati
vena, pl. venae
    v. afferentes hepatis
    v. anastomotica inferior
    v. anastomotica superior
    v. appendicularis
    venae arcuatae renis
    v. arteriosa
    v. auricularis anterior
    v. auricularis posterior
    v. axillaris
    v. azygos
    v. azygos major
    v. azygos minor inferior
    v. azygos minor superior
    v. basalis communis
    v. basalis inferior
    v. basalis superior
    v. basilica
    v. basivertebralis
    venae bronchiales

v. bulbi penis
v. canalis pterygoidei
v. cardiaca magna
v. cava anomaly
v. cava filter
v. cava inferior
v. caval foramen
v. cava superior
venae cavernosae penis
v. centralis glandulae suprarenalis
v. cephalica
v. cephalica accessoria
venae cerebelli inferiores
venae cerebelli superiores
v. cerebri anterior
venae cerebri inferiores
v. cerebri magna
venae cerebri superiores
v. cervicalis profunda
v. colica dextra
v. colica media
v. colica sinistra
venae columnae vertebralis
venae cordis anteriores
v. cordis magna
v. cordis media
venae cordis minimae
v. cordis parva
v. coronaria ventriculi
v. cystica
venae dorsales clitoridis
  superficiales
venae dorsales linguae
venae dorsales penis superficiales
v. dorsalis clitoridis profunda
v. dorsalis penis profunda
v. emissaria
v. emissaria condylaris
v. emissaria occipitalis
v. emissaria parietalis
venae epigastricae superiores
v. epigastrica inferior
v. epigastrica superficialis
venae esophageae
venae ethmoidales
v. facialis
v. facialis anterior
v. facialis communis
v. facialis posterior
v. faciei profunda
venae frontales
v. gastrica dextra

venae gastricae breves
v. gastrica sinistra
v. gastro-omentalis dextra
v. gastro-omentalis sinistra
v. hemiazygos
v. hemiazygos accessoria
venae hemorrhoidales inferiores
venae hemorrhoidales mediae
v. hemorrhoidalis superior
venae hepaticae
venae hepaticae dextrae
venae hepaticae mediae
venae hepaticae sinistrae
v. hypogastrica
v. ileocolica
v. iliolumbalis
inferior v. cava (IVC)
v. innominata
venae intercapitales
venae intercostales anteriores
venae intercostales posteriores
v. intercostalis superior dextra
v. intercostalis superior sinistra
v. intercostalis suprema
venae interlobares renis
venae interlobulares hepatis
venae interlobulares renis
v. intermedia cephalica
v. intermedia cubiti
v. intervertebralis
venae jejunales et ilei
v. jugularis anterior
v. jugularis externa
v. jugularis interna
venae labiales anteriores
venae labiales posteriores
v. labialis inferior
v. labialis superior
v. laryngea inferior
v. laryngea superior
v. lienalis
v. lingualis
v. mammaria interna
v. mediana basilica
v. mediana cephalica
v. mediana cubiti
venae mediastinales
venae meningeae
venae meningeae mediae
v. mesenterica inferior
v. mesenterica superior
venae musculophrenicae

V

NOTES

vena *(continued)*
v. nasofrontalis
v. obliqua atrii sinistri
venae occipitales
v. occipitalis
v. ovarica dextra
v. ovarica sinistra
venae pancreaticae
venae pancreaticoduodenales
venae paraumbilicales
venae parietales
venae parotidea
venae perforantes
venae pericardiacae
venae pericardiacophrenicae
venae peroneae
v. petrosa
venae pharyngeae
venae phrenicae superiores
v. phrenica inferior
v. portae hepatis
v. portalis
v. posterior ventriculi sinistri
v. preauricularis
v. prepylorica
venae profundae clitoridis
v. profunda linguae
v. profunda penis
venae pudendae externae
v. pudenda interna
venae pulmonales
v. pulmonalis inferior dextra
v. pulmonalis inferior sinistra
v. pulmonalis superior dextra
v. pulmonalis superior sinistra
venae rectae
venae rectales inferiores
venae rectales mediae
v. rectalis superior
venae renales
venae renis
v. retromandibularis
v. saphena accessoria
v. saphena magna
v. saphena parva
v. scapularis dorsalis
venae scrotales anteriores
venae scrotales posteriores
venae sigmoideae
venae spinales
venae cavernosae of spleen
v. splenica
v. sternocleidomastoidea
v. stylomastoidea
v. subclavia
venae subcutaneae abdominis
v. sublingualis
v. submentalis

superior v. cava
v. supraorbitalis
v. suprarenalis dextra
v. suprarenalis sinistra
v. suprascapularis
venae supratrochleares
V. Tech dual vena cava filter
V. Tech-LGM vena cava filter
venae temporales profundae
venae temporales superficiales
v. temporalis media
v. testicularis dextra
v. testicularis sinistra
v. thoracica interna
v. thoracica lateralis
v. thoracoacromialis
v. thoracoepigastrica
venae thymicae
v. thyroidea ima
v. thyroidea inferior
v. thyroidea media
v. thyroidea superior
venae tracheales
venae transversae colli
v. transversa faciei
v. transversa scapulae
v. umbilicalis sinistra
venae uterinae
v. vertebralis
v. vertebralis accessoria
v. vertebralis anterior
venacavaplasty
face-a-face v.
venectomy
venereal sore
venereology
venesection
Venflon needless injection port system
venipuncture
Venn-Watson classification
venoablation
percutaneous v.
venobiliary fistula
venoconstriction
mesenteric v.
reflex v.
venodilation
nitrate-induced v.
systemic v.
Venodyne external pneumatic
compression System EPS-410
venolysis
circumferential v.
venom extract
venoperitoneostomy
venostasis
venostomy
venotomy

venous
    v. access technique
    v. admixture
    v. air embolism (VAE)
    v. angioma
    v. angle
    v. blood gas
    v. circle of mammary gland
    v. circulation
    v. compression
    v. confluence
    v. cutdown
    v. foramen
    v. grooves
    v. hemorrhage
    v. insufficiency
    v. interposition graft
    v. intravasation
    v. ligament
    v. line
    v. loop
    v. malformation
    maternal v. (MV)
    v. plexus
    v. plexus of bladder
    v. plexus of foramen ovale
    v. pressure
    v. pressure gradient support
      stocking
    v. puncture
    v. saturation
    v. segments of the kidney
    v. segments of liver
    v. sheath patch
    v. sinuses
    v. stasis disease
    umbilical v.
    v. web
    v. web disease
**venous/arterial management protection
(VAMP)**
**venous-occlusion volume
plethysmography**
venous-to-venous anastomosis
venovenostomy
venovenous
    v. bypass (VVB)
    v. extracorporeal bypass
venter
    v. anterior musculi digastrici
    v. frontalis musculi occipitofrontalis
    v. inferior musculi omohyoidei

    v. occipitalis musculi
      occipitofrontalis
    v. posterior musculi digastrici
    v. propendens
    v. superior musculi omohyoidei
ventilation
    v. agent
    airway pressure release v. (APRV)
    alveolar v.
    artificial v.
    assist-control mode v.
    assisted v.
    bag-and-mask v.
    bagged mask v.
    bag-valve-mask-assisted v.
    v. circuit
    v. collateralization
    continuous-flow v.
    continuous mandatory v.
    continuous positive pressure v.
     (CPPV)
    control of v.
    controlled v.
    controlled mechanical v. (CMV)
    control-mode v.
    cuirass v.
    v. defect
    difficult v.
    emergency v.
    v. equivalent
    forced mandatory intermittent v.
    hand v.
    heart synchronized v.
    HFJ v.
    IIFO v.
    HFPP v.
    high-frequency jet v.
    high-frequency oscillation v.
    high-frequency oscillatory v.
    high-frequency percussive v.
    high-frequency positive pressure v.
    v. index (VI)
    inspired v. (VI)
    intermittent demand v.
    intermittent mandatory v. (IMV)
    intermittent mechanical v.
    intermittent positive pressure v.
     (IPPV)
    inverse ratio v.
    inverse-ratio v.
    jet v.
    Johnson method of v.

NOTES

ventilation *(continued)*
  local exhaust v.
  low-frequency jet v.
  v. lung scan
  manual v.
  v. mask
  v. by mask
  maximal voluntary v.
  maximum voluntary v. (MVV)
  mechanical v.
  minute v. (V_E)
  mouth-to-mouth v.
  neonate v.
  one-lung v. (OLV)
  oscillatory v.
  partial liquid v.
  v. peak pressure
  percutaneous transtracheal jet v.
    (PTV)
  positive pressure v. (PPV)
  positive-pressure v.
  pressure-controlled inverse ratio v.
  pressure-regulated volume control v.
  pressure support v.
  proportional assist v.
  pulmonary v.
  split-lung v.
  spontaneous v.
  spontaneous intermittent
    mandatory v. (SIMV)
  synchronized intermittent
    mandatory v. (SIMV)
  synchronized intermittent
    mechanical v.
  synchronous intermittent
    mandatory v.
  v. threshold
  time-cycled v.
  transtracheal jet v.
  triggered v.
  v. tube
  ultrahigh frequency v.
  ultrahigh-frequency v.
  volume-cycled decelerating-flow v.
ventilation/perfusion (V/Q)
  v. abnormality
  v. defect
  v. distribution
  v. imaging
  v. inequality
  v. lung scan
  v. mismatch
  v. quotient
  v. ratio
  v. relation
  v. relationship
ventilation-to-circulation

ventilator
  v. alarm
  Cicero anesthetic v.
  v. dependency
  Dräger Nrkomed II v.
  v. management
  Ohmeda model 7000 v.
  Servo v.
  Servo 900 B, C v.
  Siemens-Elema Servo 900C v.
  Siemens Servo 900 B v.
  v. support
  v. time
  v. weaning
ventilator-assisted respiration
ventilator-associated pneumonia
ventilator-induced
  v.-i. pneumopericardium
  v.-i. pneumothorax
ventilatory
  v. depression
  v. response
Ventimask
venting percutaneous gastrostomy
ventral
  v. bending technique
  v. hernia
  v. herniorrhaphy
  v. nucleus of trapezoid body
  v. plate of neural tube
  v. primary rami of cervical spinal
    nerves
  v. primary rami of lumbar spinal
    nerves
  v. primary rami of sacral spinal
    nerves
  v. primary ramus of spinal nerve
  v. root
  v. sacrococcygeal ligament
  v. sacrococcygeus muscle
  v. spinocerebellar tract
  v. spinothalamic tract
  v. tegmental decussation
ventricle
  dilation of v.
  v.'s of heart
  laryngeal v.
  left v.
  Morgagni v.
  right v.
ventricular
  v. aberration
  v. activation time
  v. band of larynx
  v. canal
  v. depolarization abnormality
  v. diastolic pressure
  v. dilation

v. endoaneurysmorrhaphy
v. endomyocardial biopsy
v. end-systolic pressure-volume relation
v. filling pressure
v. fold
v. inflow anomaly
v. inflow tract obstruction
v. ligament
v. outflow tract
v. outflow tract obstruction
v. perforation
v. peritoneal shunting
v. phonation
v. preexcitation
v. puncture
v. relaxation
v. septal defect closure
v. septal rupture
v. septum
v. tachycardia/ventricular fibrillation
ventricularization
ventricular-programmed stimulation
ventriculi (*pl. of* ventriculus)
ventriculocisternostomy
Torkildsen v.
ventriculocordectomy
ventriculomastoidostomy
ventriculoperitoneal
v. shunting
ventriculoplasty
ventriculopuncture
ventriculoscopy
ventriculostomy
straight-in v.
terminal v.
third v.
tunneled v.
ventriculotomy
encircling endocardial v.
partial encircling endocardial v.
ventriculus, pl. ventriculi
v. cordis
v. dexter
v. laryngis
v. sinister
ventrocystorrhaphy
ventroinguinal
ventroptosis
ventroscopy
ventrotomy
ventrum penis flap

vent tube
Venturi
V. bobbin myringotomy tube
V. collar-button myringotomy tube
V. grommet myringotomy tube
V. pediatric myringotomy tube
venula, pl. venulae
venulae rectae renis
venulae stellatae
v. temporalis retinae inferior
v. temporalis retinae superior
venular lesion
venule
high endothelial v.
inferior temporal v. of retina
straight v.'s of kidney
superior temporal v. of retina
temporal v.'s of retina
VePesid injection
verapamil
veratridine
veratrin
verbotonal method
Verdan
V. osteoplastic thumb reconstruction
V. technique
verge
anal v.
Verhoeff-Chandler
V.-C. capsulotomy
V.-C. operation
Verhoeff operation
vermian fossa
vermiculation
vermiform
v. appendage
v. body
v. process
vermilion border
vermilionectomy
vermix
Vermont spinal fixator articulation
Verneuil canal
vernix membrane
Vernon antral wash tube
verrucous lesion
Versed
vertebra, pl. vertebrae
basilar v.
caudal vertebrae
cervical vertebrae
vertebrae cervicales

V

NOTES

vertebra *(continued)*
    vertebrae coccygeae
    coccygeal vertebrae
    dorsal vertebrae
    false vertebrae
    vertebrae lumbales
    lumbar vertebrae
    v. magna
    picture frame v.
    v. plana fracture
    v. prominens
    sacral vertebrae
    vertebrae sacrales
    vertebrae spuriae
    tail vertebrae
    thoracic vertebrae
    vertebrae thoracicae
    true v.
    v. vera
    wedge-shaped v.

vertebral
    v. arch
    v. artery
    v. artery bypass graft
    v. body
    v. body anterior cortex
    v. body corpectomy
    v. body decompression
    v. body fracture
    v. bone mass
    v. border of scapula
    v. canal
    v. column
    v. compression
    v. corpectomy
    v. dissection
    v. epidural space
    v. exposure
    v. foramen
    v. fusion
    v. ganglion
    v. groove
    v. nerve
    v. notch
    v. osteosynthesis
    v. osteosynthesis fusion rate
    v. part of the costal surface of
      the lungs
    v. part of diaphragm
    v. plexus
    v. region
    v. resection
    v. ribs
    v. ring apophysis
    v. rotation
    v. stable burst fracture
    v. subluxation complex
    v. subluxation syndrome

    v. vein
    v. venous plexus
    v. wedge compression fracture
vertebrarium
vertebrated
vertebrectomy
    Bohlman anterior cervical v.
    cervical spondylotic myelopathy v.
vertebroarterial
    v. foramen
vertebrochondral
    v. ribs
vertebrocostal
    v. trigone
vertebrofemoral
vertebroiliac
vertebropelvic ligaments
vertebrosacral
vertebrosternal
    v. ribs
vertex, pl. vertices
    v. position
vertical
    v. angulation
    v. banded gastroplasty (VBG)
    v. banded gastroplasty pouch
    v. compression
    v. compression test
    v. condensation root canal filling
      method
    v. divergence position
    v. flap
    v. illumination
    v. index
    v. lip biopsy
    v. mattress suture
    v. maxillary excess
    v. midline incision
    v. muscle of tongue
    v. osteotomy
    v. osteotomy of ramus of
      mandible
    v. partial laryngectomy
    v. plane
    v. plate of palatine
    v. relation
    v. section
    v. shear fracture
    v. Silastic ring gastroplasty
    v. suspension reflex
    v. tooth fracture
    v. translation
    v. tube
    v. vs. horizontal preparation
vertical-cut
    v.-c. method
    v.-c. technique
vertically-acquired infection

vertices (*pl. of* vertex)
verticomental
verumontanitis
verumontanum
Verwey eyelid operation
very
    v. large scale integration
    v. late activation
Vesalius
    V. bone
    canal of V.
    V. foramen
    V. vein
vesica, pl. vesicae
    v. biliaris
    ectopia v.
    v. fellea
    v. prostatica
    v. urinaria
vesical
    v. calculus
    v. diverticulectomy
    v. fistula
    v. gland
    v. lithotomy
    v. plexus
    v. surface of uterus
    v. triangle
    v. veins
vesicalis anus
vesication
vesicle
    air v.
    brush-border membrane v.
    v. hernia
    seminal v.
vesicoabdominal
vesicoacetabular fistula
vesicobullous lesion
vesicocele
vesicocervical
    v. space
vesicoclysis
vesicocolic fistula
vesicocutaneous fistula
vesicoenteric fistula
vesicofixation
vesicointestinal
    v. fistula
vesicolithiasis
vesicomyectomy
vesicomyotomy

vesico-ovarian fistula
vesicoprostatic
vesicopubic
vesicorectal
    v. fistula
vesicorectostomy
vesicosalpingovaginal fistula
vesicosigmoid
vesicosigmoidostomy
vesicospinal
vesicostomy
    cutaneous v.
    preputial continent v.
    vaginal v.
vesicotomy
vesicoumbilical
    v. ligament
vesicoureteral
vesicourethral
    v. anastomosis
    v. canal
vesicouterine
    v. fistula
    v. ligament
    v. pouch
vesicouterovaginal
vesicovaginal
    v. fistula
    v. repair
vesicovaginorectal
    v. fistula
vesicovaginostomy
vesicovisceral
vesicula, pl. vesiculae
    v. fellis
    v. seminalis
vesicular
    v. acute inflammation
    v. appendage
    v. granulomatous inflammation
    v. venous plexus
    v. viral infection
vesiculation
vesiculectomy
    prostatoseminal v.
    total prostatoseminal v.
vesiculitis
vesiculocavernous respiration
vesiculoprostatectomy
    retropubic v.
vesiculoprostatitis
vesiculotomy

V

NOTES

Vesling line
vessel
  absorbent v.
  chyle v.
  deep lymphatic v.
  ectatic v.
  endosteal v.
  innominate v.
  lacteal v.
  v. ligation
  lymph v.'s
  lymphatic v.'s
  nutrient v.
  superficial lymphatic v.
  thoracic great v.
  tumor v.
  v.'s of vessels
vestibula (pl. of vestibulum)
vestibular
  v. blind sac
  v. canal
  v. crest
  v. fissure of cochlea
  v. fold
  v. ganglion
  v. glands
  v. labyrinth
  v. ligament
  v. membrane
  v. nerve section
  v. neurectomy
  v. veins
  v. window
vestibule
  esophagogastric v.
  gastroesophageal v.
  labial v.
  v. of larynx
  v. of omental bursa
  v. of vagina
vestibuloplasty
vestibulospinal tract
vestibulourethral
vestibulum, pl. vestibula
  v. bursae omentalis
  v. laryngis
  v. pudendi
  v. vaginae
vestige
  v. of processus vaginalis
  v. of vaginal process
vestigial muscle
vestigium
  v. processus vaginalis
vest-over-pants
  v.-o.-p. hernial repair
  v.-o.-p. herniorrhaphy

Veterans Administration Cooperative
  study
V-flap meatoplasty
V-Gan injection
VI
  inspired ventilation
  ventilation index
via
viable
  v. tissue
vial
  multidose v.
  scintillation v.
vibesate
Vibramycin injection
vibrating line
vibration
  v. condensation
  v. disease
  v. syndrome
  v. threshold test
vibrational angioplasty
vibrator hand syndrome
Vibrio fetus infection
vibroacoustic stimulation
vicarious respiration
vicious union
Vicq d'Azyr bundle
Vicryl
  V. pop-off suture
  V. Rapide suture
  V. SH suture
Victor Gomel method
Vidal-Ardrey fracture technique
video
  v. endoscopy
  v. esophagoscopy
  v. fluoroscopy
  v. small bowel enteroscopy
  v. transurethral resection technique
video-assisted
  v.-a. excisional biopsy
  v.-a. procedure
  v.-a. technique
  v.-a. thoracic surgery (VATS)
  v.-a. thoracic surgical procedure
  v.-a. thoracoscopic surgery
  v.-a. thoracoscopic thymectomy
videoendoscopy
videoesophagogoscopy
videofluoroscopic technique
videofluoroscopy
videostroboscopy
videothoracoscopy
videourodynamic evaluation
vidian
  v. canal
  v. vein

Vienna wire suture
Viers operation
Vieussens
    V. ansa
    V. ganglia
    V. limbus
    V. ring
    valve of V.
    V. veins
vigil
    coma v.
vigilance monitoring
vigorous hydration
villoma
villus, pl. villi
    intestinal villi
    villi intestinales
    peritoneal villi
    villi peritoneales
    pleural villi
    villi pleurales
    synovial villi
    villi synoviales
Vim-Silverman
    V.-S. technique
    V.-S. technique for liver biopsy
Vim thalamotomy
Vincasar PFS injection
Vincent infection
vinculum, pl. vincula
    v. linguae
    long v.
    v. longum
    v. preputii
    short v.
    vincula tendinum
    vincula of tendons
Vindelov method flow cytometry analysis
Vineberg procedure
vinorelbine tartrate
vinyl
    v. chloride exposure
    v. ether
    2,2,2-trifluoroethyl v.
    v. tube
Vinyon-N cloth tube
violaceous lesion
vipoma
Virag operation
viral respiratory infection
Virchow metastasis

Virchow-Robin
    V.-R. space
    V.-R. space dilatation
virga
virgin
    v. silk
    v. silk suture
virginal
    v. membrane
virginity
virilia
virilization
Viro-Tec suture
virtual point
virus
    Coxsackievirus A v.
    Coxsackievirus B v.
    Epstein-Barr v. (EBV)
viscera (pl. of viscus)
visceral
    v. anesthesia
    v. herniation
    v. layer of tunica vaginalis of testis
    v. lesion
    v. lymph nodes
    v. muscle
    v. nerve
    v. nodes
    v. pain
    v. pelvic fascia
    v. pericardiectomy
    v. peritoneum
    v. pleura
    v. pouch
    v. space
    v. surface of liver
    v. surface of the spleen
    v. sympathectomy
    v. traction reflex
visceralgia
viscerobronchial cardiovascular anomaly
viscerocranium
visceroinhibitory
visceroparietal
visceroperitoneal
visceropleural
visceroptosis
visceroskeletal
visceroskeleton
viscerosomatic
viscerotomy

NOTES

Viscoat solution
viscoelastic tissue
visco surgery
viscous lidocaine
viscus, pl. viscera
    intraperitoneal v.
    viscera retention
    retroperitoneal viscera
Visick dysphagia classification
visor flap
visual
    v. analog pain score (VAPS)
    v. analog scale (VAS)
    v. association area
    v. closure
    v. deprivation syndrome
    v. direction
    v. extinction
    v. fixation
    v. function evaluation
    v. laser ablation
    v. laser ablation of prostate
    v. laser assisted prostatectomy
    v. line
    v. method
    v. orientation
    v. plane
    v. point
    v. preservation
    v. projection
    v. stimulation
visualization
    contrast v.
    double-contrast v.
    fluoroscopic v.
Visual-Motor Integration Test
Vitagraft vascular graft
Vitalert 3200
vital knot
Vitallium cup arthroplasty
vitelliform degeneration of macula
vitelline
    v. duct anomaly
    v. fistula
    v. membrane
    v. sac
vitiation
Vitox femoral head
vitreal
    v. hemorrhage
    v. membrane
vitrectomy
    anterior v.
    closed-system pars plana v.
    core v.
    open-sky v.
    pars plana v.
    port v.

    posterior v.
    Weck-cel v.
vitreolysis
vitreoretinal traction syndrome
vitreoretinopathy
    exudative v.
    familial exudative v.
vitreous
    v. aspiration
    v. break-through hemorrhage
    v. cavity
    v. foreign body
    v. hernia
    v. herniation
    v. membrane
    v. neovascularization
    v. surgery
    v. table
vitreum
    stroma v.
vitrification
Viva-Drops solution
vividialysis
vividiffusion
vivification
vivo
    ex v.
Vivonex
    V. gastrostomy tube
    V. Moss tube
V-line
V-Lok disposable blood pressure cuff
VL thalamotomy
vocal
    v. cord
    v. cord injection
    v. fold approximation
    v. ligament
    v. muscle
    v. process
    v. process of arytenoid cartilage
    v. shelf
    v. tract
vocalis muscle
Vogel method
Vogt operation
voice
    v. disorders of phonation
    v. restoration
    v. termination time
    v. therapy
voiding
    v. flow rate
    v. urethral pressure measurement
Voigt line
vola
volar
    v. angulation

v. angulation deformity
v. aspect
v. epineurolysis
v. finger approach
v. interosseous artery
v. midline approach
v. midline oblique incision
v. plate arthroplasty
v. plate arthroplasty technique
   fracture-dislocation
v. plate repair
v. radial approach
v. semilunar wrist dislocation
v. synovectomy
v. ulnar approach
v. zig-zag finger incision
volaris
volarward approach
volatile
v. anesthesia
v. anesthetic
v. anesthetic agent
volatilization
Volkmann
V. canal
V. clawhand deformity
V. fracture
Volkov-Oganesian external fixation
volotrauma
Volpicelli functional ambulation scale
volsella
voltage regulator
Voltolini ear tube
volume
abdominal v.
circulation v.
compartmental v.
v. of dead space
drain v.
end-expiratory lung v. (EELV)
end-inspiratory v.
v. expansion
expiratory reserve v.
expiratory residual v.
v. of expired gas
extracellular fluid v. (ECFV)
fiber bundle v.
forced expiratory v.
intraperitoneal v.
maximal expiratory flow v.
minute v.
v. plethysmography

presystolic pressure and v.
respiratory minute v.
rib cage v.
v. segmentation
v. therapy
tidal v.
timed forced expiratory v.
tumor v.
weight-based peritoneal exchange v.
volume-assured pressure support
volume-cycled decelerating-flow ventilation
volumetric
v. capnometry
v. infusion pump
v. method
v. solution
v. technique
voluminous hiatus hernia
voluntary
v. guarding
v. sterilization
volvulus
cecal v.
gastric v.
v. reduction
sigmoid v.
Volz arthroplasty
Volz-Turner reattachment technique
vomer
v. cartilagineus
vomerine
v. canal
vomerobasilar
v. canal
vomeronasal
vomerorostral canal
vomerovaginal
v. canal
v. groove
vomicose
vomit
bilious v.
vomiting
intractable nausea and v.
postoperative nausea and v.
   (PONV)
von
V. Ammon operation
V. Blaskovics-Doyen operation
V. Claus chronometric method
V. Ebner line

NOTES

813

von *(continued)*
    v. Economo disease
    V. Eichen antral wash tube
    V. Frey test
    v. Graefe operation
    V. Haberer-Finney anastomosis
    V. Haberer-Finney gastrectomy technique
    v. Haberer gastroenterostomy
    v. Hippel operation
    v. Kossa method
    V. Langenbeck bipedicle mucoperiosteal flap
    v. Langenbeck palatal closure
    v. Langenbeck pedicle flap
    v. Noorden incision

vortex
    v. coccygeus

Vortex tracheotomy tube

Vossius lenticular ring

Vostal
    V. classification of radial fractures
    V. radial fracture classification

V-osteotomy
    Japas V.-o.
    off-set V.-o.

V-P curve

VPI nonadhesive open-end pouch

VPL pallidotomy

V/Q
    ventilation/perfusion

V-shaped
    V-s. incision
    V-s. osteotomy

V-sign of Naclerio

V-slope method

Vulpius-Compere tendon technique

Vulpius procedure

Vulpius-Stoffel procedure

vulsella

vulva, pl. vulvae
    noma v.

vulvar
    v. adenoid cystic adenocarcinoma
    v. biopsy
    v. carcinoma
    v. hematoma
    v. infection
    v. pigmented lesion
    v. slit

vulvectomy
    Basset radical v.
    Parry-Jones v.
    radical v.
    simple v.
    skinning v.

vulvitis

vulvocrural

vulvoplasty

vulvouterine

vulvovaginal
    v. carcinoma
    v. cystectomy
    v. gland
    v. lesion
    v. premenarchal infection

vulvovaginoplasty
    Williams v.

Vumon injection

VVB
    venovenous bypass

V-Y
    V-Y advancement flap
    V-Y gastrocplasty
    V-Y Kutler flap
    V-Y plasty
    V-Y procedure
    V-Y quadricepsplasty

W

W hernia
W procedure
Wachendorf membrane
Wackenheim clivus canal line
wadding
Wadsworth
W. elbow approach
W. posterolateral approach
W. technique
Wagener-Clay-Gipner classification
Wagner
W. classification
W. closed pinning
W. modification of Syme
amputation
W. open reduction technique
W. skin incision
W. two-stage Syme amputation
Wagoner
W. cervical technique
W. posterior approach
wagon-wheel fracture
Wagstaffe fracture
wake-up evaluation
Walcher position
Waldeyer
W. fossae
W. glands
W. ring lesion
W. sheath
W. space
W. throat ring
W. tonsillar ring
W. tract
Waldhauer operation
Waldhausen
W. procedure
W. subclavian flap technique
WALK
Walking with Angina–Learning is Key
WALK program
Walker tractotomy
walking
w. epidural anesthetic
w. program
w. ventilation test
W. with Angina–Learning is Key
(WALK)
wall
anterior w. of stomach
anterior w. of vagina
carotid w. of middle ear
cavity w.
chest w.

gingival cavity w.
jugular w. of middle ear
mastoid w. of middle ear
medial w. of tympanic cavity
membranous w. of trachea
nail w.
parietal w.
peripheral cavity w.
posterior w. of stomach
posterior w. of vagina
pulpal w.
w. push maneuver
splanchnic w.
thoracic w.
variceal w.
wallaby pouch
Wallace technique
wall-echo
w.-e. shadow triad
wallet stomach
Walsh
W. pressure ring
W. radical retropubic prostatectomy
Walter
W. Reed classification
W. Reed classification for HIV
infection
W Reed operation
Walther
W. canals
W. ducts
W. fracture
W. ganglion
W. plexus
waltzed flap
wand
3-dimensional reconstruction w.
flexible w.
wandering
w. abscess
w. kidney
w. liver
w. organ
Wangensteen
W. drainage
W. suction
W. suction tube
Wanger reduction technique
Wang pleural stoma
Wannagat suction tube
Wardill
W. four-flap method
W. pharyngoplasty
Wardill-Kilner
W.-K. advancement flap method

W

Wardill-Kilner *(continued)*
  W.-K. four-flap uranoplasty
  W.-K. procedure
Ward-Mayo vaginal hysterectomy
Wardrop method
Ward-Tomasin-Vander-Griend fixation
warfarin-associated subcapsular hematoma
warm
  w. condensation
  w. ischemic time
  w. saline solution
warmer
  Bair Hugger forced-air w.
  fluid w.
  high-capacity fluid w.
  HOTLINE blood and fluid w.
  Level One pressure infusion system 250 fluid w.
warming
  forced-air w.
  preanesthetic skin-surface w.
  preoperative skin-surface w.
warm-wire anemometer
Warner-Farber
  W.-F. ankle fixation
  W.-F. ankle fixation technique
Warren flap
Warren-Marshall classification
Wartenberg syndrome
Warthin-Starry staining method
wart-like excrescence
Warwick and Ashken technique
wash
  w. technique
  w. tube
washed
  w. field technique
  w. intrauterine insemination
washer
  connector with lock w.
  plate spacer w.
  rotation-stop w.
washing
  endometrial jet w.
  peritoneal w.
washout
  peritoneal w.
  seminal tract w.
  w. test
Wasmann glands
Wassel
  W. thumb duplication classification
  W. type IV thumb duplication
wasting

Watanabe
  W. classification of discoid meniscus
  W. discoid meniscus classification
water
  w. density line
  extravascular lung w.
  hydration layer w.
  lung w.
  total body w.
  w. vapor monitoring
water-based facial foundation
water-free facial foundation
Waterhouse transpubic procedure
Waterman osteotomy
Waters
  W. operation
  W. projection
water-seal chest tube
Waterston
  W. extrapericardial anastomosis
  W. method
  W. operation
Waterston-Cooley procedure
water-suppression technique
watertight closure
water-trap stomach
Watkins
  W. fusion
  W. fusion technique
Watson
  W. capsule biopsy
  W. method
  W. scaphotrapeziotrapezoidal fusion
  W. technique
Watson-Cheyne-Burghard procedure
Watson-Cheyne technique
Watson-Crick method
Watson-Jones
  W.-J. anterior approach
  W.-J. classification of tibial tubercle avulsion fracture
  W.-J. fracture repair
  W.-J. incision
  W.-J. lateral approach
  W.-J. procedure
  W.-J. reconstruction
  W.-J. tibial fracture classification
Watzke operation
Waugh-Clagett pancreaticoduodenostomy
waveform
  aortic root velocity w.
  electrical stimulator w.
  epidural pressure w. (EPWF)
  pressure w.
wavelength frequency
wavy respiration

wax
    w. expansion
    w. pattern thermal expansion
      technique
wax-matrix technique
waxy
    w. exudate
    w. kidney
    w. liver
Wayne County reduction
Way operation
weaning
    ventilator w.
wear
    three-body w.
Weavenit patch graft
Weaver-Dunn
    W.-D. acromioclavicular technique
    W.-D. procedure
    W.-D. resection
weaving
    head w.
web
    antral w.
    cell w.
    w. corn
    duodenal w.
    esophageal w.
    w. eye
    finger w.
    w. of fingers/toes
    w. formation
    hepatic w.
    intestinal w.
    laryngeal w.
    mucosal w.
    postcricoid w.
    pulmonary arterial w.
    w. space
    w. space flap
    w. space infection
    terminal w.
    thumb w.
    tracheal w.
    venous w.
webbed penis
Webb fixation
Weber
    W. classification
    W. classification of physeal injury
    W. humeral osteotomy

    W. organ
    W. point
    W. procedure
    W. subcapital osteotomy
    W. triangle
Weber-Brunner-Freuler-Boitzy technique
Weber-Brunner-Freuler open reduction
Weber-Danis ankle injury classification
Weber-Fergusson procedure
Weber-Vasey traction-absorption wiring
  technique
Webril immobilization
Webster
    W. infusion tube
    W. operation
Weck-cel vitrectomy
Weckesser technique
Weck suction tube
weddellite calculus
Wedensky facilitation
wedge
    arterial w.
    ball w.
    bone w.
    w. bone
    cast w.
    closing base w.
    compensatory w.
    w. compression fracture
    dental w.
    disconnect w.
    w. excision
    Good 'N Bed w.
    w. graft
    w. hepatic biopsy
    inner heel w.
    light-reflecting w.
    Livingston peribulbar w.
    medial heel w.
    mediastinal w.
    open w.
    w. osteotomy
    plastic w.
    w. pressure
    pulmonary artery w.
    w. resection
    self-adhering varus-valgus w.
    step w.
    temporal w.
    wooden w.
    Yancy cast w.

W

NOTES

wedge-and-groove
  w.-a.-g. joint
  w.-a.-g. suture
wedged hepatic venous pressure
wedge-shaped
  w.-s. erosion
  w.-s. fasciculus
  w.-s. osteotomy
  w.-s. tubercle
  w.-s. uncomminuted fragment
  w.-s. uncomminuted tibial plateau
    fracture
  w.-s. vertebra
Weeker operation
Weeks operation
weeping lesion
Wegner line
Weigert iodine solution
weight
  body w.
  w. estimation and assessment
  ideal body w.
  lean body w.
  low molecular w. (LMW)
  w. reduction
  w. reduction surgery
  total body w. (TBW)
weight-based peritoneal exchange
  volume
Weiland
  W. classification
  W. iliac crest bone graft
Weinberg modification of pyloroplasty
Weinstein-Ponseti technique
Weinstock desyndactylization
Weir
  W. incision
  W. operation
Weisinger operation
Weiss logarithmic method
Weissman classification
Weitbrecht
  W. cartilage
  W. cord
Welch Allyn suction tube
Welcker method
weld
  laser tissue w.
welding
  fusion w.
  laser tissue w.
  pressure w.
  tissue w.
well-circumscribed lesion
Wellcovorin injection
well-defined mass
Wells posterior rectopexy
Wendell Hughes operation

Wendl tube
Wepfer glands
Wepsic suction tube
Werb operation
Wernekinck decussation
Wernicke radiation
Wertheim-Bohlman technique
Wertheim operation
Wertheim-Schauta operation
Wesenberg-Hamazaki body
Wesolowski
  W. bypass graft
  W. Teflon graft
Wessely ring
Westberg space
Westcott Pyramid Program
Westergren sedimentation rate method
Western blot infection
"western boot" in open fracture
Westin-Hall incision
West operation
West-Soto-Hall
  W.-S.-H. patellar technique
  W.-S.-H. patellectomy
wet
  w. colostomy
  w. lung
wetting solution
Weve operation
Weyers-Thier syndrome
Wharton duct
Wharton-Jones operation
Wheeler
  W. halving repair
  W. method
  W. operation
  W. procedure
Wheeler-Reese operation
Wheelhouse operation
wheel rotation
wheezing
  expiratory w.
whewellite calculus
whiplash injury
whipping condensation
Whipple
  W. operation
  W. pancreatectomy
  W. pancreaticoduodenectomy
  W. pancreaticoduodenostomy
  W. procedure
  W. resection
whipstitch suture
whipworm infection
whistle-tip
whistling deformity
Whitaker pressure-perfusion test

white
- w. braided silk suture
- W. classification
- w. fixation
- w. graft
- w. lesion
- w. line of anal canal
- w. line response
- w. line of Toldt
- w. muscle
- w. nylon suture
- w. patch
- w. point
- W. posterior ankle fusion
- w. pulp
- w. ring
- w. ring of cornea
- W. slide procedure
- W. tube
- w. twisted suture
- w. without pressure

white-centered hemorrhage
Whitecloud-LaRocca fibular strut graft
whitegraft reaction
Whitehead
- W. classification
- W. deformity
- W. operation

Whitesides-Kelly cervical technique
Whitesides technique
white-spot lesion
Whitman
- W. femoral neck reconstruction
- W. osteotomy
- W. talectomy procedure

Whitman-Thompson procedure
Whitnall
- W. sling operation
- W. tubercle

WHO gastric carcinoma classification
whole
- w. abdominal radiation
- w. abdominopelvic irradiation
- w. blood lysis technique
- w. body cooling
- w. body radiation

whole-abdomen irradiation
whole-arm fusion
whole-body
- w.-b. extract
- w.-b. hyperthermia
- w.-b. irradiation
- w.-b. scanning
- w.-b. titration curve

whole-brain radiation therapy
whole-cell patch clamp recording
whole-gut
- w.-g. irrigation
- w.-g. lavage solution

whole-pelvis irradiation
whorl
- coccygeal w.

Wiberg patellar classification
Wicherkiewicz eyelid operation
Wick catheter technique
Wickham technique
wicking glue patch
wide
- w. elliptical anastomosis
- w. local excision
- w. plane
- w. suture

wide-field
- w.-f. radiation therapy
- w.-f. total laryngectomy

wide-mouth sac
widened retrogastric space
wide-range radiation therapy
Widman flap
width
- line w.
- pulse w.

Wiener
- W. operation
- tract of Münzer and W.

Wies
- W. operation
- W. procedure

Wigand maneuver
Wilcoxon signed-rank test
Wilde incision
Wiley-Galey classification
Wilkie artery
Wilkins classification of radial fracture
Wilkinson synovectomy
Willett-Stampfer method
William
- W. Dixon Cratex point
- W. Harvey arterial blood filter
- W. microlumbar disk excision

Williams
- W. copulating pouch operation
- W. diskectomy
- W. esophageal tube

NOTES

W

Williams *(continued)*
    W. procedure
    W. vulvovaginoplasty
Williams-Haddad technique
Willi glass crown technique
Willis
    W. centrum nervosum
    W. cords
    W. pancreas
    W. pouch
willow fracture
Willscher tube
will therapy
Willy Meyer mastectomy
Wilmer operation
Wilms
    W. amputation
    W. thoracoplasty
Wilson
    W. ankle fusion
    W. bunionectomy
    W. fracture
    W. muscle
    W. oblique displacement osteotomy
    W. procedure for extra-articular fusion of elbow
    W. technique
Wilson-Cook
    W.-C. nasobiliary tube
    W.-C. NJFT-series feeding tube
Wilson-Jacobs
    W.-J. patellar graft
    W.-J. tibial fixation
    W.-J. tibial fracture fixation technique
Wilson-McKeever
    W.-M. arthroplasty
    W.-M. shoulder technique
Wilson-White method
Wiltberger
    W. anterior cervical approach
    W. fusion
Wiltse
    W. ankle osteotomy
    W. bilateral lateral fusion
    W. system cross-bracing
    W. system double-rod construct
    W. system H construct
    W. system single-rod construct
    W. varus supramalleolar osteotomy
Wiltse-Spencer paraspinal approach
Wimberger ring
Winberger line
windblown deformity
window
    aortic-pulmonic w.
    aortopulmonary w.
    oval w.

    pericardial w.
    peritoneal w.
    soft tissue w.
    w. technique
    vestibular w.
windpipe
Windson-Insall-Vince
    W.-I.-V. bone graft
    W.-I.-V. grafting technique
windswept deformity
wing
    Badgley resection of iliac w.
    w. of crista galli
    w. excision of Littler
    greater w. of sphenoid bone
    w. of ilium
    Ingrassia w.
    lesser w. of sphenoid bone
    w. of sacrum
    w. suture
    w. of vomer
winged V double flap
Winiwarter-Buerger disease
Winkelmann rotationplasty
Winkler body
Winkler-Waldeyer
    closing ring of W.-W.
Winnie landmarks
Winograd
    W. nail plate removal
    W. partial matrixectomy
    W. technique
Winquist femoral shaft fracture classification
Winquist-Hansen femoral fracture classification
Winsburg-White bladder tube
Winslow pancreas
Winston-Lutz method
Winter
    W. classification
    W. convex fusion
    W. procedure
    W. spondylolisthesis technique
Wintrobe
    W. and Landsberg method
    W. sedimentation rate method
wire
    w. arch
    w. contour preparation
    w. extrusion
    w. insertion
    w. knot
    w. loop fixation
    w. loop test
    w. osteosynthesis
    w. passage
    w. removal technique

w. stabilization
w. Zytor suture
wire-guided
w.-g. balloon-assisted endoscopic
biliary stent exchange
w.-g. placement
wire-loop lesion
wire-wound endotracheal tube
wiring
compression w.
continuous loop w.
craniofacial suspension w.
facet fracture stabilization w.
facet subluxation stabilization w.
Ivy loop w.
multiple loop w.
Wirsung
W. canal
W. dilation
W. duct
Wirth-Jager tendon technique
with correction
withdrawal
within-list recognition (WLR)
without correction
Witzel
W. duodenostomy
W. gastrostomy
W. jejunostomy
WLR
within-list recognition
WOB
work of breathing
Wolf
W. full-thickness free graft
W. suction tube
Wolfe
W. breast carcinoma classification
W. classification of breast
carcinoma
W. method
W. ptosis operation
Wolfe-Kawamoto bone graft
Wolfe-Krause graft
wolffian
w. body
w. duct
w. duct carcinoma
Wolff-Parkinson-White bypass tract
Wölfler
W. gastroenterostomy

W. gland
W. suture technique
Wolf-Yoon ring
Womack procedure
wood
W. light examination
w. point
w. wool
Woodbridge tube
wooden wedge
Woods screw maneuver
Woodward
W. esophagogastroscopy
W. esophagogastrostomy
W. operation wound
W. procedure
W. technique
**Woofry-Chandler classification of
Osgood-Schlatter lesion**
Wookey
W. reconstruction
W. skin tube
wool
wood w.
Wooler-type annuloplasty
Woolf method
work
w. of breathing (WOB)
w. hardening program
working bite relation
World Health Organization classification
wormian bones
Woronoff ring
Worst
W. corneal contact glass
W. operation
W. suture
Worth ptosis operation
wound
abraded w.
w. approximation
avulsed w.
w. closure
crease w.
w. dehiscence
w. drainage
exit w.
w. failure
foot puncture w.
glancing w.
gunshot w.
gutter w.

NOTES

W

wound *(continued)*
    incised w.
    w. infection
    w. irrigation
    laparoscopic trocar w.
    nonpenetrating w.
    open w.
    penetrating w.
    perforating w.
    puncture w.
    w. retraction
    seton w.
    shotgun w.
    skin deficit w.
    stab w.
    sucking w.
    surgical w.
    tangential w.
    trocar w.
    Woodward operation w.
woven
    w. dacron tube
    w. Dacron tube graft
W-plasty
W-pouch
    ileal W-p.
wrap
    cardiac muscle w.
    gastric fundus w.
    Nissen fundoplication w.
    rectus fascial w.
    total gastric w.
    tunica vaginalis blanket w.
wraparound
    w. flap bone graft

    w. neurovascular composite free
       tissue transfer
    w. neurovascular free flap
    w. periapical lesion
wrapping
    valve w.
    vein valve w.
Wright
    W. maneuver
    W. operation
Wright-Giemsa evaluation
wrinkler muscle of eyebrow
wrinkling membrane
Wrisberg
    W. cartilage
    W. lesion
    W. tubercle
wrist
    w. block
    w. deformity
    w. disarticulation
    w. dislocation
    w. extensors
    w. extensor tendon
Wroblewski method
WR surgical nerve stimulator
W-shaped
    W.-s. ileal pouch-anal anastomosis
    W.-s. incision
    W.-s. pouch
Wullstein microsuction tube
Wurbs-type nasobiliary tube
Wyamine Sulfate injection
Wycillin injection

xanthoastrocytoma
xanthogranuloma
xanthoma planum
xanthomatosis
xanthosarcoma
X body
Xe
^{133}Xe intravenous injection technique
xenogeneic
  x. graft
  x. tissue
xenogenic cell therapy
xenograft
  bovine pericardial heart valve x.
  x. transplantation
xenon
  x. arc photocoagulation
  x. gas
  x. lung ventilation imaging
  x. method
xenon-washout technique
xeroma
xeroradiogram
xerosis
xerostomia
X-exotropia
xiphisternal
  x. joint
xiphisternum

xiphocostal
xiphodynia
xiphoid
  x. cartilage
  x. process
xiphoidalgia
xiphoid-to-pubis midline abdominal
  incision
xiphoid-to-umbilicus incision
Xi-scan fluoroscopy
x-line method
XM-50 Dialow membrane
Xomed
  X. endotracheal tube
  X. straight-shank tube
Xomed-Treace ventilation tube
x-radiation
x-ray
  x-r. therapy
Xylocaine
  topical X.
  X. topical anesthetic
  X. viscous solution
  X. with epinephrine
Xylocaine-MPF
xylol pulse indicator
xylonite frame
xylostyptic ether

Y

    Y body
    Y cartilage
    Y fracture
    Y graft
    Y incision

Yacoub and Radley-Smith classification

YAG
    yttrium-aluminum-garnet

Yale Optimal Observation Score

Yancey osteotomy

Yancy cast wedge

Yankauer
    Y. aspirating tube
    Y. sucker
    Y. suction
    Y. suction tube

Yankauer-type suction tube

Yasargil
    Y. craniotomy
    Y. microsuction tube
    Y. suction tube

Yates correction

Y-configuration

yeast infection

Yeder suction tube

Yee posterior shoulder approach

yellow
    y. body
    y. hepatization
    y. lesion
    y. ligament
    y. nail
    y. nail syndrome
    y. point

yellow-ochre hemorrhage

Yellow Springs Instruments thermistor

Y-fracture

Y-incision

yohimbine

yoke
    alveolar y.
    y. block
    y. bone
    cricoid y.
    y. hanger
    Y. transposition procedure

yolk
    y. membrane
    y. sac
    y. sac tumor of testis
    y. space

Yoon tubal sterilization ring

York-Mason
    Y.-M. procedure
    Y.-M. repair

Y-osteotomy
    Pauwels Y.-o.

Young
    Y. operation
    Y. pelvic fracture classification
    Y. procedure
    Y. technique
    Y. type epispadias repair

Young-Dees
    Y.-D. bladder neck reconstruction
    Y.-D. operation
    Y.-D. procedure
    Y.-D. technique

Young-Dees-Leadbetter
    Y.-D.-L. bladder neck
      reconstruction
    Y.-D.-L. operation

Youngwhich modification

Yount
    Y. fasciotomy
    Y. procedure

yo-yo weight fluctuation phenomenon

Y-piece

Y-plasty

ypsiliform

Y-shaped incision

YSI 2300 STAT Plus glucose and lactose analyzer

Y-T fracture

yttrium-90

yttrium-aluminum-garnet (YAG)

Y-type Dianeal peritoneal dialysis solution

Yu osteotomy

Y-V
    Y-V anoplasty
    Y-V plasty

Y-V-plasty incision

Z

Z direction
Z fashion
Z line
Z marginal tenotomy
Z myotomy
Z point
Z procedure
Z suture

z

z point pressure
Zadik total matrixectomy
Zaglas ligament
Zahn
anomaly of Z.
Z. lines
Zaias nail biopsy
Zancolli
Z. capsuloplasty
Z. clawhand deformity repair
Z. procedure for clawhand deformity
Z. reconstruction
Z. rerouting technique
Z. static lock procedure
Zancolli-Lasso procedure
Zang space
Zantac injection
Zariczny technique
Zarins-Rowe
Z.-R. ligament technique
Z.-R. procedure
Zavala technique
Zavanelli maneuver
Zazepen-Gamidov technique
ZEEP
zero end-expiratory pressure
Zeier transfer technique
Zeis glands
Zemuron
Zenker
Z. pouch
Z. solution
zero
z. end-expiratory pressure (ZEEP)
z. end-inspiratory pressure
z. line
zeta sedimentation ratio method
Zetran injection
zeugmatography
rotating-frame z.
Zickel
Z. classification
Z. nail fixation

Z. subtrochanteric fracture fixation
Z. subtrochanteric fracture operation
Ziegler
Z. operation
Z. puncture
Zielke technique
zig-zag
z.-z. approach
z.-z. compensatory deformity
z.-z. finger incision
zigzagplasty
Zimany bilobed flap
Zimmerman-Brittin exchange model
Zinacef injection
zinc
z. permanganate
z. sulfate
z. sulfate solution
Z-incision
zinc-sulfate flotation method
Zinn
Z. ligament
Z. membrane
Z. ring
Z. zonule
zipped canal
zipper
z. ring
z. stitch
Ziramic femoral head
Zirconia orthopaedic prosthetic head
Z-line
Zlotsky-Ballard classification of acromioclavicular injury
Zoeller-Clancy technique
Zoellner-Clancy procedure
Zofran
Zöllner line
Zollner suction tube
zona, pl. zonae
z. arcuata
z. ciliaris
z. dermatica
z. epithelioserosa
z. fasciculata
z. glomerulosa
z. hemorrhoidalis
z. medullovasculosa
z. orbicularis
z. pectinata
z. perforata
z. pupillaris
z. reticularis
z. tecta
z. vasculosa

Z

zonal anatomy
zone
> abdominal z.
> anal transitional z. (ATZ)
> arcuate z.
> barrier z.
> basement membrane z.
> calcification z.
> cervical z. of tooth
> cervical transformation z.
> ciliary z.
> dorsal root entry z. (DREZ)
> echo z.
> entry z.
> exudative z.
> gingival z.
> Head z.
> hemorrhoidal z.
> high pressure z. (HPZ)
> large loop excision of transformation z.
> normal transformation z.
> orbicular z.
> pectinate z.
> proliferation z.
> pupillary z.
> transformation z.
> vascular z.

zonoskeleton
zonula, pl. **zonulae**
> z. ciliaris

zonular
> z. band
> z. fibers

zonule
> ciliary z.
> Zinn z.

zonulolysis
> Barraquer z.
> enzymatic z.

zonulotomy
zoodermic
zoograft
zoografting
zoom
zoonotic infection
zooplastic graft
zooplasty
zoospermia
Z-osteotomy
> scarf Z-o.

Z-osteotomy/bunionectomy
> scarf Z-o.

Zovirax injection
Z-plasty
> Z-p. approach
> Broadbent-Woolf four-limb Z-p.
> Cozen-Brockway Z-p.

> four-flap Z-p.
> four-limb Z-p.
> Gudas scarf Z-p.
> Z-p. incision
> Z-p. local flap graft
> Peet Z-p.
> Z-p. procedure
> scarf Z-p.
> Spencer-Watson Z-p.
> Z-p. tenotomy
> Z-p. transposition

Z-technique
Z-type deformity
Zuckerkandl
> Z. fascia
> perforating canal of Z.
> Z. perforating canal

Zuker and Manktelow technique
zygapophyseal joints
zygapophysial
zygapophysis
zygion
zygoma
> tubercle of root of z.

zygomatic
> z. arch
> z. arch fracture
> z. bone
> z. border of greater wing of sphenoid bone
> z. branch of facial nerve
> z. fossa
> z. maxillary complex fracture
> z. nerve
> z. process of frontal bone
> z. process of maxilla
> z. process of temporal bone
> z. region

zygomaticoauricular
> z. index

zygomaticoauricularis
zygomaticofacial
> z. branch of zygomatic nerve
> z. canal
> z. foramen

zygomaticofrontal
> z. suture

zygomaticomaxillary
> z. fracture
> z. suture

zygomatico-orbital
> z.-o. artery
> z.-o. foramen

zygomaticosphenoid
zygomaticotemporal
> z. branch of zygomatic nerve
> z. canal
> z. foramen

z. space
z. suture
zygomaticus
z. major muscle
z. minor muscle
zygomaxillare

zygomaxillary
z. point
zygopodium
Zyler tube
Zylik operation
Zyranox femoral head

NOTES

Z